Veterinary Microbiology

VETERINARY MICROBIOLOGY

Dwight C. Hirsh, DVM, PhD
Professor, Department of Pathology, Microbiology, and Immunology
Chief of Service, Clinical Microbiology Laboratory
Veterinary Medical Teaching Hospital
School of Veterinary Medicine
University of California
Davis, California

Yuan Chung Zee, DVM, PhD
Professor, Department of Pathology, Microbiology, and Immunology
School of Veterinary Medicine
University of California
Davis, California

Blackwell
Science

© 1999 by Blackwell Science, Inc.

Editorial Offices:
Commerce Place, 350 Main Street, Malden,
  Massachusetts 02148, USA
Osney Mead, Oxford OX2 0EL, England
25 John Street, London WC1N 2BL, England
23 Ainslie Place, Edinburgh EH3 6AJ, Scotland
54 University Street, Carlton, Victoria 3053, Australia
Other Editorial Offices:
Blackwell Wissenschafts-Verlag GmbH, Kurfürstendamm
  57, 10707 Berlin, Germany
Blackwell Science KK, MG Kodenmacho Building, 7-10
  Kodenmacho Nihombashi, Chuo-ku, Tokyo 104,
  Japan

Distributors:
USA
  Blackwell Science, Inc.
  Commerce Place
  350 Main Street
  Malden, Massachusetts 02148
  (Telephone orders: 800-215-1000 or 781-388-8250;
    fax orders: 781-388-8270)

Canada
  Login Brothers Book Company
  324 Saulteaux Crescent
  Winnipeg, Manitoba, R3J 3T2
  (Telephone orders: 204-224-4068)

Australia
  Blackwell Science Pty, Ltd.
  54 University Street
  Carlton, Victoria 3053
  (Telephone orders: 03-9347-0300;
    fax orders: 03-9349-3016)

Outside North America and Australia
  Blackwell Science, Ltd.
  c/o Marston Book Services, Ltd.
  P.O. Box 269
  Abingdon
  Oxon OX14 4YN
  England
  (Telephone orders: 44-01235-465500;
    fax orders: 44-01235-465555)

Acquisitions: Nancy Hill-Whilton
Production: Irene Herlihy
Manufacturing: Lisa Flanagan
Typeset by Best-set Typesetter Ltd., Hong Kong
Printed and bound by Maple-Vail

Printed in the United States of America
99 00 01 02 5 4 3 2 1

The Blackwell Science logo is a trade mark of Blackwell
Science Ltd., registered at the United Kingdom Trade
Marks Registry

Library of Congress Cataloging-in-Publication Data

Veterinary microbiology / edited by Dwight C. Hirsh,
Yuan Chung Zee.
       p.   cm.
    Includes bibliographical references and index.
    ISBN 0–86542–543–4
    1. Veterinary microbiology.   I. Hirsh, Dwight C.
II. Zee, Y. C.
SF780.2.V48   1999
636.089'601 — dc21   98-30284
                                                CIP

To Lucy, Dwight, and Elizabeth for years of patience and understanding
and
To Elizabeth, Norman, and Charlie for instilling a love for all creatures

Contents

Contributors   ix

Preface   x

PART I   *INTRODUCTION*   1

Chapter 1   Parasitism and Pathogenicity   3
ERNST L. BIBERSTEIN
Chapter 2   Immune Responses to Infectious
Agents   7
LAUREL J. GERSHWIN
Chapter 3   Laboratory Diagnosis   15
DWIGHT C. HIRSH, YUAN CHUNG ZEE, AND
ANTHONY E. CASTRO
Chapter 4   Antimicrobial Chemotherapy   28
JOHN F. PRESCOTT
Chapter 5   Antimicrobial Drugs: A Strategy for
Rational Use and the Ramifications
of Misuse   46
DWIGHT C. HIRSH
Chapter 6   Vaccines   51
YUAN CHUNG ZEE AND DWIGHT C. HIRSH

PART II   *BACTERIA AND FUNGI*   59

Chapter 7   The Alimentary Canal as a Microbial
Habitat   61
DWIGHT C. HIRSH
Chapter 8   Family *Enterobacteriaceae*   65
DWIGHT C. HIRSH
Chapter 9   *Escherichia*   69
DWIGHT C. HIRSH
Chapter 10   *Salmonella*   75
DWIGHT C. HIRSH
Chapter 11   *Shigella*   80
DWIGHT C. HIRSH
Chapter 12   Non-Spore-Forming Obligate
Anaerobes of the Alimentary Tract   83
DWIGHT C. HIRSH
Chapter 13   *Serpulina*   86
DWIGHT C. HIRSH
Chapter 14   Spiral Organisms I: *Campylobacter
— Arcobacter — Lawsonia* (Digestive
Tract)   89
DWIGHT C. HIRSH
Chapter 15   Spiral Organisms II: *Helicobacter*   93
JAMES G. FOX
Chapter 16   *Pseudomonas*   100
DWIGHT C. HIRSH

Chapter 17   *Yersinia enterocolitica*   102
DWIGHT C. HIRSH
Chapter 18   *Mycobacterium avium* ssp.
*paratuberculosis (Mycobacterium
paratuberculosis)*   104
DWIGHT C. HIRSH
Chapter 19   *Candida*   109
ERNST L. BIBERSTEIN
Chapter 20   The Respiratory Tract as a Microbial
Habitat   113
ERNST L. BIBERSTEIN
Chapter 21   Staphylococci   115
ERNST L. BIBERSTEIN AND DWIGHT C. HIRSH
Chapter 22   Streptococci   120
ERNST L. BIBERSTEIN AND DWIGHT C. HIRSH
Chapter 23   Corynebacteria; *Arcanobacterium
(Actinomyces) pyogenes; Rhodococcus
equi*   127
ERNST L. BIBERSTEIN AND DWIGHT C. HIRSH
Chapter 24   *Pasteurella*   135
ERNST L. BIBERSTEIN AND DWIGHT C. HIRSH
Chapter 25   *Actinobacillus*   141
ERNST L. BIBERSTEIN AND DWIGHT C. HIRSH
Chapter 26   *Haemophilus* spp.   144
ERNST L. BIBERSTEIN
Chapter 27   *Bordetella*   148
ERNST L. BIBERSTEIN AND DWIGHT C. HIRSH
Chapter 28   *Moraxella*   151
ERNST L. BIBERSTEIN AND DWIGHT C. HIRSH
Chapter 29   *Burkholderia mallei* and
Burkholderia pseudomallei   155
ERNST L. BIBERSTEIN AND DWIGHT C. HIRSH
Chapter 30   *Mycobacterium* Species: The Agents
of Animal Tuberculosis   158
ERNST L. BIBERSTEIN AND DWIGHT C. HIRSH
Chapter 31   Mollicutes   165
RICHARD L. WALKER
Chapter 32   Chlamydiae   173
ERNST L. BIBERSTEIN AND DWIGHT C. HIRSH
Chapter 33   The Urinary Tract as a Microbial
Habitat; Urinary Tract
Infections   178
ERNST L. BIBERSTEIN AND DWIGHT C. HIRSH
Chapter 34   Leptospirae   185
RANCE B. LEFEBVRE
Chapter 35   The Genital Tract as a Microbial
Habitat   190
DWIGHT C. HIRSH

Chapter 36 *Campylobacter — Arcobacter*
            (Reproductive Tract)   192
            DWIGHT C. HIRSH
Chapter 37 *Brucella*   196
            RICHARD L. WALKER
Chapter 38 *Taylorella equigenitalis*   204
            ERNST L. BIBERSTEIN
Chapter 39 The Skin as a Microbial Habitat:
            Bacterial Skin Infections   206
            ERNST L. BIBERSTEIN
Chapter 40 Dermatophytes   214
            ERNST L. BIBERSTEIN
Chapter 41 Agents of Subcutaneous Mycoses   220
            ERNST L. BIBERSTEIN
Chapter 42 *Listeria*   225
            RICHARD L. WALKER
Chapter 43 *Erysipelothrix*   229
            RICHARD L. WALKER
Chapter 44 The Clostridia   233
            ERNST L. BIBERSTEIN AND DWIGHT C. HIRSH
Chapter 45 The Genus *Bacillus*   246
            ERNST L. BIBERSTEIN AND DWIGHT C. HIRSH
Chapter 46 Pathogenic Actinomycetes
            (*Actinomyces* and *Nocardia*)   250
            ERNST L. BIBERSTEIN AND DWIGHT C. HIRSH
Chapter 47 Agents of Systemic Mycoses   256
            ERNST L. BIBERSTEIN
Chapter 48 Mycotoxins   274
            FRANCIS D. GALEY
Chapter 49 The Yersiniae   281
            ERNST L. BIBERSTEIN AND DWIGHT C. HIRSH
Chapter 50 *Francisella tularensis*   285
            ERNST L. BIBERSTEIN
Chapter 51 *Borrelia* spp.   287
            RANCE B. LEFEBVRE
Chapter 52 *Streptobacillus moniliformis*   290
            ERNST L. BIBERSTEIN
Chapter 53 Rickettsial Agents of Animal Disease;
            the *Rickettsieae*   291
            ERNST L. BIBERSTEIN AND DWIGHT C. HIRSH
Chapter 54 *Ehrlichieae*: *Ehrlichia*, *Cowdria*, and
            Neorickettsia   294
            ERNST L. BIBERSTEIN AND DWIGHT C. HIRSH
Chapter 55 *Bartonellaceae*   299
            BRUNO B. CHOMEL
Chapter 56 *Anaplasmataceae*   304
            ERNST L. BIBERSTEIN

PART III   *VIRUSES*   309

Chapter 57 General Properties of
            Viruses   311
            JANET S. BUTEL, JOSEPH L. MELNICK,
            AND YUAN CHUNG ZEE
Chapter 58 Pathogenesis of Viral Diseases   328
            YUAN CHUNG ZEE
Chapter 59 Parvoviridae   333
            YUAN CHUNG ZEE
Chapter 60 Iridoviridae   340
            JEFFREY L. STOTT
Chapter 61 Papovaviridae   343
            YUAN CHUNG ZEE
Chapter 62 Adenoviridae   346
            YUAN CHUNG ZEE
Chapter 63 Herpesviridae   350
            ALEX A. ARDANS
Chapter 64 Poxviridae   365
            JEFFREY L. STOTT
Chapter 65 Picornaviridae   371
            JEFFREY L. STOTT
Chapter 66 Caliciviridae   379
            YUAN CHUNG ZEE
Chapter 67 Togaviridae and Flaviviridae   385
            JEFFREY L. STOTT
Chapter 68 Orthomyxoviridae   396
            ALEX A. ARDANS
Chapter 69 Paramyxoviridae   403
            YUAN CHUNG ZEE
Chapter 70 Rhabdoviridae   412
            YUAN CHUNG ZEE
Chapter 71 Coronaviridae   418
            JEFFREY L. STOTT
Chapter 72 Reoviridae   430
            JEFFREY L. STOTT
Chapter 73 Birnaviridae   439
            JEFFREY L. STOTT
Chapter 74 Retroviridae   442
            RICHARD M. DONOVAN
Chapter 75 Transmissible Spongiform
            Encephalopathies   461
            YUAN CHUNG ZEE

Index   463

Contributors

Alex A. Ardans, DVM, MS
Professor, Department of Medicine and Epidemiology
Director, California Veterinary Diagnostic Laboratory
  System
School of Veterinary Medicine
University of California
Davis, California

Ernst L. Biberstein, DVM, PhD
Professor Emeritus, Department of Pathology,
  Microbiology, and Immunology
School of Veterinary Medicine
University of California
Davis, California

Janet S. Butel, PhD
Professor of Virology
Division of Molecular Virology
Baylor College of Medicine
Houston, Texas

Anthony E. Castro, DVM, PhD
Department of Veterinary Sciences
Pennsylvania State University
University Park, Pennsylvania

Bruno B. Chomel, DVM, PhD
Associate Professor, Department of Population Health
  and Reproduction
School of Veterinary Medicine
University of California
Davis, California

Richard M. Donovan, PhD
Director of Infectious Diseases Research
Henry Ford Health Sciences Center
Detroit, Michigan

James G. Fox, DVM
Professor and Director, Division of Comparative
  Medicine
Massachusetts Institute of Technology
Cambridge, Massachusetts

Francis D. Galey, DVM, PhD
Associate Professor, Department of Molecular
  Biosciences
Section Head, Clinical Toxicology
California Veterinary Diagnostic Laboratory
School of Veterinary Medicine
University of California
Davis, California

Laurel J. Gershwin, DVM, PhD
Professor, Department of Pathology, Microbiology, and
  Immunology
Chief of Service, Clinical Immunology and Virology
  Laboratory
Veterinary Medical Teaching Hospital
School of Veterinary Medicine
University of California
Davis, California

Dwight C. Hirsh, DVM, PhD
Professor, Department of Pathology, Microbiology, and
  Immunology
Chief of Service, Clinical Microbiology Laboratory
Veterinary Medical Teaching Hospital
School of Veterinary Medicine
University of California
Davis, California

Rance B. LeFebvre, PhD
Professor, Department of Pathology, Microbiology, and
  Immunology
School of Veterinary Medicine
University of California
Davis, California

Joseph L. Melnick, PhD
Professor of Virology and Epidemiology
Baylor College of Medicine
Houston, Texas

John F. Prescott, Vet MB, PhD
Professor, Department of Pathobiology
University of Guelph
Ontario, Canada

Jeffrey L. Stott, PhD
Professor, Department of Pathology, Microbiology,
  and Immunology
School of Veterinary Medicine
University of California
Davis, California

Richard L. Walker, DVM, PhD, MPVM
Associate Professor
Department of Pathology, Microbiology, and
  Immunology
School of Veterinary Medicine;
Section Head, Bacteriology
California Veterinary Diagnostic Laboratory
University of California
Davis, California

Yuan Chung Zee, DVM, PhD
Professor, Department of Pathology, Microbiology, and
  Immunology
School of Veterinary Medicine
University of California
Davis, California

Preface

This book is intended primarily for veterinary students, to accompany and supplement their first courses in pathogenic bacteriology-mycology and virology. Its focus includes pathogenic mechanisms and processes in infectious diseases; methods of diagnosis; and principles of resistance, prevention, and therapy. A working knowledge of general microbiology is assumed.

Beyond serving as a resource for students, the book is also meant to serve as a convenient reference for veterinarians and veterinary scientists whose main line of activity and expertise is outside the areas of microbiology.

The manner of presentation, i.e., sequence and chapter organization, was determined by the way which the editors found most appropriate for teaching their respective subjects: the bacteriology-mycology portion is arranged roughly by host organ systems and other milieus that serve as sources of pathogenic agents. This approach creates a logical place to consider the various environments as microbial habitats. The virology section is organized more along taxonomic lines. Regardless of the user's preference or custom, all topics are readily located with the aid of the table of contents and the alphabetic index.

While we have included all agents likely to be encountered in veterinary practice, we have tried to avoid indiscriminate listing of conditions and microorganisms reported only exceptionally, particularly in the contemporary literature. Our objective is the main current of veterinary microbiology.

The purpose of the reference citations at the end of chapters is to guide the reader to more comprehensive sources of information rather than to document chapter content. We have therefore favored recent reviews and monographs. We believe these to be of greatest use since they will lead the interested reader to the primary sources, which considerations of brevity and economy forced us to omit.

The content of this book varies somewhat from our earlier work, *Review of Veterinary Microbiology* (1990). Most notable is the replacement of the chapters dealing with general immunology with one limited to a discussion of immunologic phenomena related to infectious agents. We have also changed the focus of the chapters dealing with antimicrobial agents to one more clinical by the addition of a chapter on the rational choice of antimicrobial agents in the treatment of an infectious disease. We have added chapters dealing with microbiological diagnosis, and one on vaccines.

We gratefully acknowledge Trudi Schuster, whose help is much appreciated. A special thank you goes to Jill Connor and Irene Herlihy of Blackwell Science, who have been unbelievably patient and extremely helpful in getting our effort to press.

D.C.H.
Y.C.Z.

PART I

Introduction

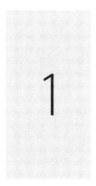

1

Parasitism and Pathogenicity

Ernst L. Biberstein

Veterinary microbiology deals with microbial agents affecting animals. Such agents are characterized according to their ecologic arrangements: *parasites* live in permanent association with, and at the expense of, animal hosts; *saprophytes* normally inhabit the inanimate environment. Parasites that cause their host no discernible harm are called *commensals*. The term *symbiosis* usually refers to reciprocally beneficial associations of organisms. This arrangement is also called *mutualism*.

Pathogenic organisms are parasites or saprophytes that cause disease. The process by which they establish themselves in a host individual is infection, but infection need not be followed by clinical illness. The term *virulence* is sometimes used to mean pathogenicity but sometimes to express degrees of pathogenicity.

SOME ATTRIBUTES OF HOST–PARASITE RELATIONSHIPS

Many pathogenic microorganisms are host-specific in that they parasitize only one or a few animal species. *Streptococcus equi* is essentially limited to horses. Others — certain *Salmonella* types, for example — have a broad host range. The basis for this difference in host specificity is incompletely understood, but it may in part be related to the need for specific attachment devices between host (receptors) and parasite (adhesins).

Some agents infect several host species but with varying effects. The plague bacillus *Yersinia pestis* behaves as a commensal parasite in many, but by no means all, small rodent species but causes fatal disease in rats and humans. Evolutionary pressure may have produced some of these differences, but not others: *Coccidioides immitis*, a saprophytic fungus requiring no living host, infects cattle and dogs with equal ease; yet it produces no clinical signs in cattle but frequently causes progressive fatal disease in dogs.

Potential pathogens vary in their effects on different tissues in the same host. The *Escherichia coli* that is commensal in the intestine can cause severe disease in the urinary tract and peritoneal cavity.

Some microorganisms that are commensal in one habitat may turn pathogenic in a habitat that is pathologically altered or otherwise compromised. Thus, oral streptococci, which occasionally enter the bloodstream, may colonize a damaged heart valve and initiate bacterial endocarditis. In the absence of such a lesion, however, they would be cleared uneventfully via the macrophage system. Similarly, the frequent entrance of intestinal bacteria into vascular channels normally leads to their disposal by humoral and cellular defense mechanisms. In immuno-incompetent hosts, however, such entrance may lead to fatal septicemia.

Transfer to a new host or tissue, or a change in host resistance, are common ways that commensal parasites are converted into active pathogens. *Commensalism* is the stable form of parasitic existence. It ensures survival of the microorganism, which active disease would jeopardize by killing the host or evoking an active immune response. Either effect deprives the agent of its habitat. Evolutionary selective pressure therefore tends to eliminate host–parasite relationships that threaten the survival of either partner. It does so by allowing milder strains of the pathogen, which permit longer survival of the host and thereby facilitate their own dissemination, to replace the more lethal ones. It also favors a resistant host population by screening out highly susceptible stock. The trend is thus toward commensalism. Most agents causing serious infections have alternative modes of survival as commensals in tissues or hosts not subject to disease (e.g., plague) or in the inanimate environment (e.g., coccidioidomycosis). Others cause chronic infections lasting months or years (tuberculosis, syphilis), during which their dissemination to other hosts ensures their survival.

CRITERIA OF PATHOGENICITY — KOCH'S POSTULATES

The presence of a microorganism in diseased individuals does not prove its pathogenic significance. To demonstrate the causal role of an agent in a disease, the following qualifications or "postulates" formulated by Robert Koch (1843–1910) should be satisfied:

1. The suspected agent is present in all cases of the disease.
2. The agent is isolated from such disease and propagated serially in pure culture, apart from its natural host.
3. Upon introduction into an experimental host, the isolate produces the original disease.
4. The agent can be reisolated from this experimental infection.

These postulates are ideals that are not satisfied in all cases of infectious diseases. The presence of some microorganisms cannot be demonstrated at the time of disease, especially in affected tissues (tetanus, botulism). Others lose virulence rapidly after isolation (*Leptospira* spp.), while still others, though indispensable for pathogenesis, require undetermined accessory factors (*Pasteurella*-related pneumonias). For some human viral pathogens (cytomegalovirus), no experimental host is known, and some agents (e.g., *Mycobacterium leprae*) have not been grown apart from their natural hosts.

ELEMENTS IN THE PRODUCTION OF AN INFECTIOUS DISEASE

Effective transmission through indirect contact occurs by ingestion; inhalation; or mucosal, cutaneous, or wound contamination. Airborne infection takes place largely via droplet nuclei, which are 0.1 to 5 mm in diameter. Particles of this size stay suspended in air and can be inhaled. Larger particles settle out but can be resuspended in dust, which may also harbor infectious agents from nonrespiratory sources (e.g., skin squames, feces, saliva). Arthropods may serve as mechanical carriers of pathogens (e.g., *Shigella*, *Dermatophilus*) or play an indispensable part in the life cycles of disease-producing agents (plague, ehrlichioses, viral encephalitides).

Attachment to host surfaces requires interaction between the agent's adhesins, which are usually proteins, and the host's receptors, which are most often carbohydrate residues. Examples of bacterial adhesins are fimbrial proteins (*Escherichia coli*, *Salmonella* spp.), P-1 protein of *Mycoplasma pneumoniae*, and afimbrial surface proteins (some streptococci). Examples of host receptor substances include fibronectin for some streptococci and staphylococci, mannose for many *E. coli* strains, and sialic acid for *M. pneumoniae*.

Attachment is inhibited by normal commensal flora that occupy or block available receptor sites and discourage colonization by excreting toxic metabolites, bacteriocins and microcins. This colonization resistance is an important defense mechanism and may be assisted by mucosal antibody and other antibacterial substances (lysozyme, lactoferrin, organic acids).

Penetration of host surfaces is a variable requirement among pathogens. Some agents, having reached a primary target cell population, penetrate no farther (e.g., enterotoxigenic *E. coli*, *Vibrio cholerae*). Others traverse surface membranes after inducing cytoskeletal rearrangements, resulting in "ruffles" that entrap adhered bacteria or passage between epithelial cells (e.g., *Salmonella*, *Yersinia*). Inhaled facultative intracellular parasites like *Mycobacterium tuberculosis* are taken up by pulmonary macrophages, in which they may multiply and travel via lymphatics to lymph nodes and other tissues. Percutaneous penetration occurs mostly through injuries, including arthropod bites.

Dissemination takes place by extension, aided perhaps by such bacterial enzymes as collagenase and hyaluronidase, which are produced by many pathogens. Microorganisms are also spread via lymph and blood vessels, the bronchial tree, bile ducts, nerve trunks, and mobile phagocytes.

Growth in or on host tissue is a prerequisite of pathogenesis for all pathogenic organisms, except the few that produce toxins in foodstuffs prior to ingestion. In order to multiply to pathogenic levels, they must be able to neutralize host defense efforts. Relevant adaptations of various bacteria include firm attachment to prevent mechanical removal; repulsion or nonattraction of phagocytes; and interference with phagocytic function by capsules and cell walls, by leukotoxic activity, or by prevention of phagocytic digestion. Some bacteria are able to digest or divert antibodies and deplete complement. Some destroy the vascular supply to tissue, shutting out defensive resources and suspending antimicrobial activity in the affected area.

With host defenses neutralized, microbial growth can proceed if nutritional supplies are adequate and the pH, temperature, and oxidation reduction potential (Eh) are appropriate. Iron is often a limiting nutrient. Microbial ability to appropriate iron from iron-binding host proteins (transferrin, lactoferrin) is a factor in virulence. Gastric acidity accounts for the resistance of the stomach to most pathogenic bacteria, although expression of alternative sigma factors when bacteria are in stationary phase results in an RNA polymerase that transcribes genes whose products help the pathogen resist an acidic environment (e.g., *Salmonella*, *E. coli*). The high body temperature of birds may explain their resistance to some diseases (e.g., anthrax, histoplasmosis), while low Eh requirements account for the restriction of anaerobic growth to devitalized (i.e., nonoxygenated) tissues or tissues in which simultaneous aerobic growth has lowered the Eh.

PATHOGENIC ACTION

Microbial disease manifests itself either as direct damage to host structures and functions by exotoxins or viruses, or as damage due to host reactions such as those triggered by endotoxin or immune responses.

Direct Damage

Exotoxins are bacterial proteins, which are often freely excreted into the environment. The differences between endotoxins and exotoxins are shown in Table 1.1.

Two types of exotoxins exist. One acts extracellularly or on cell membranes, attacking intercellular substances or cell surfaces by enzymatic or detergent-like mechanisms. It includes, for example, bacterial hemolysins, leukocidins, collagenases, and hyaluronidases, which may play an ancillary role in infections.

The other type of exotoxin consists of proteins or polypeptides that enter cells and enzymatically disrupt cellular processes. These usually consist of an A fragment, which has enzymatic activity, and a B fragment, which is

Table 1.1. Exo- and Endotoxins Compared

Exotoxins	Endotoxins
Often spontaneously diffusible	Cell-bound as part of cell wall
Proteins or polypeptides	Lipopolysaccharide (lipid A is toxic component)
Produced by gram-positive and gram-negative bacteria	Limited to gram-negative bacteria
Produce a single, pharmacologically specific effect	Produce a range of effects, largely due to host-derived mediators
Each is distinct in structure and reactivity according to its bacterial species of origin	All similar in structure and effect regardless of bacterial species of origin
Lethal in minute amounts (mice = nanograms)	Lethal in larger amounts (mice = micrograms)
Labile to heat, chemicals, storage	Very stable to heat, chemicals, storage
Convertible to toxoids (= nontoxic, immunogenic toxin-derivatives); elicit antitoxin production	Not convertible to toxoids

responsible for binding the toxin to its target cell. The enzymatic activity of many intracellular toxins entails the cleavage of ADP ribose from NAD, and its attachment — ADP-ribosylation — to a protein vital to cellular biosynthetic or metabolic processes, which are thereby brought to a halt. This mechanism was first found to operate in toxicity due to diphtheria toxin (produced by *Corynebacterium diphtheriae*), which stops protein synthesis by ADP-ribosylating elongation factor II. This factor is essential for building peptide chains. ADP-ribosylation is involved in the action of toxins produced by *Pseudomonas aeruginosa* (A, S), *Vibrio cholerae, Escherichia coli* (LT), *Bordetella pertussis* (pertussis toxin), *Clostridium botulinum* (C, D), *Clostridium spiroforme, Clostridium perfringens* (E), and *Clostridium difficile* (B). Exotoxins are encoded chromosomally, on plasmids, or on bacteriophages. The function the toxins serve the bacteria is not known.

Viruses produce injury by destroying the cells in which they replicate or by altering cell function, appearance, and growth characteristics. Virology is considered in Part III of this text.

Endotoxins are lipopolysaccharides, which are part of the gram-negative cell wall. They consist of polysaccharide surface chains, which are virulence factors and somatic (0) antigens; a core polysaccharide; and lipid A, where the toxicity resides.

Endotoxins are internalized by host cells and, particularly in macrophages, stimulate the secretion of mediator substances such as interleukin-1, tumor necrosis factor, and complement components. These substances elicit manifestations of endotoxemia, including fever, headache, hypotension, leukopenia, thrombocytopenia, intravascular coagulation, inflammation, endothelial damage, hemorrhage, fluid extravasation, and circulatory collapse. Many of these result from 1) activation of the complement cascade (by either pathway, see Chapter 2) and 2) production of arachidonic acid metabolites: prostaglandins, leukotrienes, and thromboxanes. Both events occur in endotoxemia, largely in response to macrophage-derived cytokines, the secretion of which is triggered by endotoxins (and other substances). The phenomena produced by endotoxins closely resemble aspects of gram-negative septicemias, but most of them can also be duplicated by peptidoglycans of gram-positive bacteria.

Immune-Mediated Damage

Tissue damage due to immune reactions is considered elsewhere (see Chapter 2). Complement-mediated responses (such as inflammation) and reactions resembling immediate-type allergic phenomena can occur in response to endotoxins or to peptidoglycan without preceding sensitization.

Specific immune responses participate in the pathogenesis of many infections, particularly chronic granulomatous infections such as tuberculosis. Lesions are due to cell-mediated hypersensitivity, which is established in the early weeks of infection. Cell-mediated responses intensify inflammatory responses and tissue destruction upon subsequent encounters with the agent or its protein through the release of effector substances from T-lymphocytes (e.g., cytokines, perforins).

Immune mechanisms apparently contribute to anemias seen in anaplasmosis, hemobartonellosis, and eperythrozoonosis. The antibody response to the hemoparasitism does not distinguish between the parasite and the host erythrocyte. Both are removed by phagocytosis.

SELECTED REFERENCES

Baggiolini M, Dewald B, Moser B. Human chemokines: an update. Annu Rev Immunol 1997;15:675.

Bearson S, Bearson B, Foster JW. Acid stress responses in enterobacteria. FEMS Microbiol Lett 1997;147:173.

Burnet EM, White DO. Natural history of infectious disease. London: Cambridge University, 1972.

Crosa JH. Signal transduction and transcriptional and post-transcriptional control of iron-regulated genes in bacteria. Microbiol Molec Biol Rev 1997;61:319.

Curfs JHAJ, Meis JFGM, Hoogkamp-Korstanje JAA. A primer on cytokines: sources, receptors, effects, and inducers. Clin Microbiol Rev 1997;10:742.

Falkow S. What is a pathogen? ASM News 1997;63:359.

Finlay BB, Cossart P. Exploitation of mammalian host cell functions by bacterial pathogens. Science 1997;276:718.

Finlay BB, Falkow S. Common themes in microbial pathogenicity revisited. Microbiol Molec Biol Rev 1997;61:136.

Jurado RL. Iron, infections, and anemia of inflammation. Clin Infect Dis 1997;25:888.

Kotwal GJ. Microorganisms and their interaction with the immune system. J Leukoc Biol 1997;62:415.

Mackowiak PA, Bartlett JG, Borden EC, et al. Concepts of fever: recent advances and lingering dogma. Clin Infect Dis 1997;25:119.

Mims CA. The pathogenesis of infectious disease. 3rd ed. London: Academic, 1987.

Rostand KS, Esko JD. Microbial adherence to and invasion through proteoglycans. Infect Immunol 1997;65:1.

Salyers AS, Whitt DD. Bacterial pathogenesis. Washington: ASM Press, 1994.

Schletter J, Heine H, Ulmer AJ, Rietschel ET. Molecular mechanisms of endotoxin activity. Arch Microbiol 1995;164:383.

Schluger NW, Rom WN. Early responses to infection: chemokines as mediators of inflammation. Curr Opin Immunol 1997;9:504.

van der Waaij D. Effect of antibiotics on colonization resistance. Med Microbiol 1984;4:227.

Verhoef J, Kalter E. Endotoxic effects of peptidoglycan. Prog Clin Biol Res 1985;189:101.

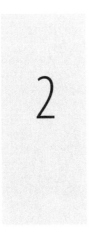

2 Immune Responses to Infectious Agents

Laurel J. Gershwin

Immunity is traditionally understood to be either *innate* or *acquired*. Innate immunity is usually thought of as those protective devices that are always present and active that each animal species possesses to protect it from the actions of infectious agents. Acquired immunity, on the other hand, makes use of antibodies and/or cell-mediated immune responses that are generated as a consequence of exposure to infectious agents.

INNATE IMMUNITY

Innate immunity is composed of physical and microbiological barriers (the normal flora), fluid phase components, and cellular constituents.

Physical Barriers

The discussion of the physical barriers and how they relate to innate immunity is included in the chapters that introduce each organ system.

Normal Flora

In order to produce disease affiliated with a mucosal surface, pathogenic microorganisms must in some way interact with a host (patient) cell comprising the surface. If that cell surface is occupied with normal flora, then association will not occur, nor will disease. Acting in this fashion, the normal flora is part of the innate immunity of the host.

The normal flora, composed of bacteria and fungi (mainly yeasts), are part of the innate host defense. These bacteria and fungi have established a unique relationship with the host, a relationship that begins as the microbiologically sterile fetus begins its journey down the birth canal. Acquisition of bacteria and fungi begins immediately, with infection (colonization) of all exposed surfaces, including mucosal surfaces (alimentary canal, upper respiratory tract, and distal genitourinary tract), with microorganisms from the birth canal and from the mother's immediate environment. The association of microbe with the host is not haphazard but rather is an association that depends upon 1) receptors (usually in the form of carbohydrates that are part of glycoproteins on the surface of the host cell) and adhesins on the microbe cell surface, 2) the chemicals in the immediate environment of the microbe–host interaction, in part due to products secreted by competing microorganisms (e.g., microcins, bacteriocins, and volatile fatty acids) and in part due to products secreted by the host (e.g., acid environment of the stomach, defensins secreted by Paneth cells, the contents of bile in the upper small intestine, or the content of sebum on the skin), and 3) the availability of nutrient substances.

The establishment of the normal flora is a dynamic one, with replacement at various exposed locations with microbes more capable of living at a particular site (niche) than the ones proceeding. In addition, the immune system appears to play some role, since it has been shown that members of the normal flora are very poorly immunogenic in the host from which the microbes are isolated. This suggests that immune responses to microbes attempting to colonize a particular location (niche) will result in the blockage of association between adhesin (microbe) with receptor (host). If a microbe cannot associate, then it will be replaced with one that will. This occurs until a strain of microbe is encountered that is more similar to the host than its predecessor, which is subsequently "accepted" as part of the normal flora of that particular animal.

The result is an ecosystem composed of numerous species of bacteria and fungi that are associated with an abundance of niches, each of which is occupied with a particular species of microbe most suited to live at that location. This "occupation" results in a barrier to colonization (infection) by microbes that are not members of the normal flora, thus the term *colonization resistance*.

Fluid Phase Constituents

There are a number of molecules in the fluid phase that exert important innate defenses against potential pathogenic microorganisms. These include complement proteins, lysozyme, acute phase proteins, interferons, and iron-binding proteins.

The complement system consists of a number of proteins that interact in a cascading, enzymatic fashion to destroy the infectious agent that instigated the cascade. Activation of the complement system without the participation of antibodies (as would be the case for innate immunity) depends on the nature of the surface upon which the activation takes place. An "activating" surface is one in which the third component of complement, C3, becomes activated and results in the covalent linkage of C3b to the surface. Complement activated in this fashion is said to be through the "alternate pathway." Activating surfaces are those present on some bacteria, fungi, and parasites. Such surfaces are characterized as lacking sialic acids residues and other inhibitory substances such as membrane cofactor protein and decay-accelerating factor — substances found on the surface of host cells.

The activation of the complement system results in the production of several important substances. Among these are C3b, an opsonin that binds to the activating surface (a bacteria or a fungus) to facilitate interaction with phagocytic cells that have surface receptors for C3b. The binding of phagocytic cells with opsonized particles greatly increases the efficiency of phagocytosis. Other important by-products of complement activation are C3a and C5a, molecules with vasoactive as well as chemotactic activity. The final product of the complement cascade is the membrane attack complex, a pore-like structure that inserts into the outer membrane of gram-negative bacteria resulting in their lysis.

Lysozyme, another important innate defense molecule, is an enzyme that is present in a wide variety of body secretions. It splits the backbone of the peptidoglycan layer of the bacterial cell wall. Gram-positive bacteria are especially vulnerable.

Acute phase proteins are normally present in very low amounts in plasma. Upon infection they increase greatly. C-reactive protein, one such molecule, recognizes and binds in a Ca^{2+} dependent manner to the surfaces of many different species of bacteria and fungi. In this fashion, C-reactive protein serves as an opsonin that facilitates phagocytosis. It also activates the complement system.

Interferons are important in viral innate immunity. Specifically the alpha and beta interferons are induced by infection of cells by certain viruses, while gamma interferon (immune interferon) is part of the acquired immune response. Virus-infected cells produce interferon, which binds to neighboring cells and confers a state of resistance.

Iron-binding proteins (lactoferrin, transferrin) found in the fluid phase limit the availability of iron. Since iron is an absolute growth requirement for bacteria and fungi, these proteins play an important role in innate immunity.

Cells of Innate Immunity

Phagocytic Cells. The polymorphonuclear leukocyte, *neutrophil*, is a bone-marrow-derived end-cell that normally comprises 30% to 70% percent of the total leukocytes in the peripheral blood of various species. The neutrophil is a granulocytic leukocyte and contains two types of granules: primary or azurophilic granules and secondary or specific granules. Neutrophils spend only about 12 hours in circulation, then go into the tissues where they survive for an additional two to three days. Within the bone marrow there is a large storage compartment for neutrophils. A bacterial infection within the body causes a rapid mobilization of this pool and the neutrophils accumulate at the site of the infectious process. They are attracted by the chemotactic factors, C3a and C5a, which are generated subsequent to activation of the complement system. The process of neutrophil accumulation begins by *adherence* of the circulating neutrophils to the vascular endothelium (margination), *extravasation* into tissue spaces, and *chemotaxis* of the cells toward the focus of injury. Invading microorganisms are ingested by neutrophils in a process called *phagocytosis* (Fig 2.1).

Phagocytosis of bacteria by neutrophils involves several steps. First, initial recognition and binding occur. This process is made more efficient by the presence of opsonins and/or immunoglobulin and complement components. Opsonization coats the surface of a particle, neutralizing the net negative charges, which might otherwise cause the neutrophil and bacterial cell to repel each other. In addition, on the cell membrane of the neutrophil, receptors are present for antibody (Fc receptors) and for complement (CR). These receptors facilitate firm attachment of the opsonized bacterium to the neutrophil. Next, pseudopodia form around the organism and then fuse to form a *phagocytic vacuole* containing the organism. Some organisms are more readily engulfed than others. For example, the presence of a polysaccharide capsule causes an organism to be resistant to phagocytosis. Such capsules have negative charges (as does the surface of phagocytic cells), as well as being relatively hydrophilic (the external membrane of phagocytic cells is relatively hydrophobic). Opsonins are particularly important for ingestion of these organisms. After engulfment, lysosomal granules fuse with the phagosome membrane to form the *phagolysosome*. The eventual elimination of the engulfed organism occurs within this structure (Fig 2.2).

Bacterial killing is accomplished by a series of metabolic and enzymatic events. Metabolic activity increases within a neutrophil during phagocytosis. Oxygen consumption increases and light energy is emitted (chemiluminescence). This metabolic or *respiratory burst* involves oxidation of glucose by the hexosemonophosphate shunt. Bactericidal products are generated. Superoxide radicals are produced and converted to H_2O_2 by superoxide dismutase. Hydrogen peroxide is toxic for bacteria that lack catalase. The enzyme myeloperoxidase, present in azurophil granules, catalyzes the oxidation of halide ions to hypohalite, which is also toxic to microorganisms. Thus the myeloperoxidase-hydrogen-peroxide-halide system is efficient in bacterial killing. Susceptible organisms are killed within minutes. Inside the primary granules of neutrophils, enzymes released during degranulation act on proteins, lipids, carbohydrates, and nucleic acids to degrade the killed bacterial cells. Some of these enzymes are collagenase, elastase, acid phosphatase, phospholipase, lysozyme, hyaluronidase, acid ribonuclease, and deoxyribonuclease. *Lysozyme* can cleave glycosyl bonds in the bacterial cell wall, making the cell susceptible to lysis. Also, lysosomes contain cationic peptides (defensins) that form lethal pores in bacteria as well as fungal cell walls.

FIGURE 2.1. *Neutrophil response to an infectious agent: A. Neutrophils are present in the circulation. B. Neutrophils express adhesin molecules (CD18) and adhere to the endothelial cells in the blood vessel. This process is called* margination. *C. Neutrophils pass through the endothelial cells by diapedesis. D. Neutrophils, now extravascular, respond and move along a chemotactic gradient.*

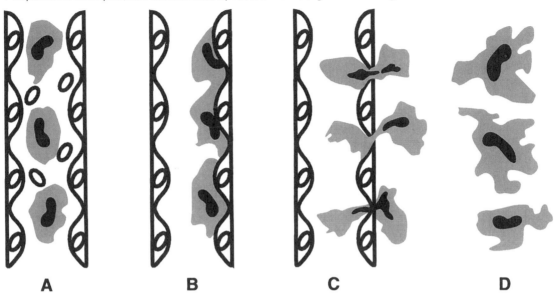

A　　　　**B**　　　　**C**　　　　**D**

FIGURE 2.2. *The process of phagocytosis: A. A bacterium is opsonized by antibody. The antibody binds to an Fc receptor on a phagocyte. B. The phagocyte begins to engulf the attached bacterium. C. The phagosome containing the bacterium fuses with lysosomes in the phagocyte cytoplasm to form a phagolysosome. D. The bacterium is killed and digested. E. The bacterial breakdown products are eliminated from the cell. Some parts of the bacterium will remain on macrophage membrane associated with MHC class II to be used in antigen presentation to T cells.*

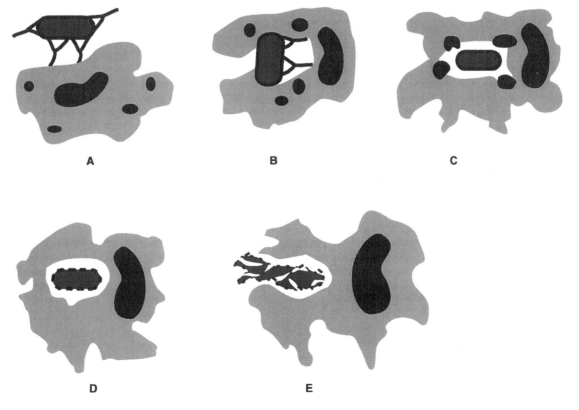

A　　　　　　**B**　　　　　　**C**

D　　　　　　**E**

Macrophage. *Macrophages*, while important in the acquired immune response, also play an essential part in innate immunity. The macrophage is a mononuclear cell derived from the bone marrow. For several days after release from the bone marrow, it circulates as a blood *monocyte* before going into the tissues, where it becomes a functional macrophage. Free macrophages are present in many parts of the body and are named accordingly, for example, alveolar macrophages (lung) and peritoneal macrophages. Fixed macrophages line sinus cavities that filter blood. These include the Kupffer cells (liver), Langerhans cells (skin), histiocytes (connective tissue), mesangial cells (kidneys), and sinus-lining cells of the spleen, lymph nodes, and bone marrow. Some of these macrophages are important in antigen processing for induction of an immune response (described later in this chapter).

As phagocytes, the macrophage and the neutrophil have similarities and differences. The macrophage differs from the neutrophil in that it has a longer life span in tissue and can reuse phagolysosomes. In addition, macrophages stimulated by cytokines (e.g., interferon) or microbial products (e.g., lipopolysaccharide) result in activation of nitric oxide synthase that catalyzes the production of nitric oxide (NO) from L-arginine. NO is toxic to many bacteria, especially those residing within macrophages (e.g., *Salmonella*, *Listeria*). The macrophage is similar to the neutrophil in that toxic oxygen metabolites are generated for bacterial killing and the lysosomes contain potent hydrolytic enzymes and cationic peptides (defensins). While the neutrophil responds to a stimulus rapidly, the macrophage is not present until later in an infectious process, often after 8 to 12 hours. In some instances, neutrophils may eliminate an organism before macrophages arrive in any great number. When tissue destruction has occurred as a result of an inflammatory response, macrophages are attracted to the area by products from dying neutrophils and bacteria. They phagocytose the debris and remove it. In some instances, macrophages may engulf particulate material that they are unable to digest. When this occurs, the macrophage may migrate to a mucosal surface such as the respiratory or gastrointestinal tract for elimination from the body.

Some microorganisms are more easily killed by phagocytes than others. Bacteria that have polysaccharide capsules are less readily engulfed than unencapsulated counterparts. Opsonizing antibody or complement components must be present to coat such organisms before phagocytes can engulf them. Some microorganisms are readily phagocytosed, but are able to grow intracellularly. For example, microorganisms such as *Listeria monocytogenes* and *Mycobacterium tuberculosis* are not killed after phagocytosis by macrophages. Organisms may produce factors that inhibit phagolysosome fusion or even escape the phagolysosome into the cytoplasm, thus preventing exposure to enzymatic degradation.

Natural Killer (NK) Cells.   The natural killer cell is a lymphoid cell with the characteristics of neither a T lymphocyte nor a B lymphocyte — i.e., it does not have a T cell receptor, CD4, CD8, or CD2 and it does not have surface immunoglobulin. The NK cell does, however, have a cell membrane receptor CD16, a low-affinity IgG receptor. This non-T, non-B cell comprises about 15% of the lymphoid cells in the peripheral blood. NK cells function to kill tumor cells, virus-infected cells, and certain bacteria; they are not MHC-restricted in their killing and they do not appear to require previous sensitization to target cells. Morphologically the NK cell is a large granular lymphocyte. Upon contact with an appropriate target, NK cells may release soluble cytotoxic factors such as perforin and tumor necrosis factors alpha and beta.

Gamma-Delta T Cells.   T cells expressing antigen-specific receptors that are composed of gamma and delta chains (gamma-delta T cells) constitute a small percentage of the circulating pool of lymphocytes in nonruminant species. In ruminants, however, gamma-delta T cells may represent up to 30% of the circulating lymphocyte pool. Most T lymphocytes, regardless of animal species, express antigen-specific receptors composed of alpha and beta chains. Gamma-delta T cells are thought to be involved in innate defense against certain bacteria. They do this by recognizing not only bacterial stress proteins (expressed by bacteria while in the host) but also cells containing facultative intracellular bacteria and some viruses. In most species, gamma-delta T cells are present in the lamina propria underlying mucosal epithelia, strategically beneficial sites for cells involved in host defense.

Inflammation

Inflammation is the term given to the response of the host to injury. Pathology textbooks classically describe four signs of inflammation: calor (heat), dolor (pain), tumor (swelling), and rubor (redness). The process that creates these clinical signs has three components: 1) increased circulation to the area, 2) increased capillary permeability, and 3) chemotaxis of neutrophils (initially) and macrophages (later) to the area. Mediators that are released in response to injury and/or an infectious process come from four enzyme systems: 1) the clotting system, 2) the kinin system, 3) the fibrinolytic system, and 4) the complement system. For example, the inflammatory response initiated following activation of the complement system leads to the production of chemotactic peptides (C3a and C5a) that cause leukocytes in the circulation to marginate, diapedese through the vascular endothelium, and migrate along a chemotactic gradient to the site of injury or infectious process. C3a and C5a also cause mast cell degranulation that results in the release of histamine followed by increased capillary permeability, which brings increased amounts of fluid to the site carrying additional factors to assist in the inflammatory response. The arrival of neutrophils and the phagocytic engulfment of microorganisms result in the formation of a purulent exudate (pus). Eventually, macrophages arrive to aid in phagocytosis and in the clean-up of cellular debris resulting from the interaction of neutrophils with the infectious agent.

One of the roles macrophages have in the response of the host to an infectious agent is to release cytokines when they encounter microbial by-products. Cytokines result in upregulation of endothelial cell adhesion molecules recognized by circulating leukocytes (IL-1, tumor necrosis factor alpha), attraction of leukocytes (IL-8), release of acute phase proteins (IL-6), and activation of effector cells such as NK cells and T cells involved with macrophage activation (IL-12).

ACQUIRED IMMUNITY

Generation of the Immune Response

The acquired immune response is instigated by the presentation of antigen to T and B cells by an antigen-presenting cell. Antigen that is taken up by macrophages from the external environment — for example, bacteria that are phagocytosed and digested in phagocytic vacuoles — is processed in phagosomes and portions of the digested antigen are brought to the surface coupled with major histocompatibility molecules (MHC class II). Recognition of the antigen/MHC class II complex by a T cell with the same MHC class II is referred to as *MHC-restriction* and is a characteristic of the acquired immune response. Production of cytokines such as interleukin-1 (IL-1) by the macrophage continues the response and is followed by production of IL-2 by the T cell. Interleukin-2 is a T cell growth factor and facilitates clonal expansion of the participating T cell. Meanwhile these T cells, which are phenotypically CD4+ and functionally called *helper T cells*, produce additional cytokines to influence the development of B cells, which are specific for the antigen. Under the influence of T cell produced IL-4, B cells develop and mature into plasma cells secreting antibodies. Helper T cells produce predominantly IL-4 (T helper 2 cells or T_{H2}), which facilitate production of IgG_1 and IgE; T cells that produce predominantly gamma interferon (T helper 1 cells or T_{H1}) facilitate cell-mediated immune responses. Hence, the ratio of T_{H2} to T_{H1} cells determines whether the immune response to a particular microorganism will be predominantly humoral (i.e., antibody) or cellular (i.e., activated macrophages). Recovery from infection is therefore frequently dependent upon the type of T cell response that is elicited upon exposure to an infectious agent.

The type of immune response that is most efficient in stopping an infectious process depends on the site of replication of the disease agent. Antibody is effective against extracellularly multiplying infectious agents, while cell-mediated immune responses are most important for those that replicate intracellularly. The site of replication also directs the way in which the immune response is stimulated. Infectious agents that replicate inside the cytoplasm of cells, such as viruses, traffic to vacuoles that intersect those containing MHC class I molecules. The distinction is important because effector cytotoxic T cells (CD8+) recognize antigen in association with MHC class I molecules.

Antibody Response

Acquired immune responses begin with the engulfment of the infectious agent by an antigen-presenting cell. Transportation of the agent to the local lymph node follows. In the lymph node, the antigen is processed and presented to lymphocytes. The immune response thus occurs locally and systemically as well because lymphatics draining the site of the infectious process carry antigen to the bloodstream and then to the spleen.

The initial introduction of antigen to a host followed by appropriate processing and T cell stimulation results in expansion of B cell clones specific to the different epitopes on the antigen. Under the influence of T cell cytokines, these B cells will differentiate into antibody-producing plasma cells. The first antibody to be produced will be of the IgM isotype and will appear in the circulation 7 to 10 days after initiation of the immune response. Next, IgG will begin to appear but will not rise to very high titers in this primary immune response. The next encounter with antigen, a secondary or anamnestic response, generates a quicker immune response and the amount of antibody produced will last longer. Most importantly, the isotype that predominates in the secondary response will be mainly IgG. This information is particularly important in evaluating the potential for a given disease agent to be the cause of clinical signs seen in a patient. It is a well-accepted diagnostic procedure to obtain acute and convalescent serum samples to be evaluated for antibody titer and sometimes isotype as well. Generally, when a disease agent is responsible for clinical signs two to three weeks after the initial appearance of signs, the titer will have increased by at least fourfold if the agent was involved in the infectious process. In an initial exposure to a disease agent, IgM is the predominant isotype, while a second or tertiary exposure (or vaccination) will elicit mostly IgG (Fig 2.3).

The antibody response that is important in defense against bacterial disease depends on the pathogenic mechanisms involved, the site of the infectious process, and the isotype of the antibody elicited (Table 2.1). If the disease is caused by an extracellular toxin, as in tetanus, then antitoxin antibodies are important to neutralize and bind the toxin before it can bind to cellular sites and initiate clinical signs. This mechanism is important in

Table 2.1. Effector Functions of Antibody

Isotype	Site of Action	Effector Functions
IgM	Intravascular	Complement fixation, agglutination
IgG	Intravascular	Complement fixation, neutralization
	Tissue spaces	Opsonization, ADCC
IgA	Secretions: respiratory, GI, salivary	Neutralization on mucosal surfaces
IgE	Subcutaneous Submucosal	Mast-cell sensitization, ADCC

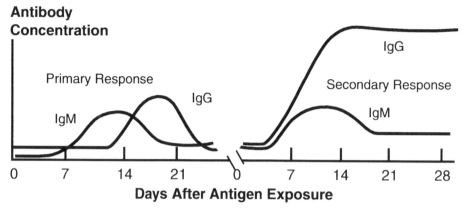

FIGURE 2.3.   *In the primary antibody response, introduction of antigen on day 0 elicits initially an IgM response followed by an IgG response. Upon secondary exposure to the antigen, there is a more rapid immune response, which is characterized by higher titers of IgG antibody that remain in the circulation longer than in the primary response.*

diseases such as tetanus, anthrax, and botulism — all toxin-mediated diseases. In some instances, when a non-immune host is at risk of developing a toxin-mediated disease, immediate administration of antitoxin (a solution containing antibodies to the toxin) is required to prevent the disease. In order to eliminate infectious agents, antibodies serve as opsonins as well as initiating the complement cascade (activation through the classical pathway). Opsonins lead to increased uptake by phagocytic cells, whereas complement activation leads to initiation of inflammation and generation of compounds that are detrimental to the infectious agent (e.g., membrane attack complex).

Generally, the IgE response is limited to parasitic infections and hypersensitivity reactions to various environmental allergens, such as pollens and grasses. Occasionally IgE is elicited in response to vaccination against infectious agents. When this occurs very serious adverse responses, such as anaphylactic shock, can result. Often there is a hereditary predisposition toward IgE production and these individuals are at increased risk of having such a vaccine reaction. For immunity to parasite infections, IgE may assist in the phenomenon of "self cure," in which large numbers of nematodes are purged from the gut by mast cell mediator induced smooth muscle contraction. Alternatively, some infestations are controlled by antibody dependent cell mediated cytotoxicity (ADCC), in which IgE binds to eosinophils by low-affinity Fc receptors and facilitates release of major basic protein and other caustic enzymes on the parasite surface.

IgA is a very desirable response to infectious agents that invade mucosal surfaces. Since secretory IgA (SIgA) is protected by secretory component from digestion in the gut by proteolytic enzymes, it is the most efficient antibody to be active in the environment of the gastrointestinal lumen. There it can neutralize virus and bacteria to prevent their respective attachment to cellular receptors. Similarly, SIgA is effective within the secretions of the respiratory tract. Before a virus or a bacterium can infect a cell it must first bind to a cell surface protein that

acts as a receptor for the infectious agent. Thus, binding of the infectious agent by antibody can inhibit binding to the receptor, and thus lower the infectivity of the agent. For example, influenza virus expresses a hemagglutinin that binds to certain glycoproteins expressed on epithelial cells in the respiratory tract. Binding of antibodies to the hemagglutinin prevents entry of the virus into these cells, and disease is prevented.

The importance of antibodies relative to cellular immune mechanisms in response to infectious agents depends on the life cycle of the agent. Antibody is extremely important in controlling agents that are extracellular, such as *Streptococcus* and *Escherichia coli*. IgG and IgM function as opsonins and work in concert with the phagocytic cells to enhance engulfment and thereby subsequent killing by mechanisms mentioned above. IgG and IgM antibody also activate the complement cascade and result in lysis of the bacteria (if gram negative). For those bacteria that are facultative intracellular dwellers, such as *Listeria* and *Mycobacterium*, antibody is relatively ineffective in achieving ultimate killing and removal of the agent, although it could be used as an indicator that exposure/infection has occurred. These types of infections require a T_{H1} response that results in production of gamma interferon. Gamma interferon, also known as *macrophage activating factor*, upregulates metabolic processes in macrophages, enabling them to kill microorganisms able to evade their killing mechanisms. Gamma interferon is also an activator of NK cells, increasing their ability to kill targets.

Antibodies are most effective against viruses that undergo a viremic phase, when there are numerous virus particles in the extracellular environment. Viruses such as influenza virus, for example, are neutralized by antibodies specific for the major surface antigens (hemagglutinin and neuraminidase). Other viruses, herpesvirus, for example, remain very closely associated with cells and do not present much opportunity for antibody-mediated inactivation. The IgA isotype is especially effective on mucosal surfaces and functions to neutralize viruses before entry into the body. Secretory IgA is an extremely effective defense against respiratory and gastrointestinal viruses as well as viruses that causes systemic disease but enter via the oral route. Virus neutralization occurs because the antibody binds to surface determinants of the virus and prevents the virus from binding to the cellular receptors to which it must attach in order to initiate the infectious process.

Cell-Mediated Immunity

Cell-mediated immune responses involve two different mechanisms: macrophage activation (sometimes referred to as *hypersensitivity*) and cytotoxic T cells (Table 2.2). Activated macrophages are useful in the destruction of intracellular infectious agents (such as *Brucella, Salmonella, Mycobacterium, Rickettsia*); cytotoxic T cells lyse host cells in which infectious agents are present (such as viral infected cells).

Macrophages are activated following the production of gamma interferon by T_{H1} cells. This subset of T helper cells is stimulated subsequent to the production of IL-12 by infected macrophages. Thus, the upregulation of macrophages results in destruction of the infectious agent

that the macrophage previously had been unable to destroy. The type of inflammatory response generated by T_{H1} cells is called *granulomatous*, describing the predominant cell types involved (mainly macrophages).

Cytotoxic T cells (CD8+) recognize antigenic determinant in the context of major histocompatibility complex class I (MHC class I). Processing of antigen (e.g., portions of a virus particle) that is in the cytoplasm of the cells results in the incorporation of a portion of the antigen in the MHC class I molecule that is displayed on the surface of the affected cell. Recognition of the combination of MHC class I and antigenic determinant by cytotoxic T cells (by way of a specific receptor) results in the release of perforins, tumor necrosis factor alpha, and activation of the Fas ligand, resulting in the death of the infected cell.

Antibody dependent cellular cytotoxicity (ADCC) occurs when antibody binds to a null cell (NK, non-T, non-B cell) by Fc receptors. The attachment of antibody to a cell that previously had no receptor for antigen renders it antigen specific and capable of binding antigen. Besides null cells, eosinophils and macrophages can also become involved in ADCC. ADCC is an effective method of killing cells infected with microorganisms (viral, bacterial, or fungal) as well as parasites. In the case of parasites, the eosinophil releases granules containing major basic protein rendering the cuticle of the parasite permeable.

CELL TRAFFIC

Recirculation of lymphocytes from the blood vascular system through the lymphoid organs and into the lymph is critical to the normal function of the immune system.

Table 2.2. Effector Functions of T Cell–Mediated Immune Responses

Effector Cell	Target	Mechanism
CD8+	MHC class I matched cell with intracellular antigen	Perforin; Fas ligand activation; TNF
CD4+	Macrophage with intracellular organisms	Gamma interferon–mediated activation of macrophage

FIGURE 2.4. *The relationship between systemic, pulmonary, and lymphatic circulation. A lymphocyte that circulates in the blood will enter the lymph tissue through postcapillary venules and will leave through the efferent lymphatics. These eventually enter the thoracic duct and then the vena cava, where they rejoin the systemic circulation. Lymphocytes in the tissues enter the lymph node through the afferent lymphatics.*

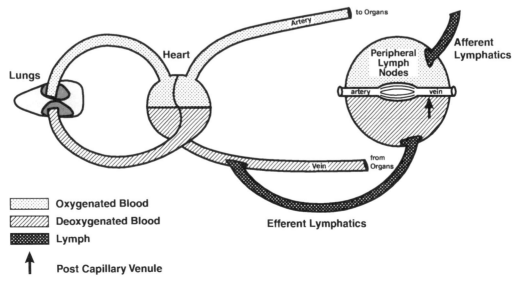

Blood leaves the left ventricle of the heart and circulates through the systemic vascular system. After returning from the tissues where oxygen is delivered, the blood enters the right ventricle and into the pulmonary circulation where reoxygenation occurs and the circuit begins again. The path taken by a lymphocyte within the blood vascular system diverges from this circuit at the postcapillary venules in lymph nodes under mucosal surfaces and the lactating mammary gland. Lymphocytes leave the blood and enter the tissue by first binding to homing receptors called *integrins*. For example, L-selectin on the lymphocyte membrane binds to a receptor on the endothelial cell of these postcapillary venules in lymph nodes, facilitating exit of the lymphocyte into the lymph node. Once in the lymph node, the lymphocyte travels to the appropriate area — paracortex for T cells and cortex for B lymphocytes. If stimulated by antigen while in the node, the cells remain, undergo clonal expansion, and become effector cells. If they do not become stimulated, they exit the lymph node through efferent lymphatics traveling eventually into the thoracic duct and then into the posterior vena cava where they once again join the systemic circulation (Fig 2.4).

The spleen is another lymphoid organ through which lymphocytes travel. While in the bloodstream, they enter the spleen and travel through the venous sinuses constituting the red pulp. If antigen has been filtered from the bloodstream, splenic lymphocytes become trapped as they traverse the sinusoids. The periarteriolar lymphatic sheath contains T cells and associated B cell follicles where immune responses to the trapped antigen occur.

Lymphocytes home to specific tissue sites depending upon where they were first stimulated. Lymphocytes stimulated by antigens that enter the body by way of a mucosal surface tend to circulate from the mucosal surface, to the bloodstream, and back to all mucosal surfaces, not just to the point of origin. Thus, a lymphocyte stimulated by antigen in the intestinal canal will recognize addressins expressed by endothelial cells on postcapillary venules traversing the lung, genitourinary tract, intestinal tract, and lactating mammary gland. Likewise, lymphocytes stimulated by antigens that enter the immune system by way of the bloodstream tend to stay within the bloodstream-lymphatic circulation and away from mucosal surfaces. Lymphocytes recognize "where they are" by possessing receptors that bind to "addressins" expressed by endothelial cells comprising postcapillary venules (e.g., L-selectin on postcapillary venules of lymph nodes).

SELECTED REFERENCES

Gershwin LJ, Krakowka S, Olsen RG. Immunology and immunopathology of domestic animals. 2nd ed. St. Louis: Mosby, 1995.

Hancock REW. Peptide antibiotics. Lancet 1997;349:418.

Janeway CA, Travers P. Immunobiology, the immune system in health and disease. 3rd ed. London: Current Biology, 1997.

MacMicking J, Xie Q, Nathan C. Nitric oxide and macrophage function. Annu Rev Immunol 1997;15:323.

Ouellette AJ, Selsted ME. Enteric defensins. Curr Opin Gastroenterol 1997;13:494.

Tizard I. Veterinary immunology: an introduction. 5th ed. Philadelphia: W.B. Saunders, 1997.

3 *Laboratory Diagnosis*

Dwight C. Hirsh   Yuan Chung Zee

Anthony E. Castro

Bacteria and Fungi

A key decision made early in the diagnostic workup is whether the patient's condition has an infectious etiology. This decision is important because drugs used to treat conditions with noninfectious etiologies — corticosteroids, for example — are often contraindicated for treatment of conditions with an infectious one, for which antibiotics are appropriate.

One of the first major goals of the microbiology laboratory is to isolate clinically significant microorganisms from an affected site and, if more than one type of microorganism is present, to isolate them in approximately the same ratio as occurs in vivo. Whether an isolate is "clinically significant" or not depends upon the circumstances of isolation. For example, the isolation of large numbers of a particular microorganism from a normally sterile site in the presence of an inflammatory cytology would be interpreted as significant.

Attention must be given to the site cultured as well as to the method of obtaining the sample for culture. The determination of significance is made a great deal easier if the sample is obtained from a normally sterile site. Obtaining a sample from the alimentary canal, and expecting meaningful answers, may be unrealistic unless one is looking for the presence or absence of a particular microorganism, for example, *Salmonella* or *Campylobacter*.

Sample Collection

Care must be given to how the sample is collected; if not, interpretation of results may be difficult. Most infectious processes arise subsequent to the contamination of a compromised surface or site by microorganisms that are also a part of the flora occurring on a contiguous mucosal surface. In other words, microorganisms isolated from an affected site are often similar (if not identical) to those found as part of the normal flora of the patient.

Transport of Samples

The sooner the sample is processed in the microbiology laboratory, the better. Realistically, the time between sample collection and processing may range from minutes to hours. Sample drying (all microorganisms) and exposure to a noxious atmosphere (oxygen for obligate anaerobes) are the major dangers in not analyzing samples promptly. For this reason, it is important that the sample be kept moist (for a syringe full of exudate, this is obviously not an important consideration) and, if conditions warrant (see below), air excluded. Moistness is maintained by placing the sample in a transport (holding) medium composed of a balanced salt solution usually in a gelled matrix. Because this medium does not contain any nutrient material, microorganisms in the sample multiply poorly if at all (and thereby relative numbers and ratios are preserved) but remain viable for a time, at least for overnight (exactly how long depends upon the microorganism involved — beta hemolytic *Streptococcus*, for example, does not survive as long as *Escherichia coli*). Swabs should always be placed in transport medium, regardless of the time elapsed between processing and collection. Fluids that may contain anaerobic bacteria (e.g., exudate from draining tracts, peritoneal and pleural effusions, abscess material) should be cultured immediately. If this material is contained in a syringe, then the air should be expelled and a sterile stopper placed over the needle. If a swab is used to collect the sample, it should be placed in an anaerobic transport medium. If a syringe full of sample cannot be processed immediately, the syringe should be emptied into an anaerobic transport medium and held at room temperature. Similarly placed swabs are treated in the same manner. Do not refrigerate samples suspected of containing anaerobes because some species do not tolerate reduced temperatures.

Demonstration of an Infectious Agent

The presence of an infectious agent is accomplished by examination of stained smears made from a portion of the clinical sample, culture techniques, molecular/immunological methods, or a combination of these methods.

Direct Smears. Information obtained from examination of a stained smear is valuable because it may be the first indication (and sometimes the only one) that an infectious agent is present. Also, what is seen (shape, gram-staining characteristics) will help guide the choice of therapy 24 hours before culture results are available. At least 10^4 microorganisms/ml or gram of material must be present in order to be readily detected microscopically.

As is the case with a sample obtained from a normally sterile site, the presence of bacteria in bladder urine is a significant finding. However, interpretation of the results of analysis of urine samples obtained by catheter or by catch is difficult because of the confounding presence of flora flushed from the distal urethra. Finding bacteria by direct smear in concentrated (the preferred) or unconcentrated urine obtained by percutaneous aspiration of bladder urine is a significant finding. Demonstration of 1 bacteria/oil field in a drop of unconcentrated urine (which has been allowed to dry and then stained) represents about 10^5 to 10^6 bacteria/ml of urine.

Two types of stains are available, the gram stain and Romanowsky-type stains such as Wright's or Giemsa. Each type of stain has advantages and disadvantages. The gram stain is useful in that the shape and the gram-staining characteristics of the agent are seen. The disadvantage of the gram stain is that the cellular content of the sample is not readily discerned. On the other hand, a Romanowsky-type stain gives the observer a feeling for the cellular nature of the sample and whether or not there is an infectious agent present. Cytologic evaluation of the sample is very important in assessing the significance of the microorganism seen and subsequently grown.

Culture Techniques.   Media are inoculated with a portion of the specimen. Inoculation should be performed in a semi-quantitative fashion (especially samples of bladder urine obtained by catheter or catch).

Determination of the relative numbers of microorganisms in a sample greatly helps interpretation of significance. Colonies of microorganisms growing on all four quadrants of a petri plate indicate that there are large numbers of microorganisms in the sample. If a sample yielded one or two colonies growing on the plate, the significance of these colonies and thus the question as to the infectious etiology of the condition would be in doubt. "Enrichment" prior to plating of a sample obtained from a normally sterile site should never be done because one microorganism can grow to numbers that equal many thousands in a very short period of time. Obviously more credence will be given to a process from which thousands of microorganisms were isolated than to a sample from which one was isolated. An important exception to this general "rule" is whether the presence or absence of a particular microorganism is significant, e.g., *Salmonella* in a fecal specimen. From a clinical perspective, the use of enrichment broths, other than for the determination of the presence or absence of a particular species of bacterium, is more trouble than it is worth. Too often, enrichment culture results lead to the unnecessary workup and treatment of a contaminating microorganism.

Determination of significance is aided by the cytology of the sample obtained from the affected site. Isolation (demonstration) of numerous microorganisms from a normally sterile site without the presence of inflammatory cells should be viewed with suspicion. The one exception to this rule is cryptococcal infection wherein the sample may contain a large number of yeast cells but very few inflammatory cells (the cryptococcal capsule is immunosuppressive). The isolation or demonstration of a "significant number" of microorganisms from a normally sterile site without evidence of an inflammatory response can be explained by contaminated collection devices, contamination of the collection device from a contiguous, normally nonsterile site, contamination of the medium inoculation device in the microbiology laboratory, or contamination of the medium before inoculation. Collection devices sterilized by liquid disinfectants quite often become contaminated by microorganisms able to live in such fluids (*Pseudomonas* is notorious for this).

Plates may be streaked in any fashion as long as individual colonies are produced after incubation. Assessing relative numbers is very subjective, and every laboratory has their own way of doing this. Relative numbers of microorganisms may be reported by noting how much growth occurs on the surface of the plate. Obviously, growth of one colony (the offspring of one bacterium) vs. growth of colonies over the whole plate would be viewed differently with respect to clinical significance. Determination of the actual numbers of bacteria present is only important when analyzing urine obtained by catch or catheter because of the problem of contamination of the sample by bacteria in the distal urethra. In this instance, disposable calibrated loops containing 0.001 or 0.01 ml of urine are used to inoculate appropriate media (blood/MacConkey, for example).

Aerobic Bacteria.   The standard medium inoculated for the isolation of facultative microorganisms is a blood agar plate. Many laboratories include a MacConkey agar plate as well (or as a "split" plate with blood agar on half and MacConkey agar on the other half). MacConkey agar is useful because enteric microorganisms (e.g., *Escherichia coli*, *Klebsiella*, *Enterobacter*) grow very well, as do the nonenteric *Pseudomonas*. Most other nonenteric gram-negative rods and all gram-positive microorganisms do not grow well on this medium. *Bordetella* grows as tiny pinpoint colonies after 24 hours, and after 48 hours of incubation, the colonies will be quite large. Assessing the growth on MacConkey agar will help greatly in determining the presence or absence of enteric organisms, the group of bacteria most difficult to deal with therapeutically.

Anaerobic Bacteria.   Anaerobic bacteria grow on blood agar that is specially prepared by ridding the medium as much as possible of oxygen and its products. The plates come from the manufacturer in sealed pouches designed to exclude air. After anaerobic plates are inoculated, they should be placed in a container of flowing oxygen-free CO_2 or placed directly into an anaerobic environment. (Note that anaerobic blood plates that have been removed from their pouches should be stored in flowing oxygen-free CO_2 or in an anaerobic environment.)

When to inoculate media for anaerobic incubation depends upon the source of the sample. Processing samples for anaerobes is time consuming and expensive.

The most common sites or conditions that contain anaerobic bacteria are draining tracts; abscesses; pleural, pericardial, and peritoneal effusions; pyometra; osteomyelitis; and lungs. Anaerobic culture of sites that contain a population of anaerobic bacteria as part of the normal flora is wasteful (e.g., feces, vagina, distal urethra, oral cavity). An exception would be culture of duodenal aspirates for assessment of bacterial overgrowth. In this instance, the relative numbers found are what are sought (overgrowth is usually considered present when the total number of bacteria, anaerobes and aerobes, exceeds 10^8/ml of contents). Anaerobic culture of the urinary tract is not routinely performed because the recovery of these microorganisms from this site is extremely rare.

Molecular/Immunologic Methods. Sometimes it is important to determine the presence or absence of a particular microorganism as quickly as possible so that appropriate measures can be taken to deal with the problem. This is especially true when infectious agents are suspected that pose a threat to other animals including human care givers (e.g., *Salmonella, Leptospira*). Likewise, some infectious agents take so long to grow in culture that formulation of a rational therapeutic strategy is difficult (e.g., some fungal agents, *Mycobacterium).* Still others are hard to detect because they are difficult to culture (e.g., *Leptospira*, rickettsias) or have not been cultured in artificial media (e.g., *Clostridium piliformis, Lawsonia intracellularis*). In these instances, various techniques are available. Immunologically based techniques make use of antibodies specific for the microorganism in question. These antibodies are usually immobilized on a solid support and are used to trap the agent. The presence of the trapped agent is then detected with specific antibody that has been labeled in some way (usually with a color reagent). Some kits making use of this approach are commercially available (e.g., *Salmonella*).

Molecular techniques utilizing DNA probes specific for a segment of DNA that is unique to the microorganism in question, or the polymerase chain reaction (PCR) using specific primers, have been designed for a number of agents, although few are commercially available.

VIRUS

General Considerations

The diagnosis of viral diseases, although tedious and time-consuming, has been enhanced by modern technology, and although an individual animal may succumb to a viral disease, most contact animals or birds can be protected from infection. In animals, viruses sometimes reside innocuously in one species but are devastating in another contact host and therefore have major health implications. Prompt diagnosis of a viral-caused disease is therefore essential for an effective course of disease prevention and control.

Proper methods of collecting and processing clinical specimens and a complete history are vital to the suc-

cessful isolation of viruses. Tissues that are autolyzed or necrotic usually do not yield infectious virus because of the susceptibility of most viruses to detrimental environmental conditions. Viral isolation and identification should be attempted in the following conditions:

1. During an existing outbreak of a vesicular disease in ruminants (e.g., foot-and-mouth disease in cattle, pigs, sheep, or goats).
2. In a feedlot or ranch situation where additional susceptible livestock or poultry are at risk.
3. Where the viral etiology is required because of zoonotic potential (e.g., bluetongue or rabies in wildlife or velogenic viscerotropic Newcastle disease in psittacines).
4. When human exposure has occurred (e.g., rabies, western or eastern encephalomyelitis virus, herpes B virus of monkeys).
5. When a prophylactic vaccination program is to be instituted in a clinically affected herd or flock.
6. In delineating epidemiologic parameters as to the incidence and prevalence of viral diseases relative to season or geography.
7. As a component part of an infectious disease in a host.

In certain instances, a diseased animal can be euthanatized for humane or diagnostic reasons and tissue specimens obtained in a fresh condition. Collection of appropriate specimens (Tables 3.1 and 3.2) during the acute phase of the disease or viremia or at necropsy, and inclusion of additional submissions from similarly affected animals, enhances isolation of viruses. The following factors should be considered in selecting clinical specimens: 1) type of disease (e.g., respiratory — lung or trachea or vesicular — vesicle or skin biopsy), 2) the age and species of the host, 3) the type of lesions in or on the animal, and 4) the size of carcasses able to be shipped on ice.

A systematic approach for the rapid laboratory diagnosis of a viral-caused disease in animals is outlined below.

1. Anamnesis and histologic examination of the diseased tissues as a presumptive diagnosis for a viral etiology.
2. Measurement of the development of viral-specific antibodies (acute and convalescent sera) during clinical disease.
3. Examination of tissue sections of 6μ by fluorescein-labeled specific antibodies to detect specific viral antigens by localization of fluorescence in specific areas in infected tissue.
4. Examination of feces, plasma, or serum by immunoassays that detect specific viral antigens (e.g., rotavirus in feces, feline leukemia virus in serum, bovine respiratory syncytial virus in lung).
5. Examination of positive- or negative-stained specimens by electron microscopy to identify the morphology of virus. This diagnostic procedure is limited by the concentration of viral particles ($>10^5$/ml) required for detection.

Table 3.1. Suggested Specimens from Mammalian Species for Virus Isolation and Identification

Type of Illness or Infection	Common Name or Associated Virus	Other Infections	Clinical Specimens to Collect	Diagnostic Identification Tests
Respiratory	Adenovirus (bovine, porcine, canine)		Nasal and ocular secretions, feces, lung, brain, tonsil	VI (CPE), HA, CF, FA, VN
	Infectious canine hepatitis (adenovirus)		Spleen, liver, lymph nodes, kidney, blood	VI (CPE), HA, FA, VN
	Bovine viral diarrhea (mucosal disease) (pestivirus)	Genital, abortions, enteric	Nasal secretions, oral lesions, lung, spleen, blood, mesenteric lymph nodes, intestinal mucosa, vaginal secretions, fetal tissues, unclotted blood	VI (CPE and virus interference), FA, VN
	Infectious bovine rhinotracheitis (herpesvirus)	Central nervous system (CNS), genital, abortions	Nasal and ocular secretions, lung, tracheal swab, tracheal segment, brain, vaginal secretions, serum, aborted fetus, liver, spleen, kidney	VI (CPE), FA, VN
	Feline rhinotracheitis (herpesvirus)		Nasal and pharyngeal secretions, conjunctival membranes, liver, lung, spleen, kidney, salivary gland, brain	VI (CPE and inclusions), FA
	Equine rhinopneumonitis (herpesvirus)	Genital, abortions	Placenta, fetus, lung, nasal secretions, lymph nodes	FA, VI (ECE and CPE), VN
	Influenza (equine, porcine) (orthomyxovirus)		Nasal and ocular secretions, lung, tracheal swab	VI (ECE), HA, HI
	Parainfluenza (bovine, equine, porcine, ovine, canine) (paramyxovirus)		Nasal and ocular secretions, lung, tracheal swab	VI (ECE), HA, HI, VN
	Bovine respiratory syncytial virus (pneumovirus)		Trachea, lung, nasal secretions, clotted blood	VI (CPE), FA, ELISA
	Bovine herpesvirus 4 (Movar, DN599)	Abortions (?)	Trachea, lung, nasal secretions, fetus, clotted blood	VI (CPE), FA, VN
	Reovirus (bovine, equine, canine, feline)		Feces, intestinal mucosa, nasal and pharyngeal secretions	VI, HA, HI
	African horse sickness (orbivirus)[a]		Whole blood in anticoagulant, lesion material, nasal and pharyngeal secretions	VI (CPE and mice), VN
	Malignant catarrhal fever[a] (herpesvirus)		Whole blood in anticoagulant, lymph nodes, spleen, lung	VI (CPE), ELISA, FA, VN, EM
	Pseudorabies[a] (herpesvirus)	CNS, genital, abortions	Nasal secretions, tonsil, lung, brain (midbrain, pons, medulla), spinal cord (sheep and cattle), spleen (swine), vaginal secretion, serum	VI (CPE and rabbits), VN, ELISA, FA
	Canine herpesvirus		Kidney, liver, lung, spleen, nasal, oropharyngeal, and vaginal secretions	VI (CPE and inclusions), FA, VN
	Porcine inclusion body rhinitis (cytomegalovirus)		Turbinate, nasal mucosa	EM, VI (CPE), FA, VN
	Equine rhinovirus		Nasal secretions, feces	VI (CPE), VN
	Maedi-Visna, ovine progressive pneumonia (retrovirus, lentivirus)	CNS	CSF, whole blood, salivary glands, lung, mediastinal lymph nodes, choroid plexus, spleen	VI (CPE and sheep), VN, CF
	Bovine rhinovirus		Nasal secretions	VI (CPE), VN
	Rift valley fever[a] (bovine, ovine) (phlebovirus)		Whole blood in anticoagulant, fetus, liver, spleen, kidney, brain	VI (CPE and mice), VN, CF, FA
Enteric	Bovine enterovirus		Feces, oropharyngeal swab	VI (CPE), VN
	Transmissible gastroenteritis (coronavirus)		Feces, nasal secretions, jejunum, ileum	VI (newborn pigs), FA, EM
	Neonatal diarrheas			
	1. Rotaviruses		Feces, small intestine	VI (CPE with trypsin), ELISA, FA, EM

Table 3.1. Continued

Type of Illness or Infection	Common Name or Associated Virus	Other Infections	Clinical Specimens to Collect	Diagnostic Identification Tests
	2. Parvoviruses	Abortion	Feces, intestinal mucosa, regional lymph nodes, brain, heart	VI (CPE), FA, EM, HA, HI, VN
	3. Coronaviruses		Feces, small intestine	VI (CPE with trypsin), FA, EM
	Picornavirus SMEDI (enterovirus)		Feces, intestine, brain, tonsil, liver	VI (CPE), VN, EM
	Polioencephalitis (Teschen, Talfan) (enterovirus)	CNS	Brain, intestine, feces	VI (CPE), VN
	Rinderpest[a] (morbillivirus)		Blood in anticoagulant, spleen, mesenteric lymph nodes	VI (CPE and cattle), AGID, CF, VN
	Peste des petits[a] ruminants[a] (morbillivirus)		Blood in anticoagulant, spleen, mesenteric lymph nodes	VI (CPE and goats), VN, CF, AGID
Central nervous system (CNS)	Rabies (lyssavirus)		Brain, salivary gland	VI (mice and inclusions), FA, VN
	Equine encephalomyelitis (VEE,[a] EEE, WEE)[b] (alphavirus)		Whole blood, brain, cerebrospinal fluid, nasal and pharyngeal secretions, pancreas	VI (ECE and mice), HA, HI, VN, CF
	Louping ill encephalomyelitis[a] (flavivirus)		Whole blood, brain, cerebrospinal fluid	VI (ECE and CPE), FA, VN, HI
	Hemagglutinating encephalomyelitis virus (coronavirus)		Brain, spinal cord, tonsil, blood	VI (CPE), HA, HAD, VN, FA
	Caprine arthritis encephalitis (retrovirus, pentivirus)	Arthritis	Blood, spinal cord	VI (CPE), AGID, ELISA
	Japanese B encephalitis[a] (flavivirus)		Brain, CSF	VI (ECE and mice), IgM, VN, CF, HI, FA, ELISA
	Borna disease (unclassified)		Brain, spinal cord	VI (ECE and rabbits), FA, CF
	Scrapie[a] (unclassified)		Brain	VI (mice and sheep)
Mucous membranes and skin	Poxviruses 1. swine pox (suipoxvirus) 2. vaccinia (orthopoxvirus) 3. cowpox (orthopoxvirus) 4. sheep and goat pox[a] (capripoxvirus)		Lesion scrapings, lesions, vesicular fluids, crusts, liver, spleen	VI (ECE, CPE, and rabbits), HA, HI, VN, FA, EM
	Foot-and-mouth[a] disease (Aphthovirus)	Enteric	Lesion material, tonsil, vesicular fluid, hoof lesions, esophageal-pharyngeal (ep) fluids, all tissues	VI (CPE and neonatal mice), CF, VN, FA, AGID, ELISA
	Bovine mammillitis (herpesvirus)		Lesion scrapings, lesions, teat swab, fluid exudates from lesion	VI (CPE), VN
	Vesicular stomatitis[a] (vesiculovirus)		Vesicular fluid, epithelial covering of lesions, whole blood, regional lymph nodes, tongue swab	VI (CPE), VN, CF
	Vesicular exanthema of swine[a] (calicivirus)		Vesicular fluid, epithelial covering of foot lesion, tonsil lymph node, serum, oral and nasal lesions	VI (CPE), CF, VN, AGID
	Swine vesicular disease[a] (enterovirus)		Vesicular fluid, epithelial covering of lesion, oral or nasal lesions	VI (CPE), VN, FA, AGID
	Papillomaviruses	Neoplasia	Lesion material, warts, skin scraping	EM, cell transformation, FA
	Contagious ecthyma ORF (parapoxvirus)		Scabs, lesions on lip	VI (ECE and CPE), VN, AGID, FA, EM
	Bovine papular stomatitis (parapoxvirus)		Lesion biopsy, scraping muzzle, mouth, teats	VI (ECE and CPE), EM
Genital and/or abortions	Enteroviruses	CNS, respiratory	Vaginal secretions, serum from dam or sow, nasal swab, tonsil, brain (swine), feces (cattle and swine)	VI (CPE), VN
	Parvovirus (swine)		Vaginal secretions, serum from dam or sow, lung (mummified fetus)	VI (CPE), FA, HA, HI

Table 3.1.   Continued

Type of Illness or Infection	Common Name or Associated Virus	Other Infections	Clinical Specimens to Collect	Diagnostic Identification Tests
	Bluetongue, Epizootic hemorrhagic disease of deer, Ibaraki (orbivirus)	Hemorrhagic syndrome, (viremia), respiratory	Serum from dam, fetal heart, heparinized blood, spleen, bone marrow, lymph nodes, lung, semen	VI (CPE and ECE), CF, AGID, FA, VN, EM
	Equine viral arteritis (Pestivirus)		Whole blood, nasal and pharyngeal secretions, placenta, fetus, spleen, nostril, lymph nodes, conjunctival sac, semen	VI (CPE), CF, AGID, FA
	Border disease (hairy shaker) (pestivirus)	CNS	Brain, spleen, blood, bone marrow	VI (CPE and interference), FA, VN
	Akabane[a] (Bunyavirus)		Placenta, fetal muscle, nerve tissues	VI (CPE and suckling mice), FA, VN, HI, HA
Hemorrhage syndrome (viremia)	Hog cholera[a] (pestivirus)		Tonsil, spleen, liver, brain, lymph nodes	VI (pigs), FA, VN
	Equine infectious anemia (retrovirus, Pentivirus)		Whole blood, spleen, lymph nodes	VI (CPE and horses), FA, VN, CF, ELISA, AGID
	African swine fever[a] (Iridovirus)		Blood in anticoagulant, spleen, liver, tonsil, lymph nodes	VI (CPE and pigs), HAD, HA, CF, FA, RIA (radioimmunoassay), ELISA, IEOP (immunoelectro-osmophoresis)
	Nairobi sheep disease[a] (Nairovirus)		Spleen, blood (plasma), mesenteric lymph nodes	VI (intracerebral suckling mice), FA
	Rift valley fever[a] (phlebovirus)		Fetus, blood in anticoagulant, liver, spleen, kidney, brain, serum	VI (CPE and suckling hamsters or mice), VN, CF, AGID, HI, FA
Neoplasia	Retrovirus (bovine, feline) (oncovirinae)	Immunodeficiency, leukemia, anemia	Lymph nodes, metastatic growths, blood in anticoagulant, serum	VI, reverse transcriptase, EM, ELISA, FA, Western immunoblot

AGID = agar gel immunodiffusion, CF = complement fixation, COFAL = complement-fixation for avian leukosis, CPE = cytopathic effect, ECE = embryonating chicken eggs, EM = electron microscopy, FA = immunofluorescence, HA = hemagglutinin, HAD = hemadsorption, HI = hemagglutination inhibition, RIA = radioimmunoassay, VI = virus isolation, VN = virus neutralization.
[a] Reportable disease or a foreign animal disease in United States.
[b] VEE = Venezuelan equine encephalomyelitis, EEE = eastern equine encephalomyelitis, WEE = western encephalomyelitis.

6. Isolation or amplification of infectious virus in cell cultures and identification of the virus propagated from the clinical submission.

Many viral diseases, such as pseudorabies in adult pigs, do not kill the host but pose a potential threat by their ability to spread to susceptible offspring and other species. Serological assays on sera from live animals determine which hosts are potential virus carriers or which are susceptible or exposed to a viral infection. Identifying these virus-infected animals permits their culling to remove a disease threat to the herd or flock. Serologic identification is also important in determining epizootiologic patterns or number of viral pathogens involved in a disease syndrome.

Isolating a virus does not necessarily implicate that virus as the causative agent in the described disease since the pathogenicity of viruses may vary from species to species. It is important, therefore, to establish that the isolated virus produces a similar disease in the same or related species. This involves inoculating susceptible or nonimmune animals. When dual viruses are isolated from a specimen, a clear interpretation of the role of each isolate in the disease process is necessary. The disease

potential of field viruses is obscured by the frequent isolation of vaccine (attenuated) strains of virus that are routinely used in most herd and flock disease prevention programs. The presence of genetic markers (e.g., plaque size, virulence, cell susceptibility, nucleic acid patterns) of these vaccine strains helps identify such viruses.

ISOLATION OF VIRUS FROM CLINICAL SPECIMENS

Cultivation in Tissue Culture

Viruses are isolated from clinical specimens by inoculating susceptible primary or continuous cell cultures derived from the host or related species, embryonated eggs, or laboratory animals. Specimens submitted for viral isolation should be placed in virus transport media (e.g., a balanced salt solution containing antibiotics) in sealed containers for safety in handling. They should be clearly identified by appropriate labeling. If histopathology (freezing destroys tissue morphology) is not required, submissions of tissues should be on ice (4°C) or frozen

T a b l e 3 . 2 .   Suggested Specimens from Avian Species for Virus Isolation and Identification

Type of Illness or Infection	Common Name or Associated Virus	Other Infections	Clinical Specimens to Collect	Diagnostic Identification Tests
Respiratory	Newcastle disease VVND[a] (paramyxovirus)	CNS	Tracheal or cloacal swabs, lung, spleen, liver, kidney, bone marrow	VI (ECE, CPE), VN, HA, HI
	Avian influenza[a] (fowl plague virus) (orthomyxovirus)	Drop in egg production, enteric	Trachea, lung, air sac, sinus exudate, liver, spleen, blood, cloacal swab	VI (ECE), HA, HI, AGP, VN
	Infectious bronchitis (coronavirus)	Nephrosis, drop in egg production	Lung, trachea, tracheal swabs	VI (ECE tracheal ring cultures), VN, HA, HI, EM
	Herpesvirus of 1. psittacines (Pacheco's Disease) 2. cranes 3. pigeons 4. owls 5. falcons		Liver, spleen, intestine	VI (ECE, birds), VN, FA, EM
	Laryngotracheitis (herpesvirus)		Trachea or tracheal exudate, lung	VI (ECE, CPE), AGP, VN, FA
	Avian adenovirus	Eggdrop syndrome, hepatitis, enteritis	Trachea, lung, air sacs, intestine, feces	VI (ECE, CPE), AGP, VN, FA
Enteric	Coronaviral enteritis of turkeys		Intestine, bursa of Fabricius, ceca	VI (ETE), FA, VN
	Reovirus		Intestine, feces	EM, VI
Central nervous system	Avian encephalomyelitis (enterovirus)		Brain	VI (chicks, ECE), VN, FA
	Alphavirus infections (eastern and western equine encephalitis viruses)		Serum, brain, heart, spleen, liver	VI (ECE, mice, CPE), VN, CF, HI
	Turkey meningoencephalitis (flavivirus)		Brain, spleen, serum	VI (ECE, mice, CPE), VN, HI
Mucous membranes and skin	Avipoxvirus 1. Pigeon pox 2. Canary pox 3. Fowl pox 4. Turkey pox		Nodular skin lesions, scab	VI (ECE, CPE), AGP, HA, VN, FA, immunoperoxidase
Hemorrhagic syndrome (viremia)	Viral arthritis (reovirus)		Synovial fluid from tibiotarsal or tibiofemoral joints, spleen swab	VI (CPE, ECE), AGP, VN, FA
	Duck plague (duck virus enteritis) (herpesvirus)		Liver, spleen, blood	VI (CPE, EDE), VN
	Hemorrhagic enteritis of turkeys or marble spleen of pheasants (adenovirus, type 2)		Intestinal contents, spleen	VI (CPE, poults), AGP, EM
	Turkey viral hepatitis (unclassified)		Liver	VI (ECE)
	Infectious bursal disease (Birnavirus)	Immunosuppression	Spleen, bursa	VI (ECE), VN, AGP
	Fledgling disease (papovavirus)		Bone marrow, kidney, heart, spleen	VI (CPE), VN, EM, FA
	Chicken anemia agent (parvovirus)	Immunosuppression, pancytopenia	Spleen, bursa, thymus, blood	VI (chicks), EM, VN, ELISA
Neoplasia	Leukosis and sarcomas (retrovirus, oncovirinae)		Whole blood, plasma, cloacal swabs, meconium, albumin, embryos, tumors	RT, VI (CPE, cell transformation, ECE), ELISA, FA, COFAL
	Reticuloendotheliosis (retrovirus, oncovirinae)	Immunosuppression, lymphoma	Spleen, tumor tissue, heparinized blood	VI (CPE, ETE), FA, RT, AGP, VN
	Marek's disease (herpesvirus)		Blood, tumor, kidney, spleen, feathers	VI (CPE, ECE), AGP, VN, FA

AGID = agar gel immunodiffusion, AGP = agar gel precipitin, CF = complement fixation, COFAL = complement-fixation for avian leukosis, CPE = cytopathic effect, ECE = embryonating chicken eggs, EDE = embryonating duck eggs, EM = electron microscopy, ETE = embryonating turkey eggs, FA = immunofluorescence, HA = hemagglutinin, HAD = hemadsorption, HI = hemagglutination inhibition, RIA = radioimmunoassay, RT = reverse transcriptase, VI = virus isolation, VN = virus neutralization, VVND = velogenic viscerotropic Newcastle disease.

FIGURE 3.1.   *Cytopathic effect (syncytial) on bovine fetal kidney cells by the herpesvirus of malignant catarrhal fever (×200).*

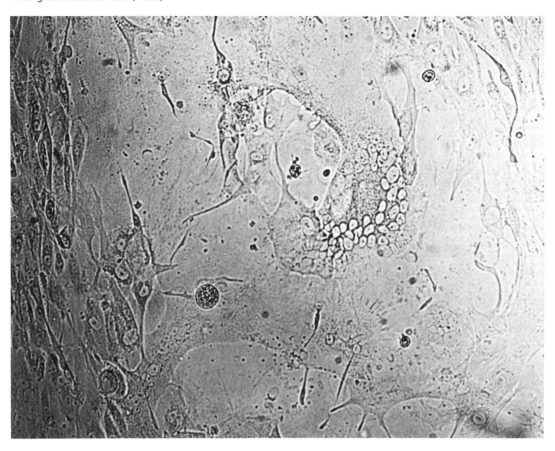

(>−20°C). Tight plastic wrapping of the specimens should be avoided because it insulates the tissues and will enhance autolysis and necrosis and decrease infectious virus.

Clinical specimens for viral isolation from a live host should be collected if possible during acute disease or prior to antibody formation. Excretions or secretions, swabs at body orifices, internal fluids (lymph or unclotted blood), and biopsy materials obtained during acute disease provide suitable specimens for viral isolation.

In the laboratory, tissue specimens are processed as a 10% or 20% (w/v) homogenate in a balanced salt solution with 200 mg of gentamicin or 100 units of penicillin and 100 mg of streptomycin per ml and filtered when grossly contaminated with other microorganisms through 0.45 μm and 0.22 μm Millipore-type filters. Cell cultures used to isolate virus should be previously tested for noncytopathic bovine viral diarrhea virus by immunofluorescence and mycoplasma by either culture or immunofluorescence.

To isolate virus, tissue homogenates are placed onto cellular monolayers, absorbed 1 hour or longer at 35°C to 37°C, and the inoculum is left on or removed and fresh media added. Inoculated and uninfected cell cultures are observed for 7 to 10 days. Viral cytopathic effect (CPE) in cells is usually evident between 24 and 72 hours for most cytopathic viruses (Fig 3.1). However, for most clinical material containing low concentrations of virus, several (>3) blind cell passages are recommended.

After a virus has been demonstrated at limiting dilution to replicate in a cell by CPE or other parameters, infectious virus is released from cells by three cycles of freeze–thaw or sonication, followed by centrifugation and storage (at −70°C) to maintain maximum infectivity. Each virus isolated should be identified as to species of origin, morphologic type, passage level, and host cell used for propagation.

Embryonated Eggs

Many avian viral pathogens can be isolated in embryonating chicken eggs (ECE). A key to successful viral isolation in ECE is the route of inoculation (Fig 3.2). Candled ECE that die within 24 hours after inoculation are considered traumatic deaths. Subsequent deaths of inoculated ECE are placed at 4°C for several hours (to avoid hemorrhages) prior to collection of fluids or visual examination of the embryos and egg membranes. Embryos that are stunted, deformed, edematous, or hem-

FIGURE 3.2.   *The chicken embryo (10 to 12 days old) and routes of inoculation to reach the various cell types (as indicated). For chorioallantoic membrane inoculation, a hole is first drilled through the egg shell and shell membrane; the shell over the air sac is then perforated, causing air to enter between the shell membrane and the chorioallantoic membrane, creating an artificial air sac, where the sample is deposited. The sample comes in contact with the chorionic epithelium. Yolk sac inoculation is usually carried out in younger (6-day-old) embryos, in which the yolk sac is larger. (Reproduced with permission from Davis BD et al. Microbiology. 2nd ed. Hagerstown, MD: Harper and Row, 1977.)*

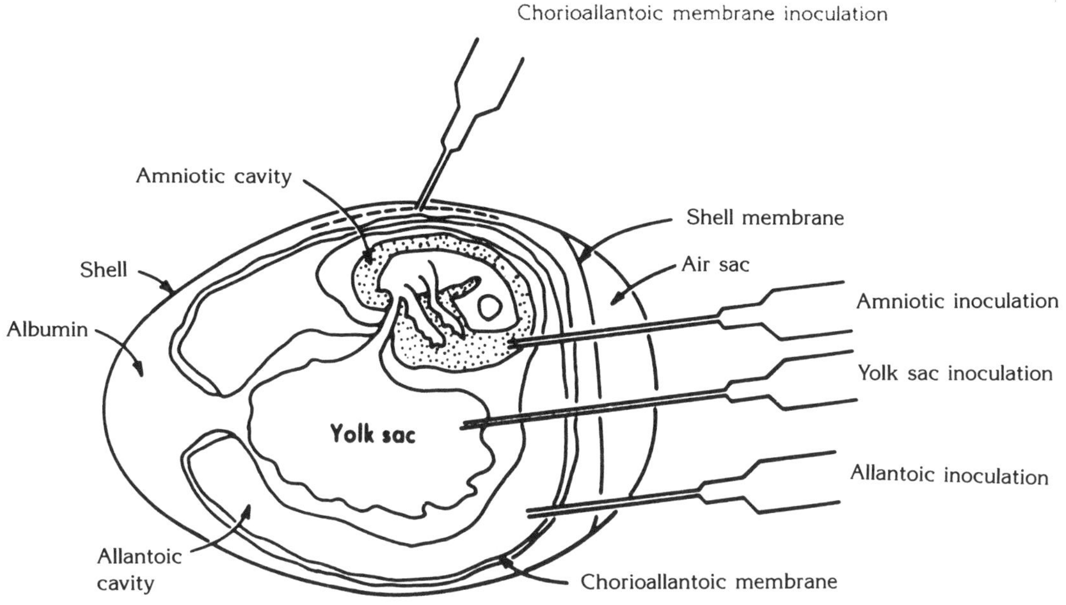

orrhagic and membranes that contain lesions (i.e., pocks) should be homogenized in a sterile balanced saline as a 10% (w/v) suspension and repassaged in ECE or cell cultures. To avoid toxicity, a dilution of the inoculum is done.

Animal Inoculation

The inoculation of animals remains a vital part of the identification procedure for a viral pathogen. Because of the unknown pathogenic effects of specific viruses on the host, inoculation of a susceptible animal provides information on tissue tropism, virulence, pathogenesis, and transmissibility of the virus. The inoculation route selected in the host usually requires knowledge of the disease (e.g., respiratory disease by nasal route or enteric disease by oral route). Certain viral diseases are known foreign animal diseases, and to prevent the spread of such viruses, appropriate containment and isolation facilities with monitored air flows and HEPA viral filters must be used when animals are inoculated with such viruses. Inoculated animals should be monitored daily and blood samples collected at routine intervals. After inoculation, animals that die are necropsied and tissues collected for viral isolation and histopathology. The carcass of the animal is incinerated to avoid the spread of viral pathogens to other susceptible hosts.

IDENTIFICATION OF VIRUSES OR VIRAL ANTIGENS IN CLINICAL SPECIMENS

Electron Microscopy

Electron microscopy (EM) identifies the morphology and size of a virus. This technique provides rapid diagnostic data on a viral isolate. Tentative diagnosis of viral diseases can be made by EM on thin sections of affected tissues and cell-free homogenates of clinical specimens. The use of EM for diagnosis is limited, however, because the method is not very sensitive ($>10^5$ virus particles/ml are required to see a single viral particle on a 200 mesh grid) and viruses from different species have similar morphology and size.

Immune Electron Microscopy

Immune electron microscopy (IEM) enhances detection of viruses in tissues, cells, or fecal specimens by reacting specific immune sera with virus. In IEM, specific antibody to a virus, preferably polyclonal, is mixed with virus for 1 hour to produce antigen-antibody complexes. These immune complexes are centrifuged at 1000 × g onto Formvar-coated grids, then stained with 4% PTA, pH 7.0, and examined by EM. The reaction of viral fluids with specific acute or convalescent serum as viewed by EM determines if a virus is associated with a specific disease. This procedure has been used successfully for viruses associated with viral-caused enteritides.

Immunofluorescence

Immunofluorescence is a visible fluorescence accentuated by ultraviolet light as a specific antibody covalently bound to a fluorochrome (e.g., fluorescein isothiocyanate, rhodamine) combines with a fixed antigen. This technique provides a sensitive and rapid method for detecting and identifying specific viruses in either tissues or cell cultures (Fig 3.3). Immunofluorescence is detectable by either a direct or indirect procedure. The direct immunofluorescence test employs a virus-specific antibody labeled with fluorescein that combines with a specific viral antigen located in cells or tissues. The indirect test requires the use of a fluorescein-labeled antiserum to a virus-specific immunoglobulin. Although the indirect assay is more sensitive, it may be less specific because most sera, except monoclonals, usually contain antibodies against more than one virus or antigen.

For each tissue examined, adequate tissue controls are necessary to distinguish autofluorescence, or nonspecific fluorescence. To determine the specificity of the immunofluorescent reaction, a blocking assay is done in which tissue antigen is exposed to a known viral antiserum and then is reacted with fluorescein-labeled anti-

serum to the virus. A decrease in the tissue fluorescence in the specific antibody-blocked sites when compared to a positive (unblocked) tissue slide indicates a specific immunofluorescence reaction.

Nucleic Acid Hybridization

Molecular hybridization techniques have led to the synthetic production of viral DNA probes. These probes, obtained by restriction endonuclease (RE) breakage of extracted viral DNA, have been used to characterize segments of viral DNA by hybridization to complementary segments peculiar to a virus. Viral DNA is produced by cloning, and such DNA is produced in an annealed segment of a bacterial plasmid, a double-stranded, covalently closed circular DNA molecule found in the cytoplasm of bacteria. The specificity of the single-stranded (ss) DNA radio-labeled probe to anneal with a complementary strand forms the basis of identifying viral sequences in cells (e.g., retroviruses). The nucleic acid hybridization technique can be applied to purified, restriction endonuclease-treated and to electrophoresed DNA or DNA from clinical tissues and is done by blotting (Southern blot) on a solid matrix (e.g., a nitrocellulose filter). After blotting, the DNA fragments are fixed to the filter and the filter is incubated with the radio-labeled or biotin-labeled DNA probe. The unbound probe is removed after extensive washing. The position (black dots) of hybridized DNA relative to the radioactive probe

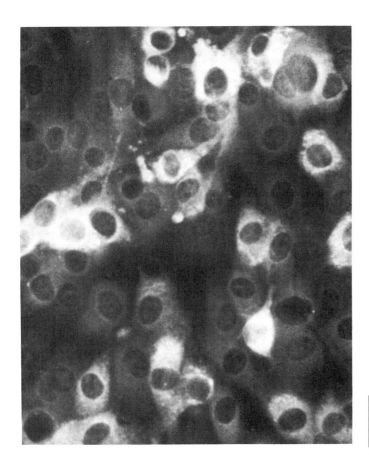

FIGURE 3.3.   *Cytoplasmic immunofluorescence in fetal bovine lung cells produced by BVD virus (×200). (Reproduced with permission from Castro AE. Bov Pract 1984;19:61.)*

or a color change on the filter is revealed, respectively, on x-ray film in contact with the filter or by spots of fluorescence on the filter.

Experimentally, this methodology has been used to delineate nucleic acid differences between strains of viruses and to locate the genes responsible for coding specific proteins and pathogenic properties of a virus. This technique is both time-consuming and labor-intensive, and currently is beyond most veterinary diagnostic laboratories. When DNA probes become routinely available, however, they will enhance the identification of viral nucleic acids in both tissues and cell cultures.

Polymerase Chain Reaction

The more recent development of the polymerase chain reaction (PCR) is unquestionably one of the most advanced techniques in molecular genetics that can be applied to the detection of extremely small amounts of viral nucleic acid in infected cells. The importance of the procedure lies in the ability to amplify impure DNA or RNA, either fragmented or intact, by the simple chemical rather than biologic proliferation of a predetermined stretch of nucleic acid. The PCR is based on the cyclic synthesis of a DNA segment limited by two specific oligonucleotides that are used as primers. Based on the nucleotide sequence of viral genomic DNA, usually a pair of 30 to 500 nucleotide primers are selected and synthesized for detecting the viral genome in infected cells using the PCR. There is little doubt that the PCR will be the diagnostic tool of the future as more viral genomes have been sequenced.

Enzyme-Linked Immunosorbent Assay

The enzyme-linked immunosorbent assay (ELISA) is a rapid, highly sensitive immunoassay adapted to measure viral antigen or antibody (see Chapter 2). ELISAs have been developed for numerous avian viral pathogens (e.g., avian laryngotracheitis virus, avian encephalitis, Newcastle disease virus, infectious bronchitis virus, and reovirus).

SEROLOGIC DETECTION OF VIRUSES

Most viruses usually elicit an immune response in the host; if an animal is infected in utero (e.g., tolerant) or is immunodeficient, however, a detectable humoral response may not occur. A humoral or cellular response is a measure of an exposure or a recent infection with a viral pathogen. Most diagnostic serologic assays measure humoral immunity in animals, and assays for measuring cellular immunity to viruses are used infrequently in veterinary diagnostic medicine.

Viruses have certain antigens that are type- or group-specific and that in part determine the serologic assay used. To establish a diagnosis by serology, acute (onset of clinical signs) and convalescent serum (10 to 28 days

later) is required. A fourfold (e.g., from 4 to ≥ 16) or higher rise in antibody titer (the reciprocal of the serum dilution) indicates an ongoing viral infection. Antibody levels in single serum samples are difficult to interpret as they pertain to the course of disease. However, in certain chronic diseases (e.g., bluetongue, bovine leukosis, caprine arthritis encephalitis, equine infectious anemia), antibody in a single serum indicates exposure to the virus and identifies a potential carrier state; therefore, culling the animal from the herd or flock is warranted.

Serology can help rapidly establish a viral diagnosis (acute or chronic) when viral isolation is negative. Serology can also definitively rule out the presence of a specific viral antigen or antigens, whereas negative viral isolation cannot. Serologic assays on single serum samples are only diagnostic on a herd or flock basis (usually sample 10% of animals at risk) to determine 1) the effectiveness of a vaccination program, or 2) exposure of a herd or flock to a viral pathogen.

Serum Virus Neutralization (SN) Test

Most viruses produce a visible cytopathic effect (CPE) in cell cultures. CPE is used to determine the presence of protective or virus-neutralizing antibodies in a serum. To quantify the amount of neutralizing antibody, serum from an animal is serially diluted by twofold dilutions and mixed with a known amount of virus (50 to 300 infectious doses of virus-$TCID_{50}$) for 1 hour at 37°C and then a uniform volume is inoculated into animals or embryonating chicken eggs (ECE) or onto cell cultures. The SN test is very specific because one antibody molecule can neutralize one infectious viral particle. Most antigenic differences between types of viruses have been determined by SN. Both IgG and IgM antibodies are measurable by this test. The SN determines the presence of a recent viral infection provided paired sera are simultaneously tested.

Hemagglutination Inhibition (HI) Test

The ability of specific viruses to hemagglutinate certain erythrocytes has been used to quantify the amount of virus. Such viruses contain a hemagglutinin protein (HA) on the virus capsid that can usually be dissociated from the viral surface by organic solvents to provide a stable HA unit. The HI can be used to identify or type a specific virus provided the hemagglutinin clumping of erythrocytes is inhibited by specific antiserum. A positive hemagglutinin reaction is seen as a button or cluster of erythrocytes in the bottom of a round microwell or tube. Gradations of hemagglutination are scored 1 through 4 to indicate the percentage of hemagglutination. If a hemagglutinating virus is isolated from an animal, the virus can be implicated in a disease by its reaction with acute and convalescent serum from the same animal. To measure viral antibodies by the HI test requires a specific type of erythrocyte, a known quantity of virus (usually 4 hemagglutinating units), a known positive and negative serum, and twofold serially diluted test sera.

Hemadsorption-Inhibition (HAD-I) Test

The HAD-I test is based on the ability of certain virus-infected cells (monolayers) to attract specific erythrocytes to their surface. The presence of hemadsorbing erythrocyte clusters on a cellular monolayer indicates that viral protein (hemagglutinin) has accumulated on the surface of the cell membrane. The hemadsorption phenomenon can be inhibited by pretreatment of virus-infected cells for 30 minutes, usually at ambient temperature with twofold dilutions of antisera followed by the addition of 0.05% to 0.5% erythrocytes. Antibody (Ab) can be quantified by comparing the observed washed virus-infected cell monolayers that contain adhered clumped erythrocytes on the surface of the cell (Ab negative) with the cell monolayers that contain free-floating erythrocytes (Ab positive).

Virus-infected cells can be recovered if the HAD-I test is done aseptically. The HAD-I assay usually can be done within 24 to 48 hours after a cellular monolayer is infected by hemadsorbing virus.

Complement Fixation

Complement fixation (CF) tests employ the cascade of complement in reactions of viral antigens that fix complement — usually guinea pig — when combined to antibody. Although CF has been used in early test tube assays to detect virus (e.g., leukemia viruses), virus-infected cells, or virus-specific antibody, the complexity of the assay and the time required have led to its replacement by simpler procedures.

Immunodiffusion

The immunodiffusion (ID) procedure is routinely used as a diagnostic tool to monitor the spread of specific viral pathogens in various animals diseases (e.g., bluetongue, equine infectious anemia, bovine leukosis, caprine arthritis, encephalitis, infectious bursal disease). The basis of the test is the ability of certain soluble viral antigens to diffuse in a semisolid medium (agar) with the formation of a precipitin line with specific antisera.

Immunoelectro-osmophoresis combines the diffusion procedure with the principle of movement of charged protein molecules in an electrical field. Since most viral antigens assume an electrically negative charge, application of an electrical current moves the viral particle to the anode (+). Following electrical migration, the antigen can be elucidated by the use of a positive antiserum that migrates toward the cathode (−). This technique has been used to detect antigens of African swine fever virus.

Radioimmunoassay

The radioimmunoassay (RIA) is an exquisitely sensitive method for quantifying antigens or antibodies when one component is radio-labeled. Although RIA has an advantage for detecting minute amounts of antibodies, the need for a scintillation counter to measure radioactivity and very pure reagents limits use of this assay to appropriately equipped diagnostic laboratories.

Enzyme-Linked Immunosorbent Assay

ELISAs are highly sensitive immunoassays in which the specificity of the reaction can be enhanced by increasing the level of purification of the antigen or antibody employed. The ELISA can detect ng levels of IgG-, IgM-, and IgA-type antibodies. ELISAs can be made quantitative

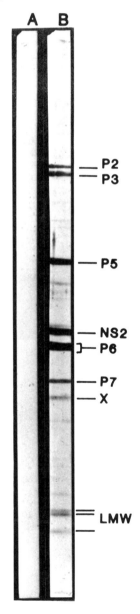

FIGURE 3.4.   *Western immunoblot of bluetongue virus proteins using serum obtained before and after natural infection with BTV serotype 17. Virus proteins identified are given in the right margin; LMW represents three low molecular weight virus proteins that have not been previously defined; X represents an additional noncharacterized virus protein; P designates specific BTV protein; NS is the nonstructural virus protein. Lanes A and B represent pre- and postinfection serum, respectively. Immune complexes were detected in lane B using a biotin-avidin-enzyme probe, e.g., biotin-labeled rabbit antisheep IgG in association with peroxidase-labeled avidin. (Reproduced with permission from MA Adkison and JL Stott.)*

if appropriate standard curves are developed. Numerous commercially available assays for avian and mammalian viruses provide qualitative information on antibody or antigens to various viruses.

Monoclonal antibody reaction in the ELISA may not always be detectable by immunofluorescence, so comparisons of antibody by ELISA to other immunoassays may not always be appropriate. A blocking assay by ELISA, in which the AgAb reaction can be blocked by another specific serum, is of interest. The amount of blocking decreases the color change and indicates the specificity of the ELISA reaction.

Western Immunoblot Assay

The Western immunoblot assay can detect antibodies to a full range of viral proteins as revealed on a strip of nitrocellulose paper as discrete bands by electrophoresis. When a serum sample is applied to the nitrocellulose strip, antibodies from animals infected with a specific virus bind to the specific viral proteins at the appropriate positions. These bands become dark and distinct when the nitrocellulose paper is treated with a reagent (Fig 3.4). Because it provides a full viral antibody profile of the serum sample, this test is the most specific viral diagnostic test currently available.

USE OF MONOCLONAL ANTIBODY FOR VIRAL DIAGNOSIS

Monoclonal antibodies have recently been applied to the characterization of viral strains and antigenic drift, and to the mapping of antigenic determinants. Monoclonal antibodies coupled to a fluorochrome have enhanced detection of viruses in tissues by immunofluorescence, especially when minimal virus is present. These techniques have provided data for separating specific serovars of viruses such as bluetongue, for which 24 different serotypes exist. Monoclonal antibodies are proving useful in the development of commercial ELISAs for viruses because they can detect minor or major viral antigenic components. Problems still associated with the use of monoclonal antibodies are the expense and the extensive development time.

Although the advent of monoclonal antibodies is a heralded event, inherent problems in their production remain. Monoclonals, however, have found initial use in veterinary virology in identifying viral morphologic types previously grouped together in a species and in developing protective subunit vaccines that circumvent problems inherent with modified-live viral vaccines.

SELECTED REFERENCES

Arnheim N, Erlich H. Polymerase chain reaction strategy. Annu Rev Biochem 1992;61:131.

Balows A, Hausler WJ, Herrmann KL, et al., eds. Manual of clinical microbiology. 5th ed. Washington: American Society for Microbiology, 1991.

Baron EJ, Finegold SM. Bailey and Scott's diagnostic microbiology. 9th ed. St. Louis: Mosby, 1994.

Crandell RA. Diagnosis of viral disease. In: Howard JL, ed. Currrent veterinary therapy food animal practice. 2nd ed. Philadelphia: WB Saunders, 1986:466–469.

Eisenstein BI. The polymerase chain reaction. New Engl J Med 1990;322:178.

Fields BN, Knipe DM, Howley PM, et al., eds. Fields virology. 3rd ed. New York: Raven Press, 1996.

Gerstman BB, Cappucci DT. Evaluating the reliability of diagnostic test results. J Am Vet Med Assoc 1986;188:248.

Johnson FB. Transport of viral specimens. Clin Microbiol Rev 1990;3:120.

Lennette EH, Halonen P, Murphy FA, eds. Laboratory diagnosis of infectious diseases: principles and practice. Vol. 2: viral, rickettsial and chlamydial diseases. New York: Springer-Verlag, 1988.

Palmer EL, Martin ML. Electron microscopy in viral diagnosis. Boca Raton: CRC, 1988.

Specter S, Lancz CJ, eds. Clinical virology manual. 2nd ed. New York: Elsevier, 1991.

Yolken RH. Enzyme immunoassays for the detection of infectious antigens in body fluids: current limitations and future projects. Rev Infect Dis 1982;4:35.

4 *Antimicrobial Chemotherapy*

JOHN F. PRESCOTT

Antimicrobial drugs exploit differences in structure or biochemical function between host and parasite. Modern chemotherapy is traced to the work of Paul Ehrlich, who devoted his life to discovering agents that possessed *selective toxicity*. The first clinically successful broad-spectrum antibacterial drugs were the sulfonamides, developed in 1935 as a result of Ehrlich's work with synthetic dyes. It was, however, the discovery of penicillin by Fleming and its development by Chain and Florey in World War II that led to the subsequent discovery of further *antibiotics*, chemical substances produced by microorganisms that at low concentrations inhibit or kill other microorganisms. The chemical modification of many of the drugs discovered early in the antibiotic revolution has led to the development of new and powerful antimicrobial drugs with properties distinct from their parents. Antibiotics and their derivatives have more importance as antimicrobial agents than do the fewer synthetic antibacterial drugs. By contrast, antiviral drugs are all chemically synthesized.

Important milestones in the development of antimicrobial drugs are shown in Figure 4.1. The therapeutic use of antimicrobial drugs in veterinary medicine has followed their use in human medicine because of the cost of their development.

SPECTRUM OF ACTION OF ANTIMICROBIAL DRUGS

Antimicrobial drugs can be classified as narrow or broad spectrum based on the following:

1. *Class of microorganism.* Penicillins are narrow spectrum because they inhibit only bacteria; trimethoprim and lincosamides are broader because they also inhibit protozoa; and tetracyclines and chloramphenicol are broad spectrum because they inhibit bacteria, mycoplasma, rickettsiae, and chlamydiae. Polyenes only inhibit fungi.
2. *Antibacterial activity.* Some antibiotics are narrow spectrum in that they inhibit only gram-positive (bacitracin, vancomycin) or gram-negative bacteria (polymyxin), whereas broad-spectrum drugs such as tetracyclines inhibit both gram-positive and gram-negative bacteria. Other drugs such as penicillin G or lincosamides are most active against gram-positive bacteria but will inhibit some gram-negatives.

3. *Bacteriostatic or bactericidal.* This distinction is an approximation that depends on drug concentrations and the organism involved. For example, penicillin is bactericidal at high concentrations and bacteriostatic at lower ones. The distinction between bactericidal and bacteriostatic is critical in certain circumstances, such as the treatment of meningitis or septicemia in neutropenic patients.

MECHANISM OF ACTION OF ANTIMICROBIAL DRUGS

The marked structural and biochemical differences between eukaryotic and prokaryotic cells give greater opportunity for selective toxicity of antibacterial drugs compared to antifungal drugs because fungi, like mammalian cells, are eukaryotic. Developing selectively toxic antiviral drugs is particularly difficult because viral replication depends largely on the metabolic pathways of the host cell. This chapter mainly discusses antibacterial drugs.

The mechanisms of action of antibacterial drugs fall into four categories: 1) inhibition of cell wall synthesis, 2) damage to cell membrane function, 3) inhibition of nucleic acid synthesis or function, and 4) inhibition of protein synthesis (Fig 4.2).

INHIBITION OF CELL WALL SYNTHESIS

Antibiotics that interfere with cell wall synthesis include penicillins and cephalosporins (beta-lactam antibiotics), cycloserine, bacitracin, and vancomycin. The bacterial cell wall is a thick envelope that gives shape to the cell. This tough wall outside the cell membrane is a major difference between bacteria and mammalian cells. In gram-positive bacteria it consists largely of a thick layer of peptidoglycan, which gives the cell rigidity and maintains a high internal osmotic pressure of about 20 atm. In gram-negative bacteria this layer is thinner and the internal osmotic pressure correspondingly lower. Peptidoglycan consists of a polysaccharide chain made up of a repeating disaccharide backbone of alternating N-acetylglucosamine-N-acetylmuramic acid in beta-1,4 linkage, a tetrapeptide attached to the N-acetylmuramic

FIGURE 4.1. *Milestones in antimicrobial therapy.*

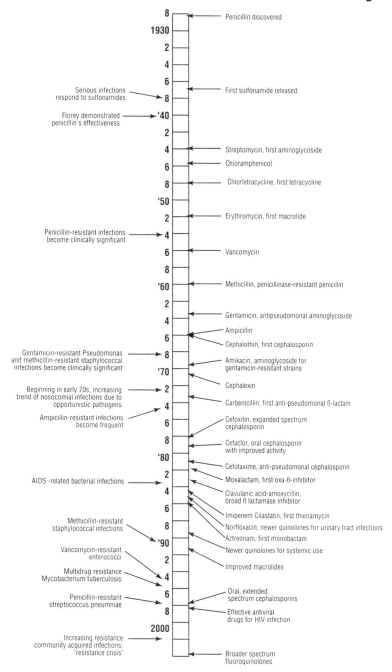

Human Infectious Disease

Antibacterial Agents

Serious infections respond to sulfonamides

Florey demonstrated penicillin's effectiveness

Penicillin-resistant infections become clinically significant

Gentamicin-resistant Pseudomonas and methicillin-resistant staphylococcal infections become clinically significant

Beginning in early 70s, increasing trend of nosocomial infections due to opportunistic pathogens

Ampicillin-resistant infections become frequent

AIDS -related bacterial infections

Methicillin-resistant staphylococcal infections

Vancomycin-resistant enterococci

Multidrug resistance Mycobacterium tuberculosis

Penicillin-resistant streptococcus pneumniae

Increasing resistance community acquired infections: "resistance crisis"

Penicillin discovered

First sulfonamide released

Streptomycin, first aminoglycoside

Chloramphenicol

Chlorletracycline, first tetracycline

Erythromycin, first macrolide

Vancomycin

Methicillin, penicillinase-resistant penicillin

Gentamicin, antipseudomonal aminoglycoside

Ampicillin

Cephalothin, first cephalosporin

Amikacin, aminoglycoside for gentamicin-resistant strains

Cephalexin

Carbenicillin, first anti-pseudomonal ß-lactam

Cefoxitin, expanded spectrum cephalosporin

Cefaclor, oral cephalosporin with improved activity

Cefotaxime, anti-pseudomonal cephalosporin

Moxalactam, first oxa-ß-inhibitor

Clavulanic acid-amoxycillin, broad ß lactamase inhibitor

Imipenem Cilastatin, first thienamycin

Norfloxacin, newer quinolones for urinary tract infections

Aztreonam, first monobactam

Newer quinolones for systemic use

Improved macrolides

Oral, extended spectrum cephalosporins

Effective antiviral drugs for HIV infection

Broader spectrum fluoroquinolones

acid, and a peptide bridge from one tetrapeptide to another, so that the disaccharide backbone is cross-linked both within and between "layers." The cross-linkage between transpeptides gives the cell wall remarkable strength. Several enzymes are involved in transpeptidation reactions.

The effect of beta-lactam antibiotics (penicillins and cephalosporins) is to prevent the final cross-linking in the cell wall, inhibiting division and creating weak points. Among the targets of these drugs are penicillin-binding proteins (PBPs), of which there are three to eight in bacteria; many of these PBPs are transpeptidase enzymes. They are responsible for the formation and remodeling of the cell wall during growth and division. Different PBPs have different affinities for drugs, which explains the variation in the spectrum of action of different beta-lactam antibiotics. Degradative mechanisms are also involved in cell wall production. These are carried out by autolysins, and some penicillins act partly by decreasing normal inhibition of the autolysins.

FIGURE 4.2.   *Mechanisms of action of antibacterial drugs.*

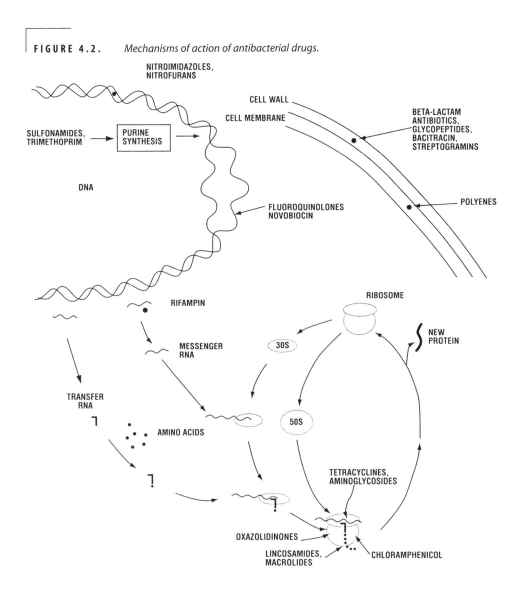

The action of beta-lactam antibiotics is thus to block peptidoglycan synthesis, which severely weakens the cell wall, and to promote the action of the autolysins, which lyse the cell. Beta-lactams are active only against actively growing cells. The greater activity of some beta-lactams against gram-positive bacteria is the result of the greater quantity of peptidoglycan and higher osmotic pressure in gram-positive bacteria, the impermeability of some gram-negative bacteria because of their lipopolysaccharide and lipid exterior, and the presence of beta-lactamase enzymes in many gram-negative organisms. The remarkable activity against gram-negatives of some of the newest penicillins and cephalosporins is due not just to their improved ability to enter gram-negative cells and bind PBPs, but to their ability to resist a variety of beta-lactamase enzymes found in the periplasmic space of gram-negative bacteria. More recently, beta-lactamase-inhibiting drugs with no intrinsic antibacterial activity, such as clavulanic acid and sulbactam, have been combined with amoxicillin or ticarcillin to expand the spectrum of activity of these latter compounds by neutralizing enzymes that might otherwise degrade them.

Bacitracin and vancomycin inhibit the early stages in peptidoglycan synthesis. They are active only against gram-positive bacteria.

Penicillins

Sir Alexander Fleming's observation that colonies of staphylococci lysed on a plate that had become contaminated with a *Penicillum* fungus was the discovery that led to the development of antibiotics. In 1940, Chain, Florey, and their associates succeeded in producing significant quantities of penicillin from *Penicillium notatum*. Almost a decade later, penicillin G became widely available for clinical use. In the years that followed, this antibiotic was found to have certain limitations: its relative instability to stomach acid, its susceptibility to inactivation by penicillinase, and its relative inactivity against most gram-negative bacteria. Isolation of the active moiety, 6-aminopenicillanic acid, in the penicillin molecule has resulted in the design and development of semisynthetic penicillins that overcome some of these limitations.

The development of the cephalosporin family, which shares with penicillin the beta-lactam ring, has led to a remarkable array of drugs with improved ability to penetrate different gram-negative bacterial species and to resist beta-lactamase enzymes. In recent years, other naturally occurring beta-lactam antibiotics have been described that lack the bicyclic ring of the classical beta-lactam penicillins and cephalosporins. Many of these new drugs have potent antibacterial activity and are highly inhibitory to beta-lactamase enzymes.

Clinically important penicillins can be divided into four groups:

1. Highest activity against gram-positive organisms, but susceptible to acid hydrolysis and beta-lactamase inactivation (e.g., penicillin G).
2. Relatively resistant to staphylococcal beta-lactamases, but of lower activity than penicillin G against susceptible gram-positive organisms and inactive against gram-negatives (e.g., oxacillin, cloxacillin, methicillin, and nafcillin).
3. Relatively high activity against both gram-negative and gram-positive organisms, but inactivated by beta-lactamases (e.g., ampicillin, amoxicillin, carbenicillin, and ticarcillin). Usually susceptible gram-negative organisms include *Escherichia coli*, *Proteus mirabilis*, and *Salmonella*. Carbenicillin and ticarcillin are considerably more active than ampicillin against *Pseudomonas aeruginosa*. These semisynthetic penicillins are less active than penicillin G against gram-positive bacteria and susceptible anaerobes.
4. Relatively stable in gastric acid and suitable for oral administration in monogastrates (e.g., penicillin V (the phenoxymethyl analogue of penicillin G), ampicillin, amoxicillin, oxacillin, and cloxacillin).

Antimicrobial Activity. Penicillin G is the most active of the penicillins against gram-positive aerobic bacteria such as non-beta-lactamase-producing *Staphylococcus aureus*, beta-hemolytic streptococci, *Bacillus anthracis* and other gram-positive rods, corynebacteria, *Erysipelothrix*, *Listeria*, and against the anaerobes. It is moderately active against the more fastidious gram-negative aerobes such as *Haemophilus*, *Pasteurella*, and some *Actinobacillus*, but it is inactive against Enterobacteriaceae, *Bordetella*, and *Pseudomonas*. The penicillinase-resistant isoxazolyl penicillins (oxacillin, cloxacillin, methicillin, and nafcillin) are resistant to *S. aureus* penicillinase, but are less active than penicillin G against other penicillin sensitive gram-positive bacteria. Ampicillin and amoxicillin are slightly less active than penicillin G against gram-positive and anaerobic bacteria and are also inactivated by penicillinase produced by *S. aureus*. They have considerably greater activity against gram-negative bacteria. They are ineffective against *Pseudomonas aeruginosa*. Carbenicillin and ticarcillin resemble ampicillin in spectrum of activity with the notable difference of having activity against *P. aeruginosa*.

Resistance. In gram-positive bacteria (particularly *S. aureus*), resistance is mainly through production of extra-cellular beta-lactamase (penicillinase) enzymes that break the beta-lactam ring of most penicillins. Resistance in gram-negative bacteria results, in part, from a wide variety of beta-lactamase enzymes and also from low bacterial permeability or lack of penicillin-binding protein receptors. Most or all gram-negative bacteria express low levels of species-specific chromosomally mediated beta-lactamase enzymes within the periplasmic space, and these sometimes contribute to resistance.

Plasmid-mediated beta-lactamase production is widespread among common gram-negative bacteria pathogens and opportunistic pathogens. The enzymes are constitutively expressed and cause high-level resistance. The majority are penicillinases rather than cephalosporinases. The most widespread are TEM-type beta-lactamases, which readily hydrolyze penicillin G and ampicillin rather than methicillin, cloxacillin, or carbenicillin. The less widespread OXA-type beta-lactamases hydrolyze isoxazolyl penicillins (oxacillin, cloxacillin, and related compounds).

A major recent advance has been the discovery of broad-spectrum inhibitors of beta-lactamase (e.g., clavulanic acid, sulbactam). These drugs have weak antibacterial activity but show extraordinary synergism when administered with penicillin G, ampicillin, or amoxicillin because they irreversibly bind the beta-lactamase enzymes of resistant bacteria.

Absorption, Distribution, and Excretion. The penicillins are organic acids that are generally available as the sodium or potassium salt of the free acid. Apart from the isoxazolyl penicillins and penicillin V, acid hydrolysis limits the systemic availability of most penicillins from oral preparations. Both ampicillin and amoxicillin are relatively stable in acid.

The penicillins are predominantly ionized in the blood plasma, have relatively small apparent volumes of distribution, and have short half-lives (0.5 to 1.2 hours) in all species of domestic animals. After absorption, penicillins are widely distributed in body fluids. Because of their high degree of ionization and low solubility in lipid, they attain only low intracellular concentrations and do not penetrate well into transcellular fluids. The relatively poor diffusibility of penicillins across cell membranes is reflected in their milk-to-plasma concentration ratios (0.3). The relatively low tissue levels attained may, however, be clinically effective because of the high sensitivity of susceptible bacteria to penicillins and their bactericidal action. Ampicillin and amoxicillin, in addition to having a wider spectrum of antimicrobial activity, penetrate cellular barriers more readily than penicillin G. Their somewhat longer half-lives might be attributed to enterohepatic circulation. Penetration to cerebrospinal fluid (CSF) is usually poor but is enhanced by inflammation. In addition, active removal of penicillin from CSF is diminished by inflammation. The penicillins are eliminated almost entirely by renal excretion, which results in very high levels in the urine. The renal excretion mechanisms include glomerular filtration and mainly proximal tubular secretion.

Adverse Effects. Penicillins are remarkably free of toxic effects, even at doses grossly in excess of those recommended. The major adverse effect is acute anaphylaxis; milder hypersensitivity reactions (urticaria, fever, angioneurotic edema) are more common. All penicillins are cross-sensitizing and cross-reacting. Anaphylactic reactions are less common after oral penicillin administration than after parenteral administration. Many of the acute toxicities reported in animals are the toxic effects of the potassium or procaine with which the penicillin is combined. The use of penicillin in guinea pigs invariably causes fatal *Clostridium difficile* colitis, and use of ampicillin in rabbits causes fatal *C. spiriforme* colitis.

Cephalosporins

Cephalosporins are natural or semisynthetic products of the fungi *Cephalsporium* spp.; the related cephamycins are derived from actinomycetes. The nucleus of the semisynthetic cephalosporins, 7-aminocephalosporanic acid, bears a close structural resemblance to that of the penicillins, which accounts for a common mechanism of action and other properties shared by these two classes of drugs. They are bactericidal. Like the penicillins, cephalosporins have short half-lives, and most are excreted unchanged in the urine. Attachment of various R groups to the cephalosporanic acid nucleus has resulted in compounds with low toxicity and high therapeutic activity. Though not an ideal description, the classification of cephalosporins as belonging to "generations" relates to their increasing spectrum of activity against gram-negative bacteria because of improved penetration of cells and their progressive resistance to the beta-lactamases of gram-negative bacteria.

Antimicrobial Activity. The first-generation cephalosporins (e.g., cephalothin, cephalexin, cephaloridine, and cefadroxil) have a similar spectrum of activity to ampicillin, with the notable difference that beta-lactamase-producing staphylococci are susceptible. They are active against a variety of gram-positive bacteria such as *S. aureus*, many streptococci (except enterococci), corynebacteria, and gram-positive anaerobes (*Actinomyces* and *Clostridium*). Among gram-negative bacteria, *Haemophilus* and *Pasteurella* are susceptible, as are some *E. coli*, *Klebsiella*, *Proteus*, and *Salmonella*. *Enterobacter* and *P. aeruginosa* are resistant. Many anaerobic bacteria, except members of the *Bacteroides fragilis* group, are susceptible. The second-generation cephalosporins (e.g., cefamandole, cefoxitin, and cefuroxime) have increased resistance to gram-negative beta-lactamases and thus broader activity against gram-negative bacteria as well as against bacteria susceptible to the first-generation drugs. They are active against some strains of *Enterobacter* and against cephalothin-resistant *E. coli*, *Klebsiella*, and *Proteus*. Some *B. fragilis* are susceptible. Like the first-generation cephalosporins, these drugs are not active against *P. aeruginosa* or *Serratia*. The third-generation cephalosporins (e.g., cefotaxime, moxalactam, and cefoperazone) are characterized by reduced activity against gram-positive bacteria, modest activity against *P. aeruginosa*, and remarkable activity against *Enterobacteriaceae*.

Resistance. The mechanisms of acquired resistance to cephalosporins are not well understood. Methicillin-resistant *S. aureus* are resistant to all generations of cephalosporins. Plasmid-mediated resistance to first- and second-generation drugs have been described in gram-negative bacteria. Emergence of resistance in *Enterobacter*, *Serratia*, and *P. aeruginosa* during treatment with third-generation drugs results from derepression of inducible, chromosomal beta-lactamase enzymes, which in turn results in broad-spectrum resistance to beta-lactam antibiotics.

Absorption, Distribution, and Excretion. Cephalosporins are water-soluble drugs. Of the first-generation cephalosporins, cephalexin and cephadroxil are relatively acid-stable and sufficiently well absorbed from the intestine to be administered orally in dogs and cats, but not in horses or ruminants. Other first-generation cephalosporins must be administered parenterally although they are often painful on intramuscular injection and irritating on intravenous injection. Second- and third-generation cephalosporins are available for oral use and could be given to dogs and cats. Following absorption from injection sites, cephalosporins are widely distributed into tissue and body fluids. Third-generation cephalosporins penetrate cerebrospinal fluid well, and because of their high activity against gram-negative bacteria, have particular potential application in the treatment of meningitis.

Adverse Effects. Cephalosporins are relatively nontoxic antibiotics in humans. Allergic reactions occur in 5% to 10% of human patients who are hypersensitive to penicillin. Intravenous and intramuscular injections of some drugs are an irritant.

Other Beta-Lactam Antibiotics

The last 15 years have seen the discovery of other naturally occurring beta-lactam antibiotics. These include the cephamycins, clavulanic acid, thienamycin, the monobactams (such as aztreonam), the carbapenems (such as imipenem), the PS-compounds, and the carpetimycins — all compounds with the basic beta-lactam ring but without the bicyclic ring structure of the classical beta-lactams. All are highly inhibitory to beta-lactamases, and many possess potent antibacterial properties or are used in combination with earlier beta-lactams for their potent beta-lactamase inhibitory effects (clavulanic acid, sulbactam).

DAMAGE TO CELL MEMBRANE FUNCTION

Antibiotics that damage cell membrane function include the polymyxins, the polyenes (amphotericin, nystatin), the imidazoles (miconazole, ketoconazole, itraconazole, fluconazole, clotrimazole), and monensin. The cell membrane lies beneath the cell wall, enclosing the cytoplasm. It controls the passage of materials into or out of the cell. If its function is damaged, cellular contents (proteins, nucleotides, ions) can leak from the cell and result in cell damage and death.

Polymyxins

The structure of the polymyxins is such that they have well-defined separate hydrophilic and hydrophobic sectors. Polymyxins act by binding to the membrane phospholipid, which results in structural disorganization, permeability damage, and cell lysis. The polymyxins are selectively toxic to gram-negative bacteria because of the presence of certain phospholipids in the cell membrane and because the outer surface of the outer membrane of gram-negative bacteria consists mainly of lipopolysaccharide. Parenteral use is associated with nephrotoxic, neurotoxic, and neuromuscular blocking effects. The major clinical applications are limited to the oral treatment of *E. coli* and *Salmonella* diarrheas and the local treatment of coliform infections.

Polyenes

The polyenes are selectively active against fungi since they only affect membranes containing sterols. Polyenes inhibit the formation of membrane lipids, forming pores through which the vital contents of the cytoplasm are lost. See the section on antifungal therapy, below.

Imidazoles

Imidazoles interfere with the biosynthesis of sterols and bind cell membrane phospholipids to cause leakage of cell contents. They are active against the fungal cell membrane. See the section on antifungal therapy, below.

INHIBITION OF NUCLEIC ACID FUNCTION

Examples of drugs that inhibit nucleic acid function are nitroimidazoles, nitrofurans, nalidixic acid, the fluoroquinolones (enrofloxacin, ciprofloxacin), novobiocin, rifampin, sulfonamides, trimethoprim, and 5-flucytosine. Because the mechanisms of nucleic acid synthesis, replication, and transcription are similar in all cells, drugs affecting nucleic acid function have poor selective toxicity. Most act by binding to DNA to inhibit its replication or transcription. Drugs with greater selective toxicity are the sulfonamides and trimethoprim, which inhibit the synthesis of folic acid.

Nitroimidazoles

Nitroimidazoles, such as metronidazole and dimetridazole, possess antiprotozoal and antibacterial properties.

Activity within bacterial cells is due to the unidentified, reduced products of the drug, which are only seen in anaerobes or microaerophiles. Nitroimidazoles cause extensive DNA strand breakage either by inhibiting the DNA repair enzyme, DNase 1, or by forming complexes with the nucleotide bases that the enzyme does not recognize. Nitroimidazoles are bactericidal to anaerobic gram-negative and many gram-positive bacteria and are active against protozoa such as *Tritrichomonas fetus*, *Giardia lamblia*, and *Histomonas meleagridis*. They are highly active against *Serpulina hyodysenteriae*, the agent of swine dysentery. Chromosomal resistance may cause slight increases in minimum inhibitory concentrations (MIC) but, as is the case for nitrofurans, plasmid-encoded resistance is rare. Nitroimidazoles are generally well absorbed after oral administration, but parenteral injection is highly irritating. They are well distributed throughout body tissues and fluids, including brain and cerebrospinal fluid. Excretion is through the urine. There are no reports of adverse effects in animals given a therapeutic dosage. The most serious potential hazard is the controversial report of carcinogenicity in laboratory animals. For this reason, these drugs are not used in food animals.

Nitrofurans

Like the nitroimidazoles, the nitrofurans are antiprotozoal but have wider antibacterial activity; they are most active under anaerobic conditions. After entry into the cell, bacterial nitroreductases produce uncharacterized unstable reduction products, which differ with each type of nitrofuran. These products cause strand breakage in bacterial DNA. The nitrofurans are synthetic 5-nitrofuraldehyde derivatives with broad antimicrobial activity. Toxicity and low tissue concentrations limit their use to the local treatment of infections and to the treatment of urinary tract infections.

Fluoroquinolones

Fluoroquinolones (ciprofloxacin, enrofloxacin, sparfloxacin) are active against gram-negative bacteria. They cause selective inhibition of bacterial DNA synthesis by inhibiting DNA gyrase. Fluoroquinolones are bactericidal drugs that inhibit DNA synthesis by a poorly understood mechanism. Nalidixic acid (which is rarely used because of toxicity) is most active against gram-negative bacteria except *P. aeruginosa*, but the newer fluoroquinolone derivatives are broader spectrum and active against some gram-positive bacteria, including mycobacteria. Activity against mycoplasma and rickettsia is also an important attribute of the newer fluoroquinolones. The fluoroquinolones are rapidly absorbed after oral administration and have half-lives in humans varying from 4 to 12 hours. They are widely distributed in tissues, and may be concentrated, for example, in the prostate. Penetration into cerebrospinal fluid is about half that of serum, which makes these drugs useful to treat meningitis. They are being introduced rapidly into veterinary use, particularly for use against gram-negative bacteria and mycoplasma. One drawback is the fairly rapid development of chromosomally mediated resistance.

Rifampin

Rifampin, which has particular activity against gram-positive bacteria and mycobacteria, has remarkable selectivity of inhibition of bacterial DNA-dependent ribonucleic acid (RNA) polymerase. Rifampin prevents initiation of transcription.

Sulfonamides and Trimethoprim

Sulfonamides are synthetic drugs with broad antibacterial and antiprotozoal properties. They interfere with the biosynthesis of folic acid and prevent the formation of purine nucleotides. Sulfonamides are functional analogues of para-aminobenzoic acid and compete with it for the same enzyme, tetrahydropteroate synthetase, forming nonfunctional folic acid analogues and inhibiting bacterial growth. Selective toxicity of sulfonamides occurs because mammalian cells have lost their ability to synthesize folic acid but rather absorb it from the intestine, whereas bacteria must synthesize it. In the bacterial cell, preformed folic acid is progressively exhausted by several bacterial divisions.

Other drugs affect folic acid synthesis by interfering with the enzyme dihydrofolate reductase. One example is trimethoprim, which is selectively toxic to bacteria rather than to mammalian cells because of greater affinity for the bacterial enzyme. The enzyme inhibits the conversion of dihydrofolate to tetrahydrofolate, producing a sequential blockade of folic acid synthesis with sulfonamides.

Sulfonamides

The sulfonamides constitute a series of weak organic acids that enter most tissues and body fluids. The degree of ionization and lipid solubility of the large number of individual sulfonamides influences absorption, determines capacity to penetrate cell membranes, and can affect the rate of elimination. Sulfonamides exert a bacteriostatic effect against both gram-positive and gram-negative bacteria and can also inhibit other microorganisms (chlamydia and some protozoa). They are available in a wide variety of preparations for either oral or parenteral use. They have largely been abandoned because of widespread resistance, difficulties in administration, and the existence of better alternatives. Certain individual sulfonamides are combined with trimethoprim in fixed ratio (5:1) combination preparations that have the advantage of both synergistic and bactericidal effects.

Individual sulfonamides are derivatives of sulfanilamide, which contains the structural prerequisites for antibacterial activity. The various derivatives differ in physicochemical and pharmacokinetic properties and in degree of antimicrobial activity. The sodium salts of sulfonamides are readily soluble in water, and parenteral preparations are available for intravenous administration. Certain sulfonamide molecules are designed for low sol-

ubility (e.g., phthalylsulfathiazole) so that they will be slowly absorbed; these are intended for use in the treatment of enteric infections.

Antimicrobial Activity. Sulfonamides are broad-spectrum antimicrobial drugs. They are active against aerobic gram-positive cocci and some rods and some gram-negative bacteria, including *Enterobacteriaceae*. Many anaerobes are sensitive.

Resistance. Resistance to sulfonamides in pathogenic and nonpathogenic bacteria isolated from animals is widespread. This situation reflects their extensive use in human and veterinary medicine for many years. Sulfonamide resistance may occur as a result of mutation causing overproduction of para-aminobenzoic acid (PABA) or as a result of a structural change in the dihydrofolic acid-synthesizing enzyme with a lowered affinity for sulfonamides. Most often, sulfonamide resistance is plasmid-mediated.

Absorption, Distribution, and Excretion. Most sulfonamides are rapidly absorbed from the gastrointestinal tract and distributed widely to all tissues and body fluids, including synovial and cerebrospinal fluid. They are bound to plasma proteins to a variable extent. In addition to differences among sulfonamides in extent of binding, there is variation among species in binding of individual sulfonamides. Extensive (80%) protein binding serves to increase half-life. They enter cerebrospinal fluid well.

Sulfonamides are eliminated by a combination of renal excretion and biotransformation processes in the liver. This combination of elimination processes contributes to the species variation in the half-life of individual sulfonamides. While a large number of sulfonamide preparations is available for use in veterinary medicine, many of these are different dosage forms of sulfamethazine. This sulfonamide is most widely used in the food-producing animals and can attain effective plasma concentrations (within the range 50 to 150 μg/ml) when administered either orally or parenterally. Due to their alkalinity, most parenteral preparations should only be administered by intravenous injection. Prolonged-release oral dosage forms of sulfamethazine are available.

Adverse Effects. The sulfonamides can produce a wide variety of side effects, some of which may have an allergic basis whereas others are due to direct toxicity. The more common adverse effects are urinary tract disturbances (crystalluria, hematuria, or even obstruction) and hematopoietic disorders (thrombocytopenia and leukopenia). Some adverse effects are associated with particular sulfonamides. Sulfadiazine and sulfasalazine given for long periods to dogs to control chronic hemorrhagic colitis have caused keratoconjunctivitis sicca.

Trimethoprim-Sulfonamide Combinations

Trimethoprim is combined with a variety of sulfonamides in a fixed ratio. The combination produces a bactericidal effect against a wide range of bacteria, with some important exceptions, and also inhibits certain other microorganisms. Veterinary preparations contain trimethoprim combined with sulfadiazine or sulfadoxine in the 1:5 ratio.

Antimicrobial Activity. Trimethoprim-sulfonamide combinations have a generally broad spectrum and usually bactericidal action against many gram-positive and gram-negative aerobic bacteria, including *Enterobacteriaceae.* The combination is active against a large proportion of anaerobic bacteria, at least under in vitro conditions. Mycoplasma and *P. aeruginosa* are resistant.

Synergism occurs when the microorganisms are sensitive to both drugs in the combination. When bacteria are resistant to sulfonamides, it may still be obtained in up to 40% of cases, even when bacteria are only moderately sensitive to trimethoprim. Due to differences between the trimethoprim and sulfonamide in distribution pattern and processes of elimination, the concentration ratios of the two drugs will differ considerably in tissues and urine from the ratio in the plasma. This variation is not important since the synergistic interaction occurs over a wide range of concentration ratios of the two drugs.

Resistance. Resistance to sulfonamides is due to structural alteration in the dihydrofolic acid synthesizing enzyme (dihydropteroate synthetase), whereas resistance to trimethoprim usually results from plasmid-encoded synthesis of a resistant dihydrofolate reductase enzyme. Bacterial resistance to the combination has progressively developed with use of these preparations in animals.

Absorption, Distribution, and Elimination. Trimethoprim is a lipid-soluble organic base that is approximately 60% bound to plasma proteins and 60% ionized in the plasma. This combination of physicochemical properties enables the drug to distribute widely, to penetrate cellular barriers by nonionic diffusion, and to attain effective concentrations in most body fluids and tissues, including brain and cerebrospinal fluid. Hepatic metabolism is the principal process for elimination of trimethoprim. The half-life and fraction of the dose that is excreted unchanged in the urine vary widely among different species. The drug is well absorbed following oral administration in dogs, cats, and horses or from injection sites in these and other species.

Adverse Effects. Serious side effects are uncommon; those that do occur can usually be attributed to the sulfonamide component. Oral trimethoprim-sulfonamide has the advantage over other oral antimicrobials of causing little disturbance among the normal intestinal anaerobic microflora.

INHIBITION OF PROTEIN SYNTHESIS

Examples of drugs that inhibit protein synthesis are tetracyclines, aminoglycosides (streptomycin, neomycin, kanamycin, gentamicin, tobramycin, and others), aminocyclitols (spectinomycin), chloramphenicol, lincosamides (lincomycin, clindamycin), and macrolides (erythromycin, tylosin, tiamulin, and others). Because of the marked differences in ribosomal structure, composition, and function between prokaryotic and eukaryotic cells, many important antibacterial drugs selectively inhibit bacterial protein synthesis. Antibiotics affecting protein synthesis can be divided into those affecting the 30S ribosome (tetracyclines, aminoglycosides, aminocyclitols) and those affecting the 50S ribosome (chloramphenicol, macrolides, lincosamides).

Tetracyclines

Tetracyclines interfere with protein synthesis by inhibiting the binding of aminoacyl tRNA to the recognition site. The various tetracyclines have similar antimicrobial activity but differ in pharmacologic characteristics.

Antimicrobial Activity. Tetracyclines are broad-spectrum drugs active against gram-positive and gram-negative bacteria, rickettsiae, chlamydiae, some mycoplasmas, and protozoa such as *Theileria*. Tetracyclines have good activity against many gram-positive bacteria, the more fastidious nonenteric bacteria such as *Actinobacillus*, *Bordetella*, *Brucella*, *Haemophilus*, some *Pasteurella*, and many anaerobic bacteria, but their activity against these bacteria and against *Enterobacteriaceae* is increasingly limited by resistance. *Pseudomonas aeruginosa* is resistant, except in urinary tract infections, where tetracyclines may be drugs of choice.

Resistance. Widespread resistance to the tetracyclines has considerably reduced their usefulness. Such resistance is high level and usually plasmid-mediated. Cross-resistance between tetracyclines is complete.

Adverse Effects. Tetracyclines are generally safe antibiotics with a reasonably high therapeutic index. The main adverse effects are associated with their severely irritant nature, with disturbances in gastrointestinal flora, with their ability to bind calcium (cardiovascular effects, teeth or bone deposition), and with the toxic effects of degradation products on liver and kidney cells. Their use in horses has largely been abandoned because of a tendency to produce broad-spectrum suppression of the normal intestinal flora and fatal superinfection with *Salmonella* or with unidentified pathogens ("Colitis X").

Chloramphenicol

Chloramphenicol is a broad-spectrum, generally bacteriostatic drug that binds the 50S ribosome, distorting the region and inhibiting the peptidyl transferase reaction. Chloramphenicol is a stable, lipid-soluble, neutral compound. It was originally produced from cultures of an actinomycete, but it is now synthesized chemically.

Antimicrobial Activity. Chloramphenicol is active against gram-positive and gram-negative bacteria, chlamydiae, rickettsiae, and some mycoplasmas. Most gram-positive and many gram-negative pathogenic aerobic and anaerobic bacteria are susceptible, though resistance is increasing in *Enterobacteriaceae*. The drug is generally bacteriostatic.

Resistance. Most chloramphenicol resistance is the result of plasmid-encoded chloramphenicol acetylase enzymes which modify chloramphenicol so that it is no longer active.

Absorption, Distribution, and Excretion. In dogs, cats, and pre-ruminants, chloramphenicol is well absorbed from the intestine; in ruminants the drug is inactivated after oral administration. Because of its low molecular weight, lipid solubility, and modest plasma protein binding, the drug is well distributed in most tissues and fluids, including the cerebrospinal fluid and aqueous humor. The half-life of chloramphenicol varies widely in animals from a low of 1 hour in horses to 5 or 6 hours in cats. In neonates the half-life is considerably longer. The drug is mainly eliminated by glucuronide conjugation in the liver.

Adverse Effects. The fatal aplastic anemia seen in 1 in 25,000 to 40,000 humans treated with chloramphenicol does not occur in animals, although prolonged high dosing may cause reversible abnormalities in bone marrow activity. The potential for nondose-related fatal aplastic anaemia in humans has led to its prohibition for use in food animals in the United States and Canada because of fear of the presence of drug residues in meat products.

Aminoglycosides and Aminocyclitols

The aminoglycosides are bactericidal. The mode of action of streptomycin is best understood. Streptomycin has a variety of complex effects in the bacterial cell: a) it binds to a specific receptor protein in the 30S ribosomal subunit, distorting the codon–anticodon interactions at the recognition site and causing misreading of the genetic code so that faulty proteins are produced; b) it binds to "initiating" ribosomes to prevent the formation of 70S ribosomes; and c) it inhibits the elongation reaction of protein synthesis. The other aminoglycosides act similarly to streptomycin in causing mistranslation of the genetic code and in irreversible inhibition of initiation, although the extent and type often differ. They have multiple binding sites on the ribosome, whereas strepto-mycin has only one, and can also inhibit the transloca-tion step in protein synthesis. Spectinomycin is a bacteriostatic aminocyclitol antibiotic that is believed to inhibit polypeptide chain elongation at the translocation step.

The aminoglycoside antibiotics are polar organic bases. Their polarity largely accounts for the similar pharmaco-kinetic properties that are shared by all members of the group. Chemically, they consist of a hexose nucleus to which amino sugars are attached by glycosidic linkages. All are potentially ototoxic and nephrotoxic. The newer aminoglycosides are more resistant to plasmid-mediated enzymatic degradation and are less toxic than the older compounds. Amikacin > tobramycin ≥ gentamicin > neomycin = kanamycin > streptomycin in potency, spec-trum of activity, and stability to plasmid-mediated resis-tance. This activity mirrors the age of introduction of the drugs, with streptomycin being the oldest of the aminoglycosides.

Antimicrobial Activity. Aminoglycosides are particularly active against gram-negative bacteria as well as against mycobacteria and some mycoplasma. Anaerobic bacteria are usually resistant. As a general rule, gram-positive bacteria are resistant to older drugs (streptomycin, neomycin) but may be inhibited by newer drugs (gen-tamicin, amikacin). A particularly useful property is the activity of newer aminoglycosides against *P. aeruginosa*. Their bactericidal action on aerobic gram-negative bacilli is markedly influenced by pH; they are most active in an alkaline environment. Increased local acidity secondary to tissue damage may account for the failure of an amino-glycoside to kill usually susceptible microorganisms at infection sites or in abscess cavities. Combinations of aminoglycosides with penicillins are often synergistic; the concurrent administration of the newer beta-lactam antibiotics with gentamicin or tobramycin has been used to treat serious gram-negative infections, for example, those caused by *P. aeruginosa*.

Resistance. Most clinically important resistance is caused by a variety of R plasmid-specified degradative enzymes located in the periplasmic space. Certain of these enzymes inactivate only the older aminoglycosides (streptomycin, or neomycin and kanamycin), but others are broader spectrum. The remarkable property of amikacin is its resistance to many of the enzymes that inactivate other aminoglycosides. Plasmid-mediated resis-tance to streptomycin is widespread and commonly linked to sulfonamides, tetracyclines, and ampicillin. Chromosomal resistance to streptomycin, but not to the other aminoglycosides, develops fairly readily during treatment.

Absorption, Distribution, and Excretion. Aminoglycosides are poorly absorbed from the gastrointestinal tract, bind to a low extent to plasma proteins, and have limited capacity to enter cells and penetrate cellular barriers. They do not readily attain therapeutic concentrations in transcellular fluids, particularly cerebrospinal and ocular fluid. Poor diffusibility can be attributed to their low degree of lipid solubility. Their apparent volumes of distribution are relatively small, and their half-lives are short (2 hours) in domestic animals. Even though these drugs have a small volume of distribution, selective binding to renal tissue (kidney cortex) occurs. Elimina-tion takes place entirely by renal excretion (glomerular filtration), and unchanged drug is rapidly excreted in the urine. Impaired renal function decreases their rate of excretion and makes adjustment of the maintenance dosage necessary to prevent accumulation with attendant toxicity.

Major changes are taking place in recommendations for intramuscular dosage with aminoglycosides, which is moving from three times daily to a single daily dosage. This has the effect of increasing therapeutic efficacy, since antibacterial activity depends on both peak concentrations and total concentration, and reducing toxicity, since the nephrotoxic effects depend on a threshold effect, concentrations above which have no further action. This dramatically changed understanding of aminoglycoside dosage will likely increase the use of the less toxic members.

Adverse Effects. All aminoglycosides can cause varying degrees of ototoxicity and nephrotoxicity. The tendency to produce vestibular or cochlear damage varies with the drug: neomycin is the most likely to cause cochlear damage and streptomycin to cause vestibular damage. Nephrotoxicity (acute tubular necrosis) occurs in association with prolonged therapy and excessive trough concentrations of the aminoglycoside (particularly gentamicin) in plasma. The aminoglycosides can produce neuromuscular blockage of the nondepolarizing type, which causes flaccid paralysis and apnea. This is most likely to occur in association with anesthesia.

Spectinomycin

Spectinomycin is an aminocyclitol antibiotic with a spectrum of activity and mechanism of action similar to that of kanamycin but without the toxic effects of the aminoglycosides. It is normally bacteriostatic and is not particularly active on a weight basis. Its activity against gram-negative bacteria is unpredictable because of naturally resistant strains. Chromosomal resistance develops readily but does not cross-react with aminoglycosides. Plasmid resistance is uncommon but often extends to streptomycin. The drug has most of the pharmacokinetic properties of aminoglycosides but appears to penetrate cerebrospinal fluid better. It has been used in agricultural practice to treat salmonellosis and mycoplasma infections.

Macrolides

Macrolide antibiotics are bacteriostatic with activity particularly against gram-positive bacteria and mycoplasma. They bind to 50S ribosome in competition with chloramphenicol and inhibit the translocation step of protein synthesis. The precise mechanism of action is unknown. Macrolide antibiotics (erythromycin, tylosin, tiamulin, azithromycin, clarithromycin, and spiramycin) have action and pharmacokinetic properties similar to the lincosamides. Like the lincosamides they are lipid soluble, basic drugs that are concentrated in tissue compared to serum and penetrate cells well.

Antimicrobial Activity. Erythromycin has an antibacterial spectrum similar to penicillin G, but it includes activity against penicillinase-producing *S. aureus, Campylobacter, Leptospira, Bordetella*, rickettsia, chlamydia, some mycoplasma, and atypical mycobacteria. It may be bactericidal at high concentrations. Tylosin and spiramycin are less active than erythromycin against bacteria but more active against a broad range of mycoplasma. Tiamulin has better activity than the other macrolides against anaerobes, including *Serpulina hyodysenteriae*, and is distinguished for its remarkable activity against mycoplasmas. Azithromycin and clarithromycin are particularly active against non-tuberculous mycobacteria.

Resistance. One-step chromosomal resistance to erythromycin develops fairly readily, even during treatment, but is generally unstable. Plasmid-mediated resistance is common. Cross-resistance between erythromycin and lincosamides and other macrolides is common. There is little information about resistance of veterinary pathogens to tylosin. Development of resistance to tiamulin appears to be relatively uncommon; organisms resistant to tiamulin show one-way cross-resistance with other macrolides.

Absorption, Distribution, and Excretion. Erythromycin stearate and estolate are well absorbed after oral administration, but the base is not. Intramuscular injection of erythromycin is very irritating. The absorption of tylosin from the intestine varies with the formulation. Tiamulin is well absorbed. These drugs are well distributed through body tissues and fluids, except the cere-brospinal fluid. Tissue concentrations often exceed serum concentrations. In the case of spiramycin, such tissue concentration is extreme and is associated with tissue binding. A large proportion of these drugs is degraded in the body, but some is excreted through the kidney and the liver.

Adverse Effects. Macrolides are generally safe drugs though painful on injection. Their potential for causing irreversible diarrhea in adult horses means that they should be avoided in this species. Tylosin and tiamulin administered intravenously to calves may produce severe nervous depression. The drugs should not be given orally to ruminants because of their potential for disturbing the rumen flora.

Lincosamides

Lincomycin and clindamycin have antibacterial activity mainly against gram-positive aerobic bacteria and against anaerobic bacteria. The drugs bind the 50S ribosomal subunits at binding sites that overlap with those of chloramphenicol and the macrolides. They inhibit the peptidyl transferase reaction. The lincosamides, lincomycin and clindamycin, are products of an actinomycete with activity and mechanism of action similar to that of the macrolides. Lincomycin is most commonly used in veterinary medicine, although it is less active on a weight basis than clindamycin. Lincosamides are active against gram-positive aerobic and all anaerobic bacteria, and against mycoplasmas; but most gram-negative aerobes are resistant. Clindamycin is more active than lincomycin against anaerobes and may be bactericidal. Chromosomal stepwise resistance develops fairly readily, and plasmid-mediated resistance is common. Cross-resistance between lincosamides is complete and commonly occurs also with macrolides. Lincomycin is readily absorbed after oral or intramuscular administration. Food delays and reduces absorption. The absorption of different clindamycin compounds is variable. The lincosamides are widely distributed in body tissues and fluids, including the prostate and milk, but cerebrospinal fluid concentrations are low. They penetrate intracellularly because of their lipophilic properties. Most excretion is through the liver. The major adverse effect of lincosamides is their ability to cause fatal diarrhea in horses, rabbits, guinea pigs, and hamsters. In rabbits, fatal diarrhea results from proliferation of *Clostridium spiroforme* or *C. difficile*. Oral lincosamides at low concentrations produce severe ruminal disturbances in adult ruminants.

ANTIMICROBIAL SUSCEPTIBILITY AND DRUG DOSAGE PREDICTION

The use of antimicrobial drugs in treating infections depends on the relation of the quantitative susceptibility of the microorganism to tissue concentrations of drug. The antimicrobial susceptibility of many veterinary pathogens is highly predictable and clinical experience has established effective dosages for infections caused by these organisms. In many bacteria, however, the presence of various mechanisms for acquiring resistance means that susceptibility to a particular antibacterial drug may need to be tested.

Antimicrobial Susceptibility Testing

There are two general methods for antimicrobial susceptibility testing in vitro: the dilution method and the diffusion method. The dilution method gives quantitative information on drug susceptibility while the diffusion method gives qualitative (or at best semiquantitative) information. The tests must be performed under standardized conditions.

Dilution Antimicrobial Tests. Antimicrobial drugs of known potency are prepared in doubling dilutions of concentrations similar to those achievable in the tissues of patients given usual drug dosages. The highest dilution at which there is no visible bacterial growth following inoculation and incubation is the minimum inhibitory concentration (MIC), which is usually less than the minimum bactericidal concentration (MBC) for drugs (Table 4.1).

The advantage of determining quantitative susceptibility of an organism is that this information can be related to knowledge of drug concentrations in particular tissues in the prediction of appropriate drug dosage. In medical practice, MIC results are usually interpreted by the system of categories suggested by the U.S. National Committee for Clinical Laboratory Standards (1997). These interpretative guidelines take into account the inherent susceptibility of the organism to each drug, the pharmacokinetic properties of the particular

Table 4.1.   Minimum Concentration of Tetracycline Inhibitory to Selected Veterinary Pathogens

	Minimum Inhibitory Concentration (μg/ml)	
	MIC$_{50}$*	MIC$_{90}$*
Bordetella bronchiseptica	1.6	1.6
Brucella canis	0.09	0.19
Corynebacterium pseudotuberculosis	0.25	0.25
Escherichia coli	4.0	64.0
Klebsiella pneumoniae	2.0	64.0
Mycoplasma canis	5.0	10.0
Pasteurella multocida	0.4	0.4

*   Highest MIC$_{50}$ of 50% of isolates tested, MIC$_{90}$ of 90% of isolates tested. The MIC of different organisms varies with strain and species.

drug, dosage, site of infection, and drug toxicity. These categories are 1) susceptible, meaning that the infecting organism is usually inhibited by concentrations of a particular antibiotic attained in tissues by usual dosage; 2) intermediately susceptible, meaning that the infecting organism is inhibited by blood or tissue concentrations achieved with maximum dosage; and 3) resistant, meaning that it is resistant to normally achievable and tolerated concentrations of antimicrobial drugs.

Diffusion Antimicrobial Tests.   A standard concentration of a pure culture of the pathogen is placed on appropriate agar and individual filter paper discs containing known concentrations of individual antibiotics are placed on the agar, which is incubated for 18 hours at 35°C. The zone of inhibition around each disc is measured and the measurement is referred to a chart that classifies the organism as being susceptible, resistant, or moderately susceptible to the particular antibiotic in each drug. Standards for performing these tests are defined. Under standard conditions, there is a linear inverse relationship between the diameter of the zone of growth inhibition and MIC. The interpretation of zone diameters as susceptible, resistant, or intermediate relates to serum drug concentrations of antibiotics in different animal species commonly achievable under standard dosage regimens. From these drug concentrations, MIC break points have been selected and extrapolated to zone diameters in providing the interpretative standards.

The description of a bacterium as "susceptible" or "resistant" to an antimicrobial drug depends ultimately on clinical success or failure of treatment. Quantitative information on susceptibility is obtained in the laboratory under artificial circumstances, which do not take into account host defenses, the dynamics of drug disposition, or the dynamics of interaction of a varying drug concentration with a bacterium in the host environment.

Design of Drug Dosage

Pharmacokinetic descriptions of drug disposition in different animal species, when combined with quantitative susceptibility (MIC) data, allow prediction of reasonable drug dosage in animals. It is generally assumed, and in some cases has been shown, that optimum drug dosage requires that tissue concentration of the drug equal or exceed the MIC of the pathogens. The extent to which tissue concentrations should exceed MIC has not been well defined for most antibiotics, although it is well recognized that high concentrations of drugs maintained for sustained periods give better effects than lower concentrations for shorter times. The tendency to try to maintain serum drug concentrations over MIC ignores the *postantibiotic effect* when, for several hours after removal of a drug present at > MIC, no bacterial growth occurs. The postantibiotic effect is observed with drugs such as aminoglycosides but not with beta-lactams, and is more marked in vivo than in vitro. The maximum interval of drug dosing should, however, preclude resumption of bacterial growth.

Factors Affecting Tissue Drug Concentrations

Dosage. The dosage regimen is made up of the *size* of the dose, which is limited by drug toxicity, and the dosage *interval*, which is determined by the half-life of the drug. The dosage interval required to maintain therapeutic tissue concentrations by intravenous dosing should not exceed twice the half-life for most antibiotics, but giving drugs by other routes lengthens the dosage interval.

Routes of Administration. Antibacterial drugs can be administered by a wide variety of routes — for example, oral, subcutaneous, intramuscular, intravenous, intramammary, intrauterine, or respiratory.

Intravenous Injection. Intravenous injection of a drug gives immediate high serum drug concentrations, which rapidly decline as the drug is distributed. Intravenous dosing may be the only way to exceed the MIC of some pathogens, but frequent dosing by this route is generally impractical in veterinary medicine.

Intramuscular Injection. Intramuscular injection is commonly used in veterinary medicine because it gives good serum concentrations within 1 to 2 hours of administration. The major advantage is that intramuscular injection gives the highest serum concentration of all routes other than intravenous, although subcutaneous injection is a reasonable alternative. Drug formulation can be prepared to give slow release of the drug after intramuscular injection and thus prolong dosage intervals to reduce handling of animals.

Oral Administration. The oral administration of antimicrobial drugs is limited to monogastric and pre-ruminant animals and to young foals. The oral dose is generally several times greater than the parenteral dose because the drug is less well absorbed. Although the oral route is often the easiest way to administer drugs, it is not always the most reliable. Some drugs (aminoglycosides, polymyxins) are not absorbed from the intestine, others are destroyed by stomach acidity (benzyl penicillin), and absorption may be impaired by food (as occurs with ampicillin, tetracyclines, lincomycin). Administration of antibiotics in water is nevertheless a particularly simple, convenient, and inexpensive way to treat livestock because it involves little if any handling of animals and avoids the expense of mixing antibiotics in feed.

Local Application. Infections of the udder, female genital tract, external ear canal, and skin are commonly treated by local application of antibiotics. High drug concentrations are obtained without systemic toxic effects.

The concentration of free drug in the serum largely determines the concentration in tissue fluids, since penetration of drugs into interstitial fluids in most tissues of the body is through pores in capillary endothelium.

Physicochemical Properties of the Drug. These characteristics largely determine the extent of the distribution of a drug in the body. Most antimicrobial drugs distribute well in extravascular tissue fluids, principally the interstitial fluid. They penetrate capillary endothelium through pores that admit molecules with a molecular weight of less than about 1000. Passage across biological membranes such as into tissue cells or across nonfenestrated capillary endothelium depends on drug ionization, lipid solubility, molecular weight, and the amount of free drug present. Lipid-soluble and nonionized drugs such as the macrolides and chloramphenicol distribute well and even concentrate in tissue, whereas ionized and weakly lipid-soluble drugs such as penicillins and aminoglycosides distribute poorly. These physicochemical differences largely determine the pharmacokinetic characteristics of the drugs; thus, aminoglycosides and penicillins have small apparent volumes of distribution and short half-lives after intravenous injection and are eliminated through the urinary tract, whereas macrolides and tetracyclines have large apparent volumes of distribution and longer half-lives and are eliminated in part through the liver. Penetration of special sites in the body such as the central nervous system, eye, and prostate (which among other differences lack capillary pores) is only by low molecular weight, lipid-soluble, nonionized drugs.

Protein Binding of Drug. In general, serum protein binding of drugs up to 90 percent is of little clinical importance. Aminoglycosides and polymyxin bind extensively to intracellular constituents and thus are inactivated by pus.

Excretion Mechanisms. These determine the concentration of drugs in the organs of excretion. Remarkably high concentrations of drugs may be achieved in urine or bile.

Physiological Barriers. Anatomic-physiologic barriers in the brain, cerebrospinal fluid, eye, and mammary gland reduce the entry of drugs from the blood. Inflammation reduces but does not abolish these barriers.

Duration of Treatment

Although it is axiomatic that a drug must be present for adequate time at the site of infection, the variables affecting time of treatment have not been defined. The response of different types of infection to antibiotics varies, and clinical experience with different types of infection is important in assessing response to treatment. In general, if no response to treatment is observed after two days, diagnosis and treatment should be reassessed. Treatment should be continued for 48 hours after symptoms have resolved, depending on the severity of infection. For serious infections, treatment should last 7 to 10 days. Some uncomplicated infections, such as cystitis in females, have been successfully treated with single doses of antibiotics.

USE OF ANTIBACTERIAL COMBINATIONS

Combinations of drugs sometimes have dramatic success where individual drugs fail. An outstanding early example is the use of penicillin-streptomycin combinations in enterococcal endocarditis in humans. However, early studies of the outcome of combination treatment of pneumococcal meningitis in humans showed the serious clinical effects of mixing bacteriostatic and bactericidal drugs. The importance of antagonistic interactions between drugs is greatest in those infections or patients where immune defenses are poor — meningitis, endocarditis, or chronic osteomyelitis — or where immunodeficiencies are present. In other patients or diseases, because of the complexity of the host-bacterial–antibiotic interaction, it is harder to detect either synergistic or antagonistic effects clinically.

A drug combination is *additive* if the combined effect of several drugs is the sum of their independent activities measured separately, *synergistic* if the combined effect is significantly greater than their independent effects, and *antagonistic* if it is significantly less than their independent effects. Synergism and antagonism are not absolute characteristics; such interactions are often difficult to predict, vary with bacterial species and strains, and may occur only over a narrow range of concentrations. No single in vitro method detects all such interactions. The methods used to determine in vitro interactions are generally time-consuming and are not often available in the laboratory.

Antimicrobial combinations are frequently synergistic if they involve the following mechanisms: 1) sequential inhibition of successive steps in metabolism (e.g., trimethoprim-sulfonamide combination), 2) sequential inhibition of cell wall synthesis (e.g., vancomycin-penicillin, mecillinam-ampicillin), 3) facilitation of drug entry of one antibiotic by another (e.g., beta-lactam-aminoglycoside, polymyxin-sulfonamide), 4) inhibition of inactivating enzymes (e.g., ampicillin-clavulanic acid), and 5) prevention of emergence of resistant populations (e.g., erythromycin-rifampin combination against *Rhodococcus equi*).

To some extent, antagonism between antibiotic combinations is a laboratory artifact that depends on the method of measurement and may thus, with some exceptions, be unimportant clinically. The antagonistic effects of some combinations are, however, detected clinically. Antagonism may occur if antimicrobial combinations involve the following mechanisms: 1) inhibition of bactericidal activity (e.g., bacteriostatic and bactericidal drugs used to treat meningitis where, depending on the time-dose relation, bactericidal effects are prevented), 2) competition for drug binding sites (e.g., macrolide-chloramphenicol combinations, which are of unclear clinical significance), 3) inhibition of cell permeability mechanisms (e.g., chloramphenicol or tetracycline-aminoglycoside combinations, which are of unclear clinical significance), and 4) derepression of resistance enzymes (e.g., new third-generation cephalosporin antibiotics with older beta-lactam drugs).

RESISTANCE TO ANTIBACTERIAL DRUGS

The potential for mutation and for genetic exchange between all types of bacteria, combined with the short bacterial generation time, is of major importance in limiting the use of antimicrobial drugs in controlling infection in animals and humans. The use of antimicrobial drugs does not induce resistance in bacteria but rather eliminates the susceptible bacteria and leaves the resistant bacteria already present in the population.

Resistance to antimicrobial drugs can be classified as constitutive or acquired.

Constitutive Resistance

Microorganisms may be resistant to certain antibiotics because the cellular mechanisms required for antibiotic susceptibility are absent from the cell. Mycoplasma, for example, are resistant to benzyl penicillin G because they lack a cell wall.

Acquired Resistance

Acquired, genetically based resistance can arise because of chromosomal mutation or, more importantly, through the acquisition of genetic material. Chromosomal mutations tend to produce changes in bacterial cell structures, whereas plasmid-mediated resistance tends to encode synthesis of enzymes that modify antibiotics. Chromosomal resistance is often a gradual, stepwise process, whereas plasmid resistance is often high-level, all or none, resistance. Examples of important mechanisms of resistance are 1) enzymatic inactivation of antibiotics, 2) failure of bacterial permeability, 3) alteration in target receptors, 4) development of by-pass mechanisms in metabolic pathways, and 5) development of enzymes with low drug affinity.

Chromosomal Mutation to Resistance. Chromosomal mutation to resistance is generally a minor problem. Mutations to antibiotic resistance are spontaneous events involving changes in chromosomal DNA sequences uninfluenced by the presence of antibiotics. Such mutations often lead to other changes that leave the cell at a disadvantage so that, in the absence of antibiotic selection, these mutants may gradually be lost. Mutation to antibiotic resistance can be dramatic, as in the case of single-step mutation to streptomycin resistance where MIC increases a thousandfold, or gradual, as in the case of chromosomal resistance to penicillin where a series of mutational events may gradually increase the MIC of the organisms. These differences occur because when antibiotics affect one target site, chromosomal mutation is a single-step process, whereas when several targets are affected, mutation to resistance is a multistep process.

The rate of mutation differs for, and is characteristic of, each antibiotic. Sometimes antibiotics are used in combination to overcome the possibility of mutation to resistance — the chance of mutation to resistance to two antibiotics is the product of the chances of mutation for each antibiotic alone. In veterinary medicine, mutational resistance has limited the use of streptomycin, novobiocin, rifampin, and, to a lesser extent, erythromycin.

A chromosomal mutation resulting in multiple antibiotic resistance has been described for clinically relevant bacteria. The region involved, Mar (multiple antibiotic resistance) locus, controls efflux systems resulting in resistance to a variety of drugs without modification of the drugs.

Transferable Drug Resistance. Genetic exchange as a cause of antibiotic resistance is of major importance in veterinary medicine. Unlike chromosomal resistance, which occurs in individual bacteria, transfer of genetic material produces *epidemic* or *infectious* resistance, often to several antibiotics at one time and even, though rarely, in the absence of antibiotic selection. The extrachromosomal elements responsible for antibiotic resistance are plasmids that in this context were sometimes called *R factors* (or *R plasmids*). The plasmid DNA responsible for resistance can reproduce itself within a cell and spread to other cells by transformation, transduction, conjugation, or transposition.

Transformation. A clinically unimportant method of gene transfer in which naked DNA passes from one cell to another, altering the genotype of the recipient. Transposons may be transferred in this way (see below).

Transduction. A process by which plasmid DNA is incorporated by a bacterial virus and then transferred to another bacterium. An example is transfer of a beta-lactamase gene from penicillin resistant to susceptible staphylococci.

Conjugation. In this common process of gene transfer, a donor bacterium synthesizes a sex pilus, which attaches to a recipient bacterium in a mating process and transfers copies of plasmid genes to the recipients. The donor retains copies of the plasmid genes but the recipient has now become a potential donor. Conjugation can occur between species of the same genera but also across genera and families.

Transposition. Short DNA sequences known as *transposons* ("jumping genes") can transpose from plasmid to plasmid, plasmid to chromosome, or chromosome to plasmid. A transposon copy remains at the original site. The frequency of transposition is characteristic of the particular transposon and bacterium. The importance of transposition as the key element in resistance transfer is that transposition is independent of the recombination process of the bacterial cell — homology with the interacting DNA is not required. Plasmids from diverse sources possess identical antibiotic inactivating genes because of transposons.

Clinical Importance of Antimicrobial Drug Resistance

Acquired drug resistance has become a major problem in pathogenic bacteria of veterinary importance. It is common in many species, although some bacteria, particularly gram-positive bacteria such as many streptococci and corynebacteria, have remained highly susceptible to commonly used drugs. Acquired resistance to penicillins is frequent in *S. aureus*, and acquired multiple antibiotic resistance to many common antibiotics seriously limits their use in *Enterobacteriaceae* such as *Salmonella*, *E. coli*, and *Proteus*. Acquired resistance is increasingly observed in nonenteric bacteria such as *Pasteurella*, *Bordetella*, and *Haemophilus* and has been identified in virtually every pathogenic bacterial genus as well as in the normal flora.

There is a causal relationship between antimicrobial drug use and the development of resistance; given the nature of the genetic elements responsible, it is inevitable. The development of resistance has been well documented among enteric bacteria in veterinary medicine. The intestine is a major site of transfer of antibiotic resistance both because of the vast numbers of bacteria present and because of the opportunities for spread of these bacteria between intensively reared animals kept in close association with their manure. While the spread of drug resistance is not so well documented in individual companion animals such as horses and dogs, analogies to the situation on farms are useful in understanding how spread occurs.

Multiple drug resistance plasmids will be maintained in a population by the use of any antibiotic to which resistance is encoded by the plasmid genes. Thus the use of almost any antibiotic will tend to promote multiple resistance.

Intestinal *Escherichia coli*. Extensive study of antimicrobial resistance in intestinal *E. coli* in animals has provided information on the mechanisms and ecology of antimicrobial resistance. These studies have shown the relationship between the extent of resistance and the degree of antimicrobial use. For example, resistance in *E. coli* from adult ruminants is slight, whereas it is pronounced in intensively reared animals where antibiotic use is common. These *E. coli* may be resistant to up to 10 clinically useful drugs as a result of plasmid-mediated resistance. Among enterotoxigenic *E. coli* from farm animals, plasmid-mediated resistance to tetracyclines, sulfonamides, and streptomycin is now practically universal, and is increasingly common to ampicillin and neomycin. Antibiotic-resistance plasmids in enterotoxigenic *E. coli* in swine and calves may also include genes for virulence determinants such as toxin production or adhesins. Antibiotic use may thus potentially promote the transfer of virulence genes between bacteria.

Within the intestine, R plasmids are found in *E. coli* and in the more dominant anaerobic flora of the large bowel. Within a short time of treating an animal with an antibiotic, the *E. coli* and much of the anaerobe population become resistant to that antibiotic, principally because of selection of resistant strains but also because of transfer of R plasmids. In the absence of antibiotics, conditions in the large bowel seem to prevent the transfer of R factors. Short-term oral use of antibiotics is followed by high levels of *E. coli* resistance, which fall once the antibiotics are removed because the majority of R plasmid bearing *E. coli* are not good intestinal colonizers. However, the continuous presence of antibiotics is associated with extensive resistance, which persists long after the antibiotic is removed since resistant *E. coli* that are good intestinal colonizers have been selected.

Salmonella typhimurium. Multiple antibiotic resistance is a major problem in *S. typhimurium*. Among *S. typhimurium* strains, certain phage types are ready recipients of R plasmids; these strains may be resistant to six or more antibiotics. The extent of resistance is most marked among calf isolates because the extensive use of antibiotics in some types of calf rearing and the nature of salmonellosis in calves apparently provide an opportunity for the development and spread of resistant *Salmonella*. The progressive development of antibiotic resistance in a certain phage-typed strain of *S. typhimurium* in calves in Britain and its spread to cause human disease have been documented by Anderson (1968) and others. Like *E. coli*, acquisition of R plasmids by certain phage types of *S. typhimurium* may confer intestinal-colonizing abilities on the recipient and permit the spread of these clones.

Hospital-Acquired Resistant Infections

Acquired antimicrobial resistance in resident hospital bacteria is a major problem. There is a causal relationship between antibiotic use in hospitals and the development of resistance in bacteria. Colonization of patients by resistant opportunist bacteria is hard to prevent because of shared air spaces and environment, utensils, and medical and nursing staff.

PUBLIC HEALTH ASPECTS OF ANTIMICROBIAL RESISTANCE IN ANIMAL PATHOGENS

The use of antimicrobial agents in animals, particularly in intensively reared livestock, can result in antibiotic-resistant bacteria reaching the human population through a variety of routes. The extent of the contribution via these routes has not been determined. Most antibiotic resistance in human pathogens comes from antibiotic use in human medicine. However, antimicrobial-resistant bacteria of animal origin, such as *E. coli*, can colonize the intestines of people. Heavily exposed humans (farmers who use feed containing antibiotics, slaughterhouse workers, cooks and other food handlers) often have a higher incidence of resistant *E. coli* in their feces than the general population. Contamination of meat by intestinal bacteria at slaughter is extensive and an important route by which resistant bacteria reach people. While many of these bacteria are nonpathogenic, many pathogenic bacterial species from the intestines of animals cause zoonotic infections in humans (e.g., *Salmonella*, *Campylobacter jejuni*) and these infections may be harder to treat because of acquired resistance. The nonpathogenic bacteria of animals acquired by humans are a potential source of resistance plasmids for human pathogenic bacteria other than the zoonotic infections.

In the mid-1960s, the British government established a commission of inquiry to assess the dangers of antibiotic feed additives in animals in promoting resistance in human pathogens. This was launched because of 1) the outbreak of antibiotic-resistant *S. typhimurium* in calves in Britain and its subsequent appearance in human infections, 2) a chloramphenicol-resistant *Salmonella typhi* outbreak in Central America, 3) evidence of resistance in the *E. coli* of intensively reared chickens and pigs routinely fed antibiotics as growth promoters, and 4) the discovery of transmissible antibiotic resistance. The landmark 1968 Swann Report recommended that antibiotics used in human medicine (such as penicillin and tetracyclines) be withdrawn from unrestricted use as growth promoters in animals. Similar measures have been adopted in the European Economic Community and Japan.

In the United States and elsewhere, many antibiotics are incorporated into feed at low levels to promote growth, and the same antibiotics are used at higher concentrations for specified therapeutic and prophylactic purposes, without veterinary prescription. The Food and Drug Administration Report (1972) investigated the problems raised in the Swann Report and concluded that there was sufficient evidence to stop the use of subtherapeutic levels of penicillin and chlortetracycline, except under veterinary prescription. The proposal has not yet been accepted.

Control of Antibiotic Resistance

Avoiding the use of a drug is almost the only way to control antibiotic resistance. The phenomenon of multiple resistance-encoding R plasmids means, however, that continued use of one antibiotic for which there are resistance genes tends to maintain resistance for all antibiotics for which the R factor encodes. In human hospitals, reducing or eliminating the use of particular antibiotics has been followed by decreased resistance to these and sometimes to other antibiotics.

ANTIFUNGAL CHEMOTHERAPY

The susceptibility of fungi to different drugs is often, but not always, predictable. Fungal drug susceptibility testing is technically complex and simple methods paralleling the disk diffusion antibacterial susceptibility test are not generally available.

Antifungal Agents for Topical Use

Many chemicals have antifungal properties and are used for topical treatment of fungal infections of the skin and sometimes of the mucosal surfaces. These include phenolic antiseptics such as hexachlorophene; iodides; quaternary ammonium antiseptics; 8-hydroxyquinoline; salicylamide; propionic, salicylic, and undecanoic acids; and chlorphenesin. Among the more effective topical broad-spectrum antifungal drugs are natamycin (a polyene antibiotic), clotrimazole (an imidazole compound), nystatin (a polyene antibiotic), and ketoconazole and miconazole (see below).

Antifungal Agents for Systemic Use

The recent development of the imidazoles (ketoconazole, itraconazole, and fluconazole) has been a major advance in systemic fungal therapy because of their oral administration, relative lack of toxicity, and effectiveness. The earlier major antifungal drug for systemic use, amphotericin B, had the disadvantages of toxicity and requiring intravenous administration, but it did have the advantage of fungicidal activity.

Griseofulvin. Griseofulvin is a fungistatic antibiotic that inhibits mitosis and is active only against dermatophytes (ringworm fungi). Resistance in some dermatophytes has been reported to develop during treatment. Griseofulvin is effective against ringworm fungi only if administered orally. The drug is incorporated into keratin in the basal cells of the epidermis and reaches the superficial dead and parasitized keratinized epithelium through progressive maturation of the basal cells.

Amphotericin. Amphotericin B is a polyene antibiotic, like nystatin, which binds ergosterol, the principal sterol of the fungal membrane, causing leakage of the cell contents. It is a broad-spectrum, generally fungicidal antibiotic. It is active against *Blastomyces dermatitidis, Histoplasma capsulatum, Cryptococcus neoformans, Candida* spp., *Sporothrix schenckii*, and *Coccidioides immitis*. Strains of filamentous fungi, though commonly sensitive, vary from extreme susceptibility to resistance.

Amphotericin B must be administered intravenously. Renal toxicity is an inevitable side effect of such treatment and must be monitored; the effect is reversible if the drug is stopped. Amphotericin is the most important drug available for treating systemic mycoses caused by dimorphic fungi and by yeasts. Its prime place is increasingly being challenged by the imidazoles, which are less toxic and easier to administer. The drug is given by slow intravenous injection, usually every other day over 6 to 10 weeks.

Lipid formulations containing amphotericin B, though expensive, show great promise clinically because of lower kidney toxicity.

Flucytosine. 5-flucytosine is deaminated in the fungal cell to 5-fluorouracil, which is incorporated into messenger RNA to produce garbled codons and faulty proteins. It has a narrow spectrum of activity, which includes most *Cryptococcus neoformans* and many *Candida*, but most filamentous fungi are resistant. Resistance develops readily during treatment. Therefore, flucytosine is often used only in combination with other drugs, usually amphotericin.

Imidazoles: Ketoconazole, Miconazole, Itraconazole, Fluconazole. Imidazoles interfere with the biosynthesis of ergosterol and bind fungal cell membrane phospholipids to cause leakage of cell contents. Ketoconazole, miconazole, itraconazole, and fluconazole are fungistatic against a wide range of yeasts, dimorphic fungi, and dermatophytes; they also have some antibacterial and antiprotozoal activity. Ketoconazole, itraconazole, and fluconazole appear to be more active than miconazole and are the favored drugs for systemic administration because they can be given orally rather than intravenously. Ketoconazole, itraconazole, and fluconazole appear to produce few significant adverse effects in humans and animals, but liver damage has been reported in people given ketoconazole. They appear to be an effective treatment for many systemic fungal infections in dogs and cats, but there has been little experience with their use in other animal species. They have the disadvantage of fungistatic action; prolonged treatment may be necessary in serious infections to prevent the relapses that have occurred, and this is expensive.

ANTIVIRAL CHEMOTHERAPY

Antiviral Drugs

The development of nontoxic chemicals for therapeutic use in viral diseases is far more difficult than the development of antibacterial drugs, but the long-term prospects for antiviral chemotherapy in animals are encouraging. HIV infection in people has led to the development and introduction of antiviral drugs effective against retroviruses. Viral replication depends largely on the active participation of the metabolic pathways of the host cell, and the balance between preventing viral

Table 4.2.   Topical Antiviral Drugs Used in Humans; Potential Veterinary Use

Drug	Human Use	Potential (Unproven) Veterinary Use
Acyclovir	First genital herpes simplex infections in otherwise healthy people; limited mucocutaneous infections in immunocompromised patients	Local herpesvirus infections — bovine vulvovaginitis and keratoconjunctivitis, bovine herpes mammillitis; equine coital exanthema; feline rhinotracheitis virus — keratoconjunctivitis
Deoxy-D-glucose	Not approved — genital herpes	Local herpes infections
Iodoxuridine	Herpes simplex keratitis	Local herpes infections
Methisazone	Not used topically	Bovine vaccinia or pseudo-cowpox teat lesions
Phosphonoformate	Not approved — genital herpes	Local herpes infections
Ribavarin		Local herpes infections (not feline); vaccinia
Vidarabine		Local bovine herpes infections; vaccinia infection of cow teats

Table 4.3.   Systemic Antiviral Agents in Clinical Use and Experimental Drugs Under Investigation in Humans; Potential Veterinary Use

Drug	Human Use	Route of Administration	Possible Veterinary Use
Acyclovir	Systemic herpes infections — prophylaxis	Intravenous	Infectious bovine rhinotracheitis, feline rhinotracheitis; Aujesky's disease — prophylaxis
Amantadine	Influenza prophylaxis, treatment	Oral	Equine influenza prophylaxis
Deoxy-D-glucose	—	Intravenous	Bovine respiratory syncytial virus, parainfluenza virus — prophylaxis
Phosphonoformate	—	Intramuscular	As Acyclovir
Ribavarin	Experimental — influenza B	Oral	Influenza; parainfluenza; bovine herpes virus; bluetongue; rotavirus
Zidovudine	Immunodeficiency virus	Oral	Retroviral infections

replication and wrecking cellular metabolism is delicate. Only a relatively small number of useful drugs have been described, and their spectrum of antiviral activity is often narrow. Work has concentrated on selective drugs that use virally encoded enzymes either as specific targets for inhibition or to activate drugs within virally infected cells. Recently these have included many drugs preferentially phosphorylated by virus-specific thymidine kinase and further phosphorylated by cellular enzymes; the resulting triphosphates of these "second generation antiviral drugs" inhibit viral DNA polymerase, act as bogus substrates for this enzyme, or both.

Antiviral drugs are generally only effective prophylactically or in the early stages of disease when viral replication is occurring. Rapid diagnosis is therefore required. Although no antiviral drugs have been approved for veterinary use, Tables 4.2 and 4.3 summarize the potential of currently available medical antiviral compounds for topical and systemic use in animals. The desirable characteristics of veterinary antiviral compounds are broad-spectrum efficacy, low cost, ease of administration, and lack of drug residues. Few of the antiviral drugs available possess these characteristics, although some of the immunomodulators may have them.

SELECTED REFERENCES

Anderson ES. Drug resistance in *Salmonella typhimurium* and its implications. Br Med J 1968;3:333.

Barry AL. Antimicrobic susceptibility tests: principles and practice. Philadelphia: Lea and Febiger, 1976.

English RB, Prescott CN. Antimicrobial therapy in the dog. II. Some practical considerations. J Small Anim Pract 1983; 24:371.

George AM. Multidrug resistance in enteric and other gram-negative bacteria. FEMS Microbiol Lett 1996;139:1.

Hays VW. Biological basis for the use of antibiotics in livestock production. In: The use of drugs in animal feeds. Washington: National Academy of Sciences, 1969:11–30.

Joint Committee on the Use of Antibiotics in Animal Husbandry and Veterinary Medicine (Swann Report). London: Her Majesty's Stationery Office, 1969.

Jolly DW, Somerville JM, eds. Medicinal feed additives for livestock. London: Association of Veterinarians in Industry, 1975.

Linton AH. Has Swann failed? Vet Rec 1981;108:328.

Lorian V, ed. Antibiotics in laboratory medicine. Baltimore: Williams and Wilkins, 1991.

McGowan JE. Antimicrobial resistance in hospital organisms and its relation to antibiotic use. Rev Infect Dis 1983;5:1033.

Mercer HD. Antimicrobial drugs in food-producing animals. Control mechanisms of governmental agencies. Vet Clin North Am 1975;5:3.

National Committee for Clinical Laboratory Standards. Performance standards for antimicrobial disk and dilution susceptibility tests for bacteria isolated from animals: tentative standard. M31-T, volume 17, no. 11. Villanova, PA: NCCLS, 1997.

Prescott JF, Baggot JD. Antimicrobial therapy in veterinary medicine. Ames, IA: Iowa State University, 1994.

Smith HW. The transfer of antibiotic resistance between strains of *Enterobacteriaceae* in chickens, calves and pigs. J Med Microbiol 1970;3:165.

Storm G, van Etten E. Biopharmaceutical aspects of lipid formulations of amphotericin B. Eur J Clin Microbiol Infect Dis 1997;16:64.

Timoney JE, Linton AH. Experimental ecological studies on H2 plasmids in the intestine and feces of the calf. J Appl Bacteriol 1982;52:417.

U.S. Food and Drug Administration. The hazard of using chloramphenicol in food animals. J Am Vet Med Assoc 1984;184:930.

Woolcock JB, Mutimer MD. Antibiotic susceptibility testing: *Caeci caecos* ducentes? Vet Rec 1983;113:125.

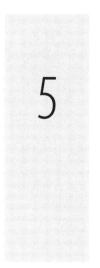

5

Antimicrobial Drugs: A Strategy for Rational Use and the Ramifications of Misuse

Dwight C. Hirsh

Antimicrobial drugs are used to treat (therapeutic) or prevent (prophylactic) disease produced by infectious bacterial agents. Most of the discussion that follows will deal with therapeutic use of these drugs, though comment will be made regarding prophylactic use when appropriate. Further, the discussion will deal with bacterial agents.

STRATEGY FOR RATIONAL USE

The decision to use antimicrobial drugs therapeutically involves the determination of whether there is an infectious agent present. Some consideration (though this rarely occurs) should be given to whether the infectious process actually poses a threat of sufficient seriousness to outweigh the risks of treatment (discussed below) and whether the infectious process will resolve without the use of this class of drug. The same comment should be made about prophylactic use: consideration should be given to whether there is an unacceptably high prevalence of infectious complications following a certain procedure to justify their use.

Central to the decision to use antimicrobial drugs is the demonstration that an infectious agent is part of the disease process under consideration. The gold standard for this determination, of course, is the results of microbiological culture. Strict application of this standard is unrealistic, however, because the decisions to use antimicrobial drugs are made several days before culture data are available. Therefore, as an aid in determining that a particular process has an infectious component, certain clues are used. The Infection Control Committee at the Veterinary Medical Teaching Hospital, University of California, has drawn up guidelines to be used as aids in the decision-making process (Table 5.1). Though these guidelines help "rule in" or "rule out" an infectious component, there is no stronger proof than the demonstration that an infectious agent is present.

The following scheme is used to justify the therapeutic use of an antimicrobial drug *the day the patient is first seen*. The whole purpose of the exercise is to answer the following questions: Is there an infectious agent present? What is the best antimicrobial drug to use?

Is There an Infectious Agent Present?

Apart from having the results of bacteriologic culture in hand, this question can be answered by experience (e.g., all similar cases have had an infectious component) or microbiologically. It is the microbiological aspect of the decision process that will be the focus of the discussion here. Unless noted otherwise, all subsequent remarks will be focused on infectious processes involving normally sterile (or nearly sterile) sites.

One of the most rewarding methods that can be used to determine the presence or absence of an infectious agent is the direct smear (see Chapter 3). Examination of a direct smear answers two very important questions: Is there an infectious agent present? And, if so, what is the agent likely to be? Answers to both of these questions help justify the use of an antimicrobial agent, and, what is equally important, help determine which one is likely to be effective.

After it has been demonstrated that an infectious agent is present, i.e., microorganisms are seen in the direct smear, the next step in the process is to make an educated guess as to their identity. This is the most important step in the process in the rational use of antimicrobial drugs — to have in mind what it is you are going to be treating. Experience and retrospective data are keys to this determination, and allow the clinician to formulate a "microbiological differential list" with the proper hierarchy. By noting the shape of the microorganisms seen in the direct smear, certain members of the differential list can be "ruled in" or "ruled out." Generally, bacteria come in two shapes: rods and cocci. Filamentous forms (*Actinomyces*, *Nocardia*) are treated as a separate category. Of course, if no infectious agents are seen but other clues point to infectious process, a microbiological differential list is still constructed, but it will be more difficult to "rule in" or "rule out" certain microorganisms or groups of microorganisms because of the lack of visual clues.

More sophisticated methods involve the detection of prokaryotic (bacterial) DNA in a normally sterile site. A

Table 5.1. Guidelines for Rational Use of Antimicrobial Agents

1. Demonstration of an infectious agent

or

2. Clinical data (at least two of the following)
   a. Fever
   b. Leukocytosis
   c. Localized inflammation
   d. Components of the sample
   e. Radiographic evidence
   f. Elevated serum fibrinogen

polymerase chain reaction (PCR) that uses universal primers for prokaryotic DNA allows for this determination. The disadvantage to such a determination is the lack of an "isolate" to identify and to test for susceptibility to antimicrobial agents.

Observation of bacteria in a direct smear may seem to result in the formulation of a microbiological differential list of endless possibilities. Experience and retrospective data allow for the paring down of the list, keeping only the most common in proper hierarchical order. For example, in samples from dogs, *Bordetella* is almost never found except from the respiratory tract, and here it is not commonly found in samples obtained from the lower tract of patients with clinical signs of pneumonia. Likewise, in samples from dogs, *Pseudomonas* is hardly ever found in locations other than the external ear or the lower urinary tract. *Bordetella* or *Pseudomonas* would be very unlikely candidates to explain the presence of rod-shaped bacteria in a sample of exudate from the peritoneal cavity of a dog. Aside from "common microbiological sense," there are other clues that are helpful. For example, misshapen or long, slender rods are almost always members of the anaerobe group (especially if seen in malodorous fluid obtained from a normally sterile site).

Alimentary Canal — A Special Case. Seeing a microorganism in a normally sterile site does not pose much of a problem in determining whether there is an infectious process present. Infectious diseases of normally contaminated sites (mouth, vagina, gastrointestinal canal), however, can pose special problems. The alimentary canal is the only contaminated site where the direct smear can help determine whether there is an infectious bacterial disease. There are three conditions in which direct smear can aid in the diagnosis and treatment: 1) diarrhea associated with *Campylobacter*, 2) *Helicobacter*-associated conditions of stomach and intestinal canal, and 3) *Serpulina*-associated diseases. In the first condition, the observation in stained smears (e.g., Wright-Giemsa) of curved rods, in the second, the observation of helical-shaped rods, and in the third, the observation of spirochetal shapes suggest that an infectious agent may be associated with the abnormal signs observed. In all three instances, the presence of a microorganism with a unique characteristic

gives the visual clue necessary to make an educated guess as to the etiology of the abnormal signs. More sophisticated techniques (PCR) have been shown to be useful in determining the presence of *Clostridium difficile* or the genes encoding its toxins.

What Is the Best Antimicrobial Agent to Use?

If an infectious agent is observed in the direct smear, the answer to the first question posed above has been answered. If none is seen, yet the other clues are present that point to an infectious process (see Table 5.1), the first question has also been answered in the affirmative. The next step in the decision-making process is to ask what antimicrobial drug should be used. To answer this question, it is important to have in mind the "microbiological target." Depending upon the site from which the sample was obtained and what was seen in the direct smear, an educated guess is made as to the identity of the agent(s) involved. Retrospective data should be used to suggest what antimicrobial agents would be effective for the microorganisms on the microbiological differential list. Then, depending upon distribution, toxicity, and expense, a final choice is made.

The next day, the microbiology laboratory should be able to furnish information that is useful in determining the appropriateness of first-day choice of antimicrobial agent(s). It can, for instance, tell you whether a rod-shaped bacteria seen in direct smear is a member of the enteric group, which is an extremely important piece of information since members of this group are unpredictable with respect to susceptibility patterns (due to the propensity of this group of microorganisms to possess R plasmids, see Chapter 4 and below) and, as a consequence, more expensive and more toxic antimicrobial drugs are used if their presence is likely.

Obligate anaerobic bacteria pose a special challenge. It is important to be led to suspect their presence early because the methods used to confirm them are lengthy; and, just as importantly, most laboratories do not perform susceptibility tests on them. Even if they did, the results would not be available for about a week after sample submission. There are, however, some clues that help determine whether members of this group are present. A major clue is odor. If an exudate or fluid smells fetid, there is a good chance that obligate anaerobes are present. Without smell, an educated guess can also be made as to their presence depending upon the site from which the sample was obtained and the shape of the microorganism (misshapen, slender rods).

RAMIFICATIONS OF MISUSE OF ANTIMICROBIAL AGENTS

In addition to obvious benefits derived from antimicrobial agents, there are risks involved with their use. These risks involve the patient as well as others that share the same environment, including ourselves. The risks concern resistance to antimicrobial agents.

Resistance

In general, there are two mechanisms whereby bacteria become resistant. They can change the target of the antimicrobial drug by mutation, a random event unrelated to the presence of the drug. Clinically relevant mutation to resistance is unusual in microorganisms isolated from veterinary sources. However, it has been recently shown that a mutation in a chromosomal gene encoding a particular transcriptional activator residing in the Mar (multiple antibiotic resistance) locus resulted in multiple drug resistance. The mechanism for this phenomenon appears to be a deregulation of control of chromosomal genes governing the flux of drugs across the bacterial cell wall. Thus, the "multidrug resistance" phenotype is due to changes in the transport systems of the cell wall, leading to resistance to just about any clinically useful antibiotic (e.g., quinolones, beta-lactams, tetracyclines, and chloramphenicol). Drugs are pumped out of the bacterial cell before they reach therapeutically useful concentrations. This phenotype has been described for *Escherichia coli*, *Salmonella*, *Pseudomonas aeruginosa*, *Proteus vulgaris*, *Klebsiella*, and *Campylobacter*.

The major way in which bacteria become resistant is through the acquisition of DNA that encodes resistance to antimicrobial drugs. These genes may contain the information for enzymes that inactivate certain antimicrobials by acetylation or phosphorylation (aminoglycoside and chloramphenicol modifying enzymes), for enzymes that inactivate by breaking bonds (beta-lactamases and cephalosporinases that inactivate penicillin/ampicillin and cephalosporins, respectively), for proteins that are involved with transport of an antimicrobial (tetracyclines), or they may encode a target protein different from the native (susceptible) one (a different tetrahydrofolate reductase is responsible for trimethoprim resistance).

DNA encoding these various enzymes can be acquired by bacteria in several ways: 1) they can take up DNA from their environment (called *transformation*); 2) they may become "infected" by a bacterial virus that contains the resistance genes the virus had acquired from a previously resistant bacterial host (called *transduction*); or 3) they can "receive" it from other bacteria by a sexual process (called *conjugation*). Although there are examples of each of these occurring in nature, the most common method of DNA acquisition is through conjugation, at least for the acquisition of resistance genes by bacteria in an environment containing antimicrobial drugs.

Acquired DNA usually exists within the bacterial cell separate from the chromosome (extrachromosomally). This extrachromosomal DNA is called a *plasmid*. If the plasmid contains genes encoding resistance to antimicrobial drugs, then these plasmids are called *R plasmids*. R plasmids may encode information for conjugation, and if so, such plasmids are transmissible and therefore have the capacity to move from one bacterium to another, either within a family (e.g., *E. coli* to *E. coli*, or *E. coli* to *Salmonella*) or outside of a family (e.g., *E. coli* to *Pasteurella*). This transmissibility has been noted for gram-positive and gram-negative bacteria, for obligate aerobes, and for facultative and obligate anaerobes. It appears to be most clinically relevant among members of the family *Enterobacteriaceae* (e.g., *E. coli*, *Salmonella*, *Klebsiella*).

A particular bacterium may contain a number of different plasmids, several of which may be R plasmids. The number of resistance genes encoded on a plasmid is variable, from two (which seems to be about the minimum) to more than seven. The genes encoding resistance to all of the commonly used antimicrobial drugs are found on plasmid DNA. The exceptions are resistance to the quinolones, the polymyxins, and metronidazole. The consequence of this is that after conjugation, a susceptible strain of bacteria may have acquired resistance to a number of antimicrobial agents and have the potential to pass these resistance genes on to yet another, while keeping a copy for itself.

In addition to being mobile by means of conjugation, resistance genes are mobile in their own right. Mobile genes, called *transposable genetic elements* or *transposons*, move from one piece of DNA to another. Most often, the information encoding resistance to a particular antimicrobial agent is on a transposon. The importance of this is that, in the hospital environment where bacteria are exposed to a number of different antimicrobial agents (and by definition they will have acquired the gene necessary to cope with *each* of these antimicrobials), the genetic pool of resistance genes is very large. And since the genes themselves are mobile, they would have the tendency to insert themselves on any number of plasmids, forming plasmids with many and varied resistance genes. Bacteria containing such R plasmids would be extremely difficult to kill or suppress with antimicrobial drugs if they were to become involved with a disease process.

R plasmids seem to be common among the enteric group. It is extremely difficult, therefore, to predict which resistance genes will be present, especially if the R plasmid has been "constructed" from the resistance gene pool in a hospital environment. For this reason, a major effort should be made in "ruling out" or "ruling in" members of this group on the microbiological differential list for a particular site or condition.

Within 24 to 48 hours after the initiation of antimicrobial therapy, dramatic changes occur in one of the major host defense systems of the patient, the normal flora. These changes are reflected in the replacement of the normal flora with bacteria resistant to the antimicrobial drug being used. To understand why this is a risk, it is important to understand the role of the normal flora as a host defense barrier.

The Risk

Colonization resistance (see Chapter 2) is a term that describes the innate immunity afforded the host by its normal flora. It is the normal flora and the mechanisms whereby the normal flora is maintained that protect the host from colonization (infection) by extraneous microorganisms. This is an important concept since prevention of colonization by agents with pathogenic potential (e.g., *Salmonella*) or prevention of colonization by resistant strains of microorganisms is key to minimizing the risk we and our patients take in living in an environment contaminated by microorganisms.

Colonization resistance can be decreased by a number of outside influences, principally stress, and by antimicrobial agents. If the colonization resistance is decreased sufficiently, then replacement will occur (a surface does not go unoccupied!).

Antimicrobial agents decrease colonization resistance. Hospitalized dogs were 38 times more likely to have acquired resistant *Salmonella* if they were first given an antibiotic. Within 24 to 48 hours after administration of an antimicrobial, the normal flora is depressed to the degree that resistant strains start to recolonize since those microorganisms that replace the normal flora will be resistant to the antimicrobial drug administered. These resistant strains may be a part of the normal flora (e.g., normal, unmedicated dogs shed large numbers of R plasmid containing *E. coli* in their feces) or from the animal's environment. In either case, the replacement strain will be resistant to the antimicrobial being used. Having resistant bacteria occupying a surface is not harmful in itself, unless the resistant strain has the ability to invade the host cell to which it has gained access. But as mentioned above, if a normally sterile site contiguous to the recolonized surface becomes compromised, bacteria (now resistant bacteria) will contaminate, and the resulting disease will be more difficult to treat. This recolonization effect is the reason behind the recommendation that prophylactic use of antimicrobial agents extend no longer than 24 to 48 hours.

Colonization resistance is reduced by the stress of illness and the stress of new social/environmental experiences. These changes occur secondary to changes in the normal flora. What appears to transpire are changes in the elements responsible for the maintenance of the stable, normal flora. Although these changes have been defined most precisely in the oral cavity, there are data that suggest that they also occur in the intestinal canal as well. In the oral cavity, the epithelial cells are coated with fibronectin, a glycoprotein. Fibronectin contains receptors for streptococci, the most abundant microorganism found on the buccal, lingual, and gingival surfaces. It is the streptococci that exclude other, potentially more dangerous microbes from associating with the oral cavity (most would agree that these would be microorganisms belonging to the enteric group such as *E. coli* or *Klebsiella*). The amount of fibronectin coating these cells decreases in the stressed animal, leaving available underlying attachment sites (for gram-negative microorganisms) either on the cells themselves or on glycoproteins that coat the cells after fibronectin is gone. It should be noted, too, that if the animal is treated with antimicrobials as well, the streptococci will also be removed since the oral streptococci are very susceptible to most antimicrobial agents. There is recent evidence that shows that some gram-negative enteric bacteria possess adhesins for receptors on fibronectin, underscoring the importance of keeping the normal flora intact. The resulting change from a flora composed of relatively innocuous bacteria

(nonhemolytic streptococci) to one with pathogenic potential (members of the enteric group) becomes an important issue if compromise occurs in a normally sterile contiguous site (e.g., the lung).

Risk to Others

Antimicrobial agents select bacteria that contain genes encoding resistance to that particular drug. Because the genes encoding resistance are almost always found on R plasmid DNA, antimicrobial use selects for resistance genes to other antibiotics as well. In the hospital environment where antimicrobials are used, the environment is contaminated with microorganisms containing very mobile genetic material encoding resistance to a variety of antimicrobial agents. We are a part of this environment, and therefore also partake in this gene pool. Even with an intact colonization resistance, we are transiently colonized with bacteria derived from animals placed in our care. Transient colonization is enough for conjugation and subsequent passage of resistance genes to our resident normal flora. If by chance the host human is also being medicated with antimicrobials, the chance of colonization with resistant animal strains increases, as does the possibility of passage of an R plasmid.

SUMMARY

In outlining the rational use of antimicrobial agents, this chapter emphasizes the importance of two questions: Is there an infectious component to the disease process under consideration? And, if so, what antimicrobial drug would be effective? The direct smear is a tool that is useful in ascertaining whether an infectious component exists. Once it has been reasonably established that there is an infectious component, a "microbiological differential list" (in hierarchical order) is created and further shaped depending upon visual clues obtained from the direct smear. Experience and retrospective susceptibility data are used to determine which antimicrobial drugs would be effective for the most likely of the constituents of the microbiological differential list. A final choice is made after considering distribution, toxicity, and cost.

Antimicrobial drugs should be treated as an environmental pollutant. They exert very powerful selective pressures on the gene pool in which we all partake. In addition to being potent selective agents, antimicrobials are a risk to those patients receiving them by diminishing host defense barriers.

SELECTED REFERENCES

Alekshun MN, Levy SB. Regulation of chromosomally mediated multiple antibiotic resistance: the mar regulon. Antimicrob Agents Chemother 1997;41:2067.

Dalton HP, Muhovich M, Escobar MR, Allison MJ. Pulmonary infection due to disruption of the pharyngeal bacterial flora by antibiotics in hamsters. Am J Pathol 1974;76:469.

Falkow S. Infectious multiple drug resistance. London: Pion, 1975.

George AM. Multidrug resistance in enteric and other gram-negative bacteria. FEMS Microbiol Lett 1996;139:1.

Hirsh DC, Burton GC, Blenden DC. The effect of tetracycline upon establishment of *Escherichia coli* of bovine origin in the enteric tract of man. J Appl Bacteriol 1974;37:327.

Hirsh DC, Ling GV, Ruby AL. Incidence of R-plasmids in fecal flora of healthy household dogs. Antimicrob Agents Chemother 1980;17:313.

Hirsh DC, Ruehl WW. Clinical microbiology as a guide to the treatment of infectious bacterial diseases of the dog and the cat. In: Scott FW, ed. Contemporary issues in small animal practice: infectious diseases. New York: Churchill Livingston, 1986:1–28.

Johanson WG. Prevention of respiratory tract infection. Am J Med 1984;15:69.

Levy SB. The antibiotic paradox. New York: Plenum, 1992.

Ling GV. Lower urinary disease of dogs and cats. St. Louis: Mosby, 1995.

MacLean LD. Host resistance in surgical patients. J Trauma 1979;19:297.

Marsh P, Martin M. Oral microbiology. In: Cole JA, Knowles CJ, Schlessinger D, eds. Aspects of microbiology. Washington: American Society for Microbiology, 1984.

Owen RH, Fullerton J, Barnum DA. Effects of transportation, surgery, and antibiotic therapy in ponies infected with *Salmonella*. Am J Vet Res 1983;44:46.

Pietsch JB, Meakins JL. Predicting infection in surgical patients. Surg Clin North Am 1979;59:185.

Tannic GW, Savage DC. Influences of dietary and environmental stress on microbial populations in the murine gastrointestinal tract. Infect Immun 1974;9:591.

Uhaa IJ, Hird DW, Hirsh DC, Jang SS. Case-control study of risk factors associated with nosocomial *Salmonella krefeld* infection in dogs. Am J Vet Res 1988;49:1501.

van der Waaij D. Antibiotic of choice: the importance of colonization resistance. Letchworth, UK: Research Studies, 1983.

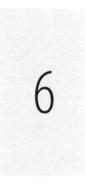

6   *Vaccines*

Yuan Chung Zee   Dwight C. Hirsh

INTRODUCTION

Vaccines are substances that are used to elicit immune responses to prevent or minimize disease produced by infectious agents. Vaccines can be composed of the infectious agent itself (either live or killed) and/or a product of the agent. Products containing a killed bacterial agent are more properly called *bacterins*. Products that have toxic activities are called *toxins*, and toxins that have been inactivated are called *toxoids*.

To be effective, vaccines must elicit an immune response that interferes with the "life style" of the infectious agent.

Humoral Immunity

Antibodies function immunologically by binding to epitopes on the surface of the infectious agent and/or one of its products. By binding to the surface of an infectious agent, antibodies interfere with attachment to host target cells by stearic interference and/or by changing the charge or hydrophobicity of the surface of the agent; interfere with viral attachment; and trigger the complement cascade generating products that are opsonic and products that are damaging to agents that have surface membranes. Antibodies that bind to products of infectious agents can block the attachment of the product to receptors on cellular targets and/or change the configuration of the product resulting in a change in binding affinity.

Cell-Mediated Immunity

Cell-mediated immunity is an immune response that results in the generation of "activated" macrophages and/or specific cytotoxic T lymphocytes. This aspect of the immune response concerns agents that live inside of cells, which are thus protected from interaction with the elements of the humoral components of the system.

Activated macrophages are mononuclear phagocytic cells that have come in contact with IL-1 and gamma interferon (INF-gamma). Such cells have increased phagocytic and enzymatic activity, contain increased amounts of nitric oxide, and have increased production of TNF, increased expression of IL-1, and increased expression of MHC-II. This increase in activity is thought to be responsible for the destruction of infectious agents that non-activated mononuclear cells cannot destroy following uptake. Some term this immune state (i.e., activation of macrophages) *cellular hypersensitivity.*

Cytotoxic T lymphocytes recognize affected host cells (e.g., cells infected with virus or bacteria). In so doing, these lymphocytes secrete substances that result in the death of the affected host cell. If the affected host cell contained an infectious agent, that agent would now be liberated and in contact with other host immune participants (e.g., antibody, complement, activated macrophages).

Generation of the Immune Response

Antibodies are elicited by antigens that are processed by antigen-processing cells via the exogenous pathway. Thus, extracelluar bacteria (live or killed), inactivated viral particles, pieces of virus, and products are processed by the exogenous pathway. Epitopes are presented to the immune system in context of MHC-II by an antigen-presenting cell that secretes IL-1 and little, if any, IL-12. T helper cells (T_{H2} subset of CD4$^+$ lymphocytes) respond to this stimulus by secreting cytokines that trigger an antibody response (IL-2, IL-4, IL-5, IL-6).

Some infectious agents replicate within cells. If the agent multiplies within a mononuclear phagocyte, then antigens are processed by way of the exogenous and/or endogenous pathways and epitopes are presented in context of MHC-II (antigen processed by exogenous pathway), but the antigen-presenting cell secretes IL-1 and IL-12. IL-12 stimulates T helper cells (T_{H1} subset) while turning off T_{H2} subset of T helper cells. T_{H1} cells secrete INF-gamma, resulting in the activation of mononuclear phagocytic cells. Some of these "intracellular" agents (some viruses, bacteria, fungi) replicate in the cytoplasm of mononuclear phagocytic cells. Antigens from these agents are processed by the endogenous pathway, as are antigens liberated within nonphagocytic cells, so that epitopes are presented to the immune system in context of MHC-I. Epitopes presented in this fashion are recognized by CD8$^+$ cytotoxic lymphocytes. These lymphocytes function by lysing infected targets, i.e., cells expressing epitope-MHC-I complexes.

To briefly summarize the generation of the immune response, the antigen is processed so that epitopes are complexed with MHC-II determinants. This means that antigen must be processed (by the exogenous pathway) by antigen-processing cells that express MHC-II determinants, i.e., macrophages (mononuclear phagocytic cells), B lymphocytes.

In order to generate activated macrophages, the antigen must not only be processed so that epitopes are complexed with MHC-II determinants, but also replicate within the antigen-processing cell.

In order to generate specific cytotoxic T lymphocytes, the antigen must be processed by the endogenous pathway. To enter the pathway the antigen must find its way into the cytoplasm of the affected cell. The easiest way to accomplish this is to escape the endosome. To achieve this, the infectious agent must be alive.

DNA VACCINES

DNA vaccines are those in which the gene encoding the antigen in question is inserted into a plasmid vector that has a strong promotor (e.g., cytomegalovirus immediate/early promotor; SV40 early promotor) that will result in expression of the target gene. The construct is injected intramuscularly. Myocytes that become transfected serve as antigen-presenting cells and express antigen in context of MHC-I (turn on CD8$^+$ T lymphocytes). It is unclear how antigen is expressed in context of MHC-II (for CD4$^+$ T lymphocytes). Possibilities include MHC-II antigen-presenting cells (macrophages/B lymphocytes) becoming transfected, or transfected myocytes transfering the plasmid construct to MHC-II antigen-presenting cells.

DNA vaccines have been successful in eliciting protective immune responses (both humoral and cellular) to a variety of bacterial, viral, and protozoal microorganisms.

ADJUVANTS

Adjuvants are used to influence the nature of the immune response elicited by an antigen. The response is influenced at various stages, depending upon the adjuvant. Some adjuvants function as depots, so that antigen is slowly released over an extended period of time to maximize the immune response. Examples include water/oil emulsions, minerals/salts (bentonite, aluminum), and inert particles (microspheres). Other adjuvants direct activity to the processing step in the initiation of the immune response. Examples include "immune stimulating complexes" (ISCOMs) composed of cholesterol-phospholipid structures that contain the immunogen, and liposomes (lipid vesicles). Immune responses can be influenced by "targeting" various components using various cytokines as adjuvants. For example, IL-1 activates T lymphocytes; IL-12 and INF-gamma influence the helper T lymphocyte subset selection; and granulocyte macrophage colony-stimulating factors activate macrophages and increase efficiency of antigen processing.

VIRAL VACCINES

Immunization of animals with viral vaccines is of utmost importance in prophylactic veterinary medicine. The basis of an effective vaccine is its ability to induce an immune response or responses capable of eliciting protection to subsequent field exposure to pathogenic organisms. A multitude of vaccine preparations have been developed and used over the years, with variable rates of success. The success of a potential vaccine hinges primarily on safety and efficacy; however, economics will play a pivotal role in vaccine design, development, and ultimate production on a commercial basis.

Various approaches have been employed over the years in vaccine development. These include 1) administering live virulent virus in an anatomical site so that the target tissue or tissues are not infected, 2) administering live virulent virus to animals at a time of relatively strong resistance to disease expression, 3) concurrent administration of live virulent virus and immune serum, 4) use of live avirulent viral strains (e.g., attenuated viruses), and 5) use of inactivated virus. In recent years, additional approaches to vaccine development have been employed. These include subunit, synthetic peptide, and recombinant products. Regardless of vaccine type, the desired result is to induce immune responses specific for viral antigens expressed on the virion surface or on the surface of infected cells, so that clinical disease is averted upon exposure to virulent virus. The rational development of an efficacious viral vaccine requires an understanding of viral pathogenesis, of protective immune responses induced following infection, and of their protein specificities. The latter point is of obvious importance for developing recombinant and synthetic peptide vaccines.

Concerning pathogenesis, the following three general types of viral infections occur:

1. Viral attachment and replication may be confined to the mucosal surfaces of the respiratory or gastrointestinal tracts. In such instances, local immunity in the form of secretory antibody (e.g., IgA) is important. The role of cell-mediated immunity (CMI) is uncertain in such infections.
2. Other viruses gain entry by similar routes but may also cause a viremia with subsequent infection of local or distant target tissue or tissues. In such cases, two lines of defense can come into play: immunity at the mucosal surface and systemic immunity.
3. Many viruses gain direct entry into the host's circulation via insect bite (arthropod-borne viruses), inadvertent inoculation, or a traumatic break in an epithelial surface. In such infections, systemic immunity is the primary line of defense.

These mechanisms of viral infection and subsequent dissemination should be considered in vaccine development and in determining route of administration.

Our discussion of viral vaccine types focuses on live virus with attenuated virulence and on inactivated virus

Table 6.1. Types of Viral Vaccines

I. Live Viral Vaccines
   A. Attenuation for low virulence of viruses that produce natural diseases.
   B. Host-range mutants — use of different viral strains infecting different host species that are related antigenically to the virus strain that produces a natural disease in the original host.
   C. Recombinant heterologous viral vector vaccines — construction of an infectious viral recombinant that expresses protective antigen(s) of another virus that produces a natural disease. Construction of a recombinant virus with insertion of genes with known antiviral activities or with known immunoregulatory functions.
   D. Recombinant homologous viral strains attenuated by targeted mutations on deletions of genes coding for specific virulence factors that produce a natural disease.
   E. Nonreplicating recombinant viral vector vaccines capable of replicating to high titer in vitro but unable to grow efficiently in vivo.

II. Inactivated Viral Vaccines
   A. Inactivated viral vaccines by chemical methods.
   B. Inactivated viral vaccines by physical methods.
   C. Purified viral antigens using monoclonal antibody immunoaffinity chromatography.
   D. Cloned viral protein subunit vaccines produced in eukaryotic or prokaryotic cells by recombinant DNA technology.
   E. Synthetic viral polypeptide vaccines representing immunologically urpident domains of viral surface antigens.
   F. Direct injection of plasmid DNA encoding viral protective antigens into tissues in vivo.
   G. Use of anti-idiotypic antibodies as antigens to induce an antiviral antibody response.

(Table 6.1). But before we begin this discussion, brief mention of additional approaches to vaccination is warranted. Concomitant administration of live virulent virus and immune serum has been practiced in the past, although it is no longer an acceptable approach. Many viruses exhibit age-dependent virulence characteristics. That is to say, at some ages, viral exposure leads to clinical disease, but at other times susceptibility to disease is negligible. Thus, there is a time period in which the animals can be immunized with live virulent virus. Intentional exposure of mature females, who are resistant to clinical disease due to age, prior to breeding may ensure the developing (avian) embryo or newborn the protection of maternal antibody. Another approach to the use of virulent virus is inoculation of an anatomical site that is isolated from the target tissue, thus inducing immunity without the risk of disease. This practice requires that the virus be strictly confined to a local infection.

Live Attenuated Viral Vaccines

The attenuated viral vaccines include artificially attenuated (modified-live) viral vaccines and naturally occurring viruses with reduced virulence for a given host. Viral isolates with reduced or no virulence have been used as vaccine material. The origin of such fortuitous isolates may be the natural host. Another source of vaccine may be a closely related virus isolated from a different host; for example, the cowpox virus was initially used to vaccinate humans against smallpox. The major requirements of such an approach are that it induce adequate immunity and that the viral avirulence be stable. The majority of vaccines currently used today in veterinary medicine are attenuated viruses. The most common approach to viral attenuation is the development of host-range mutants. Other approaches include development of temperature-sensitive and cold-adapted mutants (missense mutations), deletion mutants, and recombinant viruses (virulent X avirulence).

Host-range mutants are developed by serial passage in a host system different from the natural host to be vaccinated. Such attenuation of virulence for a given host has been routinely conducted in laboratory animals, embryonated chicken eggs, and cell cultures; the latter is gaining in popularity. Upon serial passage in such a system, the virus loses virulence for the natural host due to accumulation of missense or base substitution mutations in the viral genome that are expressed as alterations in virus-specified proteins. The basis of such attenuation is uncertain.

Conditional lethal mutants have been generated with the intent that such viruses would exhibit limited replication in the host and serve as potential vaccines. Temperature-sensitive mutants are typically created by mutagenesis and phenotypically selected on the basis of temperature. Cold-adapted mutants are generated by propagation at successively lower temperatures, the end product being incapable of replication at normal temperatures. The cold-adapted mutants typically acquire multiple mutations in genes encoding virulence and are relatively more stable than temperature-sensitive mutants.

A unique approach to expression of cloned viral genes is the use of heterologous viral expression vectors. Vaccinia virus, as an infectious vaccine expression vector, has received the most attention to date due to absence of clinical disease in animal species and the fact that at least 22 kilobases of the vaccinia genome can be deleted without loss of infectivity. The latter attribute gives researchers ample space in which to insert foreign cloned genes and has the potential to permit insertion of multiple foreign viral genes for the purpose of designing multivalent and multiviral vaccines. A major advantage of such infectious vaccine vectors is the potential for induction of CMI by inserting expressed viral proteins into the host cell membrane in context with histocompatibility antigens.

Construction of deletion mutants is another potential mechanism of virus attenuation. Theoretically, this process could be used to selectively delete genes that express factors for virulence, persistence, or immunosuppression without compromising viral replication. Realizing such an approach will require extensive information on protein function and mapping of their coding regions within the viral genome. In the light of unlimited possibilities for vaccine development, mention should be made of the newly approved pseudorabies vaccines produced by gene deletion. The thymidine kinase gene is deleted in the pseudorabies vaccine strain, which is able to induce an immune response without producing disease. Furthermore, the genes coding for virus glycoproteins gpI, gpIII, or gpx are deleted in the vaccine strain. The presence of antibody to these specific virus antigens can be used to differentiate field-strain infected animals from vaccinated animals, an immense advance in the epidemiology and control of viral disease.

The use of genetic recombination of genome segment reassortment is a potential approach to developing vaccines for viruses expressing antigenic drift. Theoretically, a standard attenuated virus could be crossed with new viral variants; avirulent virus carrying genetic information from the field virus that codes for proteins critical in induction of immunity could be subsequently selected.

Nonreplicating recombinant viral vectors that are not capable of multiplication in vivo but that can express foreign proteins during the abortive infectious stage have been shown to induce humoral and cell-mediated immunity in recipient hosts. Experimental studies show that dogs or cats are resistant to wild-type rabies viral challenge when inoculated with avian pox-rabies glycoprotein recombinant viruses. This type of viral vaccine has the distinct advantage of being safe in the immunosuppressed host.

There are advantages and disadvantages to attenuated viral vaccines. Table 6.2 illustrates such general characteristics as compared to killed viral vaccines. A major advantage of live viral vaccines is their ability to replicate within the host and thereby elicit both humoral and cellular immune responses. In the case of viral infections attaching primarily to the mucosal surfaces of the respiratory and gastrointestinal tracts, administering attenuated viruses by the nasal or oral routes provides a good stimulus of local immunity. Economic considerations also favor attenuated vaccines due to the moderate cost of production and the typical absence of a requirement for adjuvants, immunopotentiating agents, and multiple booster doses.

While attenuated viral vaccines continue to provide valuable prophylactic measures for veterinary medicine, certain disadvantages are associated with their use, some of which are proven while others remain speculative. The development of attenuated vaccines can prove to be a tedious process, and a fine line separates modification and loss of immunogenicity. Many viruses exhibit reduced immunogenicity as attenuation progresses. Assessment of viral attenuation can often be difficult, if not impossible, since consistent experimental reproduction of clinical disease is difficult with certain viruses. In such instances, a vaccine virus considered to be attenuated may produce clinical disease under special circumstances involving stress, physiologic imbalance, or concurrent infections with other organisms. Viruses that exhibit a wide host range are also problematic. Virus attenuated for one animal species may retain virulence for more susceptible species, and since attenuated viruses cause an active infection, transmission to other species may occur. Viral attenuation for the most susceptible species is an obvious approach to this dilemma, but this may result in a loss of immunogenicity for less-susceptible species.

A major concern in the use of attenuated viruses is reversion to virulence. This phenomenon has plagued vaccine development and licensing over the years. Reversion to virulence is a more serious possibility with those viruses that enjoy a wide host range or that are biologically transmitted by arthropod vectors. While the virus may appear stable in the host for which the vaccine was intended, reversion to virulence may occur in the vector or in other species. Vaccination of pregnant animals must also be of concern, since attenuated viruses may be pathogenic for the developing fetus. Vaccinating animals with reduced immunologic responsiveness can result in expression of clinical disease.

Additional negative features of attenuated virus vaccines include 1) the potential for reassortment (viruses with segmented genomes) or recombination between vaccine strains or with wild-type virus to create new viruses, 2) typical lack of a vaccine marker for serologic differentiation of vaccine and wild-type virus exposure, 3) development of persistent infections, 4) poor stability of vaccine virus, especially in hot tropical areas, and 5) replication interference between viruses in multivalent vaccines. Viruses that exhibit continued antigenic drift present a vaccine dilemma since new isolates must be continually attenuated and tested for safety and efficacy.

Inactivated Virus Vaccines

Many inactivated vaccines have been experimentally or commercially developed for use in veterinary medicine. Virus inactivation has most commonly employed formalin, beta-propiolactone, acetylethyleneimine, or binaryethyleneimine. Additional methods include ultraviolet light, gamma irradiation, psoralen compounds, and ozone gas. The primary advantage of killed virus vaccines

Table 6.2. Relative Advantages and Disadvantages of Live vs. Inactivated Virus Vaccines

Criteria	Live	Inactivated
Immunity	Long	Short
Adjuvant	No	Yes
Safety	Variable	Not applicable
Complications (potential)	Fetal infection, spread to susceptible animals	Sensitization
Potential contamination	Possible	Minimal
Interference	Possible	Minimal
Cost	Minimal	Significant
Immunomodulation	Not required	Required
Vaccine marker	Possibly genetic marker	Serologic marker
Stability	Poor	Good
CMI induction	Yes	No
Local secretory immunity	Yes	No
Reassortment/recombination	Possible	No
Persistent	Yes	No

is safety — many potential disadvantages of live-virus vaccines are eliminated since no virus replication occurs. Virus for inactivation has been produced in laboratory animals, embryonated chicken eggs, and, most commonly today, in cell cultures. From an economic viewpoint, viruses that grow to high titer in cell cultures and exhibit first-order inactivation kinetics provide the best candidates for vaccine preparation. Adjuvants are typically required to induce good immunity with killed viral products, and multiple doses are usually required. With the continued development of better adjuvants and immunopotentiating complexes (ISCOMs), inactivated vaccines will prove more effective. Inactivated vaccines are also relatively stable under adverse conditions, and their potential for strain interference in multivalent preparations is reduced compared to attenuated vaccines.

There are, however, certain disadvantages associated with the use of inactivated virus vaccines. Most inactivating agents are toxic, and some are carcinogenic. Unlike live virus, inactivated vaccine virus is not quantitatively amplified, so it requires adjuvant and multiple inoculations. Furthermore, such preparations do not induce strong CMI responses, since inducing such responses requires that the antigen be presented in association with histocompatibility antigens on cell surfaces. Nor are such vaccines associated with development of local secretory immunity, due to the usual parenteral route of vaccination.

The success of viral inactivation depends on the inactivant and viral characteristics. While most viruses can be successfully inactivated, the retention of critical antigenic integrity is variable. Antigens responsible for inducing protective immunity must be preserved. A possible complication of inactivated vaccine use is the potential for animal sensitization such that an exacerbated clinical disease is experienced upon exposure to virulent field virus. This sensitization is not well understood, but it is apparently immunologically precipitated by an unbalanced immune response such as humoral vs. cellular immunity, immune response to nonneutralizing epitopes, or preferential stimulation of IgE.

Development of subunit vaccines is currently an area of extensive research; it includes purification of viral subunits, recombinant technology, and peptide synthesis. Relative to veterinary medicine, developing such "advanced-type" vaccines is best illustrated with foot-and-mouth disease virus. The bases of a subunit vaccine are proteins (or peptide sequences) capable of eliciting protective immunity. Such proteins would typically be found on the virion surface and contain epitopes capable of inducing neutralizing antibody. Vaccines can be prepared by disruption of the virus followed by protein purification. The potential cost of such preparations has precluded their commercial development, but recent biotechnological advances have offered alternatives via recombinant DNA and peptide synthesis technologies.

The basic approach to developing recombinant vaccines involves artificial insertion of DNA that contains the desired viral genomic coding sequences into an appropriate expression vector. The DNA to be cloned can be obtained directly from the viral genome of DNA

viruses by use of restriction enzymes or indirectly by reverse transcription of mRNA or genomic segments of monocystronic RNA viruses of "positive sense." The viral or complementary DNA (cDNA) is inserted into a plasmid or bacteriophage followed by infection of susceptible prokaryotic cells such as *Escherichia coli*; more recently, yeast cells and mammalian cells are also being developed as expression vectors. Multiple strategies have been used to construct vaccine expression vectors, and most include a strong promoter (constitutive or inducible). Following infection of the cell with the plasmid, the cloned cDNA can be expressed and the desired gene product purified for vaccine use.

Recent attention has also been focused on the inoculation of plasmid DNA encoding viral antigens into tissues in vivo. Such vaccines would offer the advantages of having viral glycoproteins expressed on the surface of transfected cells and inducing immunity without interference from passively acquired viral antibodies.

Synthetic peptide vaccines are also currently receiving extensive attention. As with cloned viral vaccines, the successful development of synthetic peptide vaccines requires extensive knowledge of the viral proteins involved in inducing protective immunity. Two basic approaches are available for determining critical peptide sequences: 1) indirectly, from nucleotide sequences derived from cloned viral genes, and 2) directly, by sequencing purified peptides. The latter approach is facilitated by immunologically based peptide and epitope mapping to determine the regions involved in protective immunity. An additional approach to determining critical peptide sequences is based upon the projected tertiary structure of the viral protein, with the areas that demonstrate hydrophilic characteristics serving as candidate sequences. One major drawback of synthesizing peptide vaccines is the potential for critical epitopes to be formed by the tertiary structure (an epitope formed by juxtaposition of two separated peptide sequences). Such epitopes confound attempts to deduce the peptide sequence and realize such complex configurations in the synthetic product.

The use of anti-idiotypic antibodies as immunogens to stimulate the production of viral neutralizing antibodies has also been explored. The advantage of this type of immunogen may overcome viral variability problems by inducing broadly neutralizing antibodies. However, this type of vaccine induces only antibody responses, not cell-mediated responses.

TOXOIDS, BACTERINS, AND BACTERIAL VACCINES

As with viral vaccines, the basis of an effective toxoid, bacterin, or bacterial vaccine is the ability to induce an immune response or responses capable of eliciting protection from field exposure to the pathogenic microorganism. Most of the principles outlined above with respect to viral vaccines apply to products designed to induce protective immunity to bacterial agents. The development of an efficacious product depends on understanding the pathogenesis of the bacterial disease that is to be prevented.

In general terms, diseases produced by bacteria can be grouped into three categories: 1) those that result from association with a bacterial toxin, 2) those that result from the sequelae of extracellular multiplication of the bacterial agent, and 3) those that result from the sequelae of intracellular multiplication.

Toxoids

Bacterial toxins are of two kinds: exotoxins and endotoxins. Endotoxins are strictly defined as the lipopolysaccharide portion of the gram-negative cell wall (it is the lipid A portion that is specifically responsible for the "toxic" manifestations). Muramyl dipeptide, which is present in gram-positive cell walls and to a lesser extent in gram-negative, also has "toxic" properties. We have used quotation marks around "toxic" because both endotoxin and muramyl dipeptide elicit their "toxic" activities by inducing the production of a variety of cytokines by host cells. It is the degree of vigor of the host response that defines the "toxicity." Exotoxins are proteins that interact with host cells (usually after binding to a specific receptor) resulting in deregulation of host cell function without undue harm to the cell, interference of the normal physiology of the host cell(s), or death of the host cell.

Antibodies elicited to various epitopes on toxins that result in neutralization are sometimes called *antitoxins*. As mentioned previously, an antibody may block interaction between a toxin and its cellular receptor or change the configuration of the toxin so that it no longer has an effect on the host cell. Antibodies to exotoxins have been shown to be efficacious in preventing disease. Antibodies to endotoxins have had mixed results as far as preventing disease.

Toxoids are toxins without toxic activity that can elicit an immune response, i.e., antibodies (see above for explanation). Toxoids can be produced by chemical inactivation of the native toxin or by manipulations of the gene encoding the toxin so that the toxin is inactivated. For example, in the case of A-B toxins (see Chapter 9), where the A subunit is responsible for the toxic activity of the toxin and the B subunits are responsible for binding of the toxin to the host, the gene encoding the A subunit can be eliminated and a toxoid produced that is composed of B subunits. Antibody to lipopolysaccharide (endotoxin) is elicited by immunization with mutants (called "rough" mutants) that produce very little of the O-repeat unit of the lipopolysaccharide (see Chapter 8).

The main advantage of toxoids is that they are safe. Toxoids administered parenterally elicit antibody (IgM and IgG) that interferes with toxin-host cell interactions that are not at a mucosal surface. On the other hand, the administration of toxoids on a mucosal surface elicits antibody (sIgM and sIgA) that interferes with toxin-host cell interaction at the mucosal surface. The main disadvantage of toxoids used for immunization by way of a mucosal surface is their extremely short half-life.

Bacterins

Bacterins are killed pathogenic bacteria. They are usually produced by chemical killing of the infectious agent, with the aim to preserve bacterial structures expressing epitopes important in eliciting a protective immune response. The immune response is almost always antibody (see above for explanation).

The advantage of bacterins is that they are completely safe. If administered parenterally, the antibody elicited (IgM and IgG) will be effective if the bacterin is made from a pathogen that has an extracellular life style. If the bacterin is administered by way of a mucosal surface, the antibody elicited (sIgM and sIgA) will interfere with interactions of pathogen with host cells. The disadvantage is that the main immune response is antibody so that only antibody-mediated protection will occur. Thus, bacterins administered parenterally are not as effective against intracellular pathogens. Bacterins placed on a mucosal surface have extremely short half-lives, a serious disadvantage. Another disadvantage is that the pathogen is usually grown in vitro, and epitopes expressed in vivo may not be expressed, which can result in a product that may elicit antibodies with inappropriate specificities.

Bacterial Vaccines

Bacterial vaccines are composed of attenuated versions of the pathogen, i.e., they are live but reduced in virulence. Attenuation may be accomplished in a number of ways: selection of a naturally occurring attenuated strain; repeated passage on artificial media; or elimination of a virulence trait by mutation of the gene encoding the trait.

The major advantages of bacterial vaccines are directly related to their being alive. Live vaccines not only have longer half-lives than their dead counterparts (regardless of location), they will express epitopes that may only be expressed in vivo, thus eliciting antibody to epitopes that the pathogen will also express following infection. Another advantage is that live vaccines will elicit antibody and cellular hypersensitivity (see above for explanation). A major disadvantage is that live vaccines may produce disease, for example, through reversion to the virulent phenotype. Also, if the vaccinated host has reduced resistance, then the vaccine is more apt to produce disease.

SELECTED REFERENCES

Capron A, Locht C, Fracchia GN. Safety and efficacy of new generation vaccines. Vaccine 1994;12:667.

Condon C, Watkins SC, Celluzzi CM, et al. DNA-based immunization by in vivo transfection of dendritic cells. Nature Med 1996;2:1122.

Cox JC, Coulter AR. Adjuvants — a classification and review of their modes of action. Vaccine 1997;15:248.

Donnelly JJ, Ulmer JB, Shiver JW, Liu MA. DNA vaccines. Annu Rev Immunol 1997;15:617.

Fischetti VA, Medaglini D, Oggioni M, Pozzi G. Expression of foreign proteins on gram-positive commensal bacteria for mucosal vaccine delivery. Curr Opin Biotechnol 1993;4: 603.

Griffiths E. Environmental regulation of bacterial virulence — implication for vaccine design and production. Trends Biotechnol 1991;9:309.

Gupta RK, Relyveld EH, Lindblad EB, et al. Adjuvants — a balance between toxicity and adjuvanticity. Vaccine 1993;11:293.

Kaumaya PT, Kobs-Conrad S, Seo YH, et al. Peptide vaccines incorporating a "promiscuous" T-cell epitope bypass certain haplotype restricted immune responses and provide broad spectrum immunogenicity. J Mol Reg 1993;6:81.

Kitching RP. The application of biotechnology to the control of foot-and-mouth disease virus. Br Vet J 1992;148:375.

Liew FY. Biotechnology of vaccine development. Biotechnol Genet Engineer Rev 1990;8:53.

Moss B. Genetically engineered poxviruses for recombinant gene expression, vaccination, and safety. Proc Nat Acad Sci USA 1996;93:11341.

O'Hagan DT, Ott GS, Van Nest G. Recent advances in vaccine adjuvants: the development of MF59 emulsion and polymeric microparticles. Mol Med Today 1997;3:69.

Palese P, Zherig H, Engelhardt OG, et al. Negative-strand RNA viruses: genetic engineering and applications. Proc Nat Acad Sci USA 1996;93:11354.

Roy P. Genetically engineered particulate virus-like structures and their use as vaccine delivery systems. Intervirology 1996;39:62.

Russo S, Turin L, Zanella A, et al. What's going on in vaccine technology? Med Res Rev 1997;17:277.

Sela M, Arnon R. Synthetic approaches to vaccines for infectious and autoimmune diseases. Vaccine 1992;10:991.

Sharma A, Nagata H, Hamada N, et al. Expression of functional *Porphyromonas gingivalis* fimbrillin polypeptide domains on the surface of *Streptococcus gordoni*. App Environ Microbiol 1996;62:3933.

Shearer GM, Clerici M. Vaccine strategies: selective elicitation of cellular or humoral immunity? Trends Biotechnol 1997; 15:106.

Ulrich JT, Myers KR. Monophosphoryl lipid A as an adjuvant. Past experiences and new directions. Pharm Biotechnol 1995;6:495.

PART II

Bacteria and Fungi

7

The Alimentary Canal as a Microbial Habitat

Dwight C. Hirsh

The microbial flora inhabiting the alimentary canal are part of a complex ecosystem. The stability of the ecosystem is due to factors that are in part host-related and in part microbial. The result of interactions between host and microbe is an ecosystem comprised of many thousands of niches, each inhabited by the species or strain of microbe most aptly suited to that location, to the exclusion of others. The niche dweller has successfully competed for that particular site.

To produce disease, potentially pathogenic microorganisms must first adhere to *target cells*. If the target cell is part of a niche occupied by normal flora, the microorganisms will encounter "colonization resistance," a host defense barrier they must overcome before adhering (see Chapter 2). Adherence results from the interaction of microbial surface structures (*adhesins*) with receptors on target cells. This association is called *selective adsorption*. Some adhesins are virulence factors because most pathogens cannot produce disease without first adhering to a target cell. After adherence, the pathogen may produce disease by 1) secretion of an exotoxin, resulting, for example, in disruption of fluid and electrolyte regulation of the target cell; 2) invasion of the target cell, causing its death, usually by the action of a toxin (a cytotoxin); or 3) invasion of the target cell and the lymphatics, resulting in bacteremia. If adherence is prevented (by the normal flora or antibodies), disease does not usually result regardless of the other genetic capabilities of the pathogenic microorganism.

The fetus is microbiologically sterile as it starts down the birth canal. Microorganisms are acquired from the birth canal and, after birth, from the environment. The immediate environment of the newborn is populated with microorganisms excreted by the dam and other animals. These microbes are ingested, compete for niches, and with time become established as part of the normal flora. During the first days to months after birth, the flora is in a state of flux due to the interplay between the various microbes, the niches of the host, and the changing diet. Diet influences the nutritional environment at the level of the niche, which in turn influences the kinds of microbes that will successfully compete for these nutrients.

The microbial flora of the mouth is roughly uniform among domestic mammals. No information is available for fowl. The description that follows is general and applies to carnivores and herbivores. The buccal surface, tongue, and teeth (plaque) are inhabited by facultative and obligate aerobes. These include streptococci (alpha and nonhemolytic, see Chapter 22), *Pasteurella* spp., *Actinomyces* spp. (*A. viscosus* and *A. hordeovulneris* in the dog), enterics (*Escherichia coli* being the most common), *Neisseria* spp. (*Branhamella* spp.), EF-4 ("eugonic fermenter"), and *Simonsiella*. The flora of the gingival crevice is composed almost entirely of obligate anaerobes, the most common genera being *Bacteroides*, *Fusobacterium*, *Peptostreptococcus*, *Porphyromonas*, and *Prevotella*. Saliva contains a mixture of facultative and obligate species of anaerobes and aerobes. The esophagus does not possess a normal flora but is contaminated with organisms found in saliva. The flora of the rest of the alimentary canal varies significantly among different animals, as is shown in Tables 7.1 to 7.5.

Members of the normal flora establish themselves in a particular niche by excluding other species of microorganisms (including potential pathogens), utilizing various bacterial and host properties in the process.

BACTERIAL PROPERTIES

Structures on the surface of microorganisms living in the alimentary canal are involved in establishing the ecosystem. It is through these structures that the microorganism comes in intimate contact with the host.

Fimbrial adhesins are responsible for adherence of some bacteria to the surface of the host cell. Fimbriae are protein in nature and protrude from the surface of the bacterial cell to bind with carbohydrate moieties that are part of glycoproteins on the surface of host cells. There are different types of fimbrial adhesins defined in terms of morphology, the chemical composition of the subunits that comprise the entire structure, and the composition of the receptor on the surface of the host cell. The latter property is used to determine, in general, the types of fimbriae possessed by a particular isolate of bacteria. For this purpose, the carbohydrate receptors on the surface of red blood cells are utilized. If the red blood cells possess a receptor for the fimbria on the isolate under study, an agglutination reaction is observed after the red blood cells and the bacteria are mixed. The most

Table 7.1. Microbial Flora of the Chicken

	Number of Viable Microorganisms/Gram of Contents[a]					
	Stomach		Small Intestine		Cecum	Feces
	Crop	Gizzard	Upper	Lower		
Total	6	6	8–9	8–9	8–9	8–9
Anaerobes	3	5–6	<2	<2	8–9	7–8
Enterobacteriaceae[b]	6	<2	1–2	1–3	5–6	6–7
Streptococci/Enterococci	2	<2	4	3–5	6–7	6–7
Lactobacillus	5–6	2–3	8–9	8–9	8–9	8–9

[a] Expressed as $\log_{10}$ of the number of organisms cultured.
[b] Mainly *E. coli.*

Table 7.2. Microbial Flora of the Bovine

	Number of Viable Microorganisms/Gram of Contents[a]				
	Abomasum	Small Intestine		Cecum	Feces
		Upper	Lower		
Total	6–8	>7	6–7	8–9	9
Anaerobes	7–8	NA[c]	5–6	8–9	6–9
Enterobacteriaceae[b]	3–4	<7	5–6	4–5	5–6
Streptococci/Enterococci	6–7	2–3	3–4	4–5	4–5
Yeasts	2–3	—	<3	2	—

[a] Expressed as $\log_{10}$ of the number of organisms cultured.
[b] Mainly *E. coli.*
[c] Not available.

Table 7.3. Microbial Flora of the Horse

	Number of Viable Microorganisms/Gram of Contents[a]				
	Stomach	Small Intestine		Cecum	Feces
		Upper	Lower		
Total	7–9	NA[c]	7–8	8–9	8–9
Anaerobes	6–8	NA	6–7	8–9	8–9
Enterobacteriaceae[b]	3–5	3–4	4–6	3–4	3–5
Streptococci/Enterococci	6–7	5–6	5–6	6–7	5–6
Yeasts	—	—	—	—	<3

[a] Expressed as $\log_{10}$ of the number of organisms cultured.
[b] Mainly *E. coli.*
[c] Not available.

Table 7.4. Microbial Flora of the Pig

	Number of Viable Microorganisms/Gram of Contents[a]				
	Stomach	Small Intestine		Cecum	Feces
		Upper	Lower		
Total	3–8	3–7	4–8	4–11	10–11
Anaerobes	7–8	6–7	7–8	7–11	10–11
Enterobacteriaceae[b]	3–5	3–4	4–5	6–9	6–9
Streptococci/Enterococci	4–6	4–5	6–7	7–10	7–10
Yeasts	4–5	4	4	4	4
Spiral organisms	NA[c]	NA	NA	NA	8

[a] Expressed as $\log_{10}$ of the number of organisms cultured.
[b] Mainly *E. coli*.
[c] Not available.

Table 7.5. Microbial Flora of the Dog

	Number of Viable Microorganisms/Gram of Contents[a]				
	Stomach	Small Intestine		Cecum	Feces
		Upper	Lower		
Total	>6	>6	>7	>8	10–11
Anaerobes	1–2	>5	4–5	>8	10–11
Enterobacteriaceae[b]	1–5	2–4	4–6	7–8	7–8
Streptococci/Enterococci	1–6	5–6	5–7	8–9	9–10
Spiral organisms (relative amounts)	1+	1+	1+	4+	0

[a] Expressed as $\log_{10}$ of the number of organisms cultured.
[b] Mainly *E. coli*.

commonly found fimbriae on the surface of gram-negative bacteria have affinity for mannose-containing glycoproteins on the surface of red blood cells. These fimbriae are called *type 1 fimbriae*, but they are also known as *common* or *F1 fimbriae*. Bacteria expressing type 1 fimbriae, when mixed with red blood cells, agglutinate these cells; this agglutination is inhibited by mannose (mannose-sensitive). A fimbriated isolate can be classified as expressing a mannose-sensitive or mannose-resistant hemagglutinin.

Other structures on the surface of bacterial cells influence how the bacterium will interact with host cells. These structures are carbohydrates and influence the interaction by rendering the surface of the bacterial cell relatively hydrophilic. This hydrophilic property imparts a repulsive force relative to the host cell surface, since the host cell surface is somewhat hydrophobic. On the other hand, protein receptors on the surface of some host cells have affinity for these surface carbohydrates. The outcome of the latter interaction is adhesion.

A powerful way for bacteria to secure a particular niche against other species is to secrete antibiotic-like substances such as bacteriocins and microcins. Both of these substances are significant especially in the communities living in the oral cavity. The role of bacteriocins in the gastrointestinal tract is less clear. Microcins probably play a significant role in regulating the population composition in the gastrointestinal portion of the alimentary canal.

An important mechanism for regulating population size and ensuring niche security is fatty acid excretion by obligate anaerobes. In the gingival crevice, dental plaque, and the large bowel, the obligate anaerobes in this manner play a central role in regulating the size and composition of the normal facultative flora, the members of which may include potential pathogens. Under the conditions of the bowel (low Eh, $< -500\,\text{mv}$, and pH of 5 to 6), butyric, acetic, and lactic acids are extremely toxic to facultative anaerobes, especially members of the family *Enterobacteriaceae*.

Another way for bacteria to compete successfully is to acquire nutrients more successfully than competitors.

HOST PROPERTIES

The host contributes to the establishment of a normal flora by furnishing receptors for adhesins on the surface of prospective niche dwellers.

The epithelial cell also displays structures that serve as receptors for fimbriae expressed by enteropathogenic strains of bacteria. Just as important as the expression of adhesins by the enteropathogen is expression of the corresponding receptor by the target cell.

Peristalsis is a mechanism whereby nonadhering microorganisms are swept distally. In the small bowel, peristaltic activity plays a major role in host defense of the intestinal tract. The likelihood of disease has been shown to be related directly to the size of a population of a pathogenic species of bacteria in the small intestine. The most important regulator of the size of this population is peristaltic activity, since there are few other metabolic regulators such as those that exist in the large bowel (Eh, fatty acids, and pH).

Once the normal flora is established, it gives the animal a very potent defense barrier against microorganisms that may cause disease. Exclusion of *Salmonella* from the intestinal tract of poultry by "cocktails" containing normal flora microorganisms is an example of the effectiveness of colonization resistance. Disrupting colonization resistance puts the animal at risk by exposing receptors on potential target cells and eliminating a mechanism regulating the population size of facultative organisms, including species or strains with pathogenic potential.

Antimicrobial drugs are the single most efficient agents that decrease colonization resistance. Most antimicrobial agents affect the microbial flora of the oral cavity by depleting the numbers of streptococci that inhabit the surface of the cheeks and tongue. As a result, these areas are usually repopulated with resistant (to the antimicrobial agent being administered) members of the family *Enterobacteriaceae* within 24 to 48 hours. Resistant members of the environmental flora are also found. Members of the genus *Pseudomonas* are notorious examples of this group.

Antimicrobials also affect the members of the obligate anaerobic communities that inhabit the gingival crevice and dental plaque and those that inhabit the large bowel. Overgrowth of various members of the family *Enterobacteriaceae* results because of decreases in levels of fatty acids. Colonization by potential pathogens, e.g., *Salmonella,* is enhanced by antibiotics affecting obligate anaerobes living in the bowel.

The newborn animal is susceptible to enteric disease because it is immunologically naive as well as devoid of established flora. The most vulnerable area is the midjejunum and distal ileum. The cells of this area express receptors for the fimbrial adhesins on the surface of path-

ogenic (enterotoxigenic) strains of *E. coli.* Protection of the area is mediated by immunoglobulins in colostrum that are specific for antigenic determinants on these adhesins. Combination of such antibodies with these structures blocks attachment of the pathogen to its target cell.

Stress increases the likelihood of disease. Stress results in changes in the intestinal flora, which occur mainly as a result of a drop in the anaerobic component of the normal flora. The levels of coliform bacteria are higher after a decrease in concentration of fatty acids. The reason for the decrease in the number of obligate anaerobes is not known. In addition to these changes, the amount of fibronectin (a glycoprotein) coating epithelial cells in the oral cavity decreases. Since this glycoprotein possesses receptors for gram-positive species in the oral cavity, decrease in this population occurs with a corresponding increase in gram-negative species, especially members of the family *Enterobacteriaceae.*

SELECTED REFERENCES

Baquero E, Moreno E. The microcins. FEMS Microbiol Lett 1984;23:117.

Barnes EM, Mead CC, Barnum DA. The intestinal flora of the chicken in the period 2 to 6 weeks of age, with particular reference to the anaerobic bacteria. Br Poult Sci 1972;13:311.

Bohnhoff M, Miller CR. Enhanced susceptibility to *Salmonella* infection in streptomycin-treated mice. J Infect Dis 1962;111:117.

Braun V, Pilsl H, Groz P. Colicins: structures, modes of action, transfer through membranes, and evolution. Arch Microbiol 1994;161:199.

Hirsh DC. Fimbriae: relation of intestinal bacteria and virulence in animals. In: Cornelius CE, Simpson CE, eds. Advances in veterinary science and comparative medicine. Vol. 29. New York: Academic, 1985:207–238.

Jack RW, Tagg JR, Ray B. Bacteriocins of gram-positive bacteria. Microbiol Rev 1995;59:171.

Marsh R, Martin M. Oral microbiology. In: Aspects of microbiology. 2nd ed. Washington: American Society for Microbiology, 1984.

Meynell GG. Antibacterial mechanisms of the mouse gut. II. The role of Eh and volatile fatty acids in the normal gut. Br J Exp Pathol 1963;44:209.

Nurmi E, Nuotio L, Schneitz D. The competitive exclusion concept: development and future. Int J Food Microbiol 1992;15:237.

Que JU, Hentges DJ. Effect of streptomycin administration on colonization resistance to *Salmonella typhimurium* in mice. Infect Immun 1985;48:169.

Simpson WA, Hasty DC, Beachey EH. Binding of fibronectin to human buccal epithelial cells inhibits the binding of type 1 fimbriated *Escherichia coli.* Infect Immun 1985;48:318.

Smith HW. Observations on the flora of the alimentary tract of animals and factors affecting its composition. J Pathol Bacteriol 1965;89:95.

van der Waaij D. Antibiotic choice: the importance of colonization resistance. Chichester, UK: Research Studies, 1983.

van Houte J. Bacterial adherence in the mouth. Rev Infect Dis 1983;5:S659.

Vollaard EJ, Clasener HAL. Colonization resistance. Antimicrob Agents Chemother 1994;38:409.

8 *Family* Enterobacteriaceae

Dwight C. Hirsh

Members of the family *Enterobacteriaceae* ("enterics") cause disease in both food animals (e.g., neonatal diarrhea and salmonellosis) and companion animals (e.g., urinary tract infections, abscesses). Twenty-five genera comprise the family, but only a few are consistently involved with disease of the gastrointestinal tract. Table 8.1 lists the currently recognized genera belonging to this family.

DESCRIPTIVE FEATURES

Morphology and Staining

Members of the family are similar in morphology and staining characteristics, being pleomorphic, gram-negative, non-spore-forming rods that measure 2 to 3 μm by 0.4 to 0.6 μm. It is difficult to tell members of one genus from those of another by visual observation.

Cellular Anatomy and Composition

The cell wall is typically gram negative and consists of inner and outer membranes separated by peptidoglycan. Various proteins are found in each membrane, some traversing both. Capsules, flagella, and various adhesins are sometimes present.

The capsule (K-antigens) is the outermost structural component of the bacterial cell. Capsules of enteric organisms are composed of carbohydrates. The various types of carbohydrates, together with the types of linkages between the sugars, form the antigenic determinants that define capsular antigens. Encapsulated enteric bacteria are relatively hydrophilic, a characteristic imparted by the capsule.

The somatic antigens (O-antigens) are composed of antigenic determinants formed by the different configurations of sugar types, and the linkages between sugars found in the O-repeat portion of the lipopolysaccharide (Figs 8.1 and 8.2).

Flagella, which are cellular organelles used for locomotion, are composed of protein subunits (flagellin). Depending upon the type of flagellin, different antigenic determinants are formed. These antigenic determinants comprise the H-antigens. In cells of most *Salmonella* and some other species, one or the other of two sets ("phases") of antigenic determinants are possible. In culture, spontaneous phase variation occurs, that is, a shift from phase 1 to 2 or vice versa. The antigens of both phases, if present, help define serotypes and identify the *Salmonella* "species."

Fimbriae or pili are protein adhesins that are composed of subunits — pilin — and assembled in various configurations using different pilin molecules, which results in the generation of different types defined by their affinity for various carbohydrates. The most commonly found fimbriae have affinity for mannose-containing compounds. These fimbriae are called *type 1* or *common fimbriae* (also termed *F1*). Type 1 fimbriae have not been conclusively shown to be virulence determinants. On the other hand, a variety of other virulence-associated fimbriae have been described that agglutinate erythrocytes in the presence of mannose. Examples of such mannose resistant (MR) hemagglutinins are K88 and K99, two virulence-associated adhesins that are important in the pathogenesis of enteric disease produced by certain strains of *Escherichia coli*.

Most members of the family possess mucopeptide antigens in common, the so-called enterobacterial common antigen.

Cellular Products of Medical Interest

Cellular products of medical interest common to all or most of the members of the family are endotoxins and various siderophores.

Endotoxin is the term given the lipopolysaccharide (LPS) that is part, and extrudes from, the outer membrane of the gram-negative cell wall (see Fig 8.2). The lipid portion of this substance is embedded in the outer membrane and has the toxic properties associated with endotoxin. The most important constituent of LPS as far as the toxic manifestations of the molecule are concerned is the lipid portion, called *lipid A*. This lipid is responsible for the physiologic consequences of endotoxemia.

Siderophores (Greek for "iron bearing") are iron-carrying molecules (catechols or hydroxamates) of bacterial origin. They function in the solubilization and transport of ferric ions. There is very little free iron; nearly all is associated with the iron-binding proteins of the host (ferritin, transferrin, and lactoferrin). Since iron is an absolute requirement for almost all bacteria, parasitic strains, especially invasive ones, must compete for iron. Most utilize siderophores that remove iron from the iron-binding proteins of the host.

Some members of the family *Enterobacteriaceae* produce protein exotoxins, which will be considered with the respective species.

Table 8.1.   Genera comprising the family *Enterobacteriaceae*

Budvicia	*Kluyvera*	*Salmonella*[a]
Cedecea	*Leclercia*	*Serratia*
Citrobacter	*Leminorella*	*Shigella*[a]
Edwardsiella[a]	*Moellerella*	*Tatumella*
Enterobacter[a]	*Morganella*[a]	*Trabulsiella*
Escherichia[a]	*Pantoea*	*Yersinia*[a]
Ewingella	*Proteus*[a]	*Yokenella*
Hafnia	*Providencia*[a]	
Klebsiella[a]	*Rahnella*	

[a] Members of this genus found in pathogenic conditions of animals.

FIGURE 8.1.   *Anatomy of an enterobacterial cell showing localization of cell surface antigens of* Escherichia coli. *Only one of many peritrichous flagella is shown. (Reproduced by permission of Barnum DA, et al. Colibacillosis. CIBA Veterinary Monograph Series 1967;2:8.)*

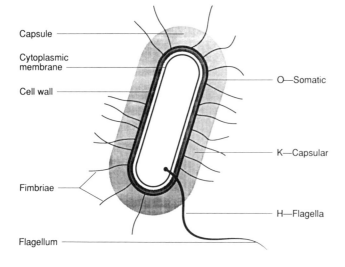

FIGURE 8.2.   *Molecular organization of the outer membrane of* Enterobacteriaceae. *The chains of rectangles represent the O-repeat units determining O-antigen specificity. They are attached to the polysaccharide core (irregular shapes), which is linked to lipid A (fringed oblongs). These three components constitute the lipopolysaccharide (LPS) of the gram-negative cell wall. With the underlying zone of phospholipid (fringed circles), LPS makes up the outer membrane, an asymmetric bilayer that also contains proteins: A — outer membrane protein A; PP — pore protein; BP — nutrient binding protein. Interior to the outer membrane lies the periplasmic space (PPS); the peptidoglycan layer (PG); and the cytoplasmic membrane (CM) with carrier protein (CP). (Reproduced by permission of Lugentberg B, Van Alphen L. Molecular architecture and function8 ing of the outer membrane of* Escherichia coli *and other gram-negative bacteria. Biochim Biophys Acta 1983;737:94.)*

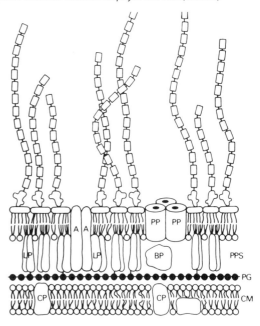

Growth Characteristics

Members of this group of microorganisms are facultative anaerobes. They utilize a variety of simple substrates for growth. Under anaerobic conditions, they are dependent upon the presence of fermentable carbohydrate. Under aerobic conditions, the range of suitable substrates includes organic acids, amino acids, and carbohydrates.

The end products of sugar fermentation are useful in making a diagnosis. Almost all members of this group ferment glucose to pyruvic acid via the Embden-Meyerhof pathway. Some, such as *E. coli* and *Salmonella*, produce succinic acid, acetic acid, formic acid, and ethanol by way of the mixed acid fermentation pathway. Others, such as *Klebsiella* and *Enterobacter*, produce butanediol from pyruvic acid, thereby reducing the relative amounts of acidic by-products.

An important diagnostically useful biochemical characteristic of all the members of the family *Enterobacteriaceae* is the absence of cytochrome c, making them oxidase negative.

Resistance

Enterobacteriaceae are killed by sunlight, drying, pasteurization, and the common disinfectants. In moist, shaded environments, such as pastures, manure, litter, and bedding, they can survive for many months. Though many are susceptible to broad-spectrum antimicrobial agents, their susceptibility is not accurately predictable and can change rapidly through acquisition of R plasmids.

Variability

Variability of one isolate of enteric as compared to another within the same species or genus depends upon the genetic basis for the trait under consideration. Differences in the capsular, somatic, or flagellar antigens account for variability among isolates of the same genus and species. Some variation among members of the same genus and species in the family, as well as among members of different genera and species, is accounted for by the presence of genes residing on plasmids encoding certain phenotypic traits. Such traits as resistance to antimicrobial agents, production of toxin, or secretion of hemolysin may be plasmid encoded and will vary depending on the presence or absence of a particular plasmid.

Transition from the smooth to the rough phenotype occurs with all members of the family. Likewise, change in the O-antigens has been shown to occur following lysogeny by certain bacteriophages (lysogenic conversion).

LABORATORY DIAGNOSIS

The family is composed of a large number of related, facultatively anaerobic, oxidase-negative, nitrate-reducing gram-negative rods. No clear divisions exist between the recognized genera. Differentiation within the family is accomplished by a combination of cultural, biochemical, and serologic tests. A number of manuals deal exclusively with this family, and because of the extreme clinical importance and prevalence of these organisms, an increasing number of programmed and/or computerized identification schemes are commercially available.

Morphology and Staining

All are gram-negative rods. All look similar in the gram-stained smear.

Cultural Characteristics

Methods used to isolate enteric pathogens vary depending upon whether the source of the sample is intestinal or extraintestinal. When the source is extraintestinal, isolating any of the family from normally sterile sites is significant. A culture medium with wide appeal is used. The medium for this purpose is an agar medium containing red blood cells (usually sheep or cow).

When the source is intestinal, two consistently pathogenic genera may occur in fecal samples: *Salmonella* and *Shigella*. Though pathogenic strains of *E. coli* might be present, there is no easy way to determine a pathogenic strain from normally occurring, nonpathogenic strains of *E. coli*.

All enteric media are devised to favor the identification of *Salmonella*, *Shigella*, or both. The bases of the media are as follows:

- An inhibitory substance, usually a bile salt or a dye. These substances inhibit gram-positive organisms from growing.
- A substrate utilized or not by *Salmonella*, *Shigella*, and by few others.
- A pH indicator to tell if the substrate has been changed.

The following are useful selective media for isolating enteric pathogens.

MacConkey Agar

Inhibitor: Bile salts and crystal violet (inhibit gram-positive microorganisms).

Substrate: Lactose — *Salmonella, Shigella,* and *Proteus* do not ferment lactose.

Neutral red: If lactose is fermented (acid), colonies will be pink; if lactose is not fermented (peptides digested — basic), colonies will be colorless.

Usefulness: Very permissive medium. *Salmonella* and *Shigella* readily grow on this medium (as do most other enterics and *Pseudomonas*).

Xylose Lysine Deoxycholate (XLD) Agar

Inhibitor: Bile salts.

Substrate: 1) Xylose — not fermented by *Shigella* (*Salmonella* ferments xylose). 2) Lysine — isolates that ferment xylose, but not lactose and sucrose, and are lysine decarboxylase negative (*Proteus mirabilis*) produce colonies that will be amber-orange. *Salmonella* decarboxylates lysine. The ratio of xylose to lysine is such that an alkaline pH predominates (more decarboxylation). *Shigella* does not decarboxylate lysine. 3) Lactose and sucrose — *Salmonella* and *Shigella* do not ferment these sugars rapidly. 4) Ferric salt — colonies of organisms producing H_2S (*Salmonella; Proteus*) will have black centers (iron sulfide).

Phenol red: Acid colonies (non-*Salmonella* or non-*Shigella*) will be yellow. Alkaline colonies (possible *Salmonella* or *Shigella*) will be red.

Usefulness: An excellent all-purpose medium for both *Salmonella* and *Shigella*.

Hektoen Enteric (HE) Agar

Inhibitor: Bile salts.

Substrate: Lactose and salicin — *Salmonella, Shigella,* and some species of *Proteus* and *Providencia* are lactose negative and salicin negative.

Ferric salt: Organisms producing H_2S will form black-centered colonies.

Bromthymol blue: Fermentors of salicin and/or lactose will form yellow to orange colonies; isolates not fermenting these sugars will form green or blue-green colonies.

Usefulness: Excellent for *Salmonella* and *Shigella*.

Brilliant Green Agar

Inhibitor: Brilliant green dye (suppresses the growth of most members of the family except *Salmonella*).

Substrate: Lactose and sucrose — *Salmonella* (and some strains of *Proteus*) does not ferment these sugars. Neither does *Shigella*, but *Shigella* will not grow on this medium.

Phenol red: If sugars are not fermented (alkaline), colonies will be red; if sugars are fermented (acid), colonies will be yellow-green (due to the color of the background dye).

Usefulness: Excellent for isolating *Salmonella*.

At times, the numbers of *Salmonella* or *Shigella* in fecal samples are too low ($<10^4$/gm) to be detected on the so-called primary plating media discussed above. Therefore, in addition to being plated directly to a selective medium, the fecal sample is also placed in an enrichment medium. To detect *Salmonella* by utilizing enrichment methods, at least 100 salmonellae/gm are needed.

For *Salmonella*, enrichment may be achieved by incubating feces for 12 to 18 hours in selenite F broth. During this time, the growth of organisms other than *Salmonella* is suppressed, whereas growth of *Salmonella* is not. After the 12 to 18 hours have elapsed, an aliquot of the broth is streaked onto a plate of selective medium (e.g., brilliant green agar).

Enrichment for *Shigella* is not easy because it is rather sensitive to commonly used inhibitory substances found in selenite F and tetrathionate broths. An enrichment broth called *gram-negative* (or *GN broth*) is used in the same manner as selenite is used for *Salmonella*.

Members of the genus *Pseudomonas* (especially *P. aeruginosa*) may be found in feces, but this is probably an insignificant finding. *Pseudomonas* has the ability to grow on enteric media. This microorganism does very little to the substrates other than the peptides and peptones and thus mimics *Salmonella* and *Shigella* on selective media. *Pseudomonas* is oxidase positive, a useful distinction.

SELECTED REFERENCES

Ewing WH. Edwards and Ewing's identification of enterobacteriaceae. 4th ed. Amsterdam: Elsevier, 1986.

Farmer JJ. Enterobacteriaceae: introduction and identification. In: Murray PR, Baron EJ, Pfaller MA, et al., eds. Manual of clinical microbiology. 6th ed. Washington: American Society for Microbiology, 1995:438.

Salyers AA, Whitt DD. Bacterial pathogenesis. Washington: American Society for Microbiology, 1994.

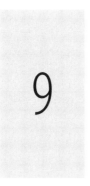

9 Escherichia

Dwight C. Hirsh

The genus *Escherichia* is composed of several species, but only *E. coli* is an important pathogen of animals. This species, the major facultative gram-negative species comprising the normal flora of the gastrointestinal tract, may be the cause of septicemic disease in foals, calves, piglets, puppies, and lambs; of enterotoxigenic diarrhea in newborn farm animals; and of edema disease in pigs. It may also be opportunistic in almost all animal species (e.g., in urinary tract disease, abscesses, and pneumonia).

DESCRIPTIVE FEATURES

Cellular Anatomy and Composition

Capsular polysaccharides (K-antigens) are important for those microorganisms that come in contact with the products and cells of the host, such as invasive strains of *E. coli*. Capsular substances protect the outer membrane from the membrane attack complex of the complement cascade and inhibit the microbe from attachment to, and ingestion by, phagocytic host cells. There are at least 80 distinct K-antigens.

The lipopolysaccharide (LPS) in the outer membrane is an important virulence determinant. Not only is the lipid A component toxic (endotoxin), but the length of the side chain in the O-repeat unit hinders the attachment of the membrane attack complex of the complement system to the outer membrane. There are approximately 165 serologically distinct O-groups.

Almost all strains of *E. coli* are motile by means of peritrichous flagella. There are at least 50 serologically different flagellar (H) antigens.

The O-, H-, and K-antigens are used in serotyping a particular isolate. For example, O141:K85:H3 describes an isolate with antigens of the 141 serogroup, capsular antigen 85, flagellar antigen 3.

Adhesins mediate adherence to target cells in the gastrointestinal tract and to cells comprising the niche for the strain. Because of their relative hydrophobicity, adhesins may also promote association with the membrane of phagocytic cells. Adhesins are important virulence factors only when the microbe is on mucosal surfaces.

Cellular Products of Medical Interest

Pathogenic strains of *E. coli* excrete at least five medically important products: enterotoxins, siderophores, shiga-like toxin (verotoxin), cytotoxic necrotizing factors, and hemolysin.

Enterotoxins are usually plasmid-encoded proteins and occur in two forms. One, labile toxin (LT), is a large heat-labile immunogenic protein of 91,000 MW that is antigenically related to cholera toxin. The other, stable toxin (ST), is a family of nonimmunogenic proteins, 1500 to 2000 MW. These protein exotoxins affect the regulation of cyclic nucleotide activity within the cell. LT affects the adenylate cyclase system; ST the guanylate cyclase system. LT is composed of two subunits, A and B. The B subunit is a multimer that binds to gangliosides on the surface of the cell, followed by translocation of the A subunit across the cell membrane. The A subunit, after activation, cleaves nicotinamide from nicotinamide adenine dinucleotide (NAD) and then couples the remaining ribosyl adenine diphosphate onto the G regulatory protein of the adenylate cyclase enzyme system. The result is deregulation of adenylate cyclase, causing overproduction of cyclic AMP (adenosine 3':5'-cyclic phosphate). This results in the opening of chloride channels in crypt cells (so-called cystic fibrosis transmembrane conductance regulator chloride channels) and the blockage of NaCl absorption in apical tip cells. As a consequence, water and electrolytes (chloride, sodium, and bicarbonate ions) are lost into the intestinal lumen. These events lead to diarrhea, hypovolemia, metabolic acidosis, and, if the acidosis is severe, hyperkalemia. There are two serologically distinct subclasses of LT. LT I is plasmid-encoded and neutralized by anticholera toxin antibodies; LT II is neither. LT I has been isolated from *E. coli* affecting humans (LTh-l) and swine (LTp-l). LT II has been isolated from cattle, water buffalo, humans, and food.

There are two kinds of ST: STa and STb. The genes encoding STa are located on a transposable element. The genes for STb are not. STa causes fluid accumulation in the intestines of suckling mice and piglets; STb causes fluid accumulation only in piglets and weaned pigs. The toxins are not related antigenically. STa affects the guanylate cyclase system by deregulating cGMP synthesis, which results in fluid and electrolyte accumulation in the bowel lumen subsequent to blockage of sodium and chloride ion (and thus water) absorption (tip cells) and loss of chloride ions (crypt cells). The receptor for STa is a membrane-bound guanylate cyclase. This receptor, when bound, results in the synthesis of cGMP. Increase in intracellular cGMP leads to the opening of chloride channels with the resultant flow of chloride and water into the intestinal lumen. The STa receptor is normally the target for guanylin (a 15 amino acid paracrine regulator), which is produced by goblet cells. Guanylin appears responsible for hydration of mucus that is also produced by goblet cells. STa and guanylin have common C-termini. The method of action of STb is unknown. In wild strains of enterotoxigenic *E. coli*, STa is more commonly found.

Siderophores (Greek for "iron bearing") allow microorganisms to acquire iron from the environment. To multiply within the host, microorganisms must acquire iron from the host iron-binding proteins because there is little free iron within the host. Siderophores that remove iron from host iron-binding proteins are necessary if a microbe is to have invasive capabilities.

Shiga-like toxins are protein toxins similar in activity to shiga toxin produced by *Shigella*. Both the shiga and the shiga-like toxins inhibit protein synthesis following interaction with the 60S ribosomal subunit. There are two types of shiga-like toxins, SLT-I and SLT-II. SLT-I is neutralized by antibody specific for the shiga toxin produced by *Shigella* spp.; SLT-II is not. SLT-I is probably identical to shiga toxin, whereas SLT-II is a variant. A family of bacteriophages has been shown to encode the shiga and shiga-like toxins. A variant of SLT-II, called *SLT-IIe*, is responsible for the vascular damage characteristic of edema disease of swine. The genes encoding SLT-IIe do not appear to be bacteriophage-associated.

E. coli may produce cytotoxic necrotizing factors (CNF), which are proteins of approximately 110 to 115 kDa in size. They interact with an epithelial cell small GTP-binding protein Rho, resulting in membrane "ruffles." There are two types of CNF, CNF1 and CNF2, which are immunologically related and similar in size. The gene encoding CNF1 is located on the chromosome in a so-called pathogenicity island, a locus that also contains the genes for a number of chromosomally encoded virulence traits, e.g., hemolysin, serum resistance, and the adherence protein Pap, needed by some strains of *E. coli* to adhere to urinary tract epithelium antecedent to urinary tract disease. The gene encoding CNF2 is plasmid-based.

E. coli produces at least two hemolysins, termed *alpha* and *beta*, that form clear zones on blood agar. The beta hemolysin is cell-bound, and little is known about its role in virulence. The alpha hemolysin is a protein (100 kDa) secreted by many virulent strains of *E. coli*. Loss or gain of the gene for a hemolysin synthesis by genetic manipulation produces corresponding changes in virulence of *E. coli* strains. The hemolysin damages cell membranes.

RNA polymerase containing RpoS (the sigma factor associated with stationary phase) preferentially transcribes genes responsible for acid tolerance (survival at pH < 5), allowing safe transit through the stomach.

ECOLOGY

Reservoir and Transmission

Strains of *E. coli* capable of producing disease reside in the lower gastrointestinal tract and are abundant in environments inhabited by animals. Transmission is through the fecal–oral route.

Pathogenesis

Enterotoxigenic Diarrhea. This disease occurs in neonatal pigs, calves, and lambs and in weanling pigs. It has been reported in dogs and horses.

Enterotoxigenic diarrhea is caused by strains of *E. coli* that produce mannose resistant adhesins (see Chapter 8) capable of attaching to glycoproteins on the surface of epithelial cells of the jejunum and ileum. Unless the ingested strain adheres to these cells, peristalsis will move it into the large bowel. The cells of the jejunum and the ileum are susceptible to the action of enterotoxin; the cells of the large bowel are not.

At least four MR adhesins may be found on enterotoxigenic *E. coli*. These proteins are designated K88, K99, 987P (also designated F4, F5, and F6, respectively), and F41, based on serologic identification. They possess some host species specificity: K88 and 987P are almost always associated with isolates from swine; K99 with isolates from cattle, sheep, and swine; and F41 with those from cattle. The epithelial cell receptors for these adhesins regulate the age incidence of this disease. In calves and lambs, the receptors appear transiently during the first week or so of life. Analogous receptors are present in pigs throughout the first six weeks of life. There are many uncharacterized adhesins that probably play a role as well.

Aside from the adhesins outlined above, some enterotoxigenic strains of *E. coli* express "curli," an adhesin with affinity for extracellular matrix proteins. So, in addition to adherence to glycoproteins on the surface of epithelial cells, some strains adhere to extracellular matrix proteins. Expression of curli may explain the increase in the window of age susceptibility to enterotoxigenic disease in animals concurrently infected with rotavirus or cryptosporidia, two agents that may cause tissue damage leading to exposure of extracellular matrix proteins.

In addition to adherence to the target tissues of the small intestine, enterotoxigenic strains must have the genetic capability of synthesizing enterotoxin. Strains producing only ST are the most common, followed by those secreting both ST and LT, and then by those secreting LT only.

Some of the adhesins and enterotoxins are encoded on plasmid DNA. As a consequence, it is difficult to predict which strain of *E. coli* possesses the genetic information necessary to produce disease. Some adhesins prefer to be associated with certain serotypes. In particular, the genes encoding the protein for the F41 adhesin are almost always found within strains of *E. coli* of the O9 and the O101 serogroups. As might be expected, the genes encoding the proteins for F41 fimbriae are located on chromosomal DNA.

Following ingestion by the host, enterotoxigenic strains of *E. coli* adhere to target cells, multiply, and secrete enterotoxin. Fluid and electrolytes accumulate in the lumen of the intestine, resulting in diarrhea, dehydration, and electrolyte imbalances. In time, the infecting strain is moved distally away from the target cell and the disease process stops, due probably in part to the cessation of expression of the adhesin along with a decrease in available substrate following the almost explosive multiplication of the strain in the small intestine. Unless steps are taken to correct the fluid and electrolyte imbalances, the disease has high mortality.

Invasive Disease. Association of susceptible animals (usually a neonate that has received inadequate amounts of colostrum or colostrum of inadequate quality) with invasive strains of *E. coli* may occur by way of the conjunctivae, inadequately treated umbilicus, or ingestion. If the invasive strain associates via ingestion, the bacteria adhere to target cells in the distal small bowel. Adherence is probably related to expression of any number of adhesins, but CS31A is one that is commonly associated with invasive *E. coli*. Likewise, the fimbrial adhesin F17 originally described on a plasmid termed *Vir* (so-called because of its association with virulent or invasive *E. coli*) is prevalent on invasive *E. coli*. Following adherence, invasive strains "induce" their own uptake by expression of either CNF1 or CNF2, which results in the formation of "ruffles" that entrap the adhering bacteria and "pull" them into the cell. Entry into the lymphatics and subsequently the bloodstream follows. Extensive multiplication within the epithelial cell probably does not occur. The mechanism by which the invasive strain gains access to lymphatics after uptake by the epithelial cell is unknown. Likewise, the mechanism of entry into lymphatics after association with conjunctivae or the umbilicus is unknown.

The infecting strain multiplies in the lymphatics and bloodstream and endotoxemia develops (Fig 9.1). Death of the host occurs if the organism is not removed by antibacterial therapy, the immune system, or both.

Invasive strains have special qualities — e.g., they must escape phagocytosis, complement-mediated lysis, and have a mechanism to acquire iron.

Capsule and various outer membrane proteins confer resistance to antibody-independent, complement-mediated lysis (serum resistance). How capsules protect the outer membrane from insertion of the membrane attack complex is not known. Certain capsules (such as K1) are chemically similar to the surface of host cells in that they are composed mainly of sialic acid. Complement components associating with surfaces composed of sialic acid are shunted to degradative pathways rather than amplification and formation of membrane attack complexes.

Escape from phagocytosis is also related to capsule and certain outer membrane proteins. The capsule is thought to endow a degree of hydrophilicity relative to the membrane of phagocytic cells. Most capsules are negatively charged, as is the membrane of phagocytic cells. How outer membrane proteins function as antiphagocytic factors is not known.

The genes encoding the adhesin (e.g., CS31A, F17) and those responsible for siderophore production reside on plasmids. As mentioned above, the genes encoding F17 have been associated with the plasmid Vir, as has the gene encoding CNF2; those responsible for siderophore production have been associated with pColV. In the latter instance, the siderophore genes are linked closely with the genes for the production of colicine V. The siderophore, aerobactin, has a high affinity for iron.

Many of the strains with invasive capability, except those from foals, produce a hemolysin and are hemolytic

FIGURE 9.1. *Cascade of biologically active mediators following interaction of lipopolysaccharide (LPS) with the body. When gram-negative microorganisms grow in the body, LPS is released (not on purpose, but when a cell makes LPS, some of it escapes). If the LPS is in the bloodstream, then a generalized cytokine "storm" plus activation of some of the enzyme cascades (complement is one) results in intravascular clotting, and increased vascular permeability → decreased organ perfusion, and multiple organ failure, and very serious pH problems. This "state" is called "septic shock" resulting from endotoxemia. (*IL-8 attracts PMNs and MCAF [macrophage chemotactic factor] attracts macrophages.)*

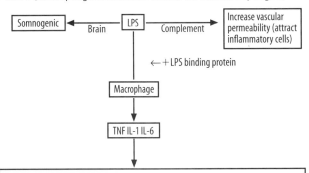

1. Increase vascular permeability–arachidonic acid pathway (TNF on endothelium)
2. Increase intravascular clotting–arachidonic acid pathway (TNF on endothelium)
3. Attract inflammatory cells–(TNF/IL-1 induce endothelium to produce IL-8 and MCAF)*
4. Release of acute phase proteins (liver) (IL-6)
5. Endogenous pyrogen (TNF, IL-1, IL-6) (brain)
6. Somnogenic (TNF, IL-1) (brain)

on blood agar. This hemolysin belongs to the RTX (repeats in toxin) family of toxins, so-called because of repeats of glycine-rich sequences within the protein. It is thought to damage phagocytic cells.

Nonenterotoxigenic Diarrheas. Enteropathogenic strains of *E. coli* (EPEC) produce diarrhea in all animal species, including human beings. EPEC do not produce ST, LT, or any other diarrhea associated toxin. They do, however, produce a characteristic lesion in the intestinal tract that is described as *attaching and effacing* lesion. The characteristic lesion occurs because of the "collapse" of the microvilli of the affected cell giving the histopathologic appearance of "effacement." The location in the tract depends upon the species of animal affected.

EPEC have a number of attributes that are involved in pathogenesis. The first is an adhesion encoded by the plasmid-based gene *bfd* (for *b*undle *f*orming *p*ilus, due to its propensity to tangle together and form "bundles"). These pili appear responsible for "targeting" the particular intestinal epithelial cell that will become involved in the process. After association with an intestinal epithelial cell, a more intimate attachment occurs (the "attaching" phase) by way of the protein *intimin* encoded by the chromosomally located gene, *eaeA* (*E. coli* *a*ttaching *effac*ing). This gene is located in a "pathogenicity island" (see above) called *LEE* (*l*ocus *e*ffacing *E. coli*). The receptor on the host cell to which intimin attaches is a protein produced by the attached EPEC strain. This protein, termed Tir (for *t*ranslocated *i*ntimin *r*eceptor), inserts into the membrane of the host cell and, following modification by the host cell, serves as receptor for intimin. Following intimate attachment, a gene product (encoded by *espA* and *espB*, for EPEC signaling *p*rotein, also located in the "pathogenicity island") activates a tyrosine phosphokinase in the affected cell resulting in cytoskeletal rearrangements leading to "collapse" of the microvilli (the "effacing" phase). Diarrhea occurs secondary to increases in intracellular calcium ions and activation of protein kinase C. Protein kinase C is responsible for phosphorylation of proteins composing the chloride channels resulting in loss of chloride and water into the intestinal lumen, as well as the phosphorylation of the membrane associated ion transport proteins resulting in blockage of absorption of NaCl.

Some attaching and effacing strains of *E. coli* are lysogenized with the bacteriophage(s) that encode the shiga-like toxins SLT-I and/or SLT-II. These strains are termed *enterohemorrhagic E. coli* (EHEC) because, in addition to producing attaching and effacing lesions, they also produce hemorrhagic diarrhea (shiga toxin is discussed in Chapter 11). The prototype EHEC is a strain of *E. coli* of the serotype O157:H7 that produces disease in human beings and calves given the strain experimentally. Following attachment (where depends upon the animal species involved [humans — large intestine]) SLT is produced. The SLTs affect endothelial cells, leading to their injury and loss of integrity. The effects of SLTs are local, i.e., the endothelial cell under the cell to which EHEC is attached, and systemic, i.e., the endothelial cells elsewhere in the body but mainly in the kidney and brain. The systemic effects of EHEC-associated disease, at least in humans, result in a syndrome called the *hemolytic uremic syndrome* (HUS), characterized by microangiopathic hemolytic anemia, glomerulonephritis, and thrombocytopenia. How SLT is absorbed locally or systemically is not understood. HUS does not appear to be a significant sequela of EHEC-based disease in nonhuman animals. Approximately 5% to 10% of human patients affected with EHEC (almost all are O157:H7) will develop HUS.

All affected animals acquire EPEC/EHEC by way of the oral route. It is not clear whether EPEC have zoonotic potential, but animals (including humans) probably acquire the infecting strain by the fecal–oral route. Strain O157:H7 is a part of the normal flora of nonhuman animals, especially bovines. Human beings become infected by ingesting contaminated food, mainly beef. At slaughter, the surface of the carcass becomes contaminated. The surfaces of cuts of meat derived from an infected carcass are readily sterilized by cooking. When the meat is ground, the microorganisms on the surface become mixed throughout. Though improper cooking will readily kill surface microorganisms, including O157:H7, those inside may not be killed.

Edema Disease. Edema disease is an acute, often fatal enterotoxemia of weaned pigs. The disease is characterized by subcutaneous and subserosal edema, caused by absorption of SLT-IIe produced by certain serotypes of *E. coli* (e.g., O141:K85, O138:K81, and O139:K82). The toxin attaches to and affects endothelial cells throughout the pig, resulting in extensive edema. The toxigenic strains

inhabit the large bowel of normal pigs, and these strains are thought to increase in numbers during nutritional, social, or physical stress.

Colibacillosis of Fowl. Colibacillosis of fowl is an economically important disease caused by invasive strains of *E. coli*. The disease takes many forms in fowl, depending upon the age of the host and mode of infection.

The egg surface can be contaminated with potentially pathogenic strains at the time of laying. The bacteria penetrate the shell and infect the yolk sac. If the bacteria grow, the embryo dies, usually late in incubation. Embryos that survive may die shortly after, with losses occurring as late as 3 weeks after hatching.

Fowl may also be infected by the respiratory tract and develop respiratory or septicemic disease. The course may be rapidly fatal or chronic, manifested by debilitation, diarrhea, and respiratory distress.

Other clinical syndromes seemingly caused by *E. coli* include cellulitis, synovitis, pericarditis, salpingitis, and panophthalmitis.

The *E. coli* responsible for this disease have been shown to possess some of the same virulence determinants as those isolated from mammals, most notably adhesins and production of aerobactin and associated iron-regulated outer membrane proteins.

IMMUNOLOGIC ASPECTS

Immunologic defense against disease produced by pathogenic *E. coli* occurs at two levels: at the site of attachment to the target cell and through destruction of the bacteria or neutralization of its products.

The neonate acquires immunity from the dam and, depending upon the isotype of the immunoglobulin — IgA, IgG, or IgM — the type of protection differs. For the first 36 hours or so of life, ingested IgG and IgM attach to receptors on the surface of epithelial cells of the small intestine. Transfer across the cell into the systemic circulation follows attachment. If the antibodies are specific for a virulence determinant, then disease may not result if the neonate encounters a pathogenic strain expressing that virulence determinant. For example, anticapsular antibodies acquired from the dam will protect the newborn from fatal invasive disease by strains of *E. coli* possessing that particular capsule. Certain isotypes prevent the attachment of a disease-producing strain to the target cell. These antibodies, sIgA and sIgM, which are found in colostrum and milk, if specific for antigenic determinants on the surface of the adhesin, will prevent the attachment of the adhesin-expressing pathogen to the target cell. Such antibodies have also been shown to promote, by an unknown mechanism, the loss of the plasmid encoding the production of the adhesin K88. Antibody to SLT-IIe will protect pigs from developing edema disease.

It is imperative therefore that the dam be exposed either naturally or artificially to the microorganism and its virulence determinants before parturition. Such exposure allows for antibodies to be made for secretion into colostrum and milk.

LABORATORY DIAGNOSIS

Demonstration of ETEC

Enterotoxigenic strains multiply to numbers approaching 10^8 to 10^9/ml of luminal contents. If the animal survives the fluid and electrolyte imbalances, large numbers are shed into the environment. Diagnosis is based on the suspicion that the disease is due to enterotoxigenic *E. coli*. The least troublesome and least invasive procedure (and also the least reliable) for verification of this suspicion is to demonstrate large numbers of fimbriae-expressing *E. coli* in the feces. Demonstration entails plating a portion of a fecal sample onto a selective medium (MacConkey agar, for example). As fimbriae are expressed poorly on selective media, a number of colonies are subcultured onto media that will promote the expression of the various fimbriae: for K88, E medium; for K99 and 987P, Minca medium; and for F41, E or Minca medium. Slide agglutination tests are run on each colony using antiserum specific for the various fimbriae. An enzyme-linked immunosorbent assay has been developed to measure directly the presence of K88 and K99 fimbriae-expressing bacteria in feces. Such a method eliminates many of the problems inherent in the analysis of feces for fimbriated bacteria.

A more reliable method to verify the clinical diagnosis of enterotoxigenic *E. coli*-induced diarrhea is to quantitate the number of *E. coli* in the small intestine. Normally, there should be very few *E. coli* in such sites, especially in the jejunum, and the presence of large numbers of bacteria in these locations is highly suggestive of enterotoxigenic *E. coli* disease. Samples are plated onto different media chosen to promote the expression of the various fimbriae, and colonies are picked and tested with the monospecific anti-fimbriae sera. Examination of stained smears of the contents of the small intestine is another method based upon the increased numbers of enterotoxigenic *E. coli* in this location; finding >100 per oil immersion field implies $>10^6$/ml of contents. Although this method lacks specificity, it strengthens the diagnosis.

Fluorescent-labeled antibody techniques provide the easiest method used and are probably the most reliable except for demonstration of the toxin. Smears of scrapings taken from the small intestine are flooded with antisera that are specific for the various fimbriae. After treatment with fluorescent-labeled secondary antiserum, preparations are examined for labeled bacteria adhering to the epithelial cells.

Enterotoxin production by isolated strains of *E. coli* is best detected by utilizing an ELISA test specific for ST and LT. This test is reputed to detect 140 pg/ml of ST (>100 times more sensitive than the suckling mouse assay) and 290 pg/ml of LT.

E. coli containing the genes encoding enterotoxin (LT, ST) can be detected by using DNA probes or polymerase chain reaction (PCR) primers specific for the corresponding base sequences encoding a specific trait (e.g., an adhesin or an enterotoxin). Such probes or primers have been used to detect the genes (in bacteria) in feces as well as in culture.

Demonstration of Attaching and Effacing Strains

The presence of genes encoding shiga-like toxins can be determined by specific DNA probes or by PCR. More cumbersome is the demonstration of cytotoxin activity for tissue culture cells (vero cells).

The demonstration of attaching and effacing strains as the cause of disease in the live animal is more difficult. Aside from biopsy of intestinal mucosa and the finding of attaching and effacing lesions, detection of genes associated with EPEC/EHEC, *eaeA*, *bfp*, or *slt* encoding intimin, bundle-forming pilus, or shiga-like toxin have been used (specific DNA probes or PCR with sequence specific primers), or function assays testing for SLT activity for tissue culture cells. Fecal isolates obtained from a selective medium (e.g., MacConkey agar) can be tested for the genes or production of shiga-like toxin in culture supernatants that are tested for cytotoxicity for tissue culture cells. Most of these isolates have been shown to produce urease, an uncommon trait for *E. coli*. *E. coli* O157:H7 does not ferment sorbitol. MacConkey agar containing this sugar instead of lactose is used to examine feces for the presence of sorbitol negative isolates, which are then tested for antiserum specific for O157 and/or H7.

Demonstration of Strains Producing Invasive Disease

The microbiological diagnosis of invasive disease is based upon the demonstration of *E. coli* in normally sterile sites or locations — joint, bone marrow, spleen, or blood. In fowl, the same sites are cultured, plus those grossly affected (lung, air sac). Dead in-shell embryos are cultured. Culture of the liver is to be avoided even though the Kupffer cells remove bacteria from the blood, because retrograde movement of enteric bacteria during the agonal stages of the disease complicates the microbiologic findings.

Demonstration of Strains Producing Edema Disease

The microbiological diagnosis of edema disease depends upon the isolation and demonstration of certain serotypes that have been shown to play a role in this disease. The characteristic gross and microscopic tissue changes make this disease relatively easier to diagnose pathologically than microbiologically.

TREATMENT, CONTROL, AND PREVENTION

Treatment of an animal that has diarrhea due to an infectious cause centers on correcting fluid and electrolyte imbalances. If the animal is in shock due to cardiovascular collapse, then the fluid and electrolytes (sodium bicarbonate, KCl) are given IV; if not, oral electrolyte solutions are given. Since the animals are acidotic, sodium bicarbonate is included. Adding glucose to oral electrolytes will enhance the absorption of the sodium ions being excreted. The use of antimicrobials is controversial. Because the concentration of antimicrobic achievable (and available) in the lumen of the bowel is not known, the results of in vitro susceptibility tests to guide therapy are of doubtful reliability. Administration of non-absorbable antimicrobics (such as neomycin) will sufficiently reduce the numbers of *E. coli* in the upper small bowel to allow correction of fluid and electrolyte imbalances. Such reduction occurs even though in vitro tests show that strains of *E. coli* commonly test "resistant" to neomycin. The fact that in vitro tests measure susceptibility to microgram amounts whereas milligram amounts may be available locally accounts for the discrepancy.

Antimicrobial agents, fluid, and electrolyte augmentation are necessary to successfully treat septicemic disease produced by invasive strains of *E. coli*. Invasive disease results in an endotoxemia progressing to a lactic acidosis because of decreased organ perfusion secondary to hypotension and disseminated intravascular coagulation. This should be taken into account when the electrolyte replacement is chosen. Antimicrobial agents should be chosen according to susceptibility trends in the practice area. Usually *E. coli* isolated from farm animals are susceptible to gentamicin or amikacin, trimethoprim-sulfonamides, and ceftiofur. They are usually resistant to tetracyclines, streptomycin, sulfonamides, ampicillin, and kanamycin. The severity of the signs of endotoxemia has been reduced experimentally by administering antibodies to the lipid A portion of the LPS.

Prevention and control of the enteric diseases produced by pathogenic strains of *E. coli* are one and the same. The key is sound husbandry practices. It is important that the dam be exposed to the antigenic determinants of the various virulence factors expressed on or by the infecting strains. Exposure can be provided naturally by placing the dam into the environment in which parturition will take place or artificially by vaccinating the dam with preparations containing the antigenic determinants perceived to be a threat to the newborn. Commercially produced preparations containing monoclonal antibodies to the adhesins (for ETEC) can be given orally to the neonatal animal. Although this practice will not significantly reduce the incidence of diarrhea, it will reduce the severity and mortality.

SELECTED REFERENCES

Bearson S, Bearson B, Foster JW. Acid stress responses in enterobacteria. FEMS Microbiol Lett 1997;147:173.

Dean-Nystrom EA, Bosworth BT, Cray WC, Moon HW. Pathogenicity of *Escherichia coli* O157:H7 in the intestines of neonatal calves. Infect Immun 1997;65:1842.

Falbo V, Pace R, Picci L, et al. Isolation and nucleotide sequence of the gene encoding cytotoxic necrotizing factor 1 of *Escherichia coli*. Infect Immun 1993;61:4909.

Fasano A. Cellular microbiology: how enteric pathogens socialize with their intestinal host. ASM News 1997;63:259.

Finlay BB, Falkow S. Common themes in microbial pathogenicity revisited. Microbiol Molec Biol Rev 1997;61:136.

Fiorentini C, Donelli G, Matarrese P, et al. *Escherichia coli* cytotoxic necrotizing factor 1: evidence for induction of actin assembly by constitutive activation of the p21 rho GTPase. Infect Immun 1995;63:3936.

Francis DH. Use of immunofluorescence, Gram's staining, histologic examination, and seroagglutination in the diagnosis of porcine colibacillosis. Am J Vet Res 1983;4:1884.

Gyimah JE, Panigraphy B. Adhesin-receptor interactions mediating the attachment of pathogenic *Escherichia coli* to chicken tracheal epithelium. Avian Dis 1988;32:74.

Holland RE. Some infectious causes of diarrhea in young farm animals. Clin Microbiol Rev 1990;3:345.

Johnson JR. Virulence factors in *Escherichia coli* urinary tract infections. Clin Microbiol Rev 1991;4:80.

Kaper JB, Morris JG, Levine MM. Cholera. Clin Microbiol Rev 1995;8:48.

Karmali MA. Infection by verotoxin-producing *Escherichia coli*. Clin Microbiol Rev 1989;2:15.

Kenny B, DeVinney R, Stein M, et al. Enteropathogenic *E. coli* (EPEC) transfers its receptor for intimate adherence into mammalian cells. Cell 1997;91:511.

Lariviere S, Lallier R, Morin M. Evaluation of various methods for the detection of enteropathogenic *Escherichia coli* in diarrheic calves. Am J Vet Res 1979;40:130.

Lee CA. Pathogenicity islands and the evolution of bacterial pathogens. Infect Agents Dis 1996;5:1.

Li Z, Taylor-Blake B, Light AR, Goy MF. Guanylin, an endogenous ligand for C-type guanylate cyclase, is produced by goblet cells in the rat intestine. Gastroenterology 1995;109:1863.

Nataro JP, Kaper JB. Diarrheagenic *Escherichia coli*. Clin Microbiol Rev 1998;11:142.

Oberman L. Enteric infections caused by non-enterotoxigenic *Escherichia coli* in animals: occurrence and pathogenicity mechanisms. A review. Vet Microbiol 1987;14:33.

Patti JM, Allen BL, McGavin MJ, Hook M. MSCRAMM-mediated adherence of microorganisms to host tissues. Annu Rev Microbiol 1994;48:585.

Sears CL, Kaper JB. Enteric bacterial toxins: mechanisms of action and linkage to intestinal secretion. Microbiol Rev 1996;60:167.

10 Salmonella

Dwight C. Hirsh

Genetically the genus *Salmonella* constitutes a single species. In recognition of its epidemiologic and pathogenic diversity, each of the more than 2000 serologic variants (serotypes, serovars) is treated and has been named like a species. Each is capable of producing disease of the gastrointestinal tract as well as septicemia.

DESCRIPTIVE FEATURES

Cellular Anatomy and Composition

There is one capsular type, Vi (for virulence), though most do not produce a capsule. The antigenic composition of the polysaccharide portion of the lipopolysaccharide (LPS) in part determines the species. The kind and number of sugars together with the linkage between them determine the antigenic determinants comprising the O-antigens of the particular isolate. The O-antigens, together with the antigenic determinants on the surface of the flagella (H-antigens) that are possessed by most salmonellae, help serologically to define an isolate as to species (Table 10.1). This classification scheme is called the *Kauffman-White* schema.

Cellular Products of Medical Interest

RNA polymerase containing RpoS preferentially transcribes genes responsible for acid tolerance (survival at pH < 5) and regulates genes found on Spv plasmids.

There are at least three different adhesins implicated in the interaction between salmonellae and the target cell (M cell, intestinal epithelial cell). These adhesins are the type 1 (so-called common fimbria encoded by the *fim* gene), the "plasmid encoded fimbria" (encoded by the *pef* gene), and the "long polar fimbriae" (encoded by the *lpf* gene). All three have been shown to be responsible for adhesion to various mammalian cell lines, with adhesin encoded by *lpf* having affinity for M cells.

"Invasin" genes encode proteins that are involved with uptake of salmonellae by the target cell(s). The gene product induces membrane "ruffles" that follow the rearrangement of the actin cytoskeleton following activation of the small GTP-binding protein, CDC42. Salmonellae become trapped in these ruffles and become interiorized. The "invasin" genes (*sip*, for *Salmonella* invasion protein) are located in a "pathogenicity island" on the *Salmonella* chromosome.

Members of the genus *Salmonella* secrete exotoxins. Three such toxins have been described, each affecting the target cell (usually an epithelial cell of the intestine). One deregulates cyclic nucleotide synthesis by ribosylation (an LT-like toxin), another interrupts protein synthesis, and a third has phospholipase A (PLA) activity. The enterotoxin, Stn (*Salmonella* enterotoxin), differs from cholera toxin and LT by being a biologically active peptide rather than being composed of subunits, even though antibodies to cholera toxin are neutralizing. Stn, however, produces increased levels of cAMP with resultant ion and fluid flow into the lumen of the bowel, resulting in diarrhea. The cytotoxin results in death of the cell target subsequent to cessation of protein synthesis. Death of the target could result in absorption and secretion abnormalities that would be manifest by diarrhea. And finally, the protein with PLA activity would result in fluid flow by virtue of its activity on the arachidonic acid pathway. The role of any of these toxins in the production of diarrhea is unclear.

Salmonellae produce siderophores when growing in iron-limiting conditions.

Plasmids of various sizes have been associated with virulence in salmonellae. The most notable is a family of large (approximately 50 to 100 kilobases [kb]) plasmids, termed *Salmonella virulence plasmids (Spv plasmids),* that are found within those species of salmonellae with potential to produce disseminated disease. Some of the genes (Spv genes) carried by these plasmids are necessary for intracellular growth and are regulated in part by RNA polymerase containing the stationary phase sigma factor, RpoS. Other genes on these plasmids are responsible for serum resistance and may be involved with adherence and invasion of the cellular target.

The transcriptional regulator, *SlyA* (for *salmolysin*), is responsible for survival of salmonellae within macrophages, perhaps affording protection from the toxic products generated by oxygen-dependent pathways.

The products of the *phoP/phoQ* operon appear responsible for resistance of salmonellae to defensins found in the lysosomal granules of phagocytic cells.

ECOLOGY

Reservoir

The reservoir for members of the genus *Salmonella* is the gastrointestinal tract of warm- and cold-blooded animals. Sources of infection include contaminated soil,

Table 10.1. Representative Antigenic Formulas for Salmonellae

O-group	Species	Antigenic Formula[a]
B	S. typhimurium	**1,4,5,12**:i:1,2
B	S. agona	**4,12**:f,g,s:-
D	S. dublin	**1,9,12**:g,p:-
E	S. anatum	**3,10**:e,h:1,6
G	S. worthington	**1,13,23**:z:1,w

[a] O-antigens: boldface numerals. Phase 1 H-antigen: lowercase letter. Phase 2 H-antigen: numeral (or lowercase letter).

vegetation, water, and components of animal feeds (such as bone meal, meat meal, and fish meal), particularly those containing milk-, meat-, or egg-derived constituents, and the feces of infected animals. Lizards and snakes (usually asymptomatic) are commonly infected, sometimes with several serotypes.

Transmission

Infection occurs following the ingestion of viable salmonellae. Disease may follow infection immediately; in an animal already infected, disease may follow a change in the intestinal environment. The outcome of the interaction between host and *Salmonella* depends upon the state of the colonization resistance of the host, the infectious dose, and the particular species of *Salmonella*.

Pathogenesis

Stationary phase salmonellae appear best suited to initiate disease, because under these conditions, RNA polymerase containing the alternative sigma factor, RpoS, initiates transcription of genes responsible for acid tolerance and subsequent survival through the stomach. Also, RNA polymerase containing RpoS is a positive regulator for the genes found on the Spv plasmids.

The target cells are primarily the M cells atop the lymphoid nodules and the epithelial cells of the distal small intestine and the upper large bowel. If the target cell is "vacant" relative to the numbers of salmonellae, disease may result. Vacancy of the target cell depends upon the status of the normal flora. If the flora is disrupted (stress, antibiotics), then the infectious dose does not have to be as high for salmonellae to gain access to the target cell. It appears that the M cell is the preferred target, and it is this cell that is affected first. Adhesion is the first step in the disease process, mediated by adhesins encoded by one or more of the described adhesins *fim, pef, lpf* or by others yet to be determined. Following adhesion, salmonellae are interiorized by the induction of membrane ruffles in the target cells that are triggered by the *sip* gene product. Ruffle formation also results in the activation of phospholipase C, subsequent increases in intracellular calcium, activation of protein kinase C, and phosphorylation of the proteins of the chloride ion channels and membrane associated ion transport proteins involved in NaCl absorption. These events lead to diarrhea. The

target cell is irreversibly damaged by this interaction, undergoing apoptosis. Salmonellae are now found in the lymph nodule and submucosal tissue. At either location, an inflammatory response is initiated with influx of polymorphonuclear neutrophil leukocytes (PMNs) and macrophages being evident. The influx may be reflected in a transient peripheral neutropenia. Macrophages within the nodule are also involved. The PMN is highly efficient in phagocytosing and destroying salmonellae, the macrophage less so. If the immune status of the host and the characteristics of the salmonellae are such, the infectious process is arrested at this stage. Diarrhea secondary to the inflammatory response, activation of protein kinase C, or as a consequence of a protein with enterotoxic-like affect (Stn, the cytotoxin, or protein with PLA activity) results. The signs are abdominal discomfort and diarrhea with evidence of cellular death (blood, cellular debris, and inflammatory cells).

If the infecting strain of *Salmonella* has properties that allow dissemination (Spv plasmid encoding ability to grow intracellularly and serum resistance; PhoQ/PhoP system allowing resistance to defensins; SlyA allowing resistance to oxygen-dependent by-products), septicemia may result. The likelihood of this occurring is increased if immune status of the host is diminished. *Salmonella* disseminate and multiply within phagocytic cells (macrophages mainly) within phagosomes. Not only are the invasive strains better able to withstand the lysosomal contents, some "sort" to phagosomes that do not fuse with lysosomes. The presenting signs are usually, but not always, septicemia and shock. Strains producing this form of disease escape destruction by the host and multiply within macrophages of the liver and spleen, as well as intravascularly. During the dissemination process, salmonellae are occasionally outside of the intracellular environment and therefore at risk from the formation of membrane attack complexes on their surfaces. This occurrence is discouraged by at least two mechanisms: a product of the Spv plasmid and the length of the O-repeat unit of the LPS (there is a direct correlation between O-repeat length and virulence).

Invasive salmonellae are capable of secreting a siderophore, enterobactin, that removes iron from the iron-binding proteins of the host, although it is doubtful whether this is needed within the cells of the host.

Multiplication of the organism results in endotoxemia (see Chapter 9), which accounts for most signs and the course of illness.

Salmonellosis is a significant disease of ruminants, mainly cattle. The disease affects young (usually 4 to 6 weeks of age) as well as adult animals. Animals in feedlots are commonly affected. The disease may be a septicemia or be limited to the enteric tract. Pneumonia, hematogenously acquired, is a common presenting sign in calves with septicemia due to *S. dublin*. Abortion may follow septicemia. *S. typhimurium, S. dublin,* and *S. newport* are the serotypes commonly isolated from cattle, *S. typhimurium* the serotype from sheep.

Salmonellosis in swine can present as an acute, fulminating septicemia or as a chronic debilitating intestinal disease. The form depends upon the strain of *Salmonella*, the dose, and the colonization resistance of the infected animal. The disease is seen most often in pigs that have been stressed. Such conditions occur often in feeder pigs, an age group in which salmonellosis commonly occurs. *S. typhimurium* and *S. cholerae-suis* are the predominant serotypes.

Adult horses are most commonly affected with *Salmonella*. The pattern is diarrhea, though septicemia is seen occasionally. Colic, gastrointestinal surgery, and antimicrobial agents predispose the horse to the development of clinical signs. The agent is either carried normally (as in approximately 3% of clinically normal horses) or acquired from other sources (e.g., a veterinary hospital). *S. typhimurium* and *S. anatum* are most commonly isolated.

Salmonellosis is uncommon in dogs and cats, although carriage is reportedly high in clinically normal pound dogs (upwards of 35%). When outbreaks occur they are usually associated with a common source, such as contaminated dog food. *Salmonella* should be high on the microbiological differential list for cats with signs of septicemia.

Epidemiology

Salmonella spp. are ubiquitous geographically and zoologically. Some serotypes are relatively host-specific (*S. dublin* — cattle; *S. typhisuis* — swine; *S. pullorum* — fowl) while others, notably *S. typhimurium, S. anatum*, and *S. newport*, affect a wide host range among which feral birds and rodents play important roles in interspecific dissemination of infection. Long periods of asymptomatic and convalescent shedding ensure widespread, unchecked distribution of the organisms.

Clinical outbreaks are correlated with depressed immune states, as in newborn animals (calves, foals) and stressed adults — for example, parturient cows, equine surgical patients, and swine with systemic viral diseases. All animals are at increased risk of developing disease if their normal flora is disrupted (stress, antibiotics). These circumstances render animals susceptible to exogenous exposure or activation of silent infections.

Humans appear to be susceptible to all *Salmonella* serotypes, the most important source for which are animals and their by-products. Poultry and poultry products (eggs) are a major source of *Salmonella* in humans. *Salmonella enteriditis* (e.g., phage type 4) is especially adapted for egg transmission. Whether a person develops disease following ingestion of salmonellae from the environment depends upon the dose of organisms, the serotype of *Salmonella,* and the colonization resistance of the infected individual. *Salmonella typhimurium* is most common, usually producing gastroenteritis. Some serotypes have greater invasion potential — for example, *S. cholerae-suis* (from swine), *S. typhimurium* DT104 (from cattle) and *S. dublin* (infected milk). Asymptomatic reptiles have become an important source of *Salmonella* in humans.

IMMUNOLOGIC ASPECTS

Protection depends upon specific and nonspecific immunological factors and microbiological defense mechanisms. At the level of the target cell, disease is prevented by an intact colonization resistance (see Chapter 2). Whether infection can be prevented is not known.

Adherence to the target cell is prevented by antibodies specific for surface structures of *Salmonella*, possibly fimbriae. The newborn is protected passively by ingesting specific sIgA or IgG_1 (bovine). The immunologically mature animal is protected by exudation of specific immunoglobulins (IgM and IgG) at the site of invasion or by the production of secretory immunoglobulins.

Another, more novel approach has been to feed animals microorganisms that out-compete salmonellae for niches along the gastrointestinal tract. *Competitive exclusion*, as this phenomenon is called, may be quite useful because, theoretically, salmonellae of any serotype would be excluded as long as they shared the same niche as the competing strain.

Antibodies in the circulation act as opsonins and promote the phagocytosis of the organism. Destruction of the salmonellae that have been phagocytosed follows the immunological activation of the macrophages by specifically stimulated lymphocytes (T cells). NK cells will lyse *Salmonella*-infected cells.

Acquired immunity revolves around activation of macrophages, which takes place as follows. After initial interaction between salmonella and macrophage, IL-12 is released by the affected macrophage. IL-12 activates the T_{H1} subset of T helper cells (see Chapter 2). This subset secretes, among other cytokines, interferon gamma, which activates macrophages. Activated macrophages are efficient killers of intracellular salmonellae.

Artificial immunization against salmonellae is difficult. Bacterins have had limited success. Apparently, they do not stimulate strong cellular immunity, even though abundant antibody is produced. Antibodies that are produced locally or passed in colostrum or milk interfere with adsorption to the target cell and protect against disease. Macrophages can be activated and antibody production stimulated in response to modified live vaccines. If given orally, these vaccines stimulate local secretory immunity and cell-mediated activation of phagocytic cells. Aromatic-dependent mutants of *Salmonella* show promise as effective modified live vaccines, especially for calves. *aroA* mutants of *Salmonella* cannot multiply within the host since vertebrate tissue does not contain the needed precursors for aromatic acid synthesis.

LABORATORY DIAGNOSIS

In cases of intestinal infection, fecal samples are collected; in systemic disease, a blood sample is collected for standard blood culture. Spleen and bone marrow are cultured for the salmonellae responsible for postmortem diagnosis of systemic salmonellosis.

Fresh samples are placed onto one or more selective media, including MacConkey agar, XLD agar, Hektoen enteric medium, and brilliant green agar. For enrichment, Selenite F, tetrathionate, or gram-negative broth (GN) is recommended.

Salmonellae appear as lactose-nonfermenting colonies on lactose-containing media (lactose-fermenting strains of *Salmonella* have been reported, but these are rarely encountered). Since most serotypes of salmonellae produce H_2S, colonies on iron-containing media (e.g., XLD agar) will have a black center. Suspicious colonies can be tested directly with polyvalent anti-*Salmonella* antiserum or inoculated into differential media and then tested with antisera.

To cultivate salmonellae from tissue, blood agar can be used.

Definitive identification involves determination of somatic and flagellar antigens and possibly bacteriophage type.

Various *Salmonella*-specific DNA probes and primers for PCR have been developed for detection in samples (food, feces, water) containing other microorganisms.

TREATMENT, CONTROL, AND PREVENTION

Nursing care is the principal treatment for the enteric form of salmonellosis. The use of antimicrobial agents is controversial. Some studies show that antibiotics do not alter the course of the disease. In addition, there is evidence that antibiotics promote the carrier state and select for resistant strains. Proponents of antibiotic usage recommend a member of the fluoroquinolone class of drug (e.g., enrofloxacin or ciprofloxacin) in nonfood animal species and human patients.

Treatment of the systemic form of salmonellosis includes nursing care and appropriate antimicrobial therapy as determined by retrospectively acquired susceptibility data. Since salmonellae survive in the phagocytic cell, the antimicrobial drug should be one that penetrates the cell. Examples of those that distribute in this manner include ampicillin, enrofloxacin, trimethoprim-sulfonamides, and chloramphenicol. Treatment options may be compromised due to acquisition of R plasmids encoding resistance to multiple antibiotics.

The disease is controlled through strict attention to protocols designed to curtail the spread to susceptible animals of any contagious agent found in feces. Artificial immunization with modified live products has shown promise (e.g., *aroA* mutants, see above). Attempts have been made to treat and prevent the endotoxemia produced by the systemic form of the disease by administering serum containing antibodies to the core LPS. Likewise, the administration of J5, a rough variant of *E. coli*, has been shown to stimulate the production of antibody to the core LPS. Both methods appear to prevent and control the signs of disease produced by systemic salmonellosis.

SALMONELLOSIS OF POULTRY

"Paratyphoid" is salmonellosis produced by any of the motile strains of *Salmonella* (all but *S. pullorum* and

S. gallinarum are motile). The disease produces its highest losses in the first 2 weeks of life as a septicemic disease. Survivors become asymptomatic excretors.

Infection is through ingestion. The source is usually feces or fecally contaminated materials (litter, fluff, water).

Diagnosis is made by culturing the organism from affected tissue (spleen, joints) from birds that had been showing clinical signs of disease. It is more difficult to detect an asymptomatic carrier because such carriers only periodically shed the organism in the feces. Some have suggested that culture of fluff and litter could be used to detect carrier flocks.

Treatment does not eliminate carriers, although it might control mortality. Treatment regimens have included araparcin, lincomycin, furazolidone, streptomycin, and gentamicin. Exclusion of salmonellae by feeding "cocktails" of normal flora has been used with some success to reduce the number of salmonellae shed by carrier birds.

Pullorum Disease

Pullorum disease, caused by *S. pullorum*, is rare in the United States but not in the rest of the world. The disease has almost been eliminated in the United States due to a breeding flock testing program.

Salmonella pullorum infects the ova of turkeys and chickens. Thus, the embryo is already infected when the egg is hatched. The hatchery environment is contaminated following hatching of an infected egg, leading to infection of other chicks and poults. Mortality is due to septicemia and is greatest in the second to third week of life. Surviving birds carry the bacterium and may pass it to their offspring. It is difficult to detect infected breeding hens by bacteriologic means. Agglutination titers, produced 3 to 10 days after infection, are used to detect carrier birds.

This disease is controlled by eliminating infected breeding birds detected serologically. Treatment with antimicrobial agents (mainly sulfonamides) reduces mortality in infected flocks.

Fowl Typhoid

Fowl typhoid, caused by *S. gallinarum*, is an acute septicemic or chronic disease of domesticated adult birds, mainly chickens. Fowl typhoid is rare now in the United States due to control programs.

The disease is diagnosed by culturing the organism from liver or spleen. It is treated with antimicrobial agents, mainly sulfonamides (sulfaquinoxaline) and nitrofurans. It is controlled by management and eliminating infected birds. A bacterin made from a rough variant of *S. gallinarum*, 9R, has been shown to decrease mortality.

Avian Arizonosis

Salmonella arizonae ("paracolon," *Arizona hinshawii*) is most often isolated from reptiles and fowl, although this species can be isolated from any animal. Turkeys are most commonly affected. There are 55 serologic types of *S. arizonae* affecting fowl, with type 7:1,7,8 most commonly isolated in the United States.

Salmonella arizonae is maintained in turkey flocks via hatching eggs, which become infected following ingestion of *S. arizonae* by the hen. It is also spread by feces.

Diagnosis is made by culturing *S. arizonae* from the liver, spleen, blood, lungs, or kidneys of affected birds, or from dead poults and hatch debris.

Most serotypes of *S. arizonae* possess R plasmids, which sometimes makes it difficult to prevent and treat this disease. Various antimicrobial agents such as furazolidone and sulfamerazine added to feed have shown some success in lowering mortality. Injection of day-old poults with gentamicin or spectinomycin decreases mortality, but survivors still harbor (and shed) the organism.

Control measures should be aimed at prevention rather than treatment. Because of the multiplicity of serotypes, no effective vaccine is available.

SELECTED REFERENCES

Bäumler AJ, Tsolis RM, Bowe FA, et al. The *pef* fimbrial operon of *Salmonella typhimurium* mediates adhesion to murine small intestine and is necessary for fluid accumulation in the infant mouse. Infect Immun 1996;64:61.

Bäumler AJ, Tsolis RM, Heffron F. Contribution of fimbrial operons to attachment to and invasion of epithelial cell lines by *Salmonella typhimurium*. Infect Immun 1996;64:1862.

Bäumler AJ, Tsolis RM, Heffron F. The *lpf* fimbrial operon mediates adhesion of *Salmonella typhimurium* to murine Peyer's patches. Proc Nat Acad Sci USA 1996;93:279.

Bearson S, Bearson B, Foster JW. Acid stress responses in enterobacteria. FEMS Microbiol Lett 1997;147:173.

Bohnhoff M, Drake BL, Miller CR. Effect of streptomycin on susceptibility of intestinal tract to experimental *Salmonella* infection. Proc Soc Exp Biol Med 1954;86:132.

Chin LM, Hobbie S, Galan JE. Requirement of CDC42 for *Salmonella*-induced cytoskeletal and nuclear responses. Science 1996;274:2115.

Cohen ND, Martin LJ, Simpson RB, et al. Comparison of polymerase chain reaction and microbiological culture for detection of salmonellae in equine feces and environmental samples. Am J Vet Res 1996;57:780.

Conlan JW. Critical roles of neutrophils in host defense against experimental systemic infections of mice by *Listeria monocytogenes*, *Salmonella typhimurium*, and *Yersinia enterocolitica*. Infect Immun 1997;65:630.

Fasano A. Cellular microbiology: how enteric pathogens socialize with their intestinal host. ASM News 1997;63:259.

Finlay BB, Falkow S. Common themes in microbial pathogenicity revisited. Microbiol Molec Biol Rev 1997;61:136.

Guiney DG, Fang FC, Krause M, Libby S. Plasmid-mediated virulence genes in non-typhoid *Salmonella* serovars. FEMS Microbiol Lett 1994;124:1.

Hermant D, Menard R, Arricau N, et al. Functional conservation of the *Salmonella* and *Shigella* effectors of entry into epithelial cells. Molec Microbiol 1985;17:781.

Hird DW, Pappaioanou M, Smith BR. Case-control study of risk factors associated with isolation of *Salmonella saintpaul* in hospitalized horses. Am J Epidemiol 1984;120:852.

Hoiseth SK, Stocker BAD. Aromatic-dependent *Salmonella typhimurium* are non-virulent and effective as live vaccines. Nature 1981;291:238.

Ikeda JS, Hirsh DC. A common plasmid encoding resistance to ampicillin, chloramphenicol, gentamicin, and trimethoprim-sulfadiazine in two serotypes of *Salmonella* isolated during an outbreak of equine salmonellosis. Am J Vet Res 1985;46:769.

Ikeda JS, Hirsh DC, Jang SS, Biberstein EL. Characteristics of *Salmonella* isolated from animals at a veterinary medical teaching hospital. Am J Vet Res 1986;47:232.

Joiner KA, Brown EJ, Frank MM. Complement and bacteria: chemistry and biology in host defense. Annu Rev Immunol 1984;2:461.

Jones BD, Falkow S. Salmonellosis: host immune responses and bacterial virulence determinants. Annu Rev Immunol 1996;14:533.

Kaufmann SHE. Immunity to intracellular bacteria. Annu Rev Immunol 1993;11:129.

Kogut MH, Tellez GI, McGruder ED, et al. Heterophils are decisive components in the early responses of chickens to *Salmonella enteritidis* infections. Microb Pathogen 1994;16:141.

Lee CA. Pathogenicity islands and the evolution of bacterial pathogens. Infect Agents Dis 1996;5:1.

Lee IS, Lin J, Hall HK, et al. The stationary-phase sigma factor σ^S (RpoS) is required for a sustained acid tolerance response in virulent *Salmonella typhimurium*. Molec Microbiol 1995;17:155.

Monack DM, Raupach B, Hromockyj AE, Falkow S. *Salmonella typhimurium* invasion induces apoptosis in infected macrophages. Proc Nat Acad Sci USA 1996;93:9833.

Mutharia LM, Crockford G, Bogard WC, Hancock REW. Monoclonal antibodies specific for *Escherichia coli* J5 lipopolysaccharide: cross-reaction with other gram-negative bacterial species. Infect Immun 1984;45:631.

Myers LL, Firehammer BD, Border MM, Shoop DS. Prevalence of enteric pathogens in the feces of healthy beef calves. Am J Vet Res 1984;45:1544.

Nurmi E, Nuotio L, Schneitz C. The competitive exclusion concept: development and future. Int J Food Microbiol 1992;15:237.

Robertsson JA, Lindberg AA, Hoiseth S, Stocker BAD. *Salmonella typhimurium* infection in calves: protection and survival of virulent challenge bacteria after immunization with live or inactivated vaccines. Infect Immun 1983;41:742.

Sears CL, Kaper JB. Enteric bacterial toxins: mechanisms of action and linkage to intestinal secretion. Microbiol Rev 1996;60:167.

Smith BR, Reina-Guerra M, Hardy AJ. Prevalence and epizootiology of equine salmonellosis. J Am Vet Med Assoc 1978;172:353.

Smith BR, Reina-Guerra M, Stocker BAD, et al. Aromatic-dependent *Salmonella dublin* as a parenteral modified live vaccine for calves. Am J Vet Res 1984;45:2231.

Stone GG, Oberst RD, Hays MP, et al. Combined PCR-oligonucleotide ligation assay for rapid detection of *Salmonella* serovars. J Clin Microbiol 1995;33:2888.

Uhaa IJ, Hird DW, Hirsh DC, Jang SS. Case control study of risk factors associated with nosocomial *Salmonella krefeld* infection in dogs. Am J Vet Res 1988;49:1501.

van der Waaij D. Antibiotic choice: the importance of colonization resistance. Chichester, UK: Research Studies, 1983.

Werner SB, Humphrey GL, Kamei I. Association between raw milk and human *Salmonella dublin* infection. Br Med J 1979;2:238.

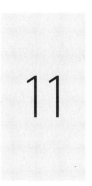

11   Shigella

Dwight C. Hirsh

Members of the genus *Shigella* cause bacillary dysentery in primates. The discussion that follows is limited to the disease in nonhuman primates. The disease occurs almost exclusively in captive primates and appears to be related to stressful situations (e.g., transportation, crowding) or immunological dysfunctions (e.g., simian acquired immunodeficiency syndrome). Humans may be affected by all four species of shigellae, whereas nonhuman primates are affected by *S. flexneri*, *S. boydii*, and *S. sonnei*.

DESCRIPTIVE FEATURES

Cellular Anatomy and Composition

Members of the genus *Shigella* do not produce a capsule nor flagella. There are four serotypes, identification of which is dependent upon the composition of the O-repeat units of the lipopolysaccharide (LPS). Each of the four serotypes has been given species designation. Within each species there are a number of serotypes (Table 11.1).

"Mannose-resistant" adhesins are produced.

Cellular Products of Medical Interest

Virulence factors produced by members of the genus *Shigella* are mainly encoded on large plasmids (termed *invasion plasmids*). These genes, for the most part, are regulated by at least six chromosomal genes. The plasmid gene products encode proteins (Mxi and Spa proteins) that are responsible for excretion of proteins (Ipa for *inva*sion *p*lasmid *a*ntigen; Ics for *inter*cellular *s*pread) that initiate *Shigella*–host cell interaction (IpaD), *Shigella*-induced uptake by the cell (IpaB, C), escape from the phagosome of affected cell (IpaB), focus of actin accumulation for intracellular spread (IcsA), and intercellular spread (IcsB).

Regulatory genes that "sense" environmental cues include *fur* (*f*erric *u*tilization *r*esponse-iron levels), temperature (*virR*, which is regulated by a "cold-shock protein," CspA), and osmotic pressure (*ompR/envZ*).

Two enterotoxins have been described, ShET1 (*Sh*igella *e*nterotoxin, chromosome) and a 63 kDa product of the *sen* gene (*S*higella *en*terotoxin, invasion plasmid). How these proteins elicit fluid secretion is not known.

Shigella dysenteriae is the only member of the group that has the genes necessary for production of shiga toxin. Shiga toxin is chromosomally encoded. The toxin is a protein of 70,000 MW composed of an A subunit (32,000 MW) and five identical B subunits (each about 7700 MW). The target cells for the toxin are the endothelial cells that line blood vessels. Receptors on these cells are recognized by the B subunit. The toxin, by way of the A subunit, inhibits peptide chain elongation at the level of the ribosome by affecting elongation factor 1-dependent processes. This action results in the death of the cell. The production of toxin is iron-regulated (by way of *fur*), more being produced in conditions of low iron concentration. The virulence of a particular strain or isolate is directly related to the amount of toxin produced.

RNA polymerase containing RpoS preferentially transcribes genes responsible for acid tolerance (survival at pH < 5), allowing safe transit through the stomach.

ECOLOGY

Reservoir

The reservoir for *Shigella* is the large bowel of clinically ill, recovered, or asymptomatic animals.

Transmission

The disease is transmitted by the fecal–oral route, but the infective dose is so small that fomites may play a role. Members of the genus *Shigella* are greatly influenced by the colonization resistance of the large bowel. Antimicrobial drugs, stress, or dietary changes will promote risk, either by promoting disease in the asymptomatic carrier animals or by lowering the oral dose needed for infection.

The mode of transmission of *S. flexneri* 4 associated with periodontal disease of nonhuman primates is unknown, but it is assumed to be feces.

Pathogenesis

Environmental cues trigger the expression and excretion of virulence proteins. The target cell appears to be the apical surface of M cells of the large intestine to which shigellae attach by way of IpaD. Cell-associated bacteria trigger uptake by initiating cytoskeletal changes by way of activation of small GTP-binding proteins of the Rho

Table 11.1.   Species of *Shigella*

Species	Group (Types)
S. dysenteriae	A (1–10)
S. flexneri	B (1–6)
S. boydii	C (1–15)
S. sonnei	D (1)

family that result in "ruffles" that entrap shigellae. Some of the shigellae within the vacuole are transported into the nodule, where the uptake is again triggered, but by macrophages within the nodule. Ingested shigellae may initiate apoptosis of the macrophage and/or other abnormalities reflected in a drop in concentration of intracellular adenosine triphosphate (ATP). Either effect results in the death of the macrophage. The liberated shigellae adhere to beta-integrins on the baso-lateral surface (the plasmid encoded adhesin, IpaD, associates with beta-integrins that are present on the baso-lateral surfaces of large intestinal epithelial cells) of the colonic epithelial cell and induce their own uptake as before. Shigellae escape the vacuole by secretion of a "hemolysin" (IpaB) that results in the deposition of the microorganism into the cytoplasm of the epithelial cell. Expression of IcsA and formation of actin at one pole of the bacterium results in intracellular movement. Movement appears to be more concentrated along actin "stress fibers" and shigellae with their actin "tails" move toward cadherin proteins marking intercellular bridges. Thus, shigellae move laterally. The double membrane resulting from movement between cells is lysed by IcsB. Cell death, by apoptosis and/or energy derangements results in inflammation. Likewise, extracellular shigellae also initiate inflammation (by virtue of their LPS). Transepithelial migration of polymorphonuclear neutrophil leukocytes (PMNs) is stimulated by LPS. NK cells have been implicated in lysis of infected epithelial cells, another inflammation-inducing process. Tissue destruction with numerous PMNs are the hallmarks of dysentery caused by shigellae. The origin of hemorrhage produced by non-shiga toxin-producing shigellae is not known.

Diarrhea is probably brought about by the activation of phospholipase C (perhaps due to "ruffle" formation) leading to increases in intracellular calcium ions, activation of protein kinase C and subsequent phosphorylation of proteins of the chloride ion channels and those of the membrane associated ion transport proteins involved in NaCl absorption.

The role of enterotoxin in this disease is unclear. The diarrhea, sometimes watery, may be caused by interactions of enterotoxin with small intestinal epithelial cells and in part be due to changes in the colonic epithelium brought about by the invasion/inflammatory process.

Shigella dysenteriae produces shiga toxin. This toxin damages submucosal endothelial cells (hemorrhage) and may cause the development of hemolytic uremic syndrome (HUS) (see Chapter 9).

Shigella flexneri 4 has been encountered in periodontal disease of monkeys. A causal role is suspected but undefined.

Epidemiology

The disease is seen almost exclusively in captive primates. Although human caretakers are susceptible to the species most often associated with nonhuman primates, there is little evidence that they become clinically ill or even infected. The reason for this apparent absence of transmission is not known.

IMMUNOLOGIC ASPECTS

Protection from bacillary dysentery is by specific secretory immunoglobulin found on the luminal side of the intestinal canal. These antibodies prevent adherence and subsequent uptake. Shigellae are serum-sensitive, and PMNs deal with them effectively. As a result, extracellular shigellae (outside of the M cell, macrophage, colonic epithelial cell) are dealt with by complement proteins in tissue fluids, and the inflammatory exudate containing complement proteins and PMNs.

Whether a nonhuman primate after infection and disease is resistant to reinfection (exacerbation) is not known. Reinfection or exacerbation occurs in human beings in stressful situations such as in prisoner-of-war camps. Bacterins given orally or parenterally have been ineffective. Some protection has been demonstrated following vaccination with avirulent, live oral vaccines. These are not universally available.

LABORATORY DIAGNOSIS

Rectal swabs or samples of feces obtained from the rectum are collected for laboratory diagnosis. Direct examination of stained smears of fecal material will reveal the presence of inflammatory cells, cellular debris, and red blood cells (RBCs). Such a finding is not diagnostic, however, since enteritis produced by *Campylobacter* results in the same signs. The presence of curved rods in the direct smear suggests that *Campylobacter* is the cause of the disease.

The sample is plated onto a selective medium that is less inhibitory than media for isolation of salmonellae. Suitable media include MacConkey agar, XLD agar, and Hektoen Enteric medium. SS agar is often too inhibitory for some strains of shigellae, and brilliant green does not work at all. For enrichment, GN broth is preferred. Selenite or tetrathionate broths do not enrich for shigellae.

Shigellae appear as lactose-nonfermenting colonies on lactose-containing media. Although some species (*S. sonnei* and *S. boydii* 9) ferment this sugar, not enough is fermented within the 24- to 48-hour incubation period to affect the selection of appropriate colonies for further testing. Suspicious colonies are tested directly with shigellae-specific antisera or inoculated into differential media and then tested with antisera.

TREATMENT, CONTROL, AND PREVENTION

Treatment of shigellosis involves nursing and supporting care. Antimicrobics are indicated in serious cases but not routinely since their use in an animal facility selects for resistant strains. Trimethoprim-sulfonamide, or a fluoroquinolone, is effective against most strains and these drugs do not disrupt the flora as much as others.

SELECTED REFERENCES

Bearson S, Bearson B, Foster JW. Acid stress responses in enterobacteria. FEMS Microbiol Lett 1997;147:173.

Beatty WL, Sansonetti PJ. Role of lipopolysaccharide in signaling to subepithelial polymorphonuclear leukocytes. Infect Immun 1997;65:4395.

Dehio C, Prévost M-C, Sansonetti PJ. Invasion of epithelial cells by *Shigella flexneri* induces tyrosine phosphorylation of cortactin by a pp60^{c-src}-mediated signalling pathway. EMBO J 1995;14:2471.

Fasano A. Cellular microbiology: how enteric pathogens socialize with their intestinal host. ASM News 1997;63:259.

Fasano A, Noriega F, Maneval D, et al. Shigella enterotoxin-1: an enterotoxin of *Shigella flexneri* 2a active in rabbit small intestine in vivo and in vitro. J Clin Invest 1995;95:2853.

Finlay BB, Falkow S. Common themes in microbial pathogenicity revisited. Microbiol Molec Biol Rev 1997;61:136.

Goldberg MB, Sansonetti PJ. *Shigella* subversion of the cellular cytoskeleton: a strategy for epithelial colonization. Infect Immun 1993;61:4941.

Griffiths E, Stevenson R, Hale TL, Formal SB. Synthesis of aerobactin and a 76,000-dalton iron regulated outer membrane protein by *Escherichia coli* K-12-*Shigella flexneri* hybrids and by enteroinvasive strains of *Escherichia coli*. Infect Immun 1985; 49:67.

Hale TL. Genetic basis of virulence in *Shigella* species. Microbiol Rev 1991;55:206.

Hentges DJ. Influence of pH on the inhibitory activity of formic and acetic acids for *Shigella*. J Bacteriol 1967;93:2029.

Lasa I, Cossart P. Actin-based bacterial motility: towards a definition of the minimal requirements. Trends Cell Biol 1996;6:109.

Nataro JP, Seriwatana J, Fasano A, et al. Identification and cloning of a novel plasmid-encoded enterotoxin of enteroinvasive *Escherichia coli* and *Shigella* strains. Infect Immun 1995;63: 4721.

O'Brien AD, Holmes RK. Shiga and shiga-like toxins. Microbiol Rev 1987;51:206.

Sansonetti RJ, Hale TL, Dammin GJ, et al. Alterations in the pathogenicity of *Escherichia coli* K-12 after transfer of plasmid and chromosomal genes from *Shigella flexneri*. Infect Immun 1983;39:1392.

Sears CL, Kaper JB. Enteric bacterial toxins: mechanisms of action and linkage to intestinal secretion. Microbiol Rev 1996;60: 167.

van der Waaij D. Antibiotic choice: the importance of colonization resistance. Chichester, UK: Research Studies, 1983.

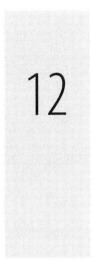

12

Non-Spore-Forming Obligate Anaerobes of the Alimentary Tract

Dwight C. Hirsh

Non-spore-forming obligate anaerobes are a component of approximately 33% of bacteriologically positive samples of pyonecrotic material obtained from normally sterile sites of animals. On average, there will be two species of obligate anaerobes admixed with facultative species in samples of such material.

Descriptive Features

Morphology and Staining

The non-spore-forming obligate anaerobes comprise a wide variety of gram-positive and gram-negative bacteria and include rods, cocci, filaments, and spiral organisms.

Cellular Anatomy and Composition

Carbohydrate-containing capsules, flagella, and fimbriae are expressed by some. The cell wall composition is the same as that of their facultative and aerobic counterparts.

Cellular Products of Medical Interest

Toxins and metabolic by-products with toxic activity have been demonstrated. These include a cytotoxin produced by *Fusobacterium necrophorum*, an enterotoxin-like entity secreted by *Bacteroides fragilis*, and succinic acid found to be inhibitory to polymorphonuclear neutrophil leukocytes (PMNs). Many produce proteolytic and other enzymes that may play a role in their pathogenic activities.

Growth Characteristics

Obligate anaerobes do not use oxygen as a final electron acceptor; in fact, molecular oxygen is toxic to this group of microbes. When exposed to molecular oxygen, obligate anaerobes form hydrogen peroxide and superoxide anions. These toxic molecules are formed from the interaction of oxygen with various flavoproteins within the bacterial cell. Unlike aerotolerant bacteria, obligate anaerobes do not produce superoxide dismutase, nor do

they usually produce catalase enzymes that break down superoxide to oxygen and hydrogen peroxide, or break down hydrogen peroxide to oxygen and water.

Ecology

Reservoir and Transmission

The non-spore-forming obligate anaerobes implicated in pyonecrotic processes are usually part of the normal flora, but they are sometimes transmitted by bites or other trauma involving contaminated fomites.

Pathogenesis

Disease results from the extension of the normal flora (both obligate and facultative anaerobic microorganisms) into a compromised site, either by contamination of a wound with nearby normal flora or from inoculation into tissue with contaminated instruments or teeth. The kind of microbes found in samples of such material reflect the site of injury or the microbial population of the inoculating agency. Proliferation of anaerobes depends on the establishment of anaerobic conditions by trauma, vascular breakdown, or concurrent infection with (facultative) aerobes.

Anaerobic bacteria cannot live in healthy tissue because they cannot survive in the presence of oxygen. In compromised tissue, inflammatory cells and co-inoculated facultative microorganisms lower the Eh (a measure of oxygen concentration) sufficiently for anaerobes to grow.

Anaerobes elicit inflammatory responses due to components of their cell wall (lipopolysaccharide, gram-negative species; peptidoglycan, gram-positive and gram-negative species). Some anaerobes produce capsules that, due to their chemistry, are potent inducers of abscess formation. There is some evidence that co-inoculated facultative microorganisms induce capsule production by anaerobes.

Synergy occurs between facultative aerobic and anaerobic microorganisms. Aside from triggering capsule

Table 12.1. Most Commonly Isolated Obligate Anaerobes

Gram-Negative Rods	Gram-Positive Cocci	Gram-Positive Rods
Bacteroides	*Peptostreptococcus*	*Clostridium*
Prevotella		
Porphyromonas		
Fusobacterium		

Table 12.2. Relative Frequency of Obligate Anaerobic Bacteria with Respect to Disease Processes

Process	Percentage with Anaerobe
Draining tract	40–50
Abscess	30–40
Pleural effusion	30–40
Pericardial effusion	30–40
Peritoneal effusion	20–30

formation, facultative species scavenge oxygen, curtail phagocytosis of the anaerobic component, and may produce enzymes (beta-lactamase, for example) that might protect a penicillin-susceptible facultative or obligate anaerobic partner (and vice versa).

The most commonly isolated species of obligate anaerobes are shown in Table 12.1. The most common sites or processes that contain obligate anaerobes are shown in Table 12.2.

Association of enterotoxin-secreting strains of *Bacteroides fragilis* with diarrhea in calves, lambs, piglets, and infant rabbits has been described.

IMMUNOLOGIC ASPECTS

Immune responses play a minor part in resolving the pyonecrotic processes involving obligate anaerobes.

LABORATORY DIAGNOSIS

Sample Collection

Anaerobic culture is time-consuming and expensive and should be used only when it holds a reasonable promise of supplying useful information. Material obtained from sites that possess a normal anaerobic flora (feces, oral cavity, vagina) is not usually cultured anaerobically. Routine anaerobic culture of urine specimens or ear, conjunctival, or nasal swabs is very rarely justified. Suppurative and necrotic processes are the most promising sources of clinically significant anaerobic bacteria.

Samples of fluids for anaerobic culture are collected in vessels containing little if any molecular oxygen. The easiest way is to collect the sample directly into a syringe and expel all the air. Materials collected onto swabs or

bronchial brushes must be placed in culture immediately or into an anaerobic environment (transport medium). Refrigeration is detrimental to recovery of anaerobic bacteria; thus, samples should not be placed at temperatures less than 4°C. However, most samples that contain obligate anaerobes contain facultative species as well. Facultative microorganisms grow in samples held at 25°C but not at 15°C (a temperature harmless to obligate anaerobes).

Direct Examination

Examination of stained smears prepared directly from the collected material may give valuable clues regarding the presence of anaerobic bacteria. Many obligate anaerobes have typical, unique morphologies: rods are usually narrow and thread-like in appearance, some having pointed ends or bulges. Most of the gram-negative species stain poorly with the saffranine used in the gram stain (thus will be pale staining in gram-stained smears). The material may have a very repugnant odor if anaerobes are present, whereas material without obligate anaerobes is usually not especially malodorous.

Isolation

Successful isolation depends on the care taken by the laboratory in shielding the bacteria from oxygen. If the sample is not processed immediately after collection, it must be held in a container free from oxygen, usually a container into which oxygen-free gas (e.g., O_2-free carbon dioxide) is flowing. The sample is plated onto a blood-containing medium (usually one with a brucella agar base) that has been freshly made and stored in an anaerobic environment. A special selective medium for isolating *B. fragilis* from feces contains polymyxin B, trichlosan, novobiocin, and nalidixic acid. After the plate has been inoculated, it is placed into an anaerobic environment and incubated at 37°C. The anaerobic environment is conveniently established by the interaction of a hydrogen-containing gas with the oxygen in the presence of a palladium catalyst in a closed container, such as in an anaerobic jar or in a glove box. A major advantage of an anaerobic glove box with a built-in incubator is that inoculated plates can be examined at any time without being exposed to oxygen.

Most obligate anaerobes grow slowly, especially during the early stages, and plates are not examined for the first 48 hours unless they can be examined in an O_2-free environment. Since facultative species will grow anaerobically, colonies growing in an anaerobic environment must be tested for aerotolerance.

Identification

After an isolate has been shown to be an obligate anaerobe, the genus to which it belongs is determined by shape, gram-staining characteristics, growth in the presence of various antibiotics, and metabolic by-products formed from various substrates, as determined by liquid-gas chromatography. Reactions in prereduced anaerobically sterilized media containing various substrates help determine the species. Miniaturized, prepared identification systems are commercially available. Gas chromatographic analysis of cell fatty acids is sometimes used to identify an isolate.

TREATMENT, CONTROL, AND PREVENTION

Treatment of infectious processes that contain an anaerobic component most importantly involve drainage and the use of antimicrobial agents.

Susceptibility data are usually not available for at least 48 to 72 hours after the sample is collected. Prior to this time, if the presence of obligate anaerobes is suggested by the clinical presentation, direct smear, and other circumstances (odor), one of the following can be used: penicillin (ampicillin, amoxicillin), chloramphenicol, tetracycline, metronidazole, and clindamycin. Though most anaerobes will test "susceptible" to trimethoprim-sulfonamides in vitro, this combination has unpredictable activity in vivo due to the presence of thymidine in necrotic material. The obligate anaerobes are resistant to all of the aminoglycoside antimicrobial agents as well as to the fluoroquinolones. Approximately 10% to 20% of the isolates, usually members of the *B. fragilis* group, will be resistant to the penicillins (penicillin G, ampicillin, amoxicillin) and first- and second-generation cephalosporins due to cephalosporinase, and often to tetracycline as well. Resistant isolates are susceptible to clavulanic acid-amoxicillin, clindamycin, metronidazole, and chloramphenicol. Antimicrobial therapy should be aimed at both the facultative and the obligate anaerobic microorganisms. Between 70% and 80% of pyonecrotic processes containing an obligate anaerobe will contain a facultative one as well. The most common are shown in Table 12.3.

Table 12.3. Facultative Microorganisms Found in Infectious Processes Containing Obligate Anaerobes

Animal Species	Facultative Microorganism
Dogs/cats	*Pasteurella*, enterics
Horse	Beta-*Streptococcus*, enterics
Ruminant	*Arcanobacterium* (*Actinomyces*) *pyogenes*, enterics

SELECTED REFERENCES

Berg JN, Fales WH, Scanlon CM. Occurrence of anaerobic bacteria in diseases of the dog and cat. Am J Vet Res 1979;40: 876.

Brook I. Pathogenesis and management of polymicrobial infections due to aerobic and anaerobic bacteria. Med Res Rev 1995;15:73.

Chambers FG, Koshy SS, Saidi RF, et al. *Bacteroides fragilis* toxin exhibits polar activity on monolayers of human intestinal epithelial cells (T84 cells) in vitro. Infect Immun 1997;65: 35612.

Chirino-Trejo JM, Prescott JE. The identification and antimicrobial susceptibility of anaerobic bacteria from pneumonic cattle lungs. Can J Comp Med 1983;47:270.

Hirsh DC, Indiveri MC, Jang SS, Biberstein EL. Changes in prevalence and susceptibility of obligate anaerobes in clinical veterinary practice. J Am Vet Med Assoc 1985;186:1086.

Hirsh DC, Jang SS. Antimicrobic susceptibility of bacterial pathogens from horses. In: Brumbaugh GW, Davis LE, eds. The veterinary clinics of North America. Philadelphia: WB Saunders, 1987:181.

Hirsh DC, Jang SS. Antimicrobial susceptibility of selected infectious agents from dogs. J Am Anim Hosp Assoc 1994;30: 487.

Indiveri MC, Hirsh DC. Susceptibility of obligate anaerobic bacteria to trimethoprim sulfamethoxazole. J Am Vet Med Assoc 1986;188:46.

Indiveri MC, Hirsh DC. Tissues and exudates contain sufficient thymidine for growth of anaerobic bacteria in the presence of inhibitory levels of trimethoprim-sulfamethoxazole. Vet Microbiol 1992;32:235.

Jang SS, Breher JE, Dabaco LA, Hirsh DC. Organisms isolated from dogs and cats with anaerobic infections and susceptibility to selected antimicrobial agents (1991–1996). J Am Vet Med Assoc 1997;210:1610.

Love DN, Johnson JL, Moore LVH. *Bacteroides* species from the oral cavity and oral-associated diseases of cats. Vet Microbiol 1989;19:275.

Myers LL, Firehammer BD, Shoop DS, Border MM. *Bacteroides fragilis*: a possible cause of acute diarrheal disease in newborn lambs. Infect Immun 1984;44:241.

Myers LL, Shoop DS, Firehammer BD, Border MM. Association of enterotoxigenic *Bacteroides fragilis* with diarrheal disease in calves. J Infect Dis 1985;152:1344.

Prescott JE. Identification of some anaerobic bacteria in non-specific anaerobic infections in animals. Can J Comp Med 1979;43:194.

Rotstein OD, Pruett TL, Fiegel VD, et al. Succinic acid, a metabolic byproduct of *Bacteroides* species, inhibits polymorphonuclear leukocyte function. Infect Immun 1985;48: 402.

13 Serpulina

Dwight C. Hirsh

Members of the genus *Serpulina* belong to the family *Spirochaetaceae*. *Serpulina hyodysenteriae*, is the causative agent of swine dysentery, a disease of actively growing pigs. *Serpulina pilosicoli* (*Anguillina coli*) is associated with intestinal spirochetosis of pigs in the post-weaning period, dogs, birds, and humans (usually those that are immunocompromised). Other serpulinas with uncertain pathogenic potential include *S. intermedius* and *S. murdochii*. *Serpulina innocens*, found in feces of symptomatic as well as asymptomatic pigs, has little if any pathogenic potential.

DESCRIPTIVE FEATURES

Morphology and Staining

Serpulina hyodysenteriae and *S. pilosicoli* are loosely coiled spirochetes, 6 to 11 μm long by 0.25 to 0.35 μm in width. Another very similar serpulina, *S. innocens* (the so-called small spirochete), is often found in the feces of pigs with signs of dysentery as well as in normal feces. *S. innocens* measures 5 to 7 μm by 0.2 μm, tightly coiled.

The serpulinas are gram negative, but this characteristic is not used to identify or detect them. Romanovsky-type stains are the most useful in demonstrating these organisms in smears.

Cellular Anatomy and Composition

Cells are typical of spirochetes. The axial filament of *S. hyodysenteriae* is made up of 8 to 12 flagella inserted at either end, *S. innocens* has 10 to 13 flagella, and *S. pilosicoli* 4 to 6.

Cellular Products of Medical Interest

The degree of hemolysis in vitro is often used to differentiate *S. hyodysenteriae*, which is strongly beta-hemolytic, from *S. innocens* (nonpathogenic) and *S. pilosicoli*. The 26.9 kDa protein responsible for the strong beta-hemolysis displayed by *S. hyodysenteriae* in vitro is a virulence determinant in vivo. Mutants that are unable to produce the cytoxin hemolysin subsequent to the "knock out" of the encoding gene, *tlyA* (for cytoxin/hemolysin), are less virulent.

Flagella, though present on virulent as well as avirulent serpulinas, appear necessary for virulence. This trait is thought to be related to movement through the intestinal mucus to gain access to target cells in the large intestine. It has also been shown that virulent strains have an affinity for intestinal mucus.

All of the serpulinas have cell wall lipopolysaccharide, a substance capable of eliciting an inflammatory response.

Growth Characteristics

All members of the genus *Serpulina* are obligate anaerobes.

Serpulina hyodysenteriae is strongly beta-hemolytic, a trait that has been used by some to differentiate it from *S. innocens* and *S. pilosicoli*, which are weakly beta-hemolytic.

Serpulina hyodysenteriae and *S. pilosicoli* are resistant to high concentrations of spectinomycin, a characteristic useful in isolating these organisms from feces. *S. hyodysenteriae* and presumably *S. pilosicoli* remain infective for long periods if enclosed within organic material in temperatures of 5°C to 25°C. They do not withstand drying or direct sunlight.

Variability

There are at least nine serotypes of *S. hyodysenteriae*. Fingerprinting isolates by means of restriction-length polymorphisms of whole-cell DNA, DNA encoding ribosomal RNA and DNA encoding specific genes (e.g., flagellin), and multilocus enzyme electrophoresis has demonstrated the heterogeneity of members of this species as well as the others (*S. innocens* and *S. pilosicoli*).

ECOLOGY

Reservoir and Transmission

The reservoir for *S. hyodysenteriae* is the gastrointestinal tract of pigs, especially asymptomatic carriers of the organism (animals recovered from the disease). The agent has been isolated from the feces of dogs, rats, and mice living on farms where the disease exists. Transmission is through the fecal–oral route.

Serpulina pilosicoli has been isolated from dogs, birds, and humans. There is evidence that humans may acquire *S. pilosicoli* from affected dogs.

Pathogenesis

Serpulina hyodysenteriae multiplies and produces disease in the colon (swine dysentery). It appears that *S. hyodysenteriae* alone will not produce disease. Other species of bacteria normally found in the colon of pigs, *Bacteroides vulgatus*, *B. fragilis*, *Fusobacterium necrophorum*, *Campylobacter coli*, a *Clostridium* sp., and *Listeria denitrificans*, have been shown to be involved in this supporting role. Superficial coagulation necrosis with epithelial cell erosion is observed. Edema, hyperemia, hemorrhage, and influx of polymorphonuclear neutrophil leukocytes (PMNs) into the mucosa and submucosa are seen. There is failure of colonic absorption, but without evidence of an active or passive secretory process. Inflammation, brought about by cytotoxin-mediated destruction of colonic target cells (goblet cells initially, then enterocytes), may induce a secretory diarrhea. DNA sequences encoding known enterotoxins have not been found in *S. hyodysenteriae*.

The signs of disease are rather typical. Affected pigs will void gray to strawberry-colored feces, become dehydrated, and, in the extreme, be acidotic and hyperkalemic. Temperature generally remains normal. Morbidity rates in susceptible pigs will be close to 90%, with mortality in untreated herds of approximately 20% to 40%. Duration of illness ranges from few days to several weeks. Survivors may be permanently stunted and remain asymptomatic shedders. There is no easy way to detect such animals.

Intestinal spirochetosis of pigs (post-weaning period), dogs, birds, and humans is associated with *S. pilosicoli*. This disease is characterized by a mild, persistent diarrhea and low mortality. Biopsies of affected colon show large clumps of spirochetes adhering "end on" to the intestinal epithelium. It is difficult to reproduce this disease by feeding pigs this microorganism. Diet and the status of the normal flora have been suggested as reasons for this difficulty.

IMMUNOLOGIC ASPECTS

Little is known about the immunologic factors of these diseases. Pigs recovered from swine dysentery are resistant to reinfection. No immunizing products are available.

LABORATORY DIAGNOSIS

Sample Collection

Fecal samples from affected animals showing signs of the disease are used to detect *S. hyodysenteriae* and *S. pilosicoli*.

Direct Examination

Smears of fecal material are stained with a Romanovsky-type stain or carbol fuchsin. Observation of large, loosely coiled spirochetes in diarrheal feces is presumptive evidence of infection with *S. hyodysenteriae* (swine dysentery) or *S. pilosicoli* (intestinal spirochetosis). *Serpulina innocens* may be present in samples from pigs with swine dysentery, but these will be smaller and have tighter coils, a distinction that is sometimes difficult to make.

Isolation/Detection

Isolation of *S. hyodysenteriae* and *S. pilosicoli* from fecal samples is accomplished by inoculation onto blood agar plates containing spectinomycin (400 μg/ml). The plates are incubated 24 to 48 hours in an anaerobic environment containing 10% carbon dioxide. Colonies of *S. hyodysenteriae* will be small and strongly beta-hemolytic; those of *S. pilosicoli* will not be as strongly hemolytic.

A multiplex polymerase chain reaction (PCR) assay using primers designed to detect the common diarrhea-associated microorganisms (*S. hyodysenteriae*, *Lawsonia intracellularis*, and *Salmonella*) has been described.

Identification

Serpulina hyodysenteriae must be differentiated from *S. innocens*. This is best done by gas chromatographic analysis of volatile fatty acids or by DNA probing/analysis. Unfortunately these techniques do not lend themselves to performance in a busy diagnostic laboratory. Therefore, observing the strength of the beta-hemolysis, fructose fermentation (*S. innocens* will be positive), and indole production (*S. hyodysenteriae* will be positive) are traits used to make the distinction. Though the hemolysis trait seems to be relatively stable, the other tests are somewhat variable and misidentifications are possible. *Serpulina pilosicoli* hydrolyzes hippurate; *S. innocens* does not.

TREATMENT, CONTROL, AND PREVENTION

Drugs shown to be effective in treating swine dysentery and intestinal spirochetosis in swine include organic arsenicals, tylosin, gentamicin, nitrofurazone, virginiamycin, and lincomycin. These have been used at low prophylactic levels, but it should be kept in mind that drugs used routinely to prevent the disease will ultimately lose their effectiveness. Metronidazole is the recommended treatment for dogs with intestinal spirochetosis.

SELECTED REFERENCES

Atyeo RF, Oxberry SL, Hampson DJ. Pulse-field gel electrophoresis for subspecies differentiation of *Serpulina pilosicoli* (formerly "*Anguillina coli*"). FEMS Microbiol Lett 1996;141:77.

Duhamel GE, Muniappa N, Mathiesen MR, et al. Certain canine weakly beta-hemolytic intestinal spirochetes are phenotypically and genotypically related to spirochetes associated with human and porcine intestinal spirochetosis. J Clin Microbiol 1995;33:2212.

Elder RO, Duhamel GE, Mathiesen MR, et al. Multiplex polymerase chain reaction for simultaneous detection of

Lawsonia intracellularis, Serpulina hyodysenteriae, and salmonellae in porcine intestinal specimens. J Vet Diagn Invest 1997;9:281.

Harris DL, Glock RD, Christensen CR, Kinyon JM. Swine dysentery. I. Inoculation of pigs with *Treponema hyodysenteriae* (new species) and reproduction of the disease. Vet Med Small Anim Clin 1972;67:61.

Hyatt DR, Huurne AAHMT, van der Zeijst BAM, Joens LA. Reduced virulence of *Serpulina hyodysenteriae* hemolysin-negative mutants in pigs and their potential to protect pigs against challenge with a virulent strain. Infect Immun 1994; 62:2244.

Joens LA, Nuessen ME. Bactericidal effect of normal swine sera on *Treponema hyodysenteriae.* Infect Immun 1986;51:282.

Kinyon JM, Harris DL. *Treponema innocens,* a new species of intestinal bacteria, and emended description of the type strain of *Treponema hyodysenteriae* Harris et al. Int J Syst Bacteriol 1979;29:102.

Lee JI, Hampson DJ. Genetic characterisation of intestinal spirochaetes and their association with disease. J Med Microbiol 1994;40:365.

Lee JI, Hampson DJ, Lymbery AJ, Harders SJ. The porcine intestinal spirochaetes: identification of a new genetic groups. Vet Microbiol 1993;34:273.

Milner JA, Sellwood R. Chemotactic response to mucin by *Serpulina hyodysenteriae* and other porcine spirochetes: potential role in intestinal colonization. Infect Immun 1994;62:4095.

Milner JA, Truelove KG, Foster FJ, Sellwood R. Use of commercial enzyme kits and fatty acid production for the identification of *Serpulina hyodysenteriae*: a potential misdiagnosis. J Vet Diagn Invest 1995;7:92.

Muir S, Koopman MBH, Libby SJ, et al. Cloning and expression of a *Serpulina (Treponema) hyodysenteriae* hemolysin gene. Infect Immun 1992;60:529.

Neef NA, Lysons RJ, Trott DT, et al. Pathogenicity of porcine intestinal spirochetes in gnotobiotic pigs. Infect Immun 1994;62:2395.

Olson LD. Survival of *Serpulina hyodysenteriae* in an effluent lagoon. J Am Vet Med Assoc 1995;207:1471.

Songer JG, Kinyon JM, Harris DL. Selective medium for isolation of *Treponema hyodysenteriae.* J Clin Microbiol 1976;4:57.

Stanton TB, Fournie-Amazouz E, Postic D, et al. Recognition of two new species of intestinal spirochetes: *Serpulina intermedius* sp. nov. and *Serpulina murdochii* sp. nov. Int J Syst Bacteriol 1997;47:1007.

Ter Huurne AAHM, Gaastra W. Swine dysentery: more unknown than known. Vet Microbiol 1995;46:347.

Trott DJ, Stanton TB, Jensen NS, et al. *Serpulina pilosicoli* sp. nov., the agent of porcine intestinal spirochetosis. Int J Syst Bacteriol 1996;46:206.

Whipp SC, Robinson IM, Harris DL, et al. Pathogenic synergism between *Treponema hyodysenteriae* and other selected anaerobes in gnotobiotic pigs. Infect Immun 1979;26:1042.

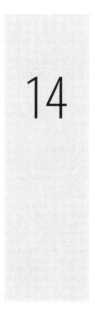

14

Spiral Organisms I: Campylobacter — Arcobacter — Lawsonia (Digestive Tract)

Dwight C. Hirsh

Members of the genera *Campylobacter, Arcobacter,* and *Lawsonia* are gram-negative, curved rods.

The family *Campylobacteriaceae* contains the genera *Campylobacter* and *Arcobacter* (previously within the genus *Campylobacter*). *Campylobacters* implicated in enteric disease of animals and humans include *C. jejuni, C. coli, C. concisus, C. helveticus, C. hyointestinalis, C. mucosalis, C. lari,* and *C. upsaliensis. Arcobacters* implicated in enteric disease of animals and humans include *A. butzleri, A. cryaerophilus,* and *A. skirrowii.*

Lawsonia intracellularis, previously known as *ileal symbiont intracellularis,* differs in many respects from members of the family *Campylobacteriaceae,* primarily in DNA relatedness (it is most similar to *Desulfovibrio*), and appears to be an obligately intracellular microorganism.

Arcobacters and campylobacters that cause genital diseases of large animals are discussed in Chapter 36.

Campylobacter jejuni and *C. coli* are major causes of gastroenteritis in people and nonhuman primates, and have been found in fecal samples from dogs and cats with diarrhea. *Campylobacter jejuni* is the more common of the two. Though *C. coli* occurs in high numbers in swine dysentery and was once thought to be the causative agent, the disease is caused by *Serpulina hyodysenteriae.* Both *C. coli* and *C. jejuni* may occur in feces of normal animals.

Campylobacter concisus has been associated with gastrointestinal disease of humans.

Campylobacter helveticus has been recovered from the feces of dogs and cats with diarrhea.

Campylobacter hyointestinalis and *C. mucosalis* were once implicated as contributors to the swine proliferative enteritis complex. This disease is now thought to be caused by *Lawsonia intracellularis,* a microorganism that produces this disease in conventional pigs in pure culture, something neither *C. hyointestinalis* nor *C. mucosalis* will do.

Campylobacter lari, isolated from the feces of asymptomatic gulls (from which it gets its name), has also been isolated from the feces of various hosts, including dogs, birds, and horses. Its role in disease is uncertain.

Campylobacter upsaliensis has been isolated from feces of dogs and cats with diarrhea. Enteric disease and abortion have been associated with this microorganism in humans.

Arcobacter butzleri, A. cryaerophilus, and *A. skirrowii* have been associated with gastrointestinal disease in domestic animals (enteritis in neonatal pigs) and humans. More serious associations have been made with respect to reproductive disease in swine and bovine species.

DESCRIPTIVE FEATURES

Morphology and Staining

Campylobacter — Arcobacter — Lawsonia are gram-negative, slender, curved rods that measure 0.2 to 0.5 μm by 0.5 to 5 μm. When two or more bacterial cells are placed together, they form S or gullwinged shapes (see Fig 36.1).

Cellular Anatomy and Composition

Campylobacter — Arcobacter — Lawsonia have a typical gram-negative cell wall, capsule, and flagella.

Cellular Products of Medical Interest

Campylobacter jejuni secretes a toxin similar in activity to cholera toxin and the heat-labile toxin (LT) of *Escherichia coli* by increasing intracellular levels of cAMP and cytoskeletal rearrangements. Both toxins are immunologically related and bind to the same ganglioside (GM_1) on the surface of the target cell. *Campylobacter coli* and *C. lari* produce uncharacterized substances with cytotonic and cytotoxic activity.

Campylobacter jejuni produces a number of proteins with cytotoxic activity. These cytotoxins include a heat and trypsin labile protein of 70 kDa in size which is neutralized by antibody to shiga-like toxin (see Chapter 11);

a protein active on Vero cells; a protein that increases intracellular cAMP followed by cell death (cytolethal distending toxin); a protein that has hemolytic activity (hemolysin); and a protein that was shown to induce hepatitis in mice (hepatotoxin). All of these toxic compounds have a tenuous association with the disease process in humans and other animals.

Campylobacter jejuni produces a mannose-resistant adhesin that binds to a fucose-containing receptor on the target cell. It also survives inside mononuclear phagocytes, implying the existence of other important, as yet unidentified surface structures.

Commonly used serological methods for typing *C. jejuni* are based upon heat-stable (presumably lipopolysaccharide) or heat-labile antigens. Both systems have described numerous serotypes and are used to determine the sources of food-borne outbreaks.

Virtually nothing is known about the cellular products of *Acrobacter* or *Lawsonia*.

Growth Characteristics

Campylobacter spp. are microaerophilic, requiring an atmosphere containing 3% to 15% oxygen and 3% to 5% carbon dioxide concentrations for growth. Some, such as *C. jejuni*, will grow at 42°C, a characteristic that is useful for its selectivity in isolation from intestinal sources. Unlike members of the family *Enterobacteriaceae*, they are oxidase positive. They do not ferment or oxidize carbohydrates, generating energy from oxidation of amino acids or tricarboxylic acid intermediates through the respiratory pathway. Though they possess catalase and superoxide dismutase, these enzymes are overwhelmed by the excess of hydrogen peroxide and superoxide anions formed when they are grown in the presence of atmospheric concentrations of oxygen.

Members of the genus *Arcobacter* are aerotolerant, a trait that separates them from *Campylobacter*. They grow over a wide temperature range, and some strains of *A. butzleri* grow at 42°C.

They are susceptible to drying, direct sunlight, and to most disinfectants. They possess R plasmids, which most commonly mediate resistance to tetracyclines.

Lawsonia intracellularis has not been grown in lifeless media.

ECOLOGY

Reservoir

Animals and animal by-products are the sources for human beings and susceptible animal species. *Campylobacter jejuni* has been found in milk, on poultry carcasses, and in feces of asymptomatic dogs and cats, as well as those with diarrhea.

Swine probably acquire *L. intracellularis* from the feces of infected pigs. Likewise, members of the genus *Arcobacter* are acquired from similarly affected animals.

The sources of *C. lari*, *C. helveticus*, and *C. upsaliensis* are not known but are presumed to be the intestinal tract of infected individuals. Feces from healthy puppies and kittens have been shown to contain *C. upsaliensis*.

Transmission

The fecal–oral route, direct or indirect, is probably the main mode of spread. Infection occurs following the ingestion of an animal product originally contaminated with infected feces.

Pathogenesis

Campylobacter jejuni adheres to cells of the small intestine, especially the distal segments. The organism multiplies and invades the target epithelial cell. It is uncertain whether the toxins elaborated by *C. jejuni* are responsible for the disease. However, the LT-like toxin is thought to deregulate the adenyl cyclase system as described for enterotoxigenic *E. coli* (see Chapter 9). At the same time, the cytotoxin destroys the mucosal epithelium. The inflammatory response elicited by *Campylobacter* interaction with the target epithelial cells probably has a lot to do with stimulating events leading to diarrhea (i.e., activation of the arachidonic acid pathway leading to production of prostaglandins and leukotrienes, and elevation of cAMP). *Campylobacter jejuni* that escape into the lymphatics and into the systemic circulation are destroyed by the bactericidal effects of serum. Diarrheal feces containing cell debris and mucus are produced, and products of the inflammatory response are seen in direct smears. Mucus and blood are sometimes seen grossly.

Swine proliferative enteritis is a disease complex involving a number of intestinal abnormalities: intestinal adenomatosis, necrotic enteritis, regional ileitis, and proliferative hemorrhagic enteropathy. The disease is characterized by a thickening of the ileal wall, but including, on occasion, segments on either side. *Lawsonia intracellularis* together with members of the normal flora is thought to be responsible for this disease complex.

Little is known regarding the interactions of other members of the genus *Campylobacter* and *Arcobacter* with the intestinal tract of the host.

Epidemiology

Human beings in developed societies acquire *C. jejuni* from symptomatic or asymptomatic companion animals (dogs and cats) and from food such as raw milk, water, and poultry products. Most sporadic cases probably arise from consumption of improperly handled poultry or contact with infected pets, whereas large outbreaks most often occur from contact with raw milk or contaminated water.

The feces of approximately 10% of asymptomatic dogs and approximately 5% of asymptomatic cats are found to contain *C. jejuni*. This percentage may be higher in animals acquired from pounds.

The ceca of approximately 50% of chickens sampled contain *C. jejuni*. At slaughter, these organisms contaminate the environment and, as a consequence, almost as many chicken carcasses found in stores will be contaminated.

From 2% to 100% of cattle may be healthy shedders of *C. jejuni*, a circumstance that may explain outbreaks of campylobacter-induced diarrheal disease following ingestion of unpasteurized milk.

IMMUNOLOGIC ASPECTS

Circulating antibody develops as a result of infection. There are no immunizing preparations available to prevent gastroenteritis.

LABORATORY DIAGNOSIS

Sample Collection

Fecal samples are taken for the diagnosis of *C. jejuni* infections. Scrapings of affected intestine are used to diagnose proliferative enteritis.

Direct Examination

Stained (gram stain with carbol fuchsin as counterstain; Romanovsky-type stain) smears of fecal material will reveal numerous slender, curved rods in most cases of diarrhea produced by *C. jejuni*. Impression smears of the intestine of swine with proliferative enteritis contain similar rods within the cells lining the area. The silver stains, such as Warthin-Starry, or a modified acid-fast stain (use 0.5% acetic acid for 30 seconds for decolorization) best demonstrate organisms in this site.

Isolation

Campylobacter jejuni and *C. coli* are best isolated from affected intestinal samples on selective media containing antimicrobial agents (e.g., Campy-CVA containing cefoperazone, vancomycin, and amphotericin B). Incubation is under increased CO_2, reduced O_2, and the plates are incubated at 37°C, or at 42°C when isolation of *C. jejuni* or *C. coli* from feces is attempted. Because the genus *Arcobacter* is aerotolerant, it does not require reduced oxygen. Its members will grow on selective media (e.g., Campy-CVA), and some will grow at increased temperature.

Immunodiagnosis

Immunodiagnosis is not used for intestinal disease produced by campylobacters. Antibody responses, measured by enzyme-linked immunosorbent assays, have been studied for epidemiologic purposes.

Molecular Diagnosis

Assays using polymerase chain reaction (PCR) have been developed to amplify DNA from feces.

TREATMENT

The enteritis produced by *C. jejuni* is most often self-limiting. Macrolide antibiotics (erythromycin, tylosin) remain the drugs of choice for treatment of *C. jejuni* diarrhea. Tetracyclines are effective when macrolides cannot be used, although tetracycline-resistant strains exist (R plasmid based). Most campylobacters from animals are susceptible to quinolone antibiotics. However, due to the high rate of mutational resistance campylobacters have to this group of antibiotics, a resistance that sometimes occurs while animals are being treated, quinolones are not the drug of choice. In addition, diarrhea due to *C. jejuni* most often occurs in younger animals, most too young to be safely treated with quinolones.

The arcobacters, *A. butzleri* and *A. cryaerophila*, are resistant to the macrolide antibiotics but susceptible to the tetracyclines and quinolones. Whether these microorganisms would have the same resistance problems as the campylobacters is unknown.

Control in the veterinary hospital and kennel requires meticulous adherence to hygienic measures such as handwashing, cleaning, and disinfection protocols.

SELECTED REFERENCES

Allos BM, Blaser MJ. *Campylobacter jejuni* and the expanding spectrum of related infections. Clin Infect Dis 1995;20:1092.

Anderson KF, Kiehlbauch JA, Anderson DC, et al. *Arcobacter* (*Campylobacter*) *butzleri*-associated diarrheal illness in a nonhuman primate population. Infect Immun 1993;61:2220.

Elder RO, Duhamel GE, Mathiesen MR, et al. Multiplex polymerase chain reaction for simultaneous detection of *Lawsonia intracellularis*, *Serpulina hyodysenteriae*, and salmonellae in porcine intestinal specimens. J Vet Diagn Invest 1997;9:281.

Fox JG, Maxwell KO, Taylor NS, et al. "*Campylobacter upsaliensis*" isolated from cats as identified by DNA relatedness and biochemical features. J Clin Microbiol 1989;27:2376.

Fox JG, Moore R, Ackerman JL. *Campylobacter jejuni*-associated diarrhea in dogs. J Am Vet Med Assoc 1983;183:1430.

Fox JG, Moore R, Ackerman JL. Canine and feline campylobacteriosis: epizootiology and clinical and public health features. J Am Vet Med Assoc 1983;183:1420.

Gebhart CJ, Edmonds R, Ward GE, et al. "*Campylobacter hyointestinalis*" sp. nov.: a new species of *Campylobacter* found in the intestines of pigs and other animals. J Clin Microbiol 1985;21:715.

Gurgan T, Diker KS. Abortion associated with *Campylobacter upsaliensis*. J Clin Microbiol 1994;32:3093.

Hald B, Madsen M. Healthy puppies and kittens as carriers of *Campylobacter* spp., with special reference to *Campylobacter upsaliensis*. J Clin Microbiol 1997;35:3351.

Kiehlbauch JA, Brenner DJ, Nicholson MA, et al. *Campylobacter butzleri* sp. nov. isolated from humans and animals with diarrheal illness. J Clin Microbiol 1991;29:376.

Lomax LG, Glock RD. Naturally occurring porcine proliferative enteritis: pathologic and bacteriologic findings. Am J Vet Res 1982;43:1608.

Munroe DL, Prescott JE, Penner JL. *Campylobacter jejuni* and *Campylobacter coli* serotypes isolated from chickens, cattle, and pigs. J Clin Microbiol 1983;18:877.

On SLW. Identification methods for campylobacters, helicobacters, and related organisms. Clin Microbiol Rev 1996;9:405.

Piddock LJV. Quinolone resistance and *Campylobacter* spp. J Antimicrob Chemother 1995;36:891.

Prescott JE, Munroe DL. *Campylobacter jejuni* enteritis in man and domestic animals. J Am Vet Med Assoc 1982;181:1524.

Reina J, Ros MJ, Serra A. Susceptibilities to 10 antimicrobial agents of 1220 *Campylobacter* strains isolated from 1987 to 1993 from feces of pediatric patients. Antimicrob Agents Chemother 1994;38:2917.

Roop EM, Smibert RM, Johnson JL, Krieg NR. DNA homology studies of the catalase-negative campylobacters and "*Campylobacter fecalis,*" an amended description of *Campylobacter sputorum*, and proposal of the neotype strain of *Campylobacter sputorum*. Can J Microbiol 1985;31:823.

Sandstedt K, Ursing J. Description of *Campylobacter upsaliensis* sp. nov. previously known as the CNW group. Syst App Microbiol 1991;14:39.

Sears CL, Kaper JB. Enteric bacterial toxins: mechanisms of action and linkage to intestinal secretion. Microbiol Rev 1996;60:167.

Stanley J, Burnens AP, Linton D, et al. *Campylobacter helveticus* sp. nov., a new thermophilic species from domestic animals: characterization, and cloning of a species-specific DNA. J Gen Microbiol 1992;138:2293.

Taylor DE, DeGradis SA, Karmali MA, Fleming RC. Transmissible plasmids from *Campylobacter jejuni*. Antimicrob Agents Chemother 1981;19:831.

Tenover EC, Williams S, Gordon KR, et al. Survey of plasmids of resistance factors in *Campylobacter jejuni* and *Campylobacter coli*. Antimicrob Agents Chemother 1985;27:37.

Vandamme P, Vancanneyt M, Pot B, et al. Polyphasic taxonomic study of the emended genus *Arcobacter* with *Arcobacter butzleri* comb. nov. and *Arcobacter skirrowii* sp. nov., an aerotolerant bacterium isolated from veterinary specimens. Int J Syst Bacteriol 1992;42:344.

Wassenaar TM. Toxin production by *Campylobacter* spp. Clin Microbiol Rev 1997;10:466.

Wempe JM, Genigeorgis CA, Farver TB, Yusufu HI. Prevalence of *Campylobacter jejuni* in two California chicken-processing plants. Appl Environ Microbiol 1983;45:355.

Wesley IV, Baetz AL, Larson DJ. Infection of Cesarean-derived colostrum-deprived 1-day-old piglets with *Arcobacter butzleri*, *Arcobacter cryaerophilus*, and *Arcobacter skirrowii*. Infect Immun 1996;64:2295.

Winkelman NL. Ileitis: an update. The Compendium (Food Animal). January, 1996:S19.

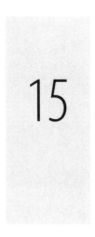

15

Spiral Organisms II: Helicobacter

James G. Fox

Gastric spiral-shaped microorganisms have been noted in animals and humans for more than a century. The first observations of gastric spiral-shaped bacteria were noted in animals. Since the discovery of *Helicobacter pylori* in diseased gastric tissue of humans in 1982, *Helicobacter* species have been cultured from the stomachs of ferrets, nonhuman primates, dogs, cats, and cheetahs. These bacteria are gram negative, microaerophilic, and curved to spiral-shaped; their isolation from gastric mucosa of humans and animals during the last 15 years has created a great deal of interest because of their causal role in gastric disease. The type species *H. pylori* colonizes the stomach of 20% to 95% of adult populations worldwide. It causes persistent, active, chronic gastritis and peptic ulcer disease in humans and also has been recently linked to the development of gastric adenocarcinoma and gastric mucosal-associated lymphoma.

In addition to the discovery of gastric helicobacters, an increasing number of *Helicobacter* spp. have been isolated from the lower gastrointestinal tract of mammals and birds. At least 17 additional *Helicobacter* spp. have now been identified and named (Table 15.1). These genera of bacteria are taxonomically distinct from *Campylobacter* spp. that also have spiral morphology, grow under microaerobic conditions, and reside in the gastrointestinal tract.

DESCRIPTIVE FEATURES

Morphology and Staining

Because many of the helicobacters observed in the stomachs of animals have been isolated only recently, many earlier studies describing these bacteria were based on morphological criteria. Three morphologically distinct organisms described in dogs are now known to be helicobacters by 16S rRNA analysis, and these early descriptions have been useful for identifying and studying similar gastric bacteria in a variety of animal species.

Flexispira rappini, now known as a *Helicobacter* sp., is a bacterium entwined with periplasmic fibers that appear to cover the entire surface of the organism. *Helicobacter felis* also has periplasmic fibers but they are sparsely distributed on the organism and can appear singly or in groups of two, three, or four. *Helicobacter heilmannii*, also known as *Helicobacter bizzozeronii*, is very tightly spiraled and does not have periplasmic fibers.

Bacteria with morphological characteristics similar to that of *H. pylori* identified in humans have been isolated from several species of nonhuman primates. More recently, *H. pylori* has been identified and subsequently cultured from commercially available cats. *H. pylori* observed in cats and primates are 0.5 to 1.0 μm by 2.5 to 5.0 μm.

A morphologically distinct bacterium has been isolated and characterized in the ferret. *Helicobacter mustelae* is rod-shaped or slightly curved and measures 0.5 by 2.0 μm; it has sheathed flagella located at both poles as well as laterally. Other gastric and intestinal helicobacters have spiral to fusiform morphologies and all except *Helicobacter pullorum* and *Helicobacter rodentium* have sheathed flagella (Table 15.2).

Cellular Products of Medical Interest

Gastric helicobacters colonize the mucosa and induce an inflammatory response. Levels of reactive oxygen species are thereby increased. The type strain, *H. pylori*, has evolved adaptive mechanisms to minimize oxidative damage by utilizing its enzymes, superoxide dismutase and catalase, and by the presence of *recA* gene products that play a role in repair of damaged DNA.

Growth Characteristics

Because *Helicobacter* spp. are fastidious, selective media are available commercially and consist of brucella agar with 10% horse blood as well as vancomycin (10 mg/l), polymyxin B (2500 U/l), and trimethoprim (5 mg/l). Fresh media are recommended for optimal growth. Specific *Helicobacter* spp. also may have different antibiotic sensitivities; therefore, selection of antibiotics in culture media may determine the success of isolation. The organisms do not grow under aerobic or anaerobic conditions and achieve optimum growth in a high humidity with microaerophilic conditions (5% CO_2, 90% N_2, 5% H_2). A flow chart outlining diagnostic schema to isolate and identify gastric helicobacters is presented in Figure 15.1.

Table 15.1. *Helicobacter* Species and Their Hosts (as of 1997)

Species	Hosts	Primary Site	Other Sites
H. pylori*	Human, macaque, cat	Stomach	
H. mustelae	Ferret, mink	Stomach	
H. felis*	Cat, dog	Stomach	
H. bizzozeronii*ᵃ	Dog, human	Stomach	
H. heilmannii*ᵃ	Dog, cat, human, monkey	Stomach	
H. nemestrinae	Pig-tailed macaque	Stomach	
H. suis	Swine	Stomach	
H. acinonyx	Cheetah	Stomach	
H. rappini*	Sheep, dog, human, mice	Intestine	Liver (sheep), stomach
H. canis*	Dog, human	Intestine	Liver (dog)
H. hepaticus	Mice	Intestine	Liver
H. bilis	Mice, dog	Intestine	Liver, stomach (dog)
H. rodentium	Mice	Intestine	
H. trogontum	Rat	Intestine	
H. muridarum	Mice, rat	Intestine	Stomach (mice)
H. cinaedi*	Human, hamster	Intestine	
H. fennelliae	Human	Intestine	
H. pullorum*	Chicken, human	Intestine	Liver (chicken)
H. pametensis	Bird, swine	Intestine	
H. cholecystus	Hamster	Liver	

* Some data suggest zoonotic potential.
ᵃ Closely related, may be same species.

Table 15.2. Characteristics That Differentiate *Helicobacter* Species*

Taxon	Catalase Production	Nitrate Reduction	Alkaline Phosphatase Hydrolysis	Urease	Indoxyl Acetate Hydrolysis	γ-Glutamyl Transpeptidase	Growth at 42°C	Growth with 1% Glycine	Susceptibility to: Nalidixic Acid (30-μg disc)	Susceptibility to: Cephalothin (30-μg disc)	Periplasmic Fibers	No. of Flagella	Distribution of Flagella	G+C Content (mol %)
H. rodentium	+	+	−	−	−	−	+	+	R	R	−	2	Bipolar	ND
H. pullorum	+	+	−	−	−	ND	+	ND	R	S	−	1	Monopolar	34–35
Helicobacter sp. CLO-3	+	−	+	−	+	−	+	+	I	R	−		ND	45
H. pylori	+	−	+	+	−	+	−	−	R	S		4–8	Bipolar	35–37
H. nemestrinae	+	−	+	+	−	ND	+	−	R	S	−	4–8	Bipolar	24
H. acinonyx	+	−	+	+	−	+	−	−	R	S	−	2–5	Bipolar	30
H. felis	+	+	+	+	−	+	+	−	R	S	+	14–20	Bipolar	42
H. fennelliae	+	−	+	−	+	−	−	+	S	S	−	2	Bipolar	35
H. trogontum	+	+	−	+	ND	+	+	ND	R	R	+	5–7	Bipolar	ND
H. muridarum	+	−	+	+	+	+	−	−	R	R	+	10–14	Bipolar	34
H. hepaticus	+	+	ND	+	+	ND	−	+	R	R	−	2	Bipolar	ND
H. canis	−	−	+	−	+	ND	+	ND	S	I	−	2	Bipolar	48
H. bilis	+	+	ND	+	−	ND	+	+	R	R	+	3–14	Bipolar	ND
"Flexispira rappini"	+	−	−	+	ND	+	+	−	R	R	+	10–20	Bipolar	34
H. cinaedi	+	+	−	−	−	−	−	+	S	I	−	1–2	Bipolar	37–38
H. pametensis	+	+	+	−	−	−	+	+	S	S	−	2	Bipolar	38
Helicobacter sp. Bird-C	+	+	+	+	+	−	+	+	S	R	−	2	Bipolar	30
Helicobacter sp. Bird-B	+	+	+	+	−	+	+	+	S	R	−	2	Bipolar	31
H. mustelae	+	+	+	+	+	+	+	−	S	R	−	4–8	Peritrichous	36
H. bizzozeronii	+	+	+	+	+	+	+	−	R	S	−	10–20	Bipolar	ND

* +: positive reaction; −: negative reaction; S: susceptible; R: resistant; I: intermediate; ND: not determined.

FIGURE 15.1.   *Diagnostic flow chart for gastric helicobacters.*

Isolation of *Helicobacter sp.* from Gastric Biopsies

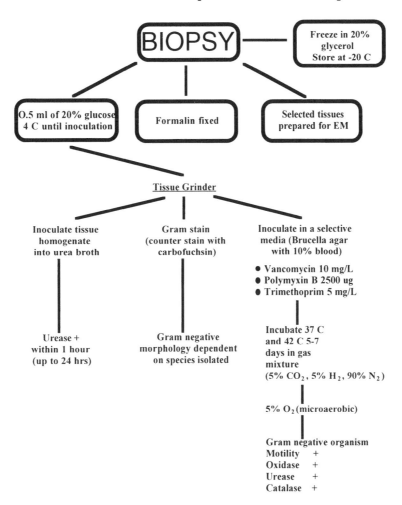

Variability

Helicobacter pylori strains exhibit a high degree of genomic heterogenicity, due in part to nucleotide substitutions among strains. However, *H. pylori* lacks an SOS mutagenesis pathway, and the large number of nucleotide substitutions are probably due to mechanisms such as replication fidelity deficiencies or mismatch repair defects.

Isolation and Identification

Helicobacters can now be isolated routinely from the gastric tissue of infected humans, ferrets, and nonhuman primates. It is more difficult to isolate *H. felis* from dogs and cats and until very recently *H. bizzozeronii* (*H. heilmannii*), the large gastric spiral, was uncultivable. This organism, however, has now been isolated from both dogs and humans. When attempting to grow *H. felis* and *H. bizzozeronii*, it is very important to use moist plates that are incubated lid uppermost. They do not form distinct colonies, but rather bacterial growth consists of a very

fine spreading film that could easily be dismissed as water stains. Another limiting factor in isolation of gastric *Helicobacter* spp. from animals and humans is the necessity of obtaining gastric biopsies. The organisms are not routinely cultured from gastric juice or feces.

Intestinal helicobacters can be isolated on the same selective antibiotic media used to isolate gastric helicobacters. Also, the use of 0.45-μ or 0.65-μ filters to selectively filter feces helps minimize contamination from other enteric organisms during primary culture on selective agar.

ECOLOGY

Reservoir

Gastric helicobacters reside in the gastric mucus layer of a variety of mammals. The ecological niche of intestinal helicobacters is the crypts of the colon and cecum; in some cases, the organism also colonizes the bile canaliculi of the liver. Animals maintained in closed colonies, reared in pounds or kennels, for example, often have prevalence rates of gastric helicobacters approaching 100%. Some *Helicobacter* spp. colonize specific hosts whereas others are capable of infecting a number of different animal species. Animals and birds, in some cases, may be reservoirs for zoonotic transmission to humans (see below).

Since the original observation of helicobacters in mice in the 1990s, it is now known that *Helicobacter* spp. are prevalent in many rodent colonies, both commercial and academic, throughout the world. Though the epizootiology of the disease is unknown, the bacteria apparently persist in the intestine for the life of the animal.

Transmission

Both oral–oral and fecal–oral routes are probably operable in transmission of gastric helicobacters. Transmission of intestinal helicobacters is via the fecal–oral route. There is continued controversy whether viable, but nonculturable, coccoid forms of helicobacter exist in the environment, and if present, whether they are important in transmission to susceptible hosts.

Pathogenesis

Although it is now known that both urease and flagella are necessary to sustain colonization of *Helicobacter* spp. in the gastric mucus, mechanisms are being actively explored to explain the chronic inflammation induced by some *Helicobacter* spp. These include several putative bacterial virulence factors (e.g., cytotoxins and urease, and certain proteins expressed by genes located on pathogenicity islands), which in the persistently infected host probably initiate sustained production of a series of inflammatory cytokines. Urease, which produces ammonia (a tissue irritant) as a by-product of urea metabolism, is an enzyme present in high levels in gastric helicobacters as well as in several species of intestinal helicobacters. The presence of these urease-producing bacteria in stomachs and liver may damage cells adjacent to the colonizing bacteria. A vacuolating cytotoxin has been suggested, based on epidemiological studies, as a potential virulence factor in *H. pylori*-induced peptic ulcer, as well as *H. pylori*-associated chronic atrophic gastritis, a precancerous gastric lesion. The purified *H. pylori* exotoxin, when inoculated directly into mouse stomachs, induced acute gastric erosions. A soluble cytotoxin exists in *H. hepaticus* that produces significant in vitro cytopathic effects in a murine hepatic cell line.

Pathology

Helicobacter felis and *H. heilmannii* (*H. bizzozeronii*) have been associated with gastric histopathology in laboratory-reared beagle dogs. When these bacteria were observed in low numbers, for example, in the fundus, the organism was considered innocuous; in large numbers, however, as seen in the cardia and fundic pyloric junction, the organism may induce lymphoreticular hyperplasia and may

cause premature senescence of parietal cells. In pet dogs and cats, the gastric *Helicobacter*-like organisms' (GHLOs') presence was often accompanied by reduction in mucus content of surface epithelia, occasional intraepithelial leukocytes, and some degenerating glands. Of the glandular epithelial cells, only the parietal cells were markedly altered. Abnormal findings included vacuolation, enlarged size, and nuclear degeneration consisting of both karyolysis and karyorrhexis. The presence of large numbers of *H. pylori* in the gastric mucosa of commercially reared cats was associated with a lymphofollicular gastritis, characterized by lymphoid aggregates and diffuse inflammation in the deep mucosa and lamina propria.

Helicobacter pylori colonized the gastrointestinal tract of gnotobiotic dogs orally challenged with *H. pylori*. The dogs were colonized with *H. pylori* in all parts of the stomach examined: cardia, fundus, antrum, and pyloric antrum; the fundus was the most heavily colonized. Focal to diffuse lymphoplasmacytic infiltrates with follicle formation and focal infiltration of neutrophils and eosinophils in the gastric lamina propria were observed. Also, gnotobiotic dogs orally inoculated with *H. felis* have the organism recovered from all areas of the stomach, with colonization being heaviest in the body and antrum. Occasionally, *H. felis* was observed within the canaliculi of gastric parietal cells.

The histopathologic changes occurring in the stomach closely coincided in topography with the presence of *H. mustelae*. A superficial gastritis present in the body of the stomach showed that *H. mustelae* was located on the surface of the mucosa but not in the crypts. In the distal antrum, inflammation occupied the full thickness of the mucosa, the so-called diffuse antral gastritis described in humans. In this location, *H. mustelae* was seen at the surface, in the pits, and on the superficial portion of the glands. In the proximal antrum and the transitional mucosa, a precancerous lesion, focal glandular atrophy, and regeneration were present, in addition to those lesions seen in the distal antrum.

The liver lesion present in naturally *H. hepaticus*-infected mice progressively increases in severity. It is an inflammatory and necrotizing lesion that involves the hepatic parenchyma, the portal triads, and importantly, the small intralobular hepatic venules. The widespread, multifocal hepatitis and single cell to coalescing hepatocellular necrosis appears to be random in distribution. Within both the parenchymal perivascular lesion and the affected portal triads, variable degrees of oval, Ito, and Kupffer cell hyperplasia are present. There is an age-associated increase in cell proliferation in infected animals that was not seen in uninfected control mice. Liver cell proliferation was more pronounced in male mice than in age-matched female mice. The increased levels of hepatocyte proliferation indices in *H. hepaticus*-infected male mice are consistent with the observation of increased hepatomas and hepatocellular carcinomas observed in *H. hepaticus*-infected aged A/JCr male mice. *Helicobacter canis* has also been observed in a dog liver with multifocal hepatitis. *Helicobacter hepaticus* and *H. bilis* infection are associated with inflammatory bowel disease in immunodeficient mice and only infrequently in *H. hepaticus*-infected immunocompetent mice.

Disease Features

Ferrets. In 1985, a gastric organism was isolated from a duodenal ulcer of a ferret (*Mustela putorius furo*) and named *Helicobacter mustelae*. Gastritis and peptic ulcers are known to be routinely present in ferrets, colonized with *H. mustelae*. Ferrets infected with *H. mustelae*, with gastric or duodenal ulcers, can be observed on endoscopy and are recognized clinically by vomiting, melena, chronic weight loss, and lowered hematocrit. Acute episodes of gastric bleeding can also be noted on occasion. *Helicobacter mustelae* has also been depicted within the pyloric mucosa of ferrets with pyloric adenocarcinoma and mucosa associated lymphoma of the stomach.

Swine. Using 16S rRNA sequencing, *Helicobacter suis*, closely related to *H. heilmannii* type 1, has been identified. Authors studying gastric disease in swine have noted a higher incidence of *H. suis* in swine with gastric ulcers located in the parsoesophagea. When these data are compared to pigs without *H. suis*, however, the data are difficult to assess because *H. suis* primarily colonizes the mucus layers and gastric pits of the antral and body mucosa.

Nonhuman Primates. Several papers have published isolation of *H. pylori* from nonhuman primates, particularly macaques. The presence of *H. pylori* in gastric mucosa of infected monkeys is often accompanied by a lymphocytic plasmacytic gastritis that apparently persists. Clinical signs have not been described.

Dogs and Cats. Clinical signs in pet animals, attributable to *Helicobacter*-associated gastritis may or may not be present. *Helicobacter pylori* was recently identified in 100% of the stomachs examined from a group of specific pathogen-free cats obtained from a commercial vendor. Clinical signs were not recognized.

Helicobacter cinaedi and *H. fennelliae* have been linked to proctitis and colitis in immunocompromised humans. Of interest is the recent isolation, based on cellular fatty acid analysis, of *H. cinaedi* from the feces of dogs and a cat. *Helicobacter fennelliae* has also been identified in the feces of a dog and macaques. *Helicobacter cinaedi* has been recovered from blood of neonates with septicemia and meningitis, and is associated with arthritis in humans.

Helicobacter canis also has been isolated from feces of normal and diarrheic dogs. It has also been isolated from the liver of a puppy diagnosed as having an active, multifocal hepatitis. *Helicobacter canis* has also been cultured from the feces of children and adult humans suffering from gastroenteritis.

Sheep. *Flexispira rappini* was first isolated in humans from a diarrheic patient; in the household, the same bacterium was isolated from the feces of a young asymptomatic dog. A similar bacterium has been cultured from aborted ovine fetuses and was given the provisional name *Flexispira*

rappini. Apparently *F. rappini* can cross the placenta in pregnant sheep, cause acute hepatic necrosis in sheep fetuses, and induce abortions. By 16S rRNA analysis, this organism also belongs in the genus *Helicobacter*. Experimentally, *F. rappini* causes similar necrotic hepatitis and abortions in guinea pigs.

Rodents. To date, eight *Helicobacter* spp. have been isolated from the intestinal tract and/or livers of rodents; two of these, *H. hepaticus* and *H. bilis*, have been isolated from the ceca and colons of mice and have also been isolated from diseased livers of infected mice. *Helicobacter muridarum* colonizes the lower intestinal tract of rats and mice, and under certain circumstances can colonize the gastric tissue of mice and induce a gastritis. *Flexispira rappini* colonizes the colons and ceca of mice; *H. cinaedi* colonizes the intestinal tract of asymptomatic hamsters. Recently, *H. trogontum* has been isolated from the colons of rats, *H. rodentium* from the colons and ceca of mice, and *H. cholecystus* has been cultured from diseased livers of hamsters. Clinical signs in infected rodents have not been noted, except in immunocompromised mice infected with *H. hepaticus* or *H. bilis*, where diarrhea and/or rectal prolapse may be present.

Birds. *Helicobacter pametensis* is a urease-negative enteric helicobacter isolated from wild bird and porcine feces. *Helicobacter pullorum* has been isolated from ceca of asymptomatic chickens, the livers and intestinal contents of chickens with hepatitis, and feces of humans with gastroenteritis. There is speculation that *H. pullorum* may be the microbial agent responsible for the syndrome termed *avian vibrionic hepatitis* described in both chickens and turkeys. Although *Campylobacter jejuni* has been raised as a possible etiological agent in this disease, studies conducted to ascertain whether *C. jejuni* (derived from humans or chickens) experimentally produces hepatopathy have failed.

Zoonotic Potential

Helicobacter pylori-infected cats have been screened by culture and polymerase chain reaction (PCR) for the presence of *H. pylori* in salivary secretions, gastric juice, gastric tissue, and feces. It was cultured from salivary secretions in 6 of 12 (50%) cats and from gastric fluid samples in 11 of 12 (91%) cats. A 298 base pair PCR product specific for an *H. pylori* 26 kDa surface protein was amplified from dental plaque samples from 5 of 12 (42%) cats and from the feces of 4 of 5 (80%) cats studied. Isolation of *H. pylori* from feline mucosal secretions suggests a zoonotic risk from exposure to personnel handling *H. pylori*-infected cats in vivaria. To date, however, there is no indication based on several epidemiological studies that pets pose increased risk of *H. pylori* transmission to humans.

Because *H. heilmannii* (*H. bizzozeronii*) and to a lesser extent *H. felis* colonize a small percentage of humans with gastritis, and no environmental source for these bacteria has been recognized, pets have been implicated in zoonotic transmission of the organisms. In Germany, a recent survey of 125 individuals infected with GHLOs provided information in a questionnaire regarding animal contact. Of these patients, 70.3% had contact with one or more animals (as compared with 37% in the "normal" population). More than a threefold preponderance of males over female patients with GHLOs was recorded.

Since *H. cinaedi* has been isolated from humans and the normal intestine flora of hamsters, it has been suggested that pet hamsters serve as a reservoir for transmission to humans. Also given that *H. canis*, *F. rappini*, and *H. pullorum* have been isolated from animals and diarrheic humans, the probability that these helicobacters are also zoonotic agents exists.

IMMUNOLOGIC ASPECTS

A variety of serologic tests have been used to measure the increased anti-*H. pylori*-specific IgG and IgA antibody found in humans with different types of gastritis and duodenal or gastric ulcers. The most popular tests have been an ELISA using glycine-extracted antigen or whole-cell sonicates of the bacteria. The severity of gastritis in terms of inflammatory response does not correlate with levels of antibody. Specific serum IgG antibodies to gastric *Helicobacter* spp. in animals have also been used to diagnose in animals both naturally and experimentally infected with *Helicobacter* spp. Analyses of serum and mucosal secretions by ELISA in cats naturally infected with *H. pylori* revealed an *H. pylori*-specific IgG response and elevated IgA anti-*H. pylori* antibody levels in salivary and local gastric secretions. As in humans, though helpful in diagnosis, neither secretory nor serum antibody responses are protective.

Helicobacter hepaticus has apparently developed strategies to evade host immune responses similar to those of gastric helicobacters. For example, *H. hepaticus* infected A/JCr mice with hepatitis have a persistent IgG antibody response to *H. hepaticus* that do not confer protection. Younger mice colonized with *H. hepaticus* in their intestinal crypts, but without appreciable hepatitis, did not have elevated IgG *H. hepaticus* antibody.

LABORATORY DIAGNOSIS

Direct Examination

In addition to using a gram stain on homogenized gastric tissue for a rapid, presumptive diagnosis, urease activity of these gastric bacteria can be utilized. A diagnostic test for urease is commercially available that detects urease activity in gastric tissue in 15 minutes to 3 hours. A gastric biopsy can be minced and placed directly into urea broth and a positive reaction obtained in 1 hour.

Gastric brushing cytology can be performed during routine endoscopy: before obtaining gastric biopsies, cells and mucus that adhere to the brush are applied to a glass slide, air dried, and stained with Giemsa stain. For identification of gastric *Helicobacter* spp., oil immersion magnification (100×) is used.

TREATMENT AND CONTROL

Various clinical trials using different antimicrobial treatments have been conducted to assess their ability to eradicate *H. pylori* in humans. A triple-therapy regimen consisting of amoxicillin and metronidazole, or tetracycline and metronidazole, in combination with bismuth subsalicylate given for 2 to 3 weeks has proven to be the most efficient in eradication of *H. pylori* in humans. Indeed, this antimicrobial regimen, plus ranitidine, has proven successful in treating patients with ulcer disease. In studies comparing this treatment to those patients receiving ranitidine alone, ulcers not only healed faster, but the recurrence of ulcers was significantly less than the antibiotic-treated group where *H. pylori* has been eradicated. Recently, therapy regimens using proton pump inhibitors (e.g., omeprazole) in combination with other antibiotics also have shown considerable efficacy in eradicating *H. pylori*. Whether antimicrobial therapy should be instituted in domestic dogs and cats with gastritis or ulcer disease is at present unknown.

Studies in ferrets indicate that the triple therapy consisting of amoxicillin (30 mg/kg), metronidazole (20 mg/kg), and bismuth subsalicylate (17.5 mg/kg) (Pepto-Bismol original formula, Proctor & Gamble) three times a day for 3 to 4 weeks has successfully eradicated *H. mustelae* from ferrets.

Mice naturally infected with *H. hepaticus* that received triple therapy consisting of amoxicillin, metronidazole, and bismuth three times daily for 2 weeks by gastric intubation had the organism successfully eradicated, as judged by the failure to isolate *H. hepaticus* from livers, ceca, or colon of these mice euthanatized four weeks after completion of antibiotic therapy. Oral gavage and dietary administration of amoxicillin triple therapy were effective in eradicating *H. hepaticus* in A/J and DBA/2 mice 6 to 10 months of age, indicating triple therapy is also effective in different strains of older mice with well-established infections.

SELECTED REFERENCES

Anderson LP, Norgaard A, Holck S, et al. Isolation of *Helicobacter heilmannii*-like organism from the human stomach (letter). Eur J Clin Microbiol 1996;15:95.

Archer JR, Romero S, Ritchie AE, et al. Characterization of an unclassified microaerophilic bacterium associated with gastroenteritis. J Clin Microbiol 1988;26:101.

Correa P, Fox JG, Fontham E, et al. *Helicobacter pylori* and gastric carcinoma: serum antibody prevalence in populations with contrasting cancer risks. Cancer 1990;66:2569.

Dewhirst FE, Seymour C, Fraser GJ, et al. Phylogeny of Helicobacter isolates from bird and swine feces and description of *Helicobacter parmetensis* sp. nov. Int J Syst Bacteriol 1994;44:553.

Erdman SE, Correa P, Coleman LA, et al. *Helicobacter mustelae*-associated gastric MALT lymphoma in ferrets. Am J Pathol 1997;151:273.

Fox JG, Chilvers T, Goodwin CS. *Campylobacter mustelae*, a new species resulting from the elevation of *Campylobacter pylori* subsp. *mustelae* to species status. Int J Syst Bacteriol 1989;39:301.

Fox JG, Dewhirst FE, Tully JG, et al. *Helicobacter hepaticus* sp. nov., a microaerophilic bacterium isolated from livers and intestinal mucosal scrapings from mice. J Clin Microbiol 1994;32:1238.

Fox JG, Dangler CA, Sager W, et al. *Helicobacter mustelae*-associated gastric adenocarcinoma in ferrets (*Mustela putorius furo*). Vet Pathol 1997;34:225.

Fox JG, Drolet R, Higgins R, et al. *Helicobacter canis* isolated from a dog liver with multifocal necrotizing hepatitis. J Clin Microbiol 1996;34:2479.

Fox JG, Perkins S, Yan L, et al. Local immune response in *Helicobacter pylori* infected cats and identification of *H. pylori* in saliva, gastric fluid and feces. Immunology 1996;88:400.

Gebhart CJ, Fennell CL, Murtaugh MP, Stamm WE. *Campylobacter cinaedi* is normal intestinal flora in hamsters. J Clin Microbiol 1989;27:1692.

Handt LK, Fox JG, Dewhirst FE, et al. *Helicobacter pylori* isolated from the domestic cat: public health implications. Infect Immun 1994;62:2367.

Hazell SL, Mendz GL. How *Helicobacter pylori* works: an overview of the metabolism of *Helicobacter pylori*. Helicobacter 1997;2:1.

Kirkbride CA, Gates CE, Collins JE. Ovine abortion associated with an anaerobic bacterium. J Am Vet Med Assoc 1985;186:789.

Lee A, Fox JG, Hazel LS. Pathogenicity of *Helicobacter pylori*: a perspective. Infect Immun 1993;61:1601.

Stanley J, Linton D, Burens AP, et al. *Helicobacter pullorum* sp. nov. — genotype and phenotype of a new species isolated from poultry and from human patients with gastroenteritis. Microbiology 1994;140:3441.

Telford JL, Ghiara P, Dell'Orco M, et al. Gene structure of the *Helicobacter pylori* cytotoxin and evidence of its key role in gastric disease. J Exp Med 1994;179:1653.

Ward JM, Fox JG, Anver MR, et al. Chronic active hepatitis and associated liver tumors in mice caused by a persistent bacterial infection with a novel *Helicobacter* species. J Nat Cancer Inst 1994;86:1222.

Ward JM, Anver MR, Haines DC, Benveniste RE. Chronic active hepatitis in mice caused by *Helicobacter hepaticus*. Am J Pathol 1994;145:959.

16 Pseudomonas

Dwight C. Hirsh

Of the many recognized species of *Pseudomonas*, only *P. aeruginosa* is of veterinary importance. Previously named pseudomonads of veterinary importance, *P. mallei* and *P. pseudomallei*, have been moved to the genus *Burkholderia* (see Chapter 29).

Pseudomonas aeruginosa is very rarely involved with primary disease, although it is extremely important in clinical medicine. Most strains are resistant to the commonly used antimicrobial agents and are therefore difficult to eliminate when they contaminate a compromised site. It is commonly found in canine otitis externa and cystitis, the uteri of mares (especially those treated with antimicrobial drugs), and the eyes of horses treated with topical steroid and antibiotic mixtures for corneal ulcers. It is an uncommon cause of bovine mastitis and septicemia in immunocompromised animals.

DESCRIPTIVE FEATURES

Morphology and Staining

The organisms are gram-negative rods, 0.5 to 1.0 μm by 1.5 to 5.0 μm. Capsules may be produced. All members are motile by means of polar flagellae. Pili are present.

Cellular Products of Medical Interest

Pseudomonas aeruginosa produces a number of protein exotoxins: exotoxin A, exotoxin S, elastase, and a number of other proteins with biological activity. Exotoxin A and exotoxin S inhibit protein synthesis by ribosylation of host cell G proteins or EF-2, respectively. Exotoxin A acts identically to diphtheria toxin. The toxins are not identical.

Pseudomonas aeruginosa produces bacteriocins (pyocins) and pigments (pyocyanins). Pyocins are useful epidemiologically for tracing epidemics within the hospital environment. Pyocyanin has toxic activity and is used as an aid in the laboratory identification of *P. aeruginosa*. Pyocyanin reacts with oxygen to form reactive oxygen radicals that are toxic to eukaryotic and prokaryotic organisms. *Pseudomonas aeruginosa* protects itself from the toxic effects of pyocyanin by increasing synthesis of catalase and superoxide dismutase.

Pseudomonas aeruginosa produces the iron-acquiring siderophores pyochelin and pyoverdin, as well as uses the siderophores produced by other bacteria living in its environment (e.g., enterobactin and aerobactin).

Growth Characteristics

Members of the genus *Pseudomonas* are obligate aerobes, deriving their energy from the oxidation of organic materials and using oxygen as a terminal electron acceptor. They grow on all common media over a wide range of temperatures: 4°C to 41°C.

ECOLOGY

Reservoir

Most members of the genus *Pseudomonas* live in soil and water. *Pseudomonas aeruginosa* may also occur in the feces of normal animals.

Transmission

Environmental or endogenous exposure is constant, and most infections are secondary to compromised host defenses.

Pathogenesis

Pseudomonas aeruginosa contaminates areas of the body that possess reduced numbers of normal flora. Disruption of the normal flora is almost always due to antimicrobial agents. Since *P. aeruginosa* is resistant to most commonly used antimicrobial agents, it will replace the normal flora. If the site colonized is compromised or contiguous to a compromised site, there is risk of infection of the site. Tissue destruction follows liberation of exotoxin(s) and pyocyanin.

Pseudomonas aeruginosa is also isolated from certain sites of animals that have no history of antimicrobial therapy.

Epidemiology

The organism is ubiquitous in the environment. Disease determinants therefore lie largely with the hosts and their immediate environment. In a veterinary hospital, however, a number of situations favor selection of this organism. *Pseudomonas aeruginosa* thrives in wet, poorly aerated environments within the hospital, especially in surgery areas within support bags that have not been properly dried, in hoses on anesthetic machines that have not been cleaned and dried properly, or in disinfectant solutions that have not been changed frequently. These situations result in an increase in the number of pseudomonads in the environment of the compromised animal (site), thereby increasing the risk of infection (contamination). *Pseudomonas aeruginosa* is a frequent cause of bacteremia in human beings with burns, leukemia, or cystic fibrosis.

IMMUNOLOGIC ASPECTS

Specific immune responses do not seem to play much of a role in pathogenesis or resistance, though artificial protection has been shown to occur in animals vaccinated with extracts of the organism or exotoxin A. The most important consideration is to decrease the risk of infection by reducing the concentration of the organism in the environment of the patient, in addition to reducing the extent of compromise, for example, by cleaning and drying an infected ear.

LABORATORY DIAGNOSIS

Pseudomonas aeruginosa grows well on blood agar medium. The colonies are somewhat large, >1 mm in diameter, gray (gunmetal), rough, usually with a zone of hemolysis. A plate containing *P. aeruginosa* has a characteristic odor, reminiscent of corn tortillas. Besides being oxidase-positive, a trait that sets it apart from members of the family *Enterobacteriaceae*, it turns triple sugar iron agar slightly alkaline (without gas), utilizes glucose oxidatively, grows at 42°C, and forms a blue-green, chloroform-soluble pigment, pyocyanin. Resistance to some antimicrobials is due to permeability barrier of the *Pseudomonas* cell wall, and to others because of inactivation due to products encoded by plasmid-based genes (R plasmids).

TREATMENT AND CONTROL

Treatment involves correction of compromise and, if necessary, the use of an antimicrobial agent. *Pseudomonas aeruginosa* is usually susceptible to gentamicin, tobramycin, amikacin, carbenicillin, ciprofloxacin, and ticarcillin clavulanic acid, and these agents are used for the treatment of soft tissue infections. In the canine urinary tract, tetracycline achieves concentrations sufficient to kill most isolates. Most pseudomonads are susceptible to levels achieved by antimicrobial agents in otic preparations: enrofloxacin, neomycin, polymyxin, chloramphenicol, and gentamicin. It should be noted that there are no in vitro tests that predict susceptibility/resistance of isolate from infectious processes that will be treated topically (e.g., the ear).

SELECTED REFERENCES

Crosa JH. Signal transduction and transcriptional and posttranscriptional control of iron-regulated genes in bacteria. Microbiol Molec Biol Rev 1997;61:319.

Hassett DJ, Charniga L, Bean K, et al. Response of *Pseudomonas aeruginosa* to pyocyanin: mechanisms of resistance, antioxidant defenses, and demonstration of a manganese-cofactored superoxide dismutase. Infect Immun 1992;60:328.

Hirsh DC, Jang SS. Antimicrobial susceptibility of selected infectious agents from dogs. J Am Anim Hosp Assoc 1994;30:487.

Iglewski B. Probing *Pseudomonas aeruginosa*, an opportunistic pathogen. ASM News 1989;55:303.

Ling GV, Creighton SR, Ruby AL. Tetracycline for oral treatment of canine urinary tract infection caused by *Pseudomonas aeruginosa*. J Am Vet Med Assoc 1981;179:578.

Middlebrook JL, Dorland RB. Bacterial toxins: cellular mechanism of action. Microbiol Rev 1984;48:199.

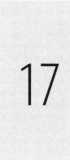

17 Yersinia enterocolitica

Dwight C. Hirsh

Yersinia enterocolitica is associated with mesenteric lymphadenitis, terminal ileitis, acute gastroenteritis, and rare septicemia in primates and occasionally in other species. Mesenteric lymphadenitis and septicemia with involvement of liver and spleen are seen in other animal species. It is a pathogen of humans, and animal products (e.g., milk, pork) are among the sources of human infection.

DESCRIPTIVE FEATURES

Cellular Anatomy

Yersinia enterocolitica is a typical member of the family *Enterobacteriaceae*. It is not encapsulated and possesses a number of temperature-regulated traits. Products formed at 22°C to 25°C (but poorly at 37°C) include flagella, O-antigens, bacteriophage receptors, and a mannose-resistant hemagglutinin. Surface fibrils are formed at 37°C but not at 22°C. These fibrils are thought to be responsible for the autoagglutination observed with virulent strains.

Cellular Products of Medical Interest

Yersinia enterocolitica produces a chromosomally encoded enterotoxin (Yst), with activity similar to the ST toxin secreted by *Escherichia coli* (see Chapter 9). The role of the enterotoxin is unclear; though it is made at 37°C, enterotoxin-negative strains produce diarrhea. Pathogenic yersiniae contain a plasmid called *pYV* (*plasmid* for *y*ersinial *v*irulence) of approximately 70 kb in size. Loss of the plasmid results in the loss of virulence, the autoagglutination trait, calcium-dependent growth at 37°C but not at 25°C, ability to survive within mononuclear phagocytes, and ability to produce keratoconjunctivitis in the guinea pig (Sereny test). The products encoded on pYV include a protein needed for adherence and uptake by target cells (*YadA*, *Y*ersinia *ad*herence; *Ail*, *a*ttachment *i*nvasion *l*ocus); antiphagocytic proteins (Yops, *Y*ersinia *o*uter *m*embrane *p*roteins — excreted proteins that are really not outer membrane bound); an outer membrane protein, invasin, that facilitates adhesion and entry into the target cell; and various regulatory proteins. Survival within macrophages is associated with the GsrA protein (*g*lobal *s*tress *r*equirement) and is induced following phagocytosis, although YopJ triggers apoptosis in this cell type.

Virulent yersiniae also make a siderophore and a hemin-binding protein (HemR) for iron uptake.

Growth Characteristics

Most of the physiological characteristics of *Y. enterocolitica* are those of the family *Enterobacteriaceae*. Some minor variations include growth at 4°C, expression of certain traits at 25°C compared to 37°C, and little or no gas production in the fermentation of glucose.

Variability

There are 34 O-antigen and 20 H-antigen serogroups. O groups 3, 5, 27, 8, and 9 are associated with classical disease of the gastrointestinal tract. There are five biotypes.

ECOLOGY

Reservoir and Transmission

Water, food, soil, fruits, vegetables, and asymptomatic individuals from humans to mollusks have been proposed as reservoirs for *Y. enterocolitica*. Expression of certain virulence determinants at 22°C to 25°C suggests that mammals acquire *Y. enterocolitica* from a "cold" source (water and food, for example) rather than a warm-blooded animal. Infection follows ingestion of organisms expressing the adhesin.

Pathogenesis

In the intraintestinal milieu, temperature and perhaps calcium ion concentration downregulate yersinia growth. In stationary phase, RpoS (the gene encoding the stationary phase sigma factor for RNA polymerase) is produced, which is necessary for optimal expression of Yst and Yops. Pathogenic yersiniae attach to M cells of lymphoid nodules of the distal small intestine following expression of the cell surface proteins invasin, Ail, and YadA. Attachment triggers actin cytoskeletal changes resulting in a "zippering" phenomenon that leads to the enclosure of the cell membrane around the attached yersiniae, resulting in their internalization. Internalized microorganisms pass through to the lymphoid nodule. At this stage, Yops are produced and secreted. These proteins interfere with phagocytosis by macrophages residing within the nodule, and induce their death by apoptosis. However, yersiniae survive to some degree within macrophages due to the expression of the GsrA protein.

Invasion of the basolateral surface of ileal epithelial cells occurs following attachment to the basolateral surface of the cell (β_1 integrins, the target for YadA and invasin, are localized on this aspect of the intestinal epithelium), and internalization follows. Inflammation induced by extracellular yersiniae, together with interferon secretion by NK and gamma delta T cell recognition of infected epithelial cells (as well as lipopolysaccharide), results in an influx of polymorphonuclear neutrophil leukocytes (PMNs), which are very efficient in killing yersiniae. Extracellular yersiniae avoid destruction by complement-mediated mechanisms by expression of Ail and YadA, both of which impart complement resistance. *Yersinia enterocolitica* produces a hemin-binding protein (HemR) and a siderophore capable of iron acquisition from transferrin and lactoferrin. Diarrhea results from secretion of the enterotoxin (Yst) and/or the consequences of an inflammatory response (activation of the arachidonic acid pathway resulting in production of prostaglandins and leukotrienes, and elevation of cAMP).

Clinical infections, which occur in chinchillas, hares, and monkeys, are enteritides potentially complicated by hematogenous spread to liver and spleen. Diarrheal disease has also been seen in pigs, goats, dogs, and cats — young animals being preferentially affected.

Epidemiology

Certain serotypes are geographically restricted. O:8 is indigenous to the United States but not the rest of the world. O:3 until recently was rarely isolated in the United States but is common in the rest of the world, and is becoming more so in the United States. O:9 has not been reported outside of Europe.

The chief interest in animal yersiniosis derives from its possible epidemiologic relation to human yersinial infections. Outbreaks linked to animals and animal products have been rare. Serotyping and biotyping suggest that there is little relationship between animal strains and human disease isolates.

IMMUNOLOGIC ASPECTS

Yersinia enterocolitica is an extracellular microorganism. It is readily destroyed by phagocytic cells, even though the microorganism excretes proteins (Yops) that interfere with this process. Most often, *Y. enterocolitica* disease is self-limiting due to the innate immune response: phagocytosis, lysis of infected epithelial cells, iron sequestration, and complement proteins.

A serologic relationship between O:9 serotype, common in swine, and *Brucella* spp. has complicated swine brucellosis eradication programs.

LABORATORY DIAGNOSIS

Samples of feces, lymph node biopsy, and biopsy from affected tissues are examined microbiologically. Selective media containing bile salts are somewhat inhibitory to *Y. enterocolitica*, especially at 37°C. MacConkey agar is least inhibitory. There are special media designed for the isolation of *Y. enterocolitica* (e.g., CIN medium). Cold enrichment of the sample at 4°C aids in attempts to isolate small numbers of *Y. enterocolitica* from a contaminated environment. Isolation from tissue necessitates the use of blood agar plates incubated at 37°C.

TREATMENT

Antimicrobial agents useful for treating disease produced by *Y. enterocolitica* are the fluoroquinolones, tetracycline, trimethoprim-sulfonamides, and chloramphenicol. R plasmids are common in *Y. enterocolitica*, and genes encoding resistance to tetracycline and streptomycin are most commonly found.

Other yersiniae are considered in Chapter 49.

SELECTED REFERENCES

Bottone EJ. *Yersinia enterocolitica*: the charisma continues. Clin Microbiol Rev 1997;10:257.

Conlan JW. Critical roles of neutrophils in host defense against experimental systemic infections of mice by *Listeria monocytogenes*, *Salmonella typhimurium*, and *Yersinia enterocolitica*. Infect Immun 1997;65:630.

Davey GM, Bruce J, Drysdale EM. Isolation of *Yersinia enterocolitica* and related species from the feces of cows. J App Bacteriol 1983;55:439.

Fasano A. Cellular microbiology: how enteric pathogens socialize with their intestinal host. ASM News 1997;63:259.

Finlay BB, Cossart P. Exploitation of mammalian host cell functions by bacterial pathogens. Science 1997;276:718.

Finlay BB, Falkow S. Common themes in microbial pathogenicity revisited. Microbiol Molec Biol Rev 1997;61:136.

Isberg RR, Nhieu GTV. Two mammalian cell internalization strategies used by pathogenic bacteria. Annu Rev Genet 1994; 27:395.

Monack DM, Mecsas J, Ghori N, Falkow S. *Yersinia* signals macrophages to undergo apoptosis and YopJ is necessary for this cell death. Proc Nat Acad Sci USA 1997;94:10385.

Neutra MR, Pringault E, Kraehenbuhl J. Antigen sampling across epithelial barriers and induction of mucosal immune responses. Annu Rev Immunol 1996;14:275.

Yamamoto T, Hanawa T, Ogata S, Kamiya S. The *Yersinia enterocolitica* GsrA stress protein, involved in intracellular survival, is induced by macrophage phagocytosis. Infect Immun 1997; 65:2190.

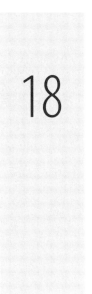

18 Mycobacterium avium *ssp.* paratuberculosis (Mycobacterium paratuberculosis)

Dwight C. Hirsh

Mycobacterium avium ssp. *paratuberculosis*, hereafter referred to as *Mycobacterium paratuberculosis*, is the causative agent of a chronic, irreversible wasting disease of ruminants called *Johne's disease*.

DESCRIPTIVE FEATURES

Morphology and Staining

Mycobacterium paratuberculosis is a rod-shaped bacillus, 1 to 2 μm by 0.5 μm. It possesses a gram-positive cell wall but, because of high lipid content, the cells are difficult to stain by the Gram method. It is acid-fast.

Cellular Anatomy and Composition

The cellular constitution is typical for the genus *Mycobacterium* (see Chapter 30).

Cellular Products of Medical Interest

Extracts of broth cultures of *M. paratuberculosis* contain the protein derivative (johnin) responsible for eliciting the delayed-type sensitivity responses that are manifest following infection with this organism.

Iron-acquiring substances exochelins and mycobactin may be responsible for intracellular growth. Exochelins are proteins that remove ferric iron from ferritin, and mycobactin is a complex lipid residing in the cell membrane of the microorganism that is responsible for transfer of iron from the exochelin to the bacterium.

Growth Characteristics

Like the rest of the genus *Mycobacterium*, *M. paratuberculosis* is an obligate aerobe. In the past, the dependency of *M. paratuberculosis* for mycobactin has been used to differentiate it from other mycobacteria. This trait has been shown to be shared, however, with other strains

of *M. avium*. The medium of choice is Herrold's egg-yolk medium. Most strains are stimulated by pyruvate.

Growth is slow. Development of visible colonies requires 8 to 12 weeks of incubation at 37°C.

Mycobacterium paratuberculosis survives many months in soil or in organic matter when protected from direct sunlight and drying.

ECOLOGY

Reservoir

Traditionally in vitro growth of most strains requires the presence of the iron-binding lipid mycobactin. This trait is also shared by other strains of *M. avium*.

The reservoir for *M. paratuberculosis* is the intestinal tract of infected animals, both the clinically affected and, more importantly, those infected but asymptomatic. In an affected herd, infected, asymptomatic fecal shedders may be 20 times more numerous than those showing clinical signs. An infected animal may also shed *M. paratuberculosis* into colostrum and milk, and may pass the organism to her fetus in utero. *Mycobacterium paratuberculosis* has been isolated from semen, seminiferous tubules, and the prostate glands of infected bulls.

Transmission

The infection is usually acquired through the ingestion of contaminated feces, but in utero infection and ingestion of contaminated colostrum or milk are also possible routes.

Pathogenesis

The pathogenic mechanisms appear to involve cell-mediated immune phenomena. The granulomatous lesions associated with clinical disease are related to cell-mediated hypersensitivity. The organism is found within macrophages in the submucosa of the ileocecal area and the adjacent lymph nodes (ileocecal) following ingestion. Extraintestinal colonization suggests the existence of a blood phase, but this probably occurs after establishment of a primary focus of infection in the intestine. Whether this occurs soon after infection or later is not known. Initially the animal shows no signs of disease. The incubation period before overt clinical disease is 12 months or longer.

After ingestion, *M. paratuberculosis* enters by means of M cells over lymphoid nodules of the ileocecal area. Shortly thereafter, macrophages within the nodule become infected, with *M. paratuberculosis* seen within phagosomes and phagolysosomes. Ingested microorganisms limit production of superoxides and discourage fusion of lysosomes with phagosomes. Those within phagolysosomes are relatively resistant to destruction (probably related to the chemistry of their cell wall). Intracellular *M. paratuberculosis* acquire iron for growth with the excretion of exochelins, which remove iron from macrophage ferritin. Iron is transported by way of exochelin-iron complexes across the mycobacterial cell wall to the cytoplasmic membrane where mycobactin transports the iron into the cell. There is evidence that iron availability dictates the distribution of *M. paratuberculosis*, with most iron available within macrophages of nodules in the ileocecal area.

Release of IL-12 by affected macrophages initiates the inflammatory and immune responses. The responses are initiated by the recruitment of specific CD4+ T_{H1} cells and subsequent release of cytokines leading to the attraction of macrophages to the site of interaction of *M. paratuberculosis* and macrophage. Normally, gamma interferon (one of the released cytokines) would activate macrophages to deal effectively with ingested mycobacteria. Activation is compromised, however, by gamma delta T lymphocytes that are cytotoxic for the specific CD4+ T_{H1} lymphocytes. This cytotoxicity is regulated by CD8+ T lymphocytes. In addition, gamma interferon released by T lymphocytes is a poor activator of *M. paratuberculosis*-infected macrophages. The interaction between all of these cell types results in the formation of a slowly progressing granulomatous reaction as evidenced by the accumulation of macrophages in the submucosal region. Some macrophages die subsequent to the multiplication of mycobacteria within them, resulting in the release of microorganisms and phagocytosis by other macrophages. The granulomatous response and cellular infiltrate lead ultimately to sloughing of the mucosal epithelium and release of infected macrophages and mycobacteria into the lumen.

The disease in some affected animals progresses to malabsorption, protein-losing enteropathy, and overt clinical disease. However, only 3% to 5% percent of the animals in an infected herd progress to clinical disease. Other economic losses are traced to breeding problems (e.g., longer calving intervals), to reduced milk production due to an increased incidence of mastitis (not caused by *M. paratuberculosis*), and to general ill thrift.

Extraintestinal localization (e.g., mammary gland, fetus, sex organs of male) suggests a blood phase. There is a direct correlation between the degree of dissemination and the numbers of *M. paratuberculosis* in feces. Infected blood monocytes have been demonstrated and may be the manner in which sites outside of the intestinal tract become infected.

Cattle. Animals showing clinical signs present with chronic weight loss, diarrhea, but normal appetite and temperature. At this stage of the disease, the submucosa of the intestinal tract, extending both cranially as well as caudally from the ileocecal area, is infiltrated with macrophages, epithelioid cells, and some giant cells that contain large numbers of *M. paratuberculosis*. The draining lymph nodes are almost always enlarged and packed with macrophages containing mycobacteria. The classical gross lesion in cattle is a permanent transverse corrugation of the intestinal mucosa caused by granulomatous inflammation within the lamina propria and submucosa (Fig 18.1). The extent of the infiltration is not always related to the severity of the clinical disease. The symptomatic disease usually progresses to a fatal outcome.

Sheep and Goats. Diarrhea is not a common clinical sign of the disease in these species. Herd unthriftiness, however, should prompt examination for *M. paratuberculosis*. Intestinal lesions in sheep and goats are less obvious than in cattle. Weight loss has been a consistent finding with affected goats.

Epidemiology

The young animal is the most susceptible to infection. Older animals can be infected only with very large inocula.

F I G U R E 1 8 . 1 . *Bovine intestine affected by Johne's disease showing permanent corrugations. (Photograph courtesy of Dr. Murray Fowler.)*

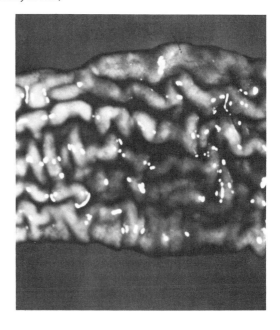

Many ruminant species are subject to infection. Clinical disease occurs mostly under conditions of domestication or captivity, especially in association with stress factors such as parturition, crowding, shipment, or faulty dietary regimes.

Genetics may play a part, as certain cattle breeds (Guernsey, Jersey, Shorthorn) seem to be preferentially affected.

High prevalence of inapparent shedders, chronicity of infection, and persistence in the environment favor dissemination of the agent. The overall prevalence in U.S. bovines is approximately 1% to 3%. The importance of transmission through milk and placenta is uncertain.

Bacteria resembling *M. paratuberculosis* have been isolated from humans with Crohn's disease (regional ileitis), a disease remarkably similar to Johne's disease.

IMMUNOLOGIC ASPECTS

The lesions and host responses are manifestations of cellular immunity. The cell-mediated immune response probably accounts for the low percentage of animals that progress to overt disease. Other problems, such as decreased milk production and increased calving intervals, may be indirectly due to the generalized immunosuppression observed in infected animals.

Artificial immunization is practiced in some areas of the world, and this practice seems to reduce the losses that occur due to this disease, but it does not eliminate the problem. In the United States, vaccination is not practiced because of its real or perceived interference with diagnostic tests (see below), since vaccinated animals will test positive for this disease and occasionally for tuberculosis as well.

LABORATORY DIAGNOSIS

Sample Collection

From cattle, samples from the ileocecal area (intestine or lymph nodes) are best, but mucosal scrapings from the rectum in the live animals are easier to obtain. Biopsies of ileocecal lymph nodes are performed on valuable cattle. In sheep and goats, examination of the ileocecal lymph nodes is the most rewarding. Samples of intestinal content or scrapings are least useful in these species.

Direct Examination

Impression smears of lymph nodes, or smears of rectal or intestinal scrapings, are stained by the Ziehl-Neelsen procedure. *Mycobacterium paratuberculosis* will stain acid-fast. They are short, slender rods, occurring in bunches (Fig 18.2). Other acid-fast staining structures in samples (saprophytic mycobacteria or bacterial endospores) will be solitary and quite large. Sections stained with hematoxylin-eosin reveal the typical granulomatous lesions. If stained by acid-fast procedure, masses of intra- and extracellular organisms can be demonstrated.

FIGURE 18.2. *Impression of mesenteric lymph node from a goat with Johne's disease, showing masses of minute intra- and extracellular acid-fast bacteria. Ziehl-Neelsen stain, about 2000×.*

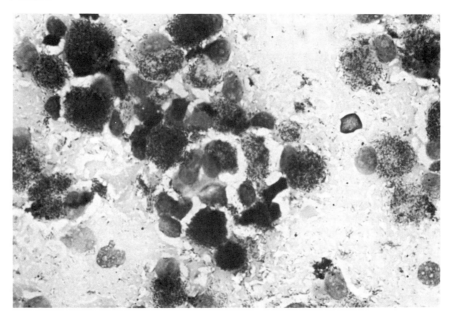

Isolation

Growth of the organism in vitro is the surest way to make the diagnosis. Fecal samples or lymph node biopsies are first decontaminated with hexadecylpyridinium chloride. The decontaminated sample is placed in egg-yolk medium containing mycobactin (mycobactin J produced by *M. paratuberculosis* is preferred). Because some strains are inhibited by sodium pyruvate, egg-yolk medium with and without this substance should be inoculated, as should the same medium with and without mycobactin. The time required to develop visible colonies is about 8 weeks. Current techniques allow for the detection of one organism per gram of material.

A radiometric procedure (BACTEC-RCM) utilizing ^{14}C-palmitic acid followed by polymerase chain reaction (PCR) amplification of the insertion sequence IS900, a *M. paratuberculosis*-specific sequence of DNA, has been described and allows detection in feces in 2 to 4 weeks.

IMMUNODIAGNOSIS

Immunodiagnostic procedures are run in parallel with cultures of the organism and examination of direct smears. Available tests rely either on the presence of antibody or on delayed-type hypersensitivity to extracts of the organism.

Delayed-Type Hypersensitivity Tests

There are three general types: an intradermal test, an IV johnin test, and a lymphocyte proliferation assay. The intradermal test requires the intradermal injection of johnin, followed by examination of the injection site for swelling 48 to 72 hours later. This test may result in as high as 75% false-positive reactors.

The IV johnin test is more specific. Reacting animals develop a fever of 1.5°F or higher following IV injection of johnin. This test detects about 80% of the cases showing clinical signs, but not asymptomatic shedders.

The third test measures the cell-mediated immune status of the animal to *M. paratuberculosis* in an in vitro lymphocyte-stimulation test. Peripheral blood lymphocytes are collected and exposed to johnin (or to its purified protein derivative). If the animal has developed cell-mediated immunity to the antigens of *M. paratuberculosis*, these lymphocytes will respond by proliferating, which is measured by the addition of a radio-labeled nucleic acid precursor. This test increases the specificity of the detection, but animals test positive at a stage when clinical signs are evident.

Serologic Tests

The complement fixation test will result in about 75% false-positive reactors. The other serological tests, the agar gel immunodiffusion (AGID) test and the enzyme-linked immunoadsorbant assay (ELISA), are more specific. ELISA detects shedders before the AGID test, which becomes positive only after large numbers of *M. paratuberculosis* are in the feces. ELISA will detect an infected animal before there are sufficient organisms in the feces for positive culture.

The usefulness of the ELISA and AGID tests for diagnosis of this disease in sheep and goats is unknown. Tests utilizing cell-mediated immune response in these species have not been useful.

Molecular Techniques

A number of DNA tests have been developed for the demonstration of the presence of *M. paratuberculosis*. All utilize a specific sequence for the development of probes or for the design of primers needed to amplify DNA by using PCR. Specific sequences that have been exploited are those found in the 16S rDNA and the insertion sequence IS900. Tests have been designed to determine the presence of *M. paratuberculosis* DNA in feces, tissue, and in blood monocytes. Methods using feces or tissue suffer from a lack of sensitivity, especially for feces, which is probably due to inhibitors found in this substance. For example, fecal analysis using probes specific for the IS900 sequence, or PCR amplification of specific sequences, results in a threshold of 10^4 to 10^5 microorganisms/gm (culture of feces can detect about 10/gm) before detection. On the other hand, PCR analysis of peripheral monocytes results in a detection level of about 1/ml to 10/ml of blood. Though molecular methods may lack some sensitivity, they are very specific.

TREATMENT, CONTROL, AND PREVENTION

At present there are no economically useful antimicrobial agents that are effective against *M. paratuberculosis* in vivo. The newer macrolides, such as clarithromycin, are effective in vitro, but are too expensive to use clinically.

The disease is best attacked by eliminating infected animals and preventing possible spread within the herd. Husbandry procedures that must be implemented include segregating the neonate from the dam and other adult animals, ensuring that parturition takes place in non-contaminated areas, and taking precautions against feeding neonates potentially infectious, unpasteurized colostrum or milk. Immunologic and cultural tests are applied to promptly identify those animals that are infected and shedding. The AGID assay detects animals shedding the organism. The ELISA detects those that are shedding numbers too low to be detected by culture. Culture is used to confirm the results of the serological assays; it is also used in vaccinated herds where serological tests are not reliable. Molecular techniques that utilize nonfecal samples (such as peripheral blood) show great promise in speeding up the process of identifying affected animals.

Prevention of the disease is difficult. Since there are few regulations governing the sale and shipment of possibly infected livestock, a producer has no way of ascertaining whether a purchased animal is uninfected except by testing. Until uniform tests and reporting procedures are established, the assurance that an animal is free of *M. tuberculosis* is not possible.

Parenteral vaccines, live and killed, are used in some countries but are not universally available.

SELECTED REFERENCES

Carrigan MJ, Seaman JT. The pathology of Johne's disease in sheep. Aust Vet J 1990;67:47.

Chiodini RJ, Davis WC. The cellular immunology of bovine paratuberculosis: the predominant response is mediated by cytotoxic gamma/delta T lymphocytes which prevent CD4+ activity. Microb Pathogen 1992;13:447.

Chiodini RJ, Davis WC. The cellular immunity of bovine paratuberculosis: immunity may be regulated by CD4+ helper and CD8+ immunoregulatory T lymphocytes which downregulate gamma/delta+ T-cell cytotoxicity. Microb Pathogen 1993;14:355.

Cocito C, Gilot P, Coene M, et al. Paratuberculosis. Clin Microbiol Rev 1994;7:328.

Davies DH, Corbeil L, Ward D, Duncan JR. A humoral suppressor of in vitro lymphocyte transformation responses in cattle with Johne's disease. Proc Soc Exp Biol Med 1974;145:1372.

Dell'Isola B, Poyart C, Goulet O, et al. Detection of *Mycobacterium paratuberculosis* by polymerase chain reaction in children with Crohn's disease. J Infect Dis 1994;169:449.

Gezon HM, Bither HD, Gibbs HC, et al. Identification and control of paratuberculosis in a large goat herd. Am J Vet Res 1988;49:1817.

Grange JM, Yates MD, Boughton E. The avian tubercle bacillus and its relatives. J App Bacteriol 1990;68:411.

Koenig GJ, Hoffsis GF, Shulaw WP, et al. Isolation of *Mycobacterium paratuberculosis* from mononuclear cells in tissues, blood, and mammary glands of cows with advanced paratuberculosis. Am J Vet Res 1993;54:1441.

Larsen AB, Stalheim QHV, Hughes DE, et al. *Mycobacterium paratuberculosis* in the semen and genital organs of a semendonor bull. J Am Vet Med Assoc 1981;179:169.

Lepper AWD, Wilks CR. Intracellular iron storage and the pathogenesis of paratuberculosis: comparative studies with other mycobacterial parasitic or infectious conditions of veterinary importance. J Comp Pathol 1988;98:31.

McClure HM, Chiodini RJ, Anderson DC, et al. *Mycobacterium paratuberculosis* infection in a colony of stumptail macaques (*Macaca arctoides*). J Infect Dis 1987;155:1011.

McFadden JJ, Butcher RD, Chiodini R, Hermon-Taylor J. Crohn's disease–isolated mycobacteria are identical to *Mycobacterium tuberculosis*, as determined by DNA probes that distinguish between mycobacterial species. J Clin Microbiol 1987;25:796.

Merkal RS. Paratuberculosis: advances in cultural, serologic, and vaccination methods. J Am Vet Med Assoc 1984;184:939.

Merkal RS, Whipple DL, Sacks JM, Snyder GR. Prevalence of *Mycobacterium paratuberculosis* in ileocecal lymph nodes of cattle culled in the United States. J Vet Med Assoc 1987;190:676.

Momotani E, Whipple DL, Thiermann AB, Cheville NF. Role of M cells and macrophages in the entrance of *Mycobacterium paratuberculosis* into domes of ileal Peyer's patches in calves. Vet Pathol 1988;25:131.

Rastogi N, Goh KS, Labrousse V. Activity of clarithromycin compared with those of other drugs against *Mycobacterium paratuberculosis* and further enhancement of its extracellular and intracellular activities by ethambutol. Antimicrob Agents Chemother 1992;36:2843.

Seitz SE, Heider BE, Hueston WD, et al. Bovine fetal infection with *Mycobacterium paratuberculosis*. J Am Vet Med Assoc 1989;194:1423.

Streeter RN, Hoffsis GF, Bech-Nielsen S, et al. Isolation of *Mycobacterium paratuberculosis* from colostrum and milk of subclinically infected cows. Am J Vet Res 1995;56:1322.

Sweeney RW, Whitlock RH, Rosenberger AE. *Mycobacterium paratuberculosis* cultured from milk and supramammary lymph nodes of infected asymptomatic cows. J Clin Microbiol 1992;30:166.

Thompson DE. The role of mycobacteria in Crohn's disease. J Med Microbiol 1994;41:74.

Thorel M, Krichevsky M, Levy-Frebault VV. Numerical taxonomy of mycobactin-dependent mycobacteria, emended description of *Mycobacterium avium* and description of *Mycobacterium avium* subsp. *avium* subsp. nov., *Mycobacterium avium* subsp. *paratuberculosis* subsp. nov., and *Mycobacterium avium* subsp. *silvaticum* subsp. nov. Int J Syst Bacteriol 1990;40:254.

van der Giessen JWB. A molecular approach to the diagnosis and control of bovine paratuberculosis. Doctoral thesis. University of Utrecht, 1993.

van der Giessen JWB, Eger A, Haagsma J, et al. Amplification of 16S ribosomal RNA sequences to detect *Mycobacterium paratuberculosis*. J Med Microbiol 1992;36:255.

Zurbrick BG, Follett DM, Czuprynski CJ. Cytokine regulation of the intracellular growth of *Mycobacterium paratuberculosis* in bovine monocytes. Infect Immun 1988;56:1692.

19 Candida

Ernst L. Biberstein

Candidiasis is usually due to the parasitic yeast *Candida albicans*, which inhabits mucous membranes of most mammals and birds. Of the more than 150 other species of *Candida* that are associated with many diverse habitats, few cause animal disease. Disease produced by members of the genus *Candida* usually occurs in an immunocompromised host.

The subsequent discussion deals with *C. albicans* unless otherwise indicated.

DESCRIPTIVE FEATURES

Cell Morphology, Anatomy, and Composition

On routine laboratory media and mucous membranes, *C. albicans* typically grows as oval budding yeast cells (blastoconidia), 3.5 μm to 6 μm × 6 μm to 10 μm in size. Under certain conditions of temperature, pH, nutrition, and atmosphere, yeast cells sprout germ tubes (Fig 19.1) that develop into septate-branching mycelium. "Pseudomycelium" is produced by elongation of the blastoconidia and their failure to separate. In vivo, mycelial or pseudomycelial growth is associated with active proliferation and invasiveness.

The so-called chlamydospore (chlamydoconidium) is a thick-walled sphere of unknown function, attached by a suspensor cell to (pseudo)mycelium and essentially confined to in vitro growth (Fig 19.2) of *C. albicans* (rarely other *Candida* spp.).

Candida cells are eukaryotes. The cell wall contains glycoproteins; the polysaccharide portions are glucans and especially mannans. Lipids and chitin are also present. Mannoproteins are found on the cell surface. Cellular products include peptidolytic enzymes, which may be virulence factors. Two major cross-reacting serogroups are recognized. These are termed *A* and *B*, and are identifiable with absorbed sera.

Candida can be stained with periodic acid Schiff (PAS), Gomori methenamine silver (GMS), and other fungal stains, but is usually studied in culture unstained. Polychrome stains (Wright's, Giemsa) are suitable for demonstrating it in tissue or exudate. With Gram stain, *Candida* cells often appear gram positive.

Growth Characteristics

Candida albicans, an obligate aerobe, grows on ordinary media over a wide range of pH and temperature. At 25°C, creamy to pasty white colonies consisting predominantly of blastoconidia appear in 24 to 48 hours. Production of (pseudo)mycelium is environmentally influenced, but the controlling factors are disputed. Incubation temperatures above 35°C, a slightly alkaline pH, and a rich, carbohydrate-free fluid medium are often recommended.

Differential ability to ferment or assimilate carbohydrates is the basis of species identification.

Candida species are killed by heat above 50°C, ultraviolet light, chlorine, and quaternary ammonium-type disinfectants. They withstand freezing and survive well in the inanimate environment. They are susceptible to polyene antimycotics, and usually to flucytosine and the azoles.

Reservoir

Candida albicans is associated with mucocutaneous areas, particularly of the alimentary and lower genital tract, of mammals and birds. Environmental sources are important especially for other *Candida* spp.

Transmission

Most *Candida* diseases arise from an endogenous source, that is, they are caused by a commensal strain. The bovine udder becomes infected via the teat canal by way of administered medication, during milking, by cow-to-cow spread, or from the environment.

Pathogenesis

Mechanisms. Chitin, mannoprotein, and lipids are possible adhesins in human candidiasis; several extracellular matrix proteins have been shown to be the receptor. Germ tube formation is correlated with experimental pathogenicity, but the role of mycelium formation in virulence is under dispute. Proteases and neuraminidase may be virulence factors. Cell wall glycoproteins have endotoxin-like activity.

Pathology. Candidiasis most frequently affects the mucous surfaces on which the agent is normally found, possibly the anterior digestive tract from mouth to stomach; it typically remains confined to areas of squamous epithelium. The genital tract, skin, and claws can be involved

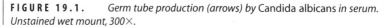

FIGURE 19.1.   *Germ tube production (arrows) by* Candida albicans *in serum. Unstained wet mount, 300×.*

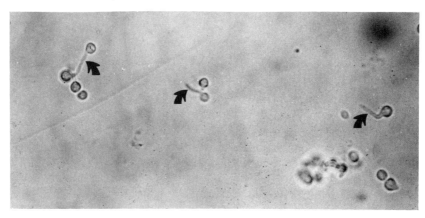

FIGURE 19.2.   Candida albicans *culture on chlamydospore agar with trypan blue, showing pseudomycelium, blastoconidia (right), and chlamydoconidia (left); 1200×.*

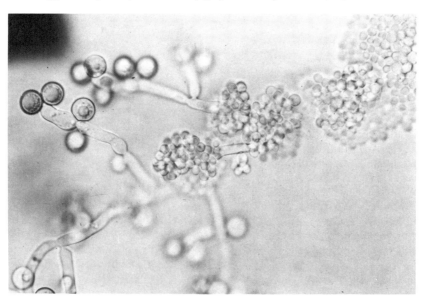

as well. Occasional respiratory, intestinal, and septicemic infections occur.

On epithelial surfaces, candidiasis forms whitish to yellow or gray plaques, marking areas of ulceration with varying degree of inflammation. Diphtheritic membranes may form in the gut or respiratory tract, and abscesses may form in the viscera. Granulomatous lesions are rare. Inflammatory responses are predominantly neutrophilic.

Disease Patterns.   Avian candidiasis affects chickens, turkeys, pigeons, and other birds. It resembles thrush of humans involving the anterior digestive tract. In the young, it can be a stunting disease and cause considerable mortality.

In the alimentary tract of foals and pigs, candidiasis causes ulcerative lesions that may lead to rupture. Equine genital infections cause infertility, metritis, and abortions.

Pneumonic, enteric, and generalized candidiasis affects calves on intensive antibiotic regimens. *Candida mastitis* in dairy cows is typically mild and self-limiting, ending in spontaneous recovery within about a week. Bovine abortions have been reported.

In the small carnivores, candidiasis produces ulcerative lesions in the digestive and genital tract. Rarely, dogs develop septicemia with lesions in muscle, bones, skin, and lower urinary tract (especially those with

FIGURE 19.3. Candida albicans *in nasal exudate from a dog. Note blastoconidia and pseudohypha. Gram stain, 1000×.*

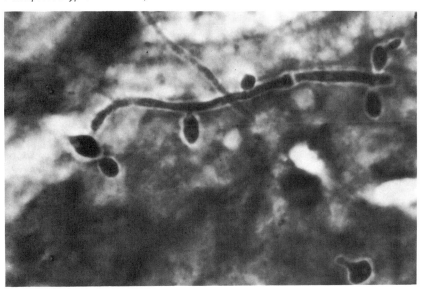

diabetes); feline pyothorax may rarely be due to *C. albicans.*

Lower primates and marine mammals may acquire mucocutaneous candidiasis.

Epidemiology

The common agents of candidiasis are commensal with most warm-blooded species. Disease is linked to immune and hormonal inadequacies, reduced colonization resistance, or intensive exposure of weakened hosts or vulnerable tissues. These conditions account for susceptibility of infants, diabetics, subjects on antibiotic and steroid regimes, patients with indwelling catheters, and mammary glands of lactating cows.

IMMUNOLOGIC ASPECTS

Immunoincompetent individuals are preferred targets for infection.

Polymorphonuclear neutrophil leukocytes (PMNs) and activated macrophages form the chief defense against candidiases. The role played by opsonins (antibody; complement) is to facilitate phagocytosis. Macrophages are activated by gamma interferon secreted by T_{H1} cells stimulated by IL-12 from phagocytizing macrophages.

There is no artificial immunization.

LABORATORY DIAGNOSIS

In exudate, *Candida* appears as blastoconidia or (pseudo)hyphae. All forms are demonstrable in unstained wet mounts and fixed smears stained with Gram, fungal, or polychrome stains (Fig 19.3).

Candida albicans grows well on blood or Sabouraud's agar, with or without inhibitors. Other *Candida* spp. may be inhibited by cycloheximide. Yeast isolates producing (pseudo)mycelium can be considered *Candida* spp. Isolation of *Candida* spp. from mucous membranes even in large numbers suggests a diagnosis of candidiasis only in the presence of compatible lesions and abundant (pseudo)hyphal forms in direct smears.

Incubation at 37°C for ≥2 hours of a lightly inoculated tube of serum will produce germ tubes if the isolate is *C. albicans* (see Fig 19.1), which also produced chlamydospores on cornmeal-tween 80 agar (see Fig 19.2). Yeast identification kits are commercially available.

DNA probes and tests for circulating antibody, antigen, and metabolites have had no adequate trial in veterinary medicine.

TREATMENT, CONTROL, AND PREVENTION

Correcting conditions underlying clinical candidiasis may in itself lead to recovery.

In poultry, copper sulfate in drinking water is a traditional treatment. Nystatin can be given in feed or water. It is also used topically in mucosal and cutaneous forms of candidiasis of mammals, as are amphotericin B and miconazole. Fluconazole (preferred) or flucytosine is useful for treating dogs or cats with lower urinary tract candidiasis.

In disseminated forms, oral fluconazole or flucytosine are drugs of choice. Susceptibility testing is advisable. Combined flucytosine-amphotericin B is sometimes used in humans and occasionally in animals.

SELECTED REFERENCES

Anderson RG, Pidgeon G. Candidiasis in a dog with parvoviral enteritis. J Am Anim Hosp Assoc 1987;23:27.

Calderone R, Diamond R, Senet J-M, et al. Host cell-fungal interactions. J Med Vet Mycol 1994;32(suppl. 1):151.

Dunn JL, Buck JD, Spotte S. Candidiasis in captive pinnipeds. J Am Vet Med Assoc 1984;185:1328.

Foley GL, Schlafer DH. *Candida* abortion in cattle. Vet Pathol 1987;24:532.

Fukazawa Y, Kagaya K. Molecular bases of adhesion of *Candida albicans*. J Med Vet Mycol 1997;35:87.

Gross TL, Mayhew IG. Gastroesophageal ulceration and candidiasis in foals. J Am Vet Med Assoc 1983;182:1370.

Kennedy MJ, Volz RA. Ecology of *Candida albicans* gut colonization: inhibition of *Candida* adhesion, colonization, and dissemination from the gastrointestinal tract by bacterial antagonism. Infect Immun 1985;49:654.

Kirk JH, Bartlett RC, Newman JR. *Candida mastitis* in a dairy herd. Compend Cont Educ Pract Vet 1986;8:F150.

Kwong-Chung KF, Lehman D, Good C, Magee PT, et al. Genetic evidence for role of extracellular proteinase in virulence of *Candida albicans*. Infect Immun 1985;49:571.

Monga DR, Tiware SC, Prasad S. Mycotic abortions in equine. Mykosen 1983;26:612.

Odds RC. *Candida* species and virulence. ASM News 1994;60:313.

Reilly LK, Palmer JE. Systemic candidiasis in four foals. J Am Vet Med Assoc 1994;205:464.

Sobel JD, Muller G, Buckley HR. Critical role of germ tube formation in the pathogenesis of candidal vaginitis. Infect Immun 1984;44:576.

Vazquez-Torres A, Balish E. Macrophages in resistance to candidiasis. Microbiol Molec Biol Rev 1997;61:170.

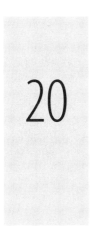

20

The Respiratory Tract as a Microbial Habitat

ERNST L. BIBERSTEIN

Breathing involves exposure of the respiratory tract to airborne agents, including microorganisms. Consequently, microorganisms are found in certain parts of the tract, while various mechanisms operate to exclude or eliminate them from other portions.

MICROBIAL FLORA OF THE RESPIRATORY TRACT

The resident flora are limited to the nose and pharynx and include consistently viridans streptococci and coagulase-negative staphylococci (see Chapters 21 and 22) along with potential pathogens that vary with the host species. As in the intestinal tract, the resident flora confers colonization resistance, which may be reduced by antibiotic treatment and other environmental changes that alter the composition of the resident flora.

Nonresident organisms may include pathogens and harmless transients. The significance of their presence in the nasopharynx is often difficult to interpret without clinical and pathologic information. The larynx, trachea, bronchi, and lungs lack a resident flora. Fluid from the distal tract may contain up to 10^3 bacteria/ml in normal animals (cats).

DEFENSES OF THE RESPIRATORY TRACT

Different protective mechanisms operate in the nasopharyngeal, tracheobronchial, and pulmonary portions of the tract, and aerodynamic filtration operates through different forces at these several levels in depositing variously sized airborne particles. Inertial forces deposit larger particles ($\geq$5 μm in diameter) in the nasopharyngeal and upper tracheobronchial section through impaction. In small bronchi and beyond, where air velocity is reduced, gravity acts to sediment particles 0.5 to 5.0 μm in size. In the smallest bronchioles and alveoli, particles measuring less than 0.5 μm gain contact with membranes through Brownian movement.

Nasopharyngeal Compartment

Vibrissae (guard hairs) around the nostrils may arrest the largest inhaled particles ($\geq$15 μm in diameter). Smaller ones may impinge on the nasal turbinates or the nasopharyngeal wall, where they encounter mucociliary action (see below) and are transported to the caudal pharynx to be swallowed and eliminated via the intestinal tract.

In the humid, warm nasal passages, particles swell through hydration, becoming more likely to impinge on a mucous membrane. Warming of air benefits cold-sensitive clearance mechanisms in the lower tract.

Pharyngeal lymphoid tissue acts in filtration of microorganisms and initiates immune responses as a constituent of the mucosa-associated lymphoid tissue (MALT, see Chapter 2).

The resident flora provides colonization resistance, while the sneeze reflex aids in clearing infectious particles.

Tracheobronchial Compartment

This compartment includes the larynx, trachea, bronchi, and bronchioles. Glottal closure during swallowing protects it from contamination, and coughing removes gross accumulations of fluids.

Particle deposition on airway membranes is favored by bronchial branching. From the caudal larynx, the tracheobronchial system is lined by mucociliary epithelium, which traps particles and transports them to the pharynx (see below). MALT is distributed along the airways and concentrated at bronchial bifurcations.

Tracheobronchial secretions contain lysozyme, which is selectively bactericidal; alpha-1 antitrypsin, an enzyme inhibitor reducing the destructive effect of inflammatory reactions; immunoglobulins; interferons; and lactoferrin, which, by binding iron, makes it unavailable to most bacteria.

Pulmonary Compartment

Clearance mechanisms at the alveolar levels of the lung consist of pulmonary alveolar macrophages (PAM) and of neutrophils and monocytes recruited from the blood. Particles are disposed of by phagocytosis. Susceptible microorganisms are killed and digested. Other particles are removed by phagocytes via mucociliary transport or lymphatics. The same protective substances as in tracheobronchial secretions operate at the pulmonary level, supplemented by those derived from alveolar macrophages.

The mucociliary apparatus and PAM constitute the main clearance mechanisms of the respiratory tract.

Mucociliary Apparatus

Ciliated and secretory cells make up the mucociliary "escalator." Ciliated cells are pseudostratified in the nasal and cranial tracheobronchial portions of the tract: simple columnar in the smaller bronchi and simple cuboidal in the smallest bronchioles. The cilia, some 200 per cell, measuring $5.0 \times 0.3\,\mu m$, resemble eukaryotic flagella and beat up to 1000 times a minute.

The secretory components are goblet cells, interspersed with ciliated cells, and, in the nose, trachea, and larger bronchi, submucosal serous and mucous glands. Serous fluid bathes the cilia, while mucus engages their tips and is propelled, along with particles trapped in it, toward the pharynx by their beat. The particle clearance rate is fastest in the trachea and slowest in the smallest airways, where goblet cells are absent, mucus is sparse, and cilia beat more slowly, an arrangement that prevents logjams in the large airways. The trachea (cat) can be cleared within an hour, and all airways within a day.

Mucociliary clearance is inhibited by temperature extremes, respiratory viral and some bacterial infections (e.g., *Bordetella*), dryness, general anesthetics, dust, noxious gases (sulfur dioxide, carbon dioxide, ammonia, tobacco smoke), and hypoxia.

Pulmonary Alveolar Macrophage

The PAM is a monocyte adapted to the lung environment and located in the alveolar space. It is a pleomorphic cell, 20 to 40 μm in diameter, with many lysosomal granules containing scores of bioactive substances, including mediator substances like complement components, interleukin 1, and tumor necrosis factor that enable it to mobilize additional cellular and humoral defenses. It is motile and phagocytic and can survive for weeks to months. Its energy is obtained mainly by oxidative phosphorylation.

Particles ingested by PAMs — other than susceptible bacteria killed upon ingestion — are removed via the mucociliary escalator or via interstitial "centripetal" or "centrifugal" lymphatics. The centripetal route leads directly to the hilar lymph nodes and may require two weeks. The centrifugal route goes via the pleura and may take months. Agents that cannot be removed are sequestered by inflammatory processes (abscesses, granulomas).

PAM activities are inhibited by sulfur dioxide, ozone, nitrogen oxide, and respiratory virus infections. Leukotoxins of *Pasteurella haemolytica* and *Actinobacillus pleuropneumoniae* destroy ruminant and porcine PAMs, respectively.

SELECTED REFERENCES

Bienenstock J, ed. Immunology of the lung and the upper respiratory tract. New York: McGraw-Hill, 1984.

Brain JD, Proctor DE, Reid LM. Respiratory defense mechanisms (in 2 parts). In: Lenfant C, ed. Lung biology in health and disease. Vol. 5. New York: Marcel Dekker, 1977.

Clarke AE. A review of environmental and host factors in relation to equine respiratory disease. Equine Vet J 1987;19:435.

Fels AOS, Cohn ZA. The alveolar macrophage. J Appl Physiol 1986;60:353.

Green GM. In defense of the lung. Am Rev Resp Dis 1970;102: 691.

Jakab GJ. Mechanisms of bacterial superinfections in viral pneumonias. Schweiz Med Wschr 1985;115:75.

McWilliam AS, Nelson DJ, Holt PG. The biology of airway dendritic cells. Immunol Cell Biol 1995;73:405.

Padrid PA, Feldman BF, Funk K, et al. Cytologic, microbiologic, and biochemical analysis of bronchoalveolar fluid attained from 24 healthy cats. Am J Vet Res 1991;52:130.

Pavia D. Lung mucociliary clearance. In: Clark SW, Pavia D, eds. Aerosols and the lung: clinical and experimental aspects. Boston: Butterworth, 1984.

Pison U, Max M, Neuendank A, et al. Host defence capacities of pulmonary surfactant: evidence for "non-surfactant" functions of the surfactant system. Eur J Clin Invest 1994;24:586.

Reynolds NY. Host defense impairments that may lead to respiratory infections. Clin Chest Med 1987;8:339.

Standiford TJ, Huffnagle GB. Cytokines in host defense against pneumonia. J Invest Med 1997;45:335.

Toews GB. Determinants of bacterial clearance from the lower respiratory tract. Semin Resp Infect 1986;1:68.

Veit H, Farrell RL. The anatomy and physiology of the bovine respiratory system relating to pulmonary disease. Cornell Vet 1978;68:555.

Wanner A. Pulmonary defense mechanisms: mucociliary clearance. In: Simmons DH, ed. Current pulmonology. Boston: Houghton Mifflin, 1980:325–350.

21 *Staphylococci*

ERNST L. BIBERSTEIN   DWIGHT C. HIRSH

Staphylococci are spherical gram-positive bacteria that divide in several planes to form irregular clusters. They are probably present in the upper respiratory tract and on other epithelial surfaces of all warm-blooded animals. Five of some 20 species are of veterinary importance: *S. aureus*, *S. intermedius*, *S. epidermidis*, *S. hyicus*, and *S. schleiferi* ssp. *coagulans*. *Staphylococcus aureus* is a common pyogenic agent in humans and several animal species. *Staphylococcus intermedius* is the leading pus-forming bacterium in dogs. *Staphylococcus epidermidis* is universally present on skin and some mucous membranes, but it is rarely pathogenic. *Staphylococcus hyicus*, which is found in several species, causes exudative epidermidis of swine and sometimes bovine mastitis. *Staphylococcus schleiferi* ssp. *coagulans* is associated with otitis externa of dogs.

DESCRIPTIVE FEATURES

Morphology and Staining

Staphylococci are 0.5 to 1.5 μm in diameter and are generally strongly gram positive. In exudates they form clusters, pairs, or short chains (Fig 21.1). Spores and flagella are absent. Encapsulation is variable.

Structure and Composition

The cell wall consists of proteins and polysaccharide. One protein ("clumping factor," "bound coagulase") is usually present in *S. aureus* and *S. intermedius*. Clumping factor interacts in vitro with fibrinogen to produce an agglutination-like reaction. Another, Protein A, produces aggregation by combining with the Fc fragment of immunoglobulins. The predominant polysaccharide is teichoic acid linked to peptidoglycan. Its alcohol moiety is ribitol in *S. aureus*, and glycerol in *S. epidermidis* and *S. intermedius*. Carotenoid pigments in the cell membrane can impart a "golden" (Latin: "aureus") color to colonies of *S. aureus*. A capsule is sometimes produced by *S. aureus*, and often times a "pseudocapsule," a loosely associated carbohydrate structure shown to be produced by strains causing bovine mastitis.

Cellular Products of Medical Interest

Staphylococcus aureus, the most intensively studied species of staphylococcus, excretes many bioactive proteins (toxins) including enzymes, such as lipase, esterase, deoxyribonuclease, staphylokinase (a plasminogen activator), hyaluronidase, and phospholipase. *Coagulase* causes plasma coagulation in vitro and identifies the pathogenic species: *S. aureus*, *S. intermedius*, *S. schleiferi* ssp. *coagulans*, and some *S. hyicus*.

Hemolytic toxins occur singly, in combination, or not at all. They differ antigenically, biochemically, and in their effect on the erythrocytes of various species. *Alpha toxin* acts on membrane lipids, is hemolytic in vitro, is mitogenic, is lethal to rabbits following intravenous injection, and is necrotizing upon intradermal injection. *Beta toxin*, a phospholipase C prevalent in animal strains, produces broad zones of "hot-cold lysis" on sheep or cattle blood agar at 37°C, a partial hemolysis that occurs and goes to completion on further incubation at lower temperatures (Fig 21.2). *Delta toxin* lyses cells of various species by a detergent-like action but is inhibited by serum. Little is known of *gamma toxin*, the activity of which is suppressed in the presence of agar.

A *leucocidin* kills neutrophils and macrophages of some species (rabbit, bovine, human) by altering cell membrane permeability, causing degranulation.

Staphylococci with pathogenic potential (coagulase-positive strains) grow better in iron-restricted conditions, as compared to those staphylococci with less potential (coagulase-negative strains). Under iron-limiting conditions, the coagulase-positive strains produce a siderophore, staphyloferrin B, which is responsible for iron acquisition from extracellular sources (e.g., transferrin).

Of mostly human medical interest is *enterotoxin*, a cause of food poisoning. It is present in many *S. aureus* and *S. intermedius* strains, is resistant to heat and digestive enzymes, and acts by reflex stimulation of the vomiting center. Six immunotypes (*A–F*) exist. *Exfoliatins* produced by some strains of *S. aureus* (staphylococcal exfoliative toxin, sET) and S. hyicus (shET) are responsible for staphylococcal scalded-skin syndrome (SSSS) in infants and may be responsible for porcine exudative dermatitis, respectively; *toxic shock syndrome toxin-1* (TSST-1; enterotoxin F, pyrogenic exotoxin C) is implicated in toxic shock syndrome, which particularly affects menstruating women using tampons. Some staphylococcal toxins are phage- or plasmid-encoded. The enterotoxins and TSST-1 are "superantigens," and part of the systemic symptomatology may be related to the cytokine "storm" that results from the interaction of T-cell receptors, macrophages, and these toxins.

FIGURE 21.1.   Staphylococcus aureus *in urinary sediment from a cat. Gram stain,
1000×.*

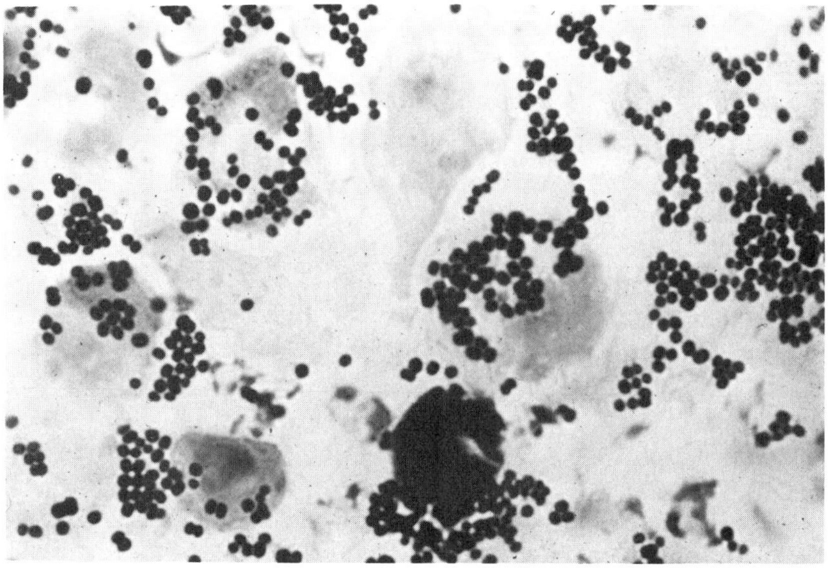

FIGURE 21.2.   Staphylococcus *sp. beta toxin activity on
bovine blood agar. For explanation, see text.*

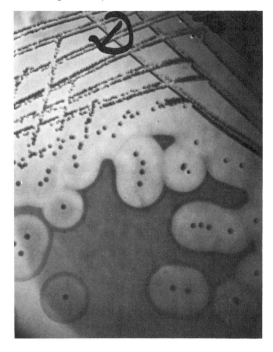

Growth Characteristics

Staphylococci grow overnight on common laboratory
media, producing on agar smooth opaque colonies over
1 mm in diameter.

Biochemical Characterization

Staphylococci are catalase-positive, facultative anaerobes
that attack carbohydrates oxidatively and fermentatively.

Resistance

Staphylococci withstand drying (especially in exudates)
for weeks, heating up to 60°C for 30 minutes, pH fluc-
tuations from 4.0 to 9.5, and salt concentrations of
7.5%, which are used in selective media for isolation of
staphylococci.

Staphylococci are inhibited by bacteriostatic dyes (e.g.,
crystal violet), bile salts, disinfectants like chlorhexidine,
and many antimicrobial drugs.

Variability

Colonies vary from smooth (S) to rough (R). G ("goni-
dial") and L (wall-less) variants reflect progressive cell wall
loss produced by unfavorable environmental conditions,
such as antibiotic treatment.

Isolates can be "typed" by their susceptibilities to bacteriophage lysis. Phage-typing sets have been developed
for human, bovine, and avian *S. aureus*.

Resistance to beta-lactam antimicrobics is most often
due to plasmid-encoded penicillinase (beta-lactamase).
Tolerance, a rarer form of penicillin resistance, is attributed to failure of autolytic cell wall enzymes. Intrinsic penicillin resistance may be due to changes in
penicillin-binding proteins (enzymes responsible for cell
synthesis).

Resistance to other antimicrobics is common.

ECOLOGY

Reservoir

Coagulase-positive species *S. aureus* and *S. intermedius* inhabit the distal nasal passages, external nares, and skin, especially near mucocutaneous borders such as the perineum, external genitalia, and bovine udder. They also occur as transients in the gastrointestinal tract.

Coagulase-negative staphylococci, especially *S. epidermidis*, are predominant among the resident skin flora but also colonize the upper respiratory tract. In swine, this generalization apparently also applies to *S. hyicus*, a species potentially pathogenic, especially for piglets.

Staphylococci are found worldwide in warm-blooded animals. Interspecies spread (e.g., humans to cows, dogs to humans) appears to be limited.

Transmission

Staphylococci spread by direct and indirect contact. Many animal infections are probably endogenous, that is, caused by a resident strain.

Pathogenesis

Mechanisms. The predominant pattern of staphylococcal pathogenesis is suppuration and abscess formation. The importance of toxins is undefined. Leukocidin may be a factor in species with susceptible leukocytes, and the cytotoxic and lethal actions of alpha toxin have parallels in some forms of the natural disease. Mutants unable to produce alpha toxin, beta toxin, or both are of lesser virulence than parenteral strains producing both toxins.

Several cell envelope constituents — capsule (and pseudocapsule), proteins, and peptidoglycan — have antiphagocytic properties. Part of the antiphagocytic effect of capsule and pseudocapsule is due to their shielding of phagocytic cells from deposited (through the alternative pathway) complement components (C3b) that may have bound to peptidoglycan. Unidentified adhesins (protein or carbohydrate) attach to host extracellular matrix proteins, for example, fibronectin.

Peptidoglycan may help trigger inflammatory responses and immobilize leukocytes at the focus of infection.

Urease activity is implicated in urolithiasis of dogs.

Cell-mediated immune phenomena intensify inflammatory responses in staphylococcal infections while spatially confining them.

In some forms of canine pyoderma (juvenile pyoderma, folliculitis), cell- and antibody-mediated hypersensitivity is thought to be induced. The toxin-caused human diseases — food poisoning and toxic shock syndrome — are not prominent in animals. The exfoliative toxins may play a role in an exudative dermatitis of pigs. A condition resembling staphylococcal scalded-skin syndrome has been described in dogs.

Pathology. The typical lesion is the *abscess*, an inflammatory focus in which participating cells have been destroyed by the combined effects of bacterial and inflammatory cell activity. This confrontation between leukocytes and microorganisms produces pus, a mixture of host cell debris and bacteria, living and dead. In an abscess, pus is surrounded by intact leukocytes and fibrin strands. Unless the pus is drained, a fibrous capsule will gradually be formed. In chronic, ulcerative staphylococcal wound infections ("botryomycosis"), fibrous elements predominate, interspersed with pockets of suppuration.

Disease Patterns. Although all warm-blooded animals can be clinically affected by coagulase-positive staphylococci, the prevalence and form of such interactions vary among host species.

1. The term *canine pyoderma* covers many clinical pictures, all of which include some degree of pyogenic skin inflammation associated with bacterial infection. *Staphylococcus intermedius* is the chief bacterium implicated. Its contribution and the degree of suppuration are variable. In chronic and recurrent forms, cell-mediated hypersensitivity and immune complexes are thought to be involved. Host aspects, including genetic, endocrine, and immunological factors, may play an important part.
2. As a leading cause of bovine mastitis, *S. aureus* rivals *Streptococcus agalactiae* (see Chapter 22). Infection occurs via the teat canal, and the course of the infection varies from subclinical to acute suppurative, gangrenous, or chronic, depending on the infecting strain, infecting dose, and host resistance. Bovine mastitis is sometimes caused by coagulase-negative staphylococci, notably *S. epidermidis*, *S. hyicus*, *S. xylosus*, and *S. sciuri*.
3. Phosphate (struvite, apatite) urolithiasis of dogs and mink is commonly associated with *S. intermedius* infections.
4. Miscellaneous pyogenic infections: coagulase-positive staphylococci affect all warm-blooded species and all organ systems. *Staphylococcus intermedius*, the chief pyogenic agent of dogs, also occurs in respiratory, genital, hemolymphatic, bone, and joint infections; wounds; and infections of eyelids and conjunctiva. *Staphylococcus intermedius* along with *S. schleiferi* ssp. *coagulans* occurs in canine otitis externa.
5. Other entities worthy of note:
   a. "Bumblefoot" of gallinaceous birds is a chronic pyogranulomatous process in the subcutaneous tissues of the foot resulting in thick-walled swellings on one or more joints.
   b. Staphylococcosis in turkeys is a bacteremia localizing in joints and tendon sheaths.
   c. Tick pyemia of lambs, resulting from inoculation of indigenous skin *S. aureus* by tick bites, may be acute with toxemic death, or chronic with disseminated abscess formation. It

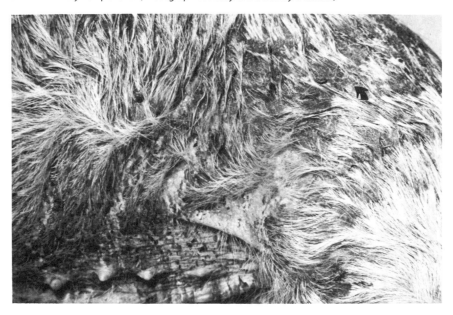

FIGURE 21.3.   *Porcine exudative epidermitis (greasy pig disease). The skin is covered and the bristles are matted by abundant brownish exudate (arrow) made up of epidermal debris and inflammatory components. (Photograph courtesy of Dr. Harvey Olander.)*

is often linked with tick-borne fever (caused by the rickettsial agent *Ehrlichia phagocytophila*).

d. Botryomycosis occurs especially in the udder of sows, mares, and cows, and in the equine spermatic cord after castration.

e. Abscess disease of sheep, resembling caseous lymphadenitis (see Chapter 23) is caused by an anaerobic subspecies of *S. aureus*.

f. Cutaneous and pyemic staphylococcoses are problems in wild and domestic rabbits.

g. Exudative epidermitis (greasy pig disease) due to *S. hyicus* affects young pigs (<7 weeks). It is often systemic and rapidly fatal, affecting the lungs, lymph nodes, kidneys, and brain. Skin lesions are characterized by a thick, grayish-brown exudate (Fig 21.3), especially around the face and ears.

Epidemiology

Staphylococcal diseases (e.g., pyoderma, otitis externa, urinary tract and wound infections) often arise endogenously. Studies on humans suggest widespread staphylococcal colonization within hours of birth. Clinical infections appear to be decisively determined by host factors.

In bovine mastitis, staphylococci may enter the gland during milking. Management practices and milking hygiene influence prevalence significantly.

Transmission of *S. aureus* between animals and humans occurs infrequently.

Prolonged environmental survival of staphylococci permits their indirect transmission.

IMMUNOLOGIC ASPECTS

Possible immune mechanisms in pathogenesis have already been cited.

Recovery and Resistance

Clearance of staphylococci depends chiefly on phagocytosis. Humoral factors are apparently important because agammaglobulinemic individuals suffer frequent infections. Cell-mediated factors contribute to localization and resolution of lesions.

Recovery from staphylococcal infection confers no lasting resistance.

Artificial Immunization

The benefits of vaccination are doubtful. Commercial or autogenous whole-culture preparations, toxoids plus bacterins, are used prophylactically on dairy cattle and sometimes in small animal dermatology to treat persistent infections. Although successes have been reported, controlled evaluations are lacking.

Use of staphylococcal phage lysates and nonspecific stimulants of cell-mediated immunity in cases of nonresponsive pyoderma awaits support by adequate clinical or experimental evidence.

LABORATORY DIAGNOSIS

Sample Collection

Aspirates from unopened lesions, in sterile syringes or sterile containers, are preferred. Swabs in transport media are acceptable. Milk is collected into containers under sterile precautions. Blood and urine culture routines are appropriate for staphylococcal isolation.

Direct Examination

On gram-stained films, staphylococci appear as gram-positive cocci in pairs, clusters, or short chains (see Fig 21.1). In specimens from skin pustules, they may be sparse.

Isolation and Identification

Bovine blood is best for the detection of beta toxin, which is diagnostic for coagulase-positive staphylococci (*S. aureus*, *S. intermedius*, and *S. schleiferi* ssp. *coagulans*; see Fig 21.2). Colonial appearance is as described.

TREATMENT AND CONTROL

Abscesses and empyemas are drained of pus. For the most superficial forms of pyoderma, topical application of mild antiseptics (3% hexachlorophene) may be adequate.

Extensive, inaccessible, and disseminated processes require systemic treatment. Staphylococci are commonly resistant to penicillin, streptomycin, and tetracycline. Usually effective antimicrobics include penicillinase-resistant penicillins, fluoroquinolones, chloramphenicol, erythromycin, cephalosporins (first generation), vancomycin, lincomycin, and trimethoprim-sulfas. Clavulanic acid inactivates the beta-lactamase produced by *S. aureus* and *S. intermedius*, therefore cell wall antibiotics containing this substance are protected (e.g., clavulanic acid/amoxicillin). Cloxacillin is effective in treating staphylococcal mastitis, especially in dry cows.

For staphylococcal cystitis, penicillins remain effective because of their high urinary concentrations. Cloxacillin is used topically and systemically on exudative epidermitis due to *S. hyicus*.

A controversial approach to prevention of staphylococcal infections in infants utilizes "bacterial interference": the implantation of a nonvirulent strain to preclude colonization by virulent staphylococci. The method shows promise for control of staphylococcosis in turkeys.

SELECTED REFERENCES

Baird-Parker AC. The staphylococci: an introduction. J Appl Bacteriol Symposium 1990;19(suppl.):1S–8S.

Baselga R, Albizu I, Amorena B. *Staphylococcus aureus* capsule and slime as virulence factors in ruminant mastitis. A review. Vet Microbiol 1994;39:195.

Bhakdi S, Tranum-Jensen J. Alpha-toxin of *Staphylococcus aureus*. Microbiol Rev 1991;55:733.

Bramley AJ, Patel AH, O'Reilly M, et al. Roles of alpha-toxin and beta-toxin in virulence of *Staphylococcus aureus* for the mouse mammary gland. Infect Immun 1989;57:2489.

Devriese LA. Staphylococci in healthy and diseased animals. J Appl Bacteriol Symposium 1990;19(suppl.):71S–80S.

Gross TL, Ihrke PJ, Walder EJ. Veterinary dermatopathology: a macroscopic and microscopic evaluation of canine and feline skin diseases. St. Louis: Mosby Year-Book, 1992.

Haag H, Fiedler HP, Meiwes J, et al. Isolation and biological characterization of staphyloferrin B, a compound with siderophore activity from staphylococci. FEMS Microbiol Lett 1994;115:125.

Henderson B, Poole S, Wilson M. Bacterial modulins: a novel class of virulence factors which cause host tissue pathology by inducing cytokine synthesis. Microbiol Rev 1996;60:316.

Horstmann RD. Target recognition failure by the nonspecific defense system: surface constituents of pathogens interfere with alternative pathway of complement activation. Infect Immun 1992;60:721.

Igimi S, Takahashi E, Mitsuoka T. *Staphylococcus schleiferi* subsp *coagulans* subsp nov isolated from the external auditory meatus of dogs with external ear otitis. Int J Syst Bacteriol 1990;40:409.

Jacoby GA, Archer GL. New mechanisms of bacterial resistance to antimicrobial agents. N Engl J Med 1991;324:601.

Lindsay JA, Riley TV. Staphylococcal iron requirements, siderophore production and iron-regulated protein expression. Infect Immun 1994;62:2309.

Lindsay JA, Riley TV, Mee BJ. Production of siderophore by coagulase-negative staphylococci and its relation to virulence. Eur J Clin Microbiol 1994;13:1063.

Ling GV. Lower urinary disease of dogs and cats. St. Louis: Mosby, 1995.

Love DN, Davis RE. Isolation of *Staphylococcus aureus* from a condition in greyhounds histologically resembling "staphylococcal scalded skin syndrome" of man. J Small Anim Pract 1980;21:351.

Patti JM, Allen BL, McGavin MJ, Hook M. MSCRAMM-mediated adherence of microorganisms to host tissues. Annu Rev Microbiol 1994;48:585.

Sato H, Tanabe T, Kuramoto M, et al. Isolation of exfoliative toxin from *Staphylococcus hyicus* subsp. *hyicus* and its exfoliative activity in the piglet. Vet Microbiol 1991;27:263.

Talan DA, Goldstein EJ, Staatz D, Overturf GD. *Staphylococcus intermedius* in canine gingiva and canine-inflicted human wound infections: laboratory characterization of a newly recognized zoonotic pathogen. J Clin Microbiol 1989;27:78.

Titball RW. Bacterial phospholipases C. Microbiol Rev 1993;57:347.

Watson DL, Watson NA. Expression of a pseudocapsule by *Staphylococcus aureus*: influence of cultural conditions and relevance to mastitis. Res Vet Sci 1989;47:152.

Zumla A. Superantigens, T cells, and microbes. Clin Infect Dis 1992;15:313.

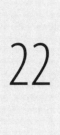

22 *Streptococci*

Ernst L. Biberstein   Dwight C. Hirsh

Streptococci are gram-positive cocci occurring in pairs and chains; they show considerable ecologic, physiologic, serologic, and genetic diversity. The main groups of streptococcal diseases are the following:

1. Upper respiratory tract infections with lymphadenitis (horses, swine, cats, guinea pigs, humans), particularly in the young.
2. Neonatal respiratory and septicemic infections of foals, piglets, pups, and infants.
3. Secondary pneumonias and complications (horses, primates, small carnivores, humans).
4. Pyogenic infections unrelated to the respiratory tract (genitourinary tract infections, bovine mastitis).

Warm-blooded animals carry a resident flora of streptococci on the mucous membranes of the upper respiratory, lower genital, and most of the alimentary tract (enterococci).

DESCRIPTIVE FEATURES

Morphology and Staining

Streptococci vary from spherical to short bacillary cells, about 1 μm in diameter. Division occurs in one plane, producing pairs and chains. Chain formation is variable, though some species (e.g., *S. equi*) are consistent chain formers (Figs 22.1, 22.2).

Young cultures are gram positive. In exudates and older cultures (>18 hours) organisms often stain gram negative.

Many species, notably *S. pneumoniae*, are encapsulated and some have fimbriae.

Structure and Composition

The cell envelope and cell wall resemble those of staphylococci. Capsules, if present, are polysaccharide and antiphagocytic. Those of *S. pyogenes* and *S. equi* consist of nonantigenic hyaluronic acid. *Streptococcus pneumoniae* and *S. agalactiae* have antigenically diverse capsules, which provide a basis for serotyping.

Various surface proteins (e.g., surface protein F) are responsible for adhesin of several streptococcal species to extracellular matrix proteins.

Of several cell wall proteins, M protein is antiphagocytic by interfering with effective deposition of complement components necessary for opsonization (*S. pyogenes*, Group E streptococci), and also may function as adhesin (*S. equi*). It is antigenically variable, forming the basis for typing in *S. pyogenes*.

"Lancefield" serologic grouping, a step in streptococcal identification, is determined by cell wall polysaccharides (C-substance, group antigen). Groups are designated by capital letters (A to V; Table 22.1).

Peptidoglycan can trigger inflammation, fever, and lymphocyte proliferation. It is dermonecrotic, and cytotoxic in vitro.

Cellular Products and Activities of Medical Interest

Exotoxins of *S. pyogenes* include hemolysins (streptolysins O and S), hyaluronidase, DNAse, NADase, protease, streptokinase (a fibrinolysin), and a phage-encoded pyrogenic toxin responsible for the rash of scarlet fever. Their pathogenic significance is poorly defined. Most evoke immune responses in the course of infection. Some comparable toxins occur in animal streptococci.

Effects on sheep or bovine blood agar are used to divide streptococci into three types:

1. Alpha-hemolytic streptococci do not destroy erythrocytes but produce a zone of green discoloration around colonies. Most commensal streptococci of animals are alpha hemolytic.
2. Beta-hemolytic streptococci destroy erythrocytes and produce zones of transparent clarity around their colonies. Most pathogenic types are beta-hemolytic.
3. Gamma streptococci are nonhemolytic. Most are nonpathogenic.

Although the word *viridans* means "greening," the viridans group of streptococci is defined by biochemical reactions and includes gamma and alpha types.

The CAMP phenomenon (named after Christie, Atkins, and Munch-Petersen) reflects hemolytic synergism between staphylococcal beta toxin and an *S. agalactiae* toxin (CAMP protein, cocytolysin). Their combined action on sheep or bovine blood agar produces larger and clearer zones of hemolysis than either agent alone (Fig 22.3). This reaction has diagnostic value.

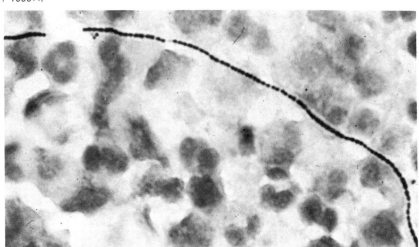

FIGURE 22.1. Streptococcus equi *in pus from lymph nodes of a horse. Gram stain,* 1000×.

Table 22.1. Streptococci of Veterinary Interest

Species	Lancefield Group	Host Species Affected[a]	Principal Diseases	Remarks
S. pyogenes	A	Humans, rodents (dairy cattle)	Pharyngotonsillitis, pyoderma, erysipelas, puerperal fever, rheumatic fever, glomerulonephritis (mastitis)	Poststreptococcal immune sequelae. More than 50 serotypes
S. agalactiae	B	Dairy cattle[b] (sheep, goats), humans[b] (cats, dogs)	Mastitis Neonatal infections	5 serotypes
S. equi[c]	C	Horses	"Strangles"	1 serotype
S. equisimilis[c]	C	Swine, horses (humans, dogs)	Miscellaneous suppurative conditions	8 serotypes
S. zooepidemicus[c]	C	Horses (fowl, dogs, ruminants, lab animals, humans)	Secondary pneumonias, miscellaneous suppurative conditions, genital and neonatal conditions	15 serotypes
S. dysgalactiae	C	Dairy cattle	Mastitis	3 serotypes
Enterococcus spp.[d]	D	All species	Many opportunistic infections, canine urinary tract infections, chicken septicemia	Normal gut flora
Group E	E	Swine	Jowl abscesses	6 serotypes
S. canis[c]	G	Carnivores	Feline lymphadenitis, miscellaneous pyogenic conditions of dogs and cats, humans[e]	
S. suis	R (=type 2) S (=type 1) RS T ungroupable	Swine (humans — R)	Neonatal infections, septicemias, pneumonia (humans — septicemia, arthritis, meningitis)	React with group D antiserum
S. uberis	—	Cattle	Mastitis	
S. pneumoniae	—	Primates (lab animals, cattle)	Pneumonia, septicemia (mastitis, calf septicemia, meningitis)	More than 80 serotypes

[a] Parentheses indicate that species is affected, but only rarely.
[b] Cattle and human strains are different.
[c] Being reclassified as a subspecies of *S. dysgalactiae*.
[d] This genus has been proposed based on nucleic acid studies. Not all group D streptococci belong to it (e.g., *S. bovis*, *S. equinus*).
[e] Canine and human strains are different.

FIGURE 22.2.   Streptococcus zooepidemicus *in cervical exudate from a mare. Gram stain, 1000×.*

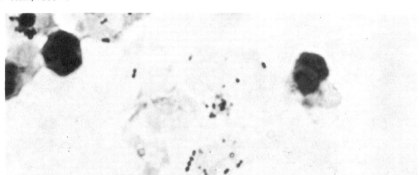

FIGURE 22.3.   *CAMP phenomenon on bovine blood agar. The dark line across the field is growth of* Staphylococcus aureus *surrounded by a zone of beta-toxin activity. Growing in lines at right angles to it are, left to right: a viridans streptococcus,* Streptococcus agalactiae, *another viridans streptococcus,* Streptococcus zooepidemicus, *and* Streptococcus agalactiae. *See text for discussion of CAMP phenomenon. (Photograph courtesy of Dr. Richard Walker.)*

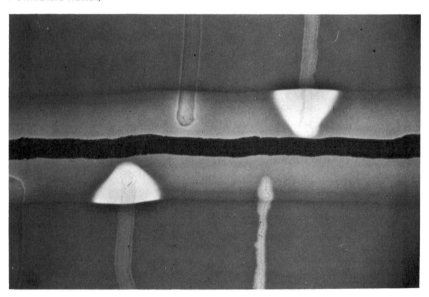

Growth Characteristics

Streptococci have fairly exacting growth needs best satisfied by media containing blood or serum. Some nutritionally variant streptococci (NVS) require, in addition, pyridoxal hydrochloride supplementation (0.002%).

After overnight incubation at 37°C, streptococci produce clear colonies, usually less than 1 mm in diameter. Capsulated forms, such as *S. equi*, produce larger, mucoid colonies.

Pathogenic species grow best at 37°C. Enterococci grow between 10°C and 45°C.

Biochemical Activities

Streptococci are catalase-negative facultative anaerobes, deriving energy from fermentation.

Resistance

Beta-hemolytic streptococci can survive in dried pus for weeks. They are killed at 55°C to 60°C in 30 minutes, and inhibited by 6.5% sodium chloride and 40% bile (except *S. agalactiae*), 0.1% methylene blue, and low (10°C) and high (45°C) temperatures. Enterococci tolerate these conditions. Viridans streptococci vary with respect to heat and bile resistance. Only *S. pneumoniae* is bile-soluble. Streptococci tolerate 0.02% sodium azide, which is used in streptococcal isolation media.

Pathogenic streptococci are usually susceptible to penicillins, cephalosporins, erythromycin, chloramphenicol, and trimethoprim-sulfonamides; they are often resistant to aminoglycosides, fluoroquinolones, and tetracycline. Enterococci are more resistant to all of these.

Variability

Serologic subdivisions exist in most streptococcal species except *S. equi* (see Table 22.1). *Streptococcus pyogenes* has some 70 immunotypes, based on M and other proteins, while *S. pneumoniae* has over 80 capsular types. Mucoid *S. equi* colonies become smooth as encapsulation is lost. In *S. pyogenes*, change from rough (matte) to smooth accompanies loss of M protein and virulence. L forms also occur.

ECOLOGY

Reservoir

Most streptococci of veterinary interest live commensally in the upper respiratory, alimentary, and lower genital tract.

Transmission

Streptococci are transmitted by inhalation or ingestion, sexually, congenitally, or indirectly via hands and fomites.

Pathogenesis

Mechanisms. The relation of streptococcal products to pathogenesis is largely speculative, with the following exceptions. The pneumococcal capsule is a proven virulence factor. M protein is an important virulence determinant, and antibody to it is protective. Other antiphagocytic cell constituents and cytotoxins of streptococci are probable virulence factors.

Surface proteins mediate adhesion of *S. pyogenes* to fibronectin on oropharyngeal cells and of Group B streptococci to infant cells. M protein is a probable adhesin of *S. equi*, and of Group B streptococci in adult humans.

Streptococci trigger inflammatory processes that may lead to suppuration and abscess formation.

Pathology. The basic pathologic process resembles that of staphylococcal infection.

Disease Patterns
1. Upper respiratory tract infections with lymphadenitis.
   a. Strangles is a contagious equine rhinopharyngitis caused by *S. equi* and marked by a serous or purulent nasal discharge, diphasic temperature rise, local pain, cough, and anorexia. In regional lymph nodes, abscesses

develop, which typically rupture and drain within two weeks. Recovery follows. The overall mortality rate is under 2%. Complications include pyemic dissemination to meninges, lungs, pericardium, and abdominal viscera, or extension to the guttural pouches. Purpura hemorrhagica, a Type III hypersensitivity manifested by subcutaneous swellings, mucosal hemorrhages, and fever, may follow the acute disease in about three weeks.
   b. Cervical lymphadenitis of swine (jowl abscess), caused by Group E streptococci, is analogous to strangles but clinically less dramatic and frequently not diagnosed until slaughter. Its most damaging aspect is carcass condemnation.
   c. Laboratory colonies of cats and guinea pigs occasionally experience cervical lymphadenitis caused by *S. canis* and *S. zooepidemicus*, respectively. (Note that *S. canis* and *S. zooepidemicus* are two of several streptococcal designations that have no official standing in bacterial taxonomy. See Table 22.1.)
2. Neonatal septicemias and respiratory tract infections are often traceable to an infected maternal genital tract.

   Streptococcus zooepidemicus is a frequent cause of equine cervicitis and metritis and of infections in newborn foals. These are often umbilical infections (navel ill, pyosepticemia, joint ill, polyarthritis) disseminated via the bloodstream and localizing in joints and renal cortex. In swine, *S. suis*, *S. equisimilis* (see Table 22.1) and Groups L and U streptococci cause neonatal septicemia, pneumonia, arthritis, and meningitis. *Streptococcus canis* is associated with septicemia in newborn puppies.
3. Secondary respiratory tract infections and sequelae include pneumonias, arthritides, and abscesses in various locations. In horses, *S. zooepidemicus* is regularly implicated in pneumonias and nonspecific pyogenic processes. In swine, *S. equisimilis*, and in dogs and cats, *S. canis*, can cause similar conditions. A pneumonia-serositis of young Peruvian alpacas is attributed to *S. zooepidemicus*.

   Streptococcus pneumoniae is a leading cause of pneumonia, septicemia, and meningitis in primates. Pneumococcal pneumonia in monkeys runs a very acute course with high mortality rates. The lesions are those of a fibrinous pleuropneumonia. Recent shipment and viral infection are common antecedents. Pneumococcal pneumonia, septicemia, and meningitis in calves have been described in Europe.
4. Miscellaneous pyogenic infections not related to the respiratory tract.
   a. Bovine mastitis. The leading agent of streptococcal mastitis is *S. agalactiae*. Less frequent causes are *S. dysgalactiae* and *S. uberis*, and rarely, enterococci, *S. pyogenes*, *S. zooepidemicus*, *S. pneumoniae*, and *S. bovis*.

Bovine *S. agalactiae* is specifically associated with the mammary gland. Infection is through the teat canal. Bacterial proliferation in lactiferous ducts and alveoli results in an acute inflammation followed by some fibrosis. Successive flare-ups cause replacement of secretory tissue by fibrous connective tissue. Eventually, entire glands may be lost.

During active phases of the chronic infection, milk yield is reduced. Milk may be abnormal and contain clots. In acute mastitis, the gland will be swollen and hot, and there may be fever and anorexia.

Mastitis due to *S. dysgalactiae* is sometimes acute and severe, while that caused by *S. uberis* is generally mild. Infections due to *S. zooepidemicus*, *S. pyogenes*, and *S. pneumoniae* can be severe and vary in acuteness.

b. Streptococci — usually enterococci — account for about 10% of canine urinary tract infections.

c. Beta-hemolytic streptococci (Groups G and C) and other streptococci may be implicated in endocarditis of dogs.

d. *Streptococcus zooepidemicus* and *Enterococcus faecalis* can cause septicemia in chickens. *Enterococcus faecalis* is often linked with endocarditis.

e. A beta-hemolytic streptococcus is responsible for a form of septicemia in freshwater aquarium fish.

f. A Group G streptococcus, *S. canis*, has been associated with a toxic shock-like syndrome and necrotizing fasciitis in dogs. No virulence-associated traits have been defined as they have for similar conditions seen in humans affected with *S. pyogenes*.

Epidemiology

All the streptococci discussed, except for *S. equi*, can be carried by healthy individuals, and many infections are probably endogenous and stress-related. Neonatal infections are commonly maternal in origin.

Strangles and porcine lymphadenitis are contagious diseases preferably affecting young animals (past infancy). *Streptococcus equi* is spread by contaminated food, drinking water, or utensils and by recovered animals, which may remain shedders for months. *Streptococcus agalactiae* among dairy cows is often spread by milking equipment, unskilled attempts at intramammary medication, and unsanitary milking practices.

Animal streptococci have limited public health significance. The Group B streptococci that cause disease in human infants are apparently distinct from bovine strains, but infections with *S. zooepidemicus* have been traced to infected milk, and *S. suis* (Group R) has caused serious infections in swine handlers. The Group G streptococci affecting dogs (*S. canis*) are apparently different from the Group G streptococci affecting human patients.

IMMUNOLOGIC ASPECTS

Immune Mechanisms of Disease

Human poststreptococcal diseases (rheumatic fever, acute glomerulonephritis) are attributed to immunopathogenic mechanisms. Similarly, equine purpura hemorrhagica following strangles is probably immune complex-mediated.

Recovery and Resistance

The main defenses against streptococcal infections are phagocytic, and antiphagocytic M protein elicits protective antibodies. Animals recovered from strangles and cervical lymphadenitis are at least temporarily immune to reinfection.

Polysaccharide capsules of *S. agalactiae* and *S. pneumoniae* evoke the formation of opsonizing antibody. In streptococcal pneumonia, their appearance determines recovery from infection. In bovine mastitis, no useful immunity develops: Cows, unless treated, remain infected. Experimental evidence suggests that anticapsular IgG_2-type antibody is protective.

All immunity is serotype-specific.

Artificial Immunization

A whole-cell bacterin and an M protein vaccine are available for vaccination against strangles. Neither is uniformly effective. An intranasal avirulent live vaccine that stimulates essential local antibody responses appears promising. Immunity to porcine jowl abscesses has been produced by feeding live avirulent cultures.

LABORATORY DIAGNOSIS

Sample Collection

The same kinds of samples and collection procedures described for staphylococci (see Chapter 21) are appropriate for streptococci.

Direct Examination

Smears of exudates or sediments of suspect fluids are fixed and gram stained. Streptococci appear as gram positive cocci in pairs, short chains, and in some instances very long chains (typically seen in pus aspirated from cervical lymph nodes of horses infected with *S. equi* — see Fig 22.1). Streptococci have a tendency to lose their gram-positivity and sometimes stain weakly gram positive or gram negative.

Culture

Exudates, milk, tissue, urine, transtracheal aspirates, and cerebrospinal fluid are cultured directly on cow or sheep blood agar. Incubation at 37°C in 3% to 5% CO_2 is preferable. Streptococcal colonies, smooth or mucoid, will appear in 18 to 48 hours. It is sometimes difficult to distinguish alpha from beta hemolysis. Intact erythrocytes remain adjacent to alpha- but not to beta-hemolytic colonies. Beta-hemolytic strains consistently lyse red cells in blood broth; alpha-hemolytic strains of animal origin generally do not.

Identification requires Lancefield grouping and biochemical tests. Commercial kits are available for both purposes. Other useful diagnostic tests include the following:

1. The CAMP phenomenon. Inoculate a beta toxin-producing staphylococcus across the equator of a sheep or bovine blood agar plate. At right angles to this line, and 0.5 cm from it, inoculate suspect *S. agalactiae*. After incubation, hemolysis by CAMP-positive bacteria will be enhanced in the beta-toxin zone (see Fig 22.3).
2. Bacitracin sensitivity. Bacitracin disks (0.04 units) inhibit growth of *S. pyogenes* on blood agar. This reaction is not entirely consistent or specific.
3. Bile esculin agar tests the ability of 40% bile-salt-tolerant bacteria to hydrolyze esculin, a characteristic of those belonging to Lancefield Group D.
4. Optochin sensitivity. Growth of *S. pneumoniae*, but not other alpha-hemolytic streptococci, is inhibited around disks impregnated with optochin (ethyl hydrocuprein hydrochloride).

TREATMENT AND CONTROL

Localized suppurative conditions are handled like those caused by staphylococci.

A preventive regime for cervical lymphadenitis of swine consists of tetracycline administered in feed (220 mg/kg feed).

For systemic treatment, penicillin G and ampicillin are effective on most beta-hemolytic and viridans streptococci. Cephalosporins, chloramphenicol, and trimethoprim-sulfas are alternatives. Enterococci are susceptible to trimethoprim-sulfas, although some strains are effective scavengers of thymidine found in exudates. Streptococcal endocarditis is treated with combined penicillin and gentamicin. Susceptibility to fluoroquinolones is unpredictable.

Penicillin (intramammary) is effective for treating mastitis due to *S. agalactiae* and most other streptococci. For the many available alternatives, a specialty text should be consulted. Important aspects of mastitis control lie in the area of sanitation and herd management.

For strangles, it is most beneficial to treat exposed and affected animals prior to abscess formation and to continue treatment past the febrile stage. Inappropriate or inadequate therapy of strangles is blamed for prolonging the illness and causing "bastard strangles" (widespread abscess formation with systemic manifestations). Populations at risk may be vaccinated. Affected or suspected horses should be rigorously isolated.

SELECTED REFERENCES

Bernheimer AW, Linder R, Avigad LS. Nature and mechanism of action of the CAMP protein of Group B streptococci. Infect Immun 1979;23:838.

Bruckner DA, Colonna P. Nomenclature for aerobic and facultative bacteria. Clin Infect Dis 1995;21:263.

Chanter N, Jones PW, Alexander TJL. Meningitis in pigs caused by *Streptococcus suis* — a speculative review. Vet Microbiol 1993;36:39.

Farrow JAE, Collins MD. Taxonomic studies on streptococci of serological groups C, G, and L and possibly related toxa. Syst Appl Microbiol 1984;5:483.

Finch LA, Martin DR. Human and bovine group B streptococci: two distinct populations. J Appl Bacteriol 1984;57:273.

Fischetti VA. Streptococcal M protein. Sci Am 1991;6:58.

Frick IM, Crossin KL, Edelman GM, Bjorck L. Protein H — a bacterial surface protein with affinity for both immunoglobulin and fibronectin type III domains. EMBO J 1995;14:1674.

Hamlen HJ, Timoney JF, Bell RJ. Epidemiologic and immunologic characteristics of *Streptococcus equi* infection in foals. J Am Vet Med Assoc 1994;204:768.

Hanski E, Caparon M. Protein F, a fibronectin-binding protein, is an adhesin of the group A streptococcus *Streptococcus pyogenes*. Proc Nat Acad Sci USA 1992;89:6172.

Hasty DL, Ofek I, Courtney HS, Doyle RJ. Multiple adhesins of streptococci. Infect Immun 1992;60:2147.

Joiner KA, Brown EJ, Frank MM. Complement and bacteria: chemistry and biology of host defense. Annu Rev Immunol 1984;2:461.

McDonald JS. Streptococcal and staphylococcal mastitis. Vet Clin N Am Large Anim Pract 1985;6:269.

Miller CW, Prescott JF, Mathews KA, et al. Streptococcal toxic shock syndrome in dogs. J Am Vet Med Assoc 1996;209:1421.

Molinari G, Talay SR, Valentin-Weigand P, et al. The fibronectin-binding protein of *Streptococcus pyogenes*, SfbI, is involved in the internalization of group A streptococci by epithelial cells. Infect Immun 1997;65:1357.

Patti JM, Allen BL, McGavin MJ, Hook M. MSCRAMM-mediated adherence of microorganisms to host tissues. Annu Rev Microbiol 1994;48:585.

Pedersen KB, Kjems E, Perch B, Slot P. Infection with RS streptococci in pigs. Acta Pathol Microbiol Scand B 1981;80:161.

Romer O. Pneumococcus infections in animals. In: Bulletin 371 of the State Veterinary Serum Laboratory. Copenhagen: C. E. Mortensen, 1962.

Srivastava SK, Barnum DA. Adherence of *S. equi* on tongue, cheek and mouth epithelial cells of ponies. Vet Microbiol 1983;8:493.

Sweeney CR, Benson CE, Whitlock RH. *Streptococcus equi* infection in horses. Compend Cont Educ Pract Vet 1987;9:689, 845 (2 parts).

Talay SR, Ehrenfeld E, Chatwal GS, Timmis KN. Expression of the fibronectin-binding components of *Streptococcus pyogenes* in *Escherichia coli* demonstrates that they are proteins. Molec Microbiol 1991;5:1727.

Talay SR, Valentin-Weigand P, Jerlstrom PG, et al. Fibronectin-binding protein of *Streptococcus pyogenes* sequence of the binding domain involved in adherence of streptococci to epithelial cells. Infect Immun 1992;60:3837.

Tamura GS, Rubens CE. Group B streptococci adhere to a variant of fibronectin attached to a solid phase. Molec Microbiol 1995;15:581.

Tillman RC, Dodson ND, Indiveri M. Group G streptococcal epizootic in a closed cat colony. J Clin Microbiol 1982;16:1057.

Timoney JE, Galan JE. The protective response of the horse to an avirulent strain of *Streptococcus equi*. In: Kimura Y, Kotami S, Shiokowa Y, eds. Recent advances in streptococci and streptococcal diseases. Chertsey Surrey, UK: Reedbooks, 1985.

Tomai M, Kotb M, Majumdar G, Beachey EH. Superantigenicity of streptococcal M protein. J Exp Med 1990;172:359.

Uchiyama T, Yan X, Imanishi K, Yagi J. Bacterial superantigens-mechanism of T cell activation by the superantigens and their role in the pathogenesis of infectious diseases. Microbiol Immunol 1994;38:245.

van Heyningen T, Fogg G, Yates D, et al. Adherence and fibronectin binding are environmentally regulated in the group A streptococci. Molec Microbiol 1993;9:1213.

Wessman GE. Biology of group E streptococci. A review. Vet Microbiol 1986;12:297.

Westerlund B, Korhonen TK. Bacterial proteins binding to the mammalian extracellular matrix. Molec Microbiol 1993;9:687.

Zumla A. Superantigens, T cells, and microbes. Clin Infect Dis 1992;15:313.

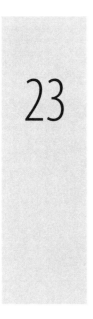

23

Corynebacteria; Arcanobacterium *(Actinomyces) pyogenes;* Rhodococcus equi

Ernst L. Biberstein   Dwight C. Hirsh

Corynebacteria are pleomorphic, non-spore-forming, nonmotile gram-positive bacilli with cell walls containing meso-diamino-pimelic acid (DAP), arabinogalactan, and mycolic acids. These ingredients are typical of "coryneform" bacteria, which also include mycobacteria and nocardiae. *Arcanobacterium (Actinomyces) pyogenes* and *Rhodococcus equi*, although not corynebacterium in the chemical sense, are "coryneform" in shape and for convenience will be considered here. *Corynebacterium renale* group is discussed in association with the urinary tract (Chapter 33).

Corynebacteria occur in packets of parallel ("palisades") or criss-crossing cells ("Chinese letters") that include coccoid, rod, club, and filamentous shapes. This pattern is called *diphtheroid* after the type species *C. diphtheriae*, which is the cause of human diphtheria.

Many corynebacteria contain metachromatic granules (Babes-Ernst granules), which are high-energy phosphate stores.

Four species of diphtheroids are prominent animal pathogens: 1) *Arcanobacterium (Actinomyces) pyogenes* is involved in suppurative processes of ruminants and swine, 2) *C. pseudotuberculosis* causes caseous abscesses in ruminants and horses, 3) *Rhodococcus equi* produces a suppurative pneumonia of young foals, and 4) *C. renale* colonizes the urogenital tract and is considered under that system (see Chapter 33).

Arcanobacterium (Actinomyces) pyogenes

Descriptive Features

Morphology and Staining

Arcanobacterium pyogenes is a small, gram-positive rod (0.5 μm × up to 2 μm; Fig 23.1) that lacks capsules and metachromatic granules. The instability of the gram-positive reaction is comparable to that of streptococci.

Structure and Composition

Its cell wall lacks the coryneform constituents but contains lysine, rhamnose, and glucose.

Cellular Products of Medical Interest

A 58 kDa hemolytic exotoxin (pyolysin) lyses red blood cells (RBCs) in vitro and kills mice and rabbits on intravenous injection. Pyolysin is similar to thio-activated cytolysins produced by other gram-positive species (e.g., *Clostridium* and *Listeria*).

Growth Characteristics

Arcanobacterium pyogenes is a facultative anaerobe requiring enriched media and up to 40 hours to produce discernible colonies on blood agar. Growth occurs optimally at 37°C and produces translucent, hemolytic colonies up to 1 mm in size.

Biochemical Activities

Arcanobacterium pyogenes is catalase negative, ferments lactose, and digests protein (gelatin, casein, coagulated serum).

Resistance

Arcanobacterium pyogenes is susceptible to drying, heat (60°C), disinfectants, and beta-lactam antibiotics; it is also resistant to sulfonamides.

Ecology

Reservoir

Arcanobacterium pyogenes is found on mucous membranes and the skin of susceptible species.

FIGURE 23.1. Arcanobacterium pyogenes *in pus from sheep lung. Gram stain, 1000×.*

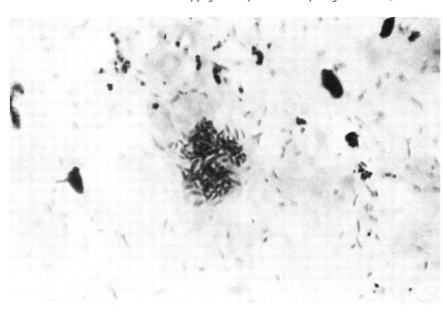

Transmission

Most infections are probably endogenous. In "summer mastitis," cow-to-cow spread, aided by flies, is thought to occur.

Pathogenesis

Mechanisms. *Arcanobacterium pyogenes* causes suppurative processes, usually complicated by other potentially pathogenic commensals, especially non-spore-forming anaerobes (*Bacteriodes, Fusobacterium, Porphyromonas, Prevotella, Peptostreptococcus*). Pyolysin is though to be a major virulence determinant (supported by the finding that antipyolysin antibodies are protective in experimental animals).

Pathology. The lesions are abscesses, empyemas, or pyogranulomas. Abscesses are often heavily encapsulated. Any offensive odors are contributions of anaerobic participants.

Disease Patterns. In cattle, *A. pyogenes* is involved in most purulent infections of traumatic or opportunistic origins, which may be local, regional, or metastatic. Common localizations are the lung, pericardium, endocardium, pleura, peritoneum, liver, joints, uterus, renal cortex, brain, bones, and subcutaneous tissues. In other susceptible species (sheep, goats, wild ruminants, swine) similar lesions may be found.

Arcanobacterium pyogenes causes abortion and mastitis in cattle. "Summer mastitis" is a communicable disease among pastured dairy cattle during their dry period. It often takes a destructive course, causing abscess formation and sloughing. Bacteria implicated in its etiology include *A. pyogenes, Streptococcus dysgalactiae*, and non-spore-forming anaerobes.

Arcanobacterium pyogenes has been recovered occasionally from suppurative conditions in humans. Circumstances pointed to opportunistic infections.

Epidemiology

Because *A. pyogenes* is a permanent resident of susceptible species, disease prevalence is sporadic and governed by precipitating stress or trauma.

"Summer mastitis" is most prevalent in northern Europe. It is spread by flies attracted to traumatized teats. Fly-borne *A. pyogenes* can survive for over two weeks.

IMMUNOLOGIC ASPECTS

Immune responses to *A. pyogenes* are not well understood. Infection or vaccination confers no useful resistance. The usefulness of pyolysin as a vaccine remains to be demonstrated.

LABORATORY DIAGNOSIS

Gram-stained films from tissues or exudates reveal gram-positive diphtheroids (see Fig 23.1) often mixed with other bacteria.

Material suspected of containing *A. pyogenes* is cultured on blood agar.

FIGURE 23.2. Corynebacterium pseudotuberculosis *in pus from an equine chest abscess. Note club shapes, palisading, "Chinese letter" patterns, pleomorphism. Gram stain, 1000×.*

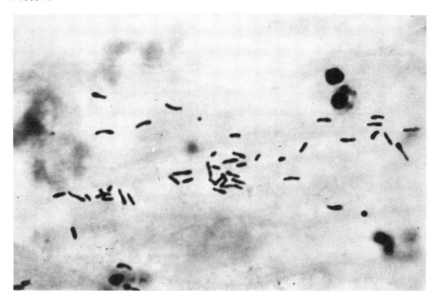

TREATMENT AND CONTROL

Incision and drainage of abscesses are essential. Although many antibiotics, including all penicillins, are active in vitro, medical treatment alone is usually disappointing due to inadequate drug delivery to the lesions.

CORYNEBACTERIUM PSEUDOTUBERCULOSIS

DESCRIPTIVE FEATURES

Morphology and Staining

Corynebacterium pseudotuberculosis (Fig 23.2) is a typical diphtheroid (syn. *C. ovis*). The cells range from coccoid to filamentous, 0.5 μm × >3.0 μm, are non-acid-fast, nonencapsulated, and often contain granules.

Structure and Composition

The cell wall is typically corynebacterial. Its high lipid contents make the cells hydrophobic and may contribute to their intraphagocytic survival and leukotoxicity.

Cellular Products of Medical Interest

An exotoxin with phospholipase D activity 1) lyses sheep and bovine erythrocytes and endothelial cells, 2) inhibits beta toxin of *Staphylococcus aureus* (Fig 23.3) and *Clostridium perfringens* alpha toxin, 3) potentiates hemolytic activity of "*R. equi* factors" (Fig 23.4), 4) produces dermal

FIGURE 23.3. *Inhibition of staphylococcal beta toxin (phospholipase C) activity on bovine blood agar by Corynebacterium pseudotuberculosis exotoxin (phospholipase D).*

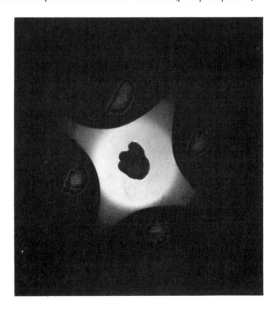

necrosis in rabbits, and 5) is lethal to various experimental animals. A 40kDa serine protease known as *CP40* (corynebacterial *p*rotease 40) is also produced.

Growth Characteristics

Corynebacterium pseudotuberculosis grows best on media containing blood or serum. At 48 hours on blood agar,

FIGURE 23.4. *Synergistic hemolysis by* Corynebacterium pseudotuberculosis *(center) and* Rhodococcus equi *(periphery). Hemolysis is maximal where the diffusion zones of the two organisms overlap.*

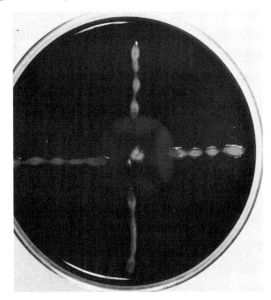

colonies are off-white, dull, faintly hemolytic, and about 1 mm in diameter. They can be pushed across the agar without disintegrating and disperse poorly in liquids.

Biochemical Activities

The agent is catalase positive and facultatively anaerobic. Some carbohydrates are fermented.

Resistance

Disinfectants and heat (60°C) kill *C. pseudotuberculosis*, but organisms survive well where moisture and organic matter abound. Penicillins (including ceftiofur), erythromycin, chloramphenicol, lincomycin, tetracycline, enrofloxicin, and trimethoprim-sulfonamide are inhibitory in vitro. The agent is resistant to aminoglycosides.

Variability

There are two biotypes that differ biochemically, serologically, and epidemiologically: 1) equine and most bovine isolates reduce nitrates to nitrites, while 2) ovine and caprine ones do not.

ECOLOGY

Reservoir

Corynebacterium pseudotuberculosis is found in lesions, the gastrointestinal tract of normal sheep, and the soil of sheep pens. The reservoir of the equine type is not known.

Transmission

Sheep become infected through breaks in the skin (e.g., wounds acquired during shearing).

Pathogenesis

Mechanisms. Virulence is attributed to the exotoxin (and perhaps the serine protease) and cell wall lipids. *Corynebacterium pseudotuberculosis* is a facultatively intracellular parasite whose resistance to phagolysosomal disposal is related to its surface lipids.

Following infection, abscesses form but remain localized when exotoxin and/or protease are absent or neutralized.

Pathology. Neutrophilic infiltration and endothelial damage characterize early changes. The lesions are abscesses. Distribution, progress, and appearance differ with species and routes of inoculation, but lymphatic involvement is consistent. The nature of the pus varies largely with age of the lesion, which grossly appears creamy to dry and crumbly ("cheesy"). Old abscesses consist of dead macrophages with peripheral neutrophils, giant cells, and fibrous tissue. Lesions almost always contain just *C. pseudotuberculosis*.

Disease Patterns. Most forms of infection are chronic. Caseous lymphadenitis of sheep and goats is usually traced to a skin infection. After introduction, the agent elicits a diffuse inflammation, followed by the formation of an abscess that coalesces and undergoes encapsulation. Inflammatory cells traverse the capsule peripherally, adding a layer of suppuration and a new capsule. Several such cycles give the lesions, especially in sheep, an "onion ring" appearance (Fig 23.5). Old lesions acquire thick, fibrous capsules. The general health is unaffected unless dissemination occurs to other lymph nodes, viscera, or the central nervous system, causing progressive debilitation (thin ewe syndrome).

Ulcerative lymphangitis of horses (rarely cattle) ascends the lymphatics, usually of the hind limbs of horses, starting at the fetlock. Its progress toward the inguinal region is marked by swelling and abscesses, which rupture to leave ulcers along its course. Hematogenous dissemination is rare. Areas other than extremities are occasionally affected. Contagious acne (Canadian horse pox) is an uncommon equine folliculitis due to *C. pseudotuberculosis* infection.

Corynebacterium pseudotuberculosis also causes abscesses, usually in the muscles of the chest and caudal abdominal region of horses ("pigeon fever," breastbone fever). The infective mechanism is not understood, but the seasonal peak (autumn) and geographic restriction (mainly California) suggest an arthropod vector. The lesions of cutaneous ventral habronemiasis and a midventral dermatitis due to horn fly (*Haematobius irritans*) activity are possible portals of entry. Signs such as swelling, pain, and lameness depend on the location and size of the abscesses. Septicemia occurs rarely, but may result in abortions, renal abscesses, debilitation, and

FIGURE 23.5.   *Caseous lymphadenitis in a sheep. Lymph nodes, lungs, spleen. Note abscesses with concentric ring pattern, especially in the lymph node, top right. (Photograph courtesy of Dr. Corrie Brown.)*

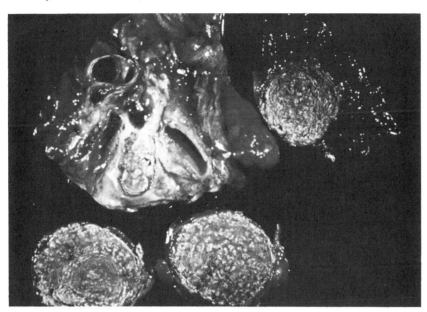

death. The superficial lesions resolve slowly after drainage.

Cattle occasionally develop skin infections with lymph node involvement. Such episodes are often acute and can be epidemic. The most common site is the lateral body wall, suggesting that trauma initiates the disease by producing breaks in the skin.

The few known human infections generally followed animal contact and were mostly benign lymphadenitides.

Epidemiology

The current view is that *C. pseudotuberculosis* is an animal parasite and only an accidental soil inhabitant. In sheep, shearing, docking, and dipping are significant factors in the spread of infection. In goats, direct contact, ingestion, and arthropod vectors must be considered. The prevalence of infection increases with age. Caseous lymphadenitis is one of the important bacterial infections of small ruminants.

The hypotheses concerning equine exposure have been considered. No age predilection has been noted. Ulcerative lymphangitis is thought to reflect poor management and is uncommon nowadays. "Pigeon fever" is limited to the far western United States. Annual prevalence varies, seeming highest after a wet winter.

IMMUNOLOGIC ASPECTS

The roles of antibody and cell-mediated responses that occur during infections are undefined. Antitoxin limits dissemination of abscesses. Caseous lymphadenitis can be progressive, and equine abscesses recur.

Bacterin-toxoid combinations prevent dissemination (not infection) in sheep for at least a year and evoke protective responses in goats and horses. Purified CP40 in adjuvant elicits a protective response in sheep. Mutants constructed by knocking out specific genes that encode products related to virulence (e.g., phospholipase D; aromatic amino acid production) result in a modified live product that elicits antibody and cell-mediated immune responses. These modified live vaccines are effective immunizing products.

LABORATORY DIAGNOSIS

Intracellular or extracellular diphtheroid-shaped organisms may be demonstrable in stained direct smears of material from lesions (see Fig 23.2).

Blood agar plates inoculated with abscess material and incubated for 24 to 48 hours produce small, off-white, faintly hemolytic colonies that can be pushed intact over the agar surface.

Inhibition of staphylococcal beta toxin (see Fig 23.3) and synergistic hemolysis with *R. equi* (see Fig 23.4) confirm identification of *C. pseudotuberculosis*. Suppression of these reactions by antibody forms the basis of serodiagnostic tests (synergistic hemolysis inhibition test).

Other tests utilize agglutination, complement fixation, indirect hemagglutination, hemolysis inhibition, gel diffusion, and toxin neutralization.

Treatment and Control

In sheep and goats, antibiotic treatment is ineffective. Control is aimed at limiting exposure by segregation or culling of affected animals and at scrupulous sanitary care during activities like shearing, dipping, and surgical procedures. Bacterin-toxoid combinations may be helpful in limiting infections. Modified-live products show promise.

Equine abscesses are handled surgically. Prolonged penicillin therapy is used to prevent or treat disseminated disease.

Erythromycin was effective in a reported case of human pneumonia.

Rhodococcus equi

Descriptive Features

Morphology and Staining

Rhodococcus equi cells measure about $1\,\mu m \times$ up to $5\,\mu m$. They pass through a cycle from coccal to bacillary forms. They are encapsulated, and are sometimes weakly acid-fast.

Structure and Products

Cell-wall ingredients are characteristic of the corynebacteria group.

The capsules are polysaccharide and form the basis of type specificity within the species. Diffusible "R. equi factors" (a phospholipase C and cholesterol oxidase) lyse erythrocytes in synergy with phospholipase D of *C. pseudotuberculosis* (see Fig 23.4).

Growth Characteristics

Rhodococcus equi grows aerobically over a wide temperature range (starting at 10°C) on most media. Mucoid colonies develop in about 48 hours, may reach large sizes (<70 mm), and may acquire a pink pigmentation.

Biochemical Activities

The agent is catalase, urease, and nitrate positive but does not acidify routine fermentation media.

Resistance

The organism withstands up to 2.5% oxalic acid and 5% sulfuric acid for 60 and 45 minutes, respectively, a feature utilized in attempts at isolation from soil and feces. It is killed at 60°C within an hour.

Rhodococcus equi is susceptible to rifampin, erythromycin, gentamicin, and usually to chloramphenicol, tetracycline, and trimethoprim-sulfonamides, but not to beta-lactam antibiotics. The combination of rifampin and erythromycin is synergistic in vitro, forming the basis for the use of this combination for treating affected animals.

Variability

Twenty-seven capsular types are described. Their prevalence varies somewhat geographically.

Ecology

Reservoir

Rhodococcus equi occurs in soil and animal manure and — perhaps secondarily — the intestine of mammals and birds.

Disease is seen most frequently in horses, less frequently in swine, and rarely in cattle, sheep, goats, cats, humans, crocodilians, koalas, buffalo, and llamas.

Transmission

Infection is acquired by inhalation, ingestion, or congenitally via umbilical or mucous membrane exposure.

Pathogenesis

Mechanisms. *Rhodococcus equi* is a facultative intracellular parasite, surviving in macrophages through suppression of phagolysosomal fusion and evoking a pyogranulomatous response. The capsule, cell wall constituents, and "*R. equi* factors" probably play a role in pathogenesis.

Virulent strains contain a high molecular weight plasmid (85–90 kb) correlated with a cell surface protein of about 15–17 kDa (called Vap, for *v*irulence *a*ssociated *p*rotein). The function of Vap is unknown.

Pathology. The organism is a parasite of macrophages. Unlike other encapsulated bacteria, *R. equi* is opsonized by complement components (C3b) generated by the alternate pathway. Opsonized *R. equi* associates with macrophages by way of the Mac-1 complement receptor. Once inside the macrophage, it survives within phagosomes by inhibiting phagolysosome fusion.

The lesions of *R. equi* infection are abscesses and granulomas. Elements of granulomatous inflammation include macrophages and giant cells, with neutrophils predominating in the caseopurulent portions.

Disease Patterns. Foal pneumonia is the most significant manifestation. The agent affects mainly foals aged 1 to 6 months and causes a suppurative bronchopneumonia, producing large abscesses in the lungs and hilar lymph nodes. Occasionally there is localization in joints, skin, and spleen. Ulcerative intestinal lesions with abscesses in mesenteric lymph nodes are common.

The prognosis varies indirectly with the age of the foal at the time of onset and is poorest for those affected at less than two months of age. The case fatality rate exceeds 50%.

Extrapulmonary disease occurs in foals and older horses. Rare uterine infections in mares are possibly related to perinatal exposure of foals.

Rhodococcus equi is recovered from both tuberculosis-like lesions in cervical lymph nodes of swine and normal nodes. Its pathogenic role is disputed.

Sporadic suppurative diseases have been described in diverse mammals. They are commonly localized in lymph nodes, lungs, and uterus. Fulminating bacteremias were observed in a crocodile and an American alligator.

In humans, *R. equi* pneumonia is seen in immuno-suppressed individuals. Affected foals are an uncommon source for humans.

Epidemiology

Rhodococcus equi is part of the equine environment. Its concentration varies with the history of equine use of the premises. On problem farms, it is highest in the foaling and rearing areas. Susceptibility coincides with the fading of maternally transmitted immunity and precedes natural immunization by subclinical exposures.

The seasonal peak in summer is attributed to the abundance of 1) susceptible foals and 2) heat and dust, which impose added burdens on respiratory tract defenses.

Human infections are not uniformly linked to animal contact.

IMMUNOLOGIC ASPECTS

Functional CD4$^+$T cells (T$_{H1}$) are necessary for protective immunity by "activating" macrophages by way of gamma interferon. Antibody, perhaps to the virulence-associated proteins (Vap), are needed since maternally derived antibody as well as passively administered antibody appear to be protective. Thus, both cell-mediated and humoral immunity are important.

Horses past infancy show signs of immunizing exposures to *R. equi*, resulting in humoral and cell-mediated responses. Both appear to be involved in enabling macrophages to kill infecting organisms. Antibody, detectable by enzyme-linked immunoadsorbent assay (ELISA), appears at five months and is passed by colostrum from mare to foal. Such passively acquired antibody declines by age 6 to 12 weeks, which is roughly the time of the highest prevalence of disease.

No immunizing products are commercially obtainable. Attempts at immunization with Vap have been disappointing.

LABORATORY DIAGNOSIS

Demonstration of *R. equi* in samples from respiratory tracts of pneumonic foals constitutes a diagnosis of *R. equi* pneumonia. In smears, organisms appear as intracellular and extracellular clusters of gram-positive cocci or rods (Fig 23.6). The identity of typical growth on blood agar is confirmed morphologically, biochemically, and by synergistic hemolysis (see Fig 23.4).

TREATMENT AND CONTROL

The prognosis in *R. equi* foal pneumonia is always guarded. Chest radiographs give valuable prognostic

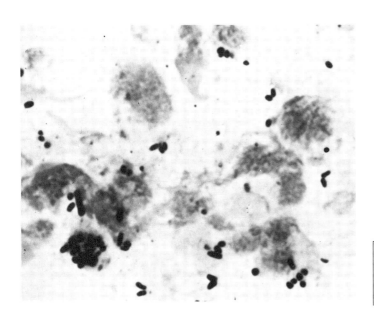

FIGURE 23.6. *Rhodococcus equi in transtracheal aspirate from a pneumonic foal. Note coccal and bacillary shapes. Cluster on lower left is suggestive of intracellular colonization. Gram stain, 1000×.*

clues. Animals with nodular or cavitary lung patterns and hilar lymph node enlargement respond less frequently to therapy than those with diffuse alveolar or interstitial reactions. The preferred treatment is erythromycin combined with rifampin.

Preventive measures include colostrum intake, dust control, and removal of foals from contaminated grounds. Prophylactic antimicrobic treatment is justifiable in epidemic situations.

SELECTED REFERENCES

Barksdale L, Lindar R, Sulea IT, Pollice M. Phospholipase D activity of *Corynebacterium pseudotuberculosis* (*Corynebacterium ovis*) and *Corynebacterium ulcerans*, a distinctive marker within the genus *Corynebacterium*. J Clin Microbiol 1981;13:335.

Billington SJ, Jost BH, Cuevas WA, et al. *Arcanobacterium* (*Actinomyces*) *pyogenes* hemolysin, pyolysin, is a novel member of the thiol-activated cytolysin family. J Bacteriol 1997;179:6100.

Brown CC, Olander HS. Caseous lymphadenitis in goats and sheep: a review. Vet Bull 1987;57:1.

Giguere S, Prescott JF. Clinical manifestation, diagnosis, treatment, and prevention of *Rhodococcus equi* infections in foals. Vet Microbiol 1997;56:313.

Hietala SK, Ardans AA. Interaction of *Rhodococcus equi* with phagocytic cells from *R. equi* exposed and nonexposed foals. Vet Microbiol 1987;14:307.

Hietala SK, Ardans AA, Sansome A. Detection of *Corynebacterium equi* antibody in horses in ELISA assay. Am J Vet Res 1985;46:13.

Hillerton JE, Bramley AJ, Watson CA. The epidemiology of summer mastitis: a survey of clinical cases. Br Vet J 1987;143:520.

Hinton M. Bovine abortion associated with *Corynebacterium pyogenes*. Vet Bull 1972;42:753.

Hodgson ALM, Krywult J, Corner LA, et al. Rational attenuation of *Corynebacterium pseudotuberculosis*: potential cheesy gland vaccine and live delivery vehicle. Infect Immun 1992;60:2900.

Hodgson ALM, Tachedjian M, Corner LA, Radford AJ. Protection of sheep against caseous lymphadenitis by use of a single oral dose of live recombinant *Corynebacterium pseudotuberculosis*. Infect Immun 1994;62:5275.

Hondalus MK, Diamond MS, Rosenthal LA, et al. The intracellular bacterium *Rhodococcus equi* requires Mac-1 to bind to mammalian cells. Infect Immun 1993;61:2919.

Kanaly ST, Hines SA, Palmer GH. Cytokine modulation alters pulmonary clearance of *Rhodococcus equi* and development of granulomatous pneumonia. Infect Immun 1995;63:3037.

Kanaly ST, Hines SA, Palmer GH. Failure of pulmonary clearance of *Rhodococcus equi* infection in CD4+ T-lymphocyte-deficient transgenic mice. Infect Immun 1993;61:4929.

Knight HD. A serologic method for the detection of *Corynebacterium pseudotuberculosis* infections in horses. Cornell Vet 1978;68:220.

Leamaster BR. Efficacy of *Corynebacterium pseudotuberculosis* bacterin for the immunologic protection of sheep against development of caseous lymphademitis. Am J Vet Res 1987;48:869.

Miers KC, Ley WB. *Corynebacterium pseudotuberculosis* in the horse: study of 117 clinical cases and consideration of etiopathogenesis. J Am Vet Med Assoc 1980;177:250.

Muckle CA, Gyles CL. Relation of lipid content and exotoxin production to virulence of *Corynebacterium pseudotuberculosis* in mice. Am J Vet Res 1983;44:1149.

Nicholson VM, Prescott JF. Restriction enzyme analysis of the virulence plasmids of VapA-positive *Rhodococcus equi* strains isolated from humans and horses. J Clin Microbiol 1997;35:738.

Prescott JF. Epidemiology of *Rhodococcus equi* infection in horses. Vet Microbiol 1987;14:211.

Prescott JF. *Rhodococcus equi*: an animal and human pathogen. Clin Microbiol Rev 1991;4:20.

Prescott JF, Nicholson VM, Patterson MC, et al. Use of *Rhodococcus equi* virulence-associated protein for immunization of foals against *R. equi* pneumonia. Am J Vet Res 1997;58:356.

Ramos CP, Foster G, Collins MD. Phylogenetic analysis of the genus *Actinomyces* based on 16S rRNA gene sequences: description of *Arcanobacterium phocae* sp. nov., *Arcanobacterium bernardiae* comb. nov., and *Arcanobacterium pyogenes* comb. nov. Int J Syst Bacteriol 1997;47:46.

Simmons CP, Hodgson ALM, Strugnell RA. Attenuation and vaccine potential of *aroQ* mutants of *Corynebacterium pseudotuberculosis*. Infect Immun 1997;65:3048.

Songer JG. Biochemical and genetic characterization of *Corynebacterium pseudotuberculosis*. Am J Vet Res 1988;49:223.

Takai S, Watanabe Y, Ikeda T, et al. Virulence-associated plasmids in *Rhodococcus equi*. J Clin Microbiol 1993;31:1726.

Wilson MJ, Brandon MR, Walker J. Molecular and biochemical characterization of a protective 40-kilodalton antigen from *Corynebacterium pseudotuberculosis*. Infect Immun 1995;63:206.

Woolcock JB, Mutimer MD, Bowles PM. The immunological response of foals to *Rhodococcus equi*. A review. Vet Microbiol 1987;14:215.

24 Pasteurella

ERNST L. BIBERSTEIN   DWIGHT C. HIRSH

Pasteurella is part of the family *Pasteurellaceae*, which comprises three genera: *Pasteurella*, *Actinobacillus*, and *Haemophilus*, consisting of gram-negative, nonmotile coccobacilli. They are facultative anaerobes, typically oxidase positive, that reduce nitrates and attack carbohydrates fermentatively. Most are commensal parasites of animals.

There are 19 recognized and proposed species of *Pasteurella* (Table 24.1). *Pasteurella piscicida* has been reclassified as *Photobacterium damsela* ssp. *piscicida* and *Pasteurella anatipestifer* as *Riemerella anatipestifer* (see Chapter 28).

DESCRIPTIVE FEATURES

Morphology and Staining

Cells measure 0.2 μm × up to 2.0 μm. Bipolarity, that is, the staining of only the tips of cells, is demonstrable with polychrome stains (e.g., Wright's stain). The capsules of *P. multocida*, *P. haemolytica*, and *P. trehalosi* are the basis for type specificity.

Structure and Composition

Capsules contain acidic polysaccharides, in *P. multocida* type A, hyaluronic acid. Some *P. multocida* and *P. haemolytica* strains express adhesins.

Cell walls consist mainly of lipopolysaccharides and proteins. Some of the latter are iron-regulated (i.e., they are expressed under iron-poor conditions).

Cell Products of Medical Interest

Members of the genus *Pasteurella* produce a number of substances that are associated with the pathogenicity of this group of microorganisms. Among the most important are the capsule, lipopolysaccharide, iron-regulated outer membrane proteins, toxic outer membrane proteins, adhesins, leukotoxins, and enzymes that may be involved in disease production (hyaluronidase, neuraminidase).

The capsule plays many roles, the most important of which are the interference with phagocytosis (antiphagocytic) and the protection of the outer membrane from the deposition of membrane attack complexes generated by activation of the complement system. The amount of capsule produced is inversely proportional to the amount of available iron. In vivo, where the amount of available iron is very low, the amount of capsule formed would be less (but sufficient to protect the microorganism from phagocytosis and complement-mediated lysis). The hyaluronic acid capsule serves as an adhesin for respiratory tract epithelial cells in the case of some avian strains of *P. multocida*.

Lipopolysaccharide (LPS) elicits an inflammatory response following its interaction with LPS-binding protein and receptors on the surface of macrophages. In addition, LPS is directly toxic to respiratory tract endothelial cells.

Some, and probably all, pasteurellae produce adhesins (and possibly more than one kind). A type 4 fimbria has been described for avian strains of *P. multocida*. As with other microorganisms, the expression of adhesins probably depends upon environmental cues. That is, adhesins are expressed while the microorganism inhabits an epithelial surface, but repressed when the microorganism is inside the host where adherence to a phagocytic cell would be disadvantageous.

Because iron is an absolute growth requirement, pasteurellae must acquire this substance if they are to exist within the host. Some avian strains of *P. multocida* produce a siderophore, multicidin, which is neither a phenolate nor hydroxynate type siderophore. Siderophores have not been demonstrated in pasteurellae from other sources or species. However, all pasteurellae bind transferrin-iron complexes by virtue of iron-regulated outer membrane proteins that are expressed under iron-poor conditions. Iron is probably acquired from the transferrin-iron complexes that bind to the surface of the microorganism.

Pasteurella haemolytica produces a leukotoxin that is important in the pathogenesis of disease associated with this microorganism. Leukotoxin (Lkt) is a 104-kDa protein toxin belonging to the RTX (repeats in *toxin*) family of toxins, so-called because of the common feature of repeats of glycine-rich sequences within the protein. Interestingly, the hemolysin of *Escherichia coli* is also an RTX-type toxin (see Chapter 9). Lkt produces a number of biological effects. These include cytotoxic effects upon leukocytes (Lkt in high concentration), activation of leukocytes (Lkt in low concentration), death of leukocytes by apoptosis, and the downregulation of MHC II proteins on the surface of macrophages affecting their ability to present antigen. Activation of macrophages results in the release of the proinflammatory cytokines TNF and IL-1,

Table 24.1. Members of the Genus *Pasteurella* and Their Usual Source or Associated Condition

Species	Usual Source or Associated Condition
P. aerogenes	Associated with gastroenteritis in swine; abortion in swine
P. anatis	Intestinal contents of normal ducks
P. avium	Respiratory tract of fowl
P. bettyae (CDC Group HB-5)	Human Bartholin gland abscess; septicemia in immunocompromised human patients; periparturient septicemia in human infants
P. caballi	Pneumonia and associated conditions in horses
P. canis	Pneumonia in dogs; other "mouth" related conditions in dogs
P. dagmatis	Respiratory tract of dogs
P. gallinarum	Respiratory tract of fowl
P. haemolytica	Pneumonia in ruminants
P. langaa	Respiratory tract of fowl
P. lymphangitidis	Bovine lymphangitis
P. mairi	Abortion in swine; septicemia in piglets
P. multocida	Pneumonia and respiratory condition in ruminants, swine, and cats; other "mouth" related conditions of cats
P. pneumotropica	Pneumonia in rodents
P. stomatis	Pneumonia in dogs; other "mouth" related conditions in dogs
P. testudinis	Respiratory tracts of Desert Tortoise and Box turtles
P. trehalosi (*P. haemolytica* T-strains)	Pneumonia/septicemia in ruminants
P. ureae	Respiratory tract of human beings
P. volantium	Wattles of fowl

and the stimulation of polymorphonuclear leukocytes leading to the release of H_2O_2, which in turn is converted by alveolar endothelial cells in the presence of Fe^{2+} to hydroxyl radicals. Hydroxyl radicals kill the cell, resulting in accumulation of edema fluid and fibrin.

Pasteurella multocida, mainly those expressing type D capsule type, produce a toxin (*P. multocida* toxin or Pmt, also known as dermonecrotic toxin, osteolytic toxin, or turbinate atrophy toxin) that has significant homology to cytotoxic necrotizing factors (CNF-1, CNF-2) of *E. coli* (see Chapter 9). These factors interact with cellular Rho proteins (small GTP-binding proteins) controlling the cellular actin cytoskeleton. Pmt is a mitogen for osteoblasts.

Some avian strains of *P. multocida* express an outer-membrane protein that is toxic to phagocytic cells. It is unclear what role this protein might have in the pathogenesis of disease. If capsule formation is downregulated in vivo due to low available iron concentrations, then the toxic outer-membrane protein might serve to protect the microorganism from phagocytosis.

Strains of *P. multocida* may produce hyaluronidase and neuraminidase. The role played by these enzymes in the pathogenesis of disease is unclear. It is tempting to speculate that hyaluronidase is active in vivo and may be responsible for the microorganism's ability to "spread" through tissue. Neuraminidase has been postulated to play a role in the colonization of epithelial surfaces by removing terminal sialic acid residues from mucin, thereby modifying normal host innate immunity.

Growth Characteristics

Pasteurellae grow best in the presence of serum or blood. After overnight incubation, colonies are about 1 mm in diameter, clear, and smooth or mucoid. *Pasteurella haemolytica* and *P. trehalosi* produce hemolysis on ruminant blood agar.

Resistance

Cultures die within 1 or 2 weeks. Disinfectants, heat (50°C for 30 minutes), and ultraviolet light are promptly lethal. Yet *P. multocida* survives for months in bird carcasses.

Pasteurella spp., especially from food animals, have become increasingly resistant to penicillins, tetracyclines, and sulfonamides, to which they were originally susceptible. The gene encoding tetracycline resistance is unique to pasteurellae. Resistance encoding genes are frequently associated with R plasmids.

Variability

In *P. multocida*, five capsular (A, B, D, E, F) and 11 somatic (1–11) serotypes occur in 20 different combinations. Another approach, utilizing agar gel immunodiffusion, has identified 16 types. Serotypes are often related to host specificity and pathogenicity.

Some biotypes of *Pasteurella* are distinct enough to qualify as subspecies or species (see Table 24.1 and the references for this chapter).

Previously, *P. haemolytica* was differentiated into two biotypes: A (ferments arabinose) and T (ferments trehalose), which differ with regard to reservoir, pathogenicity, antimicrobial susceptibility, cultural and serologic traits, and genetic relatedness. Type A consists of 12 capsular types, type T of 4. Type T has been renamed *P. trehalosi*.

ECOLOGY

Reservoir

Pasteurellae are carried on mucous membranes of susceptible host species. Carriage may be widespread, as with *P. multocida* in carnivores, or exceptional, as with fowl cholera or hemorrhagic septicemia. In fowl cholera, one host species may serve as reservoir for another.

Transmission

Infection is by inhalation, ingestion, or bites and scratch wounds. Many infections are probably endogenous. In bovine hemorrhagic septicemia and fowl cholera, environmental contamination contributes to indirect transmission.

Pathogenesis

Mechanisms. Capsules and leukotoxins may subvert phagocytic and inflammatory responses. Lesions suggest endotoxic activity.

Pmt of *P. multocida* is responsible for the lesions seen in pigs with atrophic rhinitis.

Pathology. Lesions vary with site of infection, virulence of strains, and host resistance. In septicemias of ruminants and acute pasteurellosis of birds, vascular damage results in hemorrhage and fluid loss but little cellular inflammatory response. Focal necrosis in parenchymatous organs or ulcerations of mucous membranes may occur. Mammals develop generalized hemorrhagic lymphadenopathy.

In most pneumonias, inflammatory cells are prominent, with erythrocytes, neutrophils, and mononuclear cells appearing and predominating successively. The tissue appearance changes accordingly from reddish-black to red, pink, and gray. Necrosis, abscess formation, and fibrin deposition vary in severity. In chronic fowl cholera, caseopurulent inflammation occurs in joints, middle ear, ovaries, or wattles.

Atrophic rhinitis of pigs (see also under *Bordetella bronchiseptica*, Chapter 27) is a chronic rhinitis accompanying disturbed osteogenesis adjacent to the inflamed areas. Increased osteoclastic and diminished osteoblastic activity destroys the turbinates and bones of the snout, resulting in distortions of facial structures. Histologically, fibrous tissue replaces osseous tissue. Bone atrophy is accompanied by inflammation of varying acuteness.

Disease Patterns

Cattle. Hemorrhagic septicemia is an acute systemic infection with *P. multocida*, serotype 6:B (Southeast Asia) or 6:E (Africa), occurring in tropical areas as seasonal epidemics with high morbidity and mortality. Signs include high fever, depression, subcutaneous edema, hypersalivation and diarrhea, or sudden death. All excretions and secretions are highly infectious.

The most common form of bovine pasteurellosis, involving *P. haemolytica*, biotype A, serotype 1 (A1), or *P. multocida*, type A, is shipping fever, a fibrinous pleuropneumonia or bronchopneumonia seen wherever cattle, especially calves, are transported, assembled, and handled under stressful conditions. While the ultimate cause is uncertain (Table 24.2), the agents producing severe illness and death are bacteria, most commonly and acutely *P. haemolytica* A1.

The onset, 1 to 2 weeks after stress, is marked by fever, inappetence, and listlessness. Respiratory signs (nasal discharge, cough) are few and variable. At more advanced stages, the fever may drop but respiratory distress will be obvious. Abnormal lung sounds can be detected, especially over the apical lobes, which are first and most severely affected.

Table 24.2. Etiologic and Possible Contributory Factors in Bovine Shipping Fever (after C. A. Hjerpe)

Bacteria[a]	Mycoplasmas	Viruses[b]	Environmental Stress
P. haemolytica	*M. bovis*	IBR	Exhaustion, starvation, dehydration, weaning, ration changes, overcrowding, chilling, overheating, excess or irregular high-energy feed, poor ventilation, excess humidity, nonrespiratory disease, castration, dehorning, social maladjustment
P. multocida	*M. dispar*	PI-3	
H. somnus	*Ureaplasma*	BRSV	

[a] Other bacteria uncommonly associated: *Salmonella, Streptococcus, S. aureus, E. coli, A. pyogenes*, obligate anaerobes, *Chlamydia*.
[b] Other viruses uncommonly associated: BVD, adenovirus, rhinovirus, reovirus, herpesvirus, enterovirus, calicivirus, and coronavirus.

Pasteurella haemolytica can cause mastitis with much tissue destruction, hemorrhage, and systemic toxic complications, which are often fatal. A somewhat less severe form is caused by *P. multocida*.

Sheep and Goats. Septicemic pasteurellosis, almost always due to *P. trehalosi* (biotype T *P. haemolytica*) in feeder lambs and *P. haemolytica* (biotype A) in nursing lambs, resembles bovine hemorrhagic septicemia, although intestinal involvement is often absent and the morbidity rate is much lower.

Enzootic pneumonia of sheep is the ovine equivalent of bovine shipping fever. *Pasteurella haemolytica*, biotype A, is most often involved.

Gangrenous mastitis due to *P. haemolytica* (usual) or *P. trehalosi* occurs late in lactation, when large lambs bruise the udder and provide the inoculum from their oropharyngeal flora. Acute systemic reactions accompany disease of the udder, parts of which undergo necrosis ("blue bag") and may slough.

Swine. A fibrinous pneumonia, associated with *P. multocida*, often follows viral infections.

Atrophic rhinitis (AR) of young pigs (3 weeks to 7 months) leading to turbinate destruction and secondary complications results from synergistic nasal infection by *P. multocida* and *Bordetella bronchiseptica*. Toxigenic *P. multocida*, especially type D, excretes Pmt capable of producing the lesions after irritation of the nasal mucosa. *Bordetella bronchiseptica* produces this irritation by virtue of an unrelated dermonecrotic toxin (see Chapter 27). In addition, ammonia (in concentrations sometimes found in swine-rearing houses) acts synergistically with Pmt-secreting *P. multocida*.

Signs include sneezing, epistaxis, and staining of the face due to tear-duct obstruction. Skeletal abnormalities produce lateral deviation of the snout or wrinkling due to rostrocaudal compression. Secondary pneumonia is due in part to the elimination of the turbinates as defenses of the respiratory tract.

Rabbits. Snuffles, a mucopurulent rhinosinusitis of rabbits due to *P. multocida*, develops under stress of pregnancy, lactation, or mismanagement. Complications include bronchopneumonia, middle and inner ear infection, conjunctivitis, and septicemia. In the genital tract, *P. multocida* may cause orchitis, balanoposthitis, and pyometra.

Fowl. Fowl cholera, a systemic infection due to *P. multocida* (most commonly capsule type A), is acquired by ingestion or inhalation and affects mainly turkeys, waterfowl, and chickens. The peracute form can kill about 60% of infected birds without preceding signs of illness. The acute type, marked by listlessness, anorexia, diarrhea, and nasal and ocular discharges, may last several days and be about 30% lethal. The subacute form is mostly respiratory and is manifested by rales and mucopurulent nasal discharges. In chronic fowl cholera, there is localization of caseous lesions. *Pasteurella gallinarum* is sometimes isolated from chronic cases.

Dogs and Cats. *Pasteurella multocida* (cats) and *P. canis* (dogs) are found alongside predominantly anaerobic flora in wound infections, serositides (e.g., feline pyothorax), and foreign body lesions.

Horses. *Pasteurella caballi* occurs in equine respiratory disease, usually in association with *Streptococcus zooepidemicus*.

Small Laboratory Rodents. *Pasteurella pneumotropica*, a common commensal, may contribute to opportunistic infections such as pneumonia. Phenotypically similar organisms in other hosts probably belong to different species (e.g., *P. dagmatis*).

Humans. *Pasteurella multocida* (and rarely other pasteurellae) causes wound infections in humans resulting from animal bites or scratches. A second form, inflammatory processes, especially in the respiratory tract, is usually not directly traceable to animal sources.

Epidemiology

Table 24.3 shows the relative roles of exogenous reservoir, dissemination, and stress in various pasteurelloses. In fowl cholera, feral sources are sometimes implicated.

IMMUNOLOGIC ASPECTS

Basis of Immunity

Circulating antibody is significant in protection against hemorrhagic septicemia and fowl cholera. The type-specific capsular antigens are essential immunogens in hemorrhagic septicemia. With other forms of pasteurellosis, the picture is less clear. Both antitoxic and antibacterial antibody are important in protection.

Artificial Immunization

Pasteurella adjuvant bacterins are effective in preventing bovine hemorrhagic septicemia, conferring protection

Table 24.3. The Relative Roles of Stress, Agent Introduction, and Agent Dissemination in Various Types of *Pasteurella* Infections

	Importance of:		
	Introduction of Agent into Population	Dissemination of Agent within Population	Environmental or Individual Stress or Injury
Avian cholera	+++	++++	?
Bovine hemorrhagic septicemia	+++	++++	+
Bovine shipping fever, ovine enzootic pneumonia, ovine septicemic pasteurellosis, rabbit pasteurellosis	+	++	+++
Human pasteurellosis	+?	−	++++
Sporadic pneumonia in ruminants, *Pasteurella* infection in dogs and cats	−	−	++++

Legend: − = irrelevant; + = contributory; ++ = significant; +++ = critical; ++++ = paramount.

for up to 2 years. Antiserum is useful for short-term protection.

The essential attributes of an effective fowl cholera vaccine are not known. Field performance of bacterins has been inconsistent, even with autogenous preparations. Most promising have been live vaccines containing attenuated organisms (e.g., CU or M-9). Attenuation appears inversely related to immunogenicity.

Most shipping fever vaccines are bacterins of *P. haemolytica* and *P. multocida* combined with suspect viruses and other bovine bacterial pathogens. Benefits are inconsistent. Vaccination of calves with bacterins prepared from *P. haemolytica* reduced the degree of colonization of the upper respiratory tract by this organism. The effectiveness of modified live pasteurella vaccines awaits field confirmation. Recombinant Lkt alone does not protect cattle from *P. haemolytica*-induced pneumonia.

Pasteurella multocida and *B. bronchiseptica* bacterins with toxoid are valuable in the control of atrophic rhinitis.

LABORATORY DIAGNOSIS

Direct Examination

Exudates, tissue impressions, sediments of transtracheal aspirates, and, in birds, blood smears can be stained with a polychrome stain (e.g., Giemsa, Wright's, Wayson's) and examined for bipolar organisms. Their presence is suggestive but not unique to *Pasteurella*. On Gram stain, pasteurellae do not look distinctive.

Isolation and Identification

Pasteurellae grow overnight on bovine or sheep blood agar and are identified using differential tests. Serotyping is done in a reference laboratory. .

TREATMENT AND CONTROL

Pasteurelloses respond to timely antimicrobial therapy. Strains from carnivores and humans are generally susceptible to almost all antimicrobials. Most pasteurellae show moderate resistance to aminoglycosides, which is probably not significant clinically. Those from food-producing animals vary. In these species, cost and withdrawal requirements before slaughter are additional considerations. Consequently, sulfonamides, penicillin G, ceftiofur, tilmicosin, florfenicol, and tetracyclines are preferred. Their appropriateness should be confirmed by susceptibility tests. Sulfonamides, penicillin G, quinolones, and tetracycline are used to treat fowl cholera.

Sulfonamides and tetracyclines — in swine and poultry, penicillin also — are suitable for mass medication via feed or water, therapeutically or prophylactically.

Management practices directed at reducing stress are important in preventing pasteurellosis in livestock.

Immunization has been dependable only in bovine hemorrhagic septicemia and atrophic rhinitis control.

GROUP EF-4 (EUGONIC FERMENTOR)

A gram-negative nonmotile bacterium, superficially resembling *Pasteurella* spp., occurs in the mouth of carnivores and sporadically causes apparently endogenous fatal, acute focal, pyogranulomatous pneumonias. In humans it is implicated in animal bite wound infections.

It is oxidase, catalase, and nitratase positive; it ferments glucose slowly and has no other diagnostically dependable characteristics.

Isolates from humans stemming from animal bites test susceptible to the macrolides (erythromycin, clarithromycin, azithromycin), cephalosporins, ampicillin, tetracycline, aminoglycosides, and fluoroquinolones.

SELECTED REFERENCES

Biberstein EL. Biotyping and serotyping of *Pasteurella haemolytica*. In: Bergen T, Norris JR, eds. Methods in microbiology. Vol. 10. New York: Academic, 1978:253–269.

Biberstein EL, Jang SS, Kass PH, Hirsh DC. Distribution of indole-positive urease-negative pasteurellas in animals. J Vet Diagn Invest 1991;3:319.

Breider MA, Kumar S, Corstvet RE. Bovine pulmonary endothelial cell damage mediated by *Pasteurella haemolytica* pathogenic factors. Infect Immun 1990;58:1671.

Brogden KA, Packer RA. Comparison of *Pasteurella multocida* serotyping systems. Am J Vet Res 1979;40:1332.

Carter GR. Pasteurellosis: *Pasteurella multocida* and *Pasteurella haemolytica*. Adv Vet Sci 1967;11:321.

Chang YE, Young RY, Post D, Struck DK. Identification and characterization of the *Pasteurella haemolytica* leukotoxin. Infect Immun 1987;55:2348.

Confer AW. Immunogens of *Pasteurella*. Vet Microbiol 1993;37:353.

Confer AW, Panciera RJ, Mosier DA. Bovine pneumonic pasteurellosis: immunity to *Pasteurella haemolytica*. J Am Vet Med Assoc 1988;193:1308.

Conlon JA, Shewen PE, Lo RYC. Efficacy of recombinant leukotoxin in protection against pneumonic challenge with live *Pasteurella haemolytica* A1. Infect Immun 1991;59:587.

Deneer HG, Potter AA. Iron-repressible outer-membrane proteins of *Pasteurella haemolytica*. J Gen Microbiol 1989;135:435.

Done JT. Porcine atrophic rhinitis — an update. Vet Annual 1985;25:180.

Frank GH, Briggs RE, Loan RW, et al. Respiratory tract disease and mucosal colonization by *Pasteurella haemolytica* in transported cattle. Am J Vet Res 1996;57:1317.

Gaillot O, Guilbert L, Maruejouls C, et al. In-vitro susceptibility to thirteen antibiotics of *Pasteurella* spp. and related bacteria isolated from humans. J Antimicrob Chemother 1995;36:878.

Gilmour NJL, Angus KW. Pasteurellosis. In: Martin WB, ed. Diseases of sheep. Oxford, UK: Blackwell Scientific, 1983:3–7.

Goldstein EJC, Citron DM, Gerardo SH, et al. Activities of HMR 3004 (RU 64004) and HMR 3647 (RU 66647) compared to those of erythromycin, azithromycin, clarithromycin, roxithromycin, and eight other antimicrobial agents against unusual aerobic and anaerobic human and animal bite pathogens isolated from skin and soft tissue infections in humans. Antimicrob Agents Chemother 1998;42:1127.

Hamilton TDC, Roe JM, Webster JF. Synergistic role of gaseous ammonia in etiology of *Pasteurella multocida*-induced atrophic rhinitis in swine. J Clin Microbiol 1996;34:2185.

Hansen LM, Blanchard PC, Hirsh DC. Distribution of *tet(H)* among *Pasteurella* isolates from the United States and Canada. Antimicrob Agents Chemother 1996;40:1558.

Hansen LM, Hirsh DC. Serum resistance is correlated with encapsulation of avian strains of *Pasteurella multocida*. Vet Microbiol 1989;21:177.

Hirsh DC, Martin LD, Rhoades KR. Resistance plasmids of *Pasteurella multocida* isolated from turkeys. Am J Vet Res 1985;46:1490.

Hjerpe CA. Bovine respiratory disease complex. Curr Vet Ther 1986;2:670.

Homchampa P, Strugnell RA, Adler B. Molecular analysis of the *aroA* gene of *Pasteurella multocida* and vaccine potential of a constructed *aroA* mutant. Molec Microbiol 1992;6:3585.

Hu S, Felice SJ, Sivanandan V, Maheswaran SK. Siderophore production by *Pasteurella multocida*. Infect Immun 1986;54:804.

Hughes HPA, Campos M, McDougall L, et al. Regulation of major histocompatibility complex class 2 expression by *Pasteurella haemolytica* leukotoxin. Infect Immun 1994;62:1609.

Ikeda JS, Hirsh DC. Antigenically related iron regulated outer membrane proteins produced by different somatic serotypes of *Pasteurella multocida*. Infect Immun 1988;56:2499.

Isaacson RE, Trigo E. Pili of *Pasteurella multocida* of porcine origin. FEMS Microbiol Lett 1995;132:247.

Jacques M, Belanger M, Diarra MS, et al. Modulation of *Pasteurella multocida* capsular polysaccharide during growth under iron-restricted conditions and in vivo. Microbiology 1994;140:263.

Kadel WL, Chengappa MM, Herren CE. Field trial evaluation of a *Pasteurella* vaccine in preconditioned and nonpreconditioned lightweight calves. Am J Vet Res 1985;46:1944.

Kobisch M, Pennings A. An evaluation in pigs of Nobi-Vac AR and an experimental atrophic rhinitis vaccine containing *P. multocida* DNT-toxoid and *B. bronchiseptica*. Vet Rec 1989;124:57.

Maheswaran SK, Kannan MS, Weiss DJ, et al. Enhancement of neutrophil-mediated injury to bovine pulmonary endothelial cells by *Pasteurella haemolytica* leukotoxin. Infect Immun 1993;61:2618.

McParland RJ. Pathological changes associated with Group EF-4 bacteria in the lungs of a dog and a cat. Vet Rec 1982;111:336.

Mullan PB, Lax AJ. *Pasteurella multocida* toxin is a mitogen for bone cells in primary culture. Infect Immun 1996;64:959.

Musser J, Mechor GD, Grohn YT, et al. Comparison of tilmicosin with long-acting oxytetracycline for treatment of respiratory tract infection in calves. J Am Vet Med Assoc 1996;208:102.

Mutters R, Ihm P, Pohl S, et al. Reclassification of the genus *Pasteurella trevisan* 1887 on the basis of deoxyribonucleic acid homology, with proposals for the new species *Pasteurella dagmatis*, *Pasteurella canis*, *Pasteurella stomatis*, *Pasteurella anatis*, and *Pasteurella langaa*. Int J Syst Bacteriol 1985;35:309.

Namioka S. *Pasteurella multocida*-biochemical characteristics and serotypes. In: Bergan T, Norris JR, eds. Methods in microbiology. Vol. 10. New York: Academic, 1978:271–292.

Ogunnariwo JA, Alcantara J, Schryvers AB. Evidence for non-siderophore-mediated acquisition of transferrin-bound iron by *Pasteurella multocida*. Microb Pathogen 1991;11:47.

Ogunnariwo JA, Schryvers AB. Iron acquisition in *Pasteurella haemolytica*: expression and identification of a bovine specific transferrin receptor. Infect Immun 1990;58:2091.

Prescott JF, Yielding KM. In vitro susceptibility of selected veterinary bacterial pathogens to ciprofloxacin, enrofloxacin, and norfloxacin. Can J Vet Res 1990;54:195.

Pruimboom IM, Rimler RB, Ackermann MR, Brogden KA. Capsular hyaluronic acid-mediated adhesion of *Pasteurella multocida* to turkey air sac macrophages. Avian Dis 1996;40:887.

Reissbrodt R, Erler W, Winkelmann G. Iron supply of *Pasteurella multocida* and *Pasteurella haemolytica*. J Basic Microbiol 1994;34:K61.

Rhodes MB. *Bordetella bronchiseptica* and toxigenic type D *Pasteurella multocida* as agents of severe atrophic rhinitis of swine. Vet Microbiol 1987;13:179.

Ruffolo CG, Tennent JM, Michalski WP, Adler B. Identification, purification, and characterization of the type 4 fimbriae of *Pasteurella multocida*. Infect Immun 1997;65:339.

Schiefer B, Ward GE, Moffatt RE. Correlation of microbiological and histological findings in bovine fibrinous pneumonia. Vet Pathol 1978;15:313.

Schlater KL, Brenner DJ, Steigerwalt WG, et al. *Pasteurella caballi*, a new species from equine clinical specimens. J Clin Microbiol 1989;27:2169.

Sneath PHA, Stevens M. *Actinobacillus rossii* sp. nov., *Actinobacillus seminis* sp. nov., nom. rev., *Pasteurella bettii* sp. nov., *Pasteurella lymphanditidis* sp. nov., *Pasteurella mairi* sp. nov., and *Pasteurella trehalosi* sp. nov. Int J Syst Bacteriol 1990;40:148.

Snipes KP, Hansen LM, Hirsh DC. Plasma and iron regulated expression of high molecular weight outer membrane proteins by *Pasteurella multocida*. Am J Vet Res 1988;49:1336.

Stevens PK, Czuprynski CJ. *Pasteurella haemolytica* leukotoxin induces bovine leukocytes to undergo morphologic changes consistent with apoptosis in vitro. Infect Immun 1996;64:2687.

Sutherland AD, Donachie W, Jones GE, Quirie M. A crude cytotoxin vaccine protects sheep against experimental *Pasteurella haemolytica* A2 infection. Vet Microbiol 1989;19:175.

Truscott WM, Hirsh DC. Demonstration of an outer membrane protein with antiphagocytic activity from *Pasteurella multocida* of avian origin. Infect Immun 1988;56:1538.

Watts JL, Yancey RJ Jr, Salmon SA, Case CA. A 4-year survey of antimicrobial susceptibility trends for isolates from cattle with bovine respiratory disease in North America. J Clin Microbiol 1994;32:725.

Williams P, Griffiths E. Bacterial transferrin receptors-structure, function and contribution to virulence. Med Microbiol Immunol 1992;81:301.

25 Actinobacillus

ERNST L. BIBERSTEIN   DWIGHT C. HIRSH

Although they are genetically distinct, the genera *Actinobacillus* and *Pasteurella* overlap phenotypically.

Actinobacillus lignieresii is the agent of pyogranulomatous processes, mainly of ruminants. *Actinobacillus equuli* causes neonatal septicemia of foals and occasionally of pigs and calves; it rarely affects older horses. *Actinobacillus suis* is seen in swine with respiratory, septicemic, and localized infections. A similar agent (*Actinobacillus suis*-like) occurs in horses, particularly in respiratory tract infections. *Actinobacillus pleuropneumoniae*, which requires nicotinamide adenine dinucleotide (NAD) and was originally classified as a *Haemophilus,* is the agent of porcine pleuropneumonia. All are frequent commensals on mucous membranes. *Actinobacillus capsulatus* causes arthritis of rabbits. *Actinobacillus salpingitidis* found in the respiratory tract and oviduct of chickens can produce salpingitis and peritonitis. *Actinobacilllus seminis* inhabits the lower genital tract of sheep and may cause epididymitis in lambs. Both agents are genetically unrelated to *Actinobacillus* spp.

DESCRIPTIVE FEATURES

Morphology, Staining, and Composition

Actinobacilli are gram-negative coccobacilli, approximately 0.5 µm wide and variable in length.

A surface slime found on *A. suis, A. equuli,* and A. *lignieresii* and linked to a heat-labile antigen may be related to the stickiness of their colonies on agar. *Actinobacillus pleuropneumoniae* is encapsulated.

Cell Products of Medical Interest

Actinobacillus suis, A. equuli, and A. *lignieresii* possess the genes encoding an RTX (repeats in *to*xin) membrane-active toxin (see hemolysin, *Escherichia coli*, Chapter 9; *Pasteurella haemolytica,* Chapter 24). *Actinobacillus pleuropneumoniae* produces three different RTX-type hemolysins: Apx I, Apx II, and Apx III (pleurotoxin). *Actinobacillus equuli* and A. *lignieresii* produce very small amounts of this toxin so that colonies growing on blood agar plates are not overtly hemolytic, and the organisms are not especially leukocytotoxic as compared to other microorganisms that produce this class of toxin, for example, hemolytic *E. coli, P. haemolytica, A. suis,* and A. *pleuropneumoniae.* RTX toxins kill macrophages and neu-

trophils at high concentrations and stimulate an oxidative burst at lower concentrations.

Actinobacillus pleuropneumoniae is piliated and may be the structure responsible for specific adherence to alveolar epithelia and the cilia of terminal bronchioles. In addition, the lipopolysaccharide (LPS) of *A. pleuropneumoniae* has adhesive properties that are responsible for adherence to tracheal epithelium.

Actinobacillus pleuropneumoniae produces outer membrane proteins that bind transferrin-iron complexes (a source of iron needed for growth). A periplasmic iron-binding protein, AfuA (for *A*ctinobacillus *f*erric *u*ptake) is involved in iron transport.

Growth Characteristics

Actinobacilli grow on blood and serum-containing media at 20°C to 42°C. Colony sizes at 24 hours reach 12 mm. *Actinobacillus suis* is hemolytic on ruminant blood agar.

Carbohydrates are fermented without gas production. Urease, orthonitrophenyl-beta-D-galactopyranosidase (ONPGase, "beta-galactosidase"), and nitratase are typically present. No indole is produced, and most strains grow on MacConkey agar (but poorly). Cultures die within a week.

Resistance

Actinobacillus pleuropneumoniae contains R plasmids encoding resistance to sulfonamides, tetracycline, and penicillin.

Variability

Actinobacillus lignieresii and *A. equuli* are antigenically diverse. The six somatic types of *A. lignieresii* have some relation to geographic and host species predilection. There are 12 serotypes of *A. pleuropneumoniae* (1–12).

ECOLOGY

Reservoir

Actinobacilli (except possibly *A. capsulatus*) are commensal parasites on mucous membranes. *Actinobacillus pleuropneumoniae* are more closely associated with the respiratory tracts of sick or recovered animals.

Transmission

Except in neonates, most actinobacilloses are probably endogenous infections. Neonatal foals acquire *A. equuli* before, at, or shortly after birth from their dams, commonly via the umbilicus.

Pathogenesis

Mechanisms. RTX toxins, if produced, probably play a role in the pathogenesis of disease. At low concentrations, this class of toxin increases the activity (as measured by the oxidative burst) of phagocytic cells, which may lead to damage to surrounding cells that in turn triggers inflammation. At higher concentrations, RTX toxins damage the membrane of macrophages and neutrophils. Actinobacilli are gram negative, thus have LPS that induces an inflammatory response after binding to LPS-binding protein and macrophages with subsequent release of proinflammatory cytokines IL-1 and TNF. The antiphagocytic capsule of *A. pleuropneumoniae* is a suspected virulence factor.

Actinobacillus pleuropneumoniae adheres to ciliated epithelium in the distal bronchioles and to alveolar epithelium.

Pathology. Lesions are suppurative to granulomatous resembling actinomycosis (see Chapter 46). "Wooden tongue" is a chronic granuloma in the bovine tongue. At its center is a colony of *A. lignieresii*, ringed by eosinophilic, club-like processes forming a "rosette." The complex is surrounded by neutrophils and granulation tissue containing macrophages, plasma cells, lymphocytes, giant cells, and fibroblasts. Plant fibers are often present. Through coalescence, larger granulomas (1 cm or more in diameter) may be formed. Infection spreads to lymph nodes, producing granulomas along the way. The proliferative tissue reaction causes the tongue to protrude from the mouth. Other tissues in the vicinity, and occasionally along the gastrointestinal tract, may be involved, along with adjacent lymph nodes. Superficial lesions often ulcerate. In sheep, suppurative infections occur around the head and neck and in the skin and mammary gland. Tongue involvement is not typical.

In acute umbilical infections of newborn foals ("navel ill") by *A. equuli*, only enteritis may be present. In less acute cases, suppurative multifocal nephritis, tenovaginitis, and arthritis develop. Enteritis also occurs in calves.

Actinobacillus suis in swine and a similar agent in horses (*A. suis*-like) are associated with various inflammatory processes.

Actinobacillus pleuropneumoniae, the agent of porcine pleuropneumonia, produces a necrotizing process.

Disease Patterns. Actinobacillosis involving *A. lignieresii* occurs in ruminants and, rarely, dogs and horses. In ruminants, the agent is probably inoculated by trauma (plant fibers), initiating the process described. The course is protracted and healing slow. Interference with feed intake causes weight loss and dehydration.

Foal septicemia due to *A. equuli* ("navel ill," "sleepy foal disease") occurs within a few days of birth and is marked by fever, inappetence, prostration, and diarrhea. Animals surviving the first day typically develop lameness due to (poly)arthritis.

Actinobacillus equuli occasionally causes septicemic disease or enteritis in pigs and calves.

Actinobacillus pleuropneumoniae causes a primary pneumonia of swine, particularly young pigs 2 to 6 months old. Spread is favored by crowding and poor ventilation. Early signs include fever and reduced appetite, followed within a day by acute respiratory distress. Animals may die within 24 hours. Morbidity may reach 40%, with mortality up to 24%. Survivors show intermittent cough and unsatisfactory weight gains. Chronic infections, often without preceding acute episodes, are the source of persistent herd problems. Lesions consist of fibrinous pneumonia and pleuritis. Arthritis, meningitis, and abortion occur as complications.

Septicemia of young pigs and arthritis, endocarditis, or pneumonia in older animals may be caused by *A. suis*.

In horses, *A. suis*-like organisms occur in respiratory and sometimes genital tract infections, often alongside *Streptococcus zooepidemicus*.

Actinobacillus seminis, a commensal inhabitant of the ovine prepuce, is occasionally involved in suppurative epididymitis-orchitis and polyarthritis in lambs.

Epidemiology

Actinobacilli are opportunistic pathogens producing disease when their host's integrity is compromised, as by trauma, immaturity, or other stress. Trauma to mucous membranes of ruminants by rough feed may cause herd outbreaks suggestive of transmissible diseases.

Chronic asymptomatic carriers are the apparent reservoirs of swine pleuropneumonia (commensal carriage of serotype 2 strains of *A. pleuropneumoniae* is reported from Japan) and infectious coryza. Disease occurs when nonimmune animals are exposed to subclinically infected individuals. That prevalence is highest in the colder months is due probably more to management (i.e., the mixing of individuals with different exposure histories) than climatic factors.

IMMUNOLOGIC ASPECTS

The pathology of "wooden tongue" suggests a cell-mediated hypersensitivity. Antibodies of no known protective function appear during infection. The benefits of bacterins have not been established. Antibody to *A. pleuropneumoniae* is opsonizing and colostrum protects piglets. Antibody to RTX-type toxin is protective. Immunoprophylaxis is used to control porcine pleuropneumonia.

LABORATORY DIAGNOSIS

Actinobacilli can often be demonstrated in gram-stained exudates. They grow best on blood agar under increased amounts of carbon dioxide. Colonies are often sticky. Speciation is accomplished by cultural and biochemical tests.

TREATMENT AND CONTROL

Penicillin G, tetracycline, and ceftiofur are effective in septicemia therapy if given early. Gentamicin, kanamycin, cephalosporins, and trimethoprim-sulfas are generally effective on beta-lactamase-producing *A. pleuropneumoniae*.

In "wooden tongue," iodides given orally or intravenously promptly reduce the inflammatory swelling, which is the main clinical problem.

Avoidance of harsh, dry feed reduces the likelihood of ruminant infection. Good foaling hygiene, including navel disinfection, reduces the likelihood of foal septicemia.

Actinobacillus suis-like infections respond to most antimicrobics.

An approach to control of porcine pleuropneumonia consists of the serologic identification and elimination of infected breeding animals. In exposed herds, following removal of seroreactors, mass medication (trimethoprim-sulfa) can eradicate the infection.

Complement fixation, 2-mercaptoethanol agglutination, and enzyme-linked immunoadsorbent assay (ELISA) tests are used to detect *A. pleuropneumoniae* infection in swine. They are serotype specific.

SELECTED REFERENCES

Arseculeratne SN. Actinobacillosis in joints of rabbits. J Comp Pathol 1962;72:41.

Belanger D, Dubreuil D, Harel J, et al. Role of lipopolysaccharides in adherence of *Actinobacillus pleuropneumoniae* to porcine tracheal rings. Infect Immun 1990;58:3523.

Bisgaard M, Piechulla K, Ying YT, et al. Prevalence of organisms described as *Actinobacillus suis* or haemolytic *Actinobacillus equuli* in the oral cavity of horses. Acta Pathol Microbiol Immunol Scand Sec B 1984;92:291.

Burrows LL, Lo RYC. Molecular characterization of an RTX toxin determinant from *Actinobacillus suis*. Infect Immun 1992;60:2166.

Chin N, Frey J, Chang C, Chang Y. Identification of a locus involved in the utilization of iron by *Actinobacillus pleuropneumoniae*. FEMS Microbiol Lett 1996;143:1.

Devenish J, Rosendal S, Bosse JT. Humoral antibody response and protective immunity in swine following immunization with the 104 kilodalton hemolysin of *Actinobacillus pleuropneumoniae*. Infect Immun 1990;58:3829.

Dom P, Haesebrouck F, Ducatelle R, Charlier G. In vivo association of *Actinobacillus pleuropneumoniae* serotype 2 with the respiratory epithelium of pigs. Infect Immun 1994;62:1262.

Gonzalez GC, Caamano DL, Schryvers AB. Identification and characterization of a porcine specific transferring receptor in *Actinobacillus pleuropneumoniae*. Molec Microbiol 1990;4:1173.

Jang SS, Biberstein EL, Hirsh DC. *Actinobacillus suis*-like organisms in horses. Am J Vet Res 1987;48:1036.

Jansen R, Briaire J, Smith HE, et al. Knockout mutants of *Actinobacillus pneumoniae* serotype 1 that are devoid of RTX toxins do not activate or kill porcine neutrophils. Infect Immun 1995;63:27.

Mair NS, Randall CJ, Thomas GW, et al. *Actinobacillus suis* infection in pigs. J Comp Pathol 1974;84:113.

Mraz O, Valdik R, Bohacek J. Actinobacilli in domestic fowl. Zbl Bakt Hyg I Orig A 1976;236:294.

Rycroft AN, Williams D, Cullen JML, Macdonald J. The cytotoxin of *Actinobacillus pleuropneumoniae* (pleurotoxin) is distinct from the haemolysin and is associated with a 120 kDa polypeptide. J Gen Microbiol 1991;137:561.

Smits MA, Briaire J, Jansen R, et al. Cytolysins of *Actinobacillus pleuropneumoniae* serotype 9. Infect Immun 1991;59:4497.

Sneath PHA, Stevens M. *Actinobacillus rosii* sp. nov., *Actinobacillus seminis* sp. nov., nom. rev., *Pasteurella betii* sp. nov., *Pasteurella lymphangitidis* sp. nov., *Pasteurella mairi* sp. nov., and *Pasteurella trehalosi* sp. nov. Int J Syst Bacteriol 1990;40:148.

Sponenberg DR. Suppurative epididymitis in a ram infected with *Actinobacillus seminis*. J Am Vet Med Assoc 1993;182:920.

Thwaits RN, Kadis S. Immunogenicity of *Actinobacillus pleuropneumoniae* outer membrane proteins and enhancement of phagocytosis by antibodies to the proteins. Infect Immun 1991;59:544.

Udeze FA, Kadis S. Effects of *Actinobacillus pleuropneumoniae* hemolysin of porcine neutrophil function. Infect Immun 1992;60:1558.

Williams P, Griffiths E. Bacterial transferrin receptors-structure, function and contribution to virulence. Med Microbiol Immunol 1992;181:301.

26 Haemophilus *spp.*

Ernst L. Biberstein

Haemophilus spp., beyond sharing the family traits of *Pasteurellaceae*, require for propagation one or both of two growth factors: porphyrins or nicotinamide adenine dinucleotide (NAD, NADP), originally called X (heat-stable), and V (heat-labile) factor, respectively. Some members of the family *Pasteurellaceae* showing these needs are genetically unrelated to the type species *H. influenzae*.

Haemophilus parasuis, a resident of the normal nasopharynx of swine, can cause septicemic disease (Glässer's disease, polyserositis) or secondary respiratory infections. *Haemophilus paragallinarum* causes infectious coryza in chickens. "*Haemophilus somnus*" causes septicemic, respiratory, and genital infections in cattle. It resembles "*Histophilus ovis*" and "*Haemophilus agni*," which produce similar conditions in sheep.

DESCRIPTIVE FEATURES

Morphology and Staining

Haemophilus spp. are less than a micrometer wide and 1 to 3 μm long, but sometimes form longer filaments. Some species (*H. influenzae*, *H. paragallinarum*) are encapsulated. Pili have been described in *H. influenzae*.

Cellular Constituents and Products

The cell wall resembles that of other gram-negative bacteria. Capsules consist of polysaccharides.

Heat-labile toxins have been found in *H. paragallinarum*.

Cellular Products of Medical Interest

"*Haemophilus somnus*" produces outer-membrane proteins that bind transferrin-iron complexes, a source of iron needed for growth.

Virulent strains of "*H. somnus*" are resistant to killing by complement proteins (serum resistant) whereas commensal strains are not. Evidence suggests that serum resistance is related to the presence of immunoglobulin-binding proteins and surface fibrils.

The lipopolysaccharide (after binding to lipopolysaccharide-binding protein) of all the haemophili and hemophilus-like microorganisms initiates release of proinflammatory cytokines IL-1 and TNF from macrophages.

Growth Characteristics

Haemophilus spp. on adequate media produce within 24 to 48 hours turbidity in broth and colonies 1 mm in diameter on agar. Growth factors may be supplied as hemin and NAD (about 10 μg/ml of each). A medium naturally containing them is chocolate agar, a blood agar prepared by addition of blood when the melted agar is at 75 to 80°C (rather than 50°C when making regular blood agar). This procedure liberates NAD from cells and inactivates enzymes destructive to NAD.

Alternatively, a "feeder" bacterium (e.g., *Staphylococcus*) may be inoculated across plates where *Haemophilus* has been streaked. On otherwise inadequate media, growth occurs only near the feeder streak, a phenomenon called *satellitism* (Fig 26.1). It may be duplicated by commercially prepared X and V factor-impregnated filter papers placed on the inoculated area (Fig 26.2).

For the X and V factor requirements of *Haemophilus* spp. see Table 26.1.

Biochemical Activities

Haemophilus spp. of animals are oxidase and nitratase positive and ferment carbohydrates.

Resistance

Haemophilus spp. are readily killed by heat and die rapidly in culture and storage unless freeze dried or stored at −70°C. At cool temperatures, *H. paragallinarum* survive in exudate for several days.

Variability

Serotypes may differ in pathogenicity and geographic prevalence, and determine the specificity of bacterin-induced immunity. There are three serotypes (A–C, or I–III) of *H. paragallinarum* and at least seven of *H. parasuis*.

ECOLOGY

Reservoir

Haemophilus parasuis lives in the nasopharynx of normal swine. *Haemophilus paragallinarum* is more closely associated with the respiratory tracts of sick or recovered animals.

Haemophilus haemoglobinophilus, *"H. somnus,"* and *"Histophilus ovis"* inhabit the normal lower genital tract. *"Haemophilus somnus"* is also found in normal bovine respiratory tracts.

FIGURE 26.1. *Satellitic growth of* Haemophilus *on a feeder streak of* Staphylococcus *sp.* Haemophilus *was inoculated evenly over the entire surface. The staphylococcus was then inoculated in a single streak.*

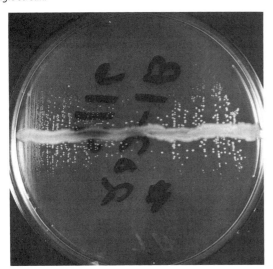

Transmission

Transmission of hemophili and related agents is probably airborne or by close contact. Indirect transmission is likely during epidemics.

Pathogenesis

Mechanisms.   The antiphagocytic capsules and heat-labile cytotoxic factors of *H. paragallinarum* are suspected virulence factors. The lesions of *Haemophilus* infections also suggest endotoxin involvement.

"Haemophilus somnus" adheres to epithelium and endothelium, is toxic to endothelial cells, is resistant to serum and phagocytic killing, and binds immunoglobulins like staphylococcal protein A.

Pathology.   All infections have suppurative components. Infection of lungs, body cavities, and joints tends to be serofibrinous to fibrinopurulent. Bacterial colonization of the meningeal vessels produces a thrombotic vasculitis leading to encephalitis and meningitis. Hemorrhagic necrotizing processes are caused by *"H. somnus."*

Fowl coryza is marked by catarrhal inflammation with heterophil exudates.

Disease Patterns.   In swine, *H. parasuis* can cause bronchopneumonia secondary to virus infections (e.g., swine influenza). Other bacteria (e.g., *Pasteurella* spp. and *Mycoplasma* spp.) may also participate.

In young weaned pigs, *H. parasuis* also causes Glässer's disease (polyserositis), an acute inflammation affecting pleura, peritoneum, mediastinum, pericardium, joints,

FIGURE 26.2. *Determination of cofactor needs with (left to right) XV, V, and X factor-impregnated filter paper discs. Growth has occurred around the XV and X discs (lower left and right), but not the V disc (top center). The organism accordingly was identified as* Haemophilus haemoglobinophilus, *which requires X but not V factor.*

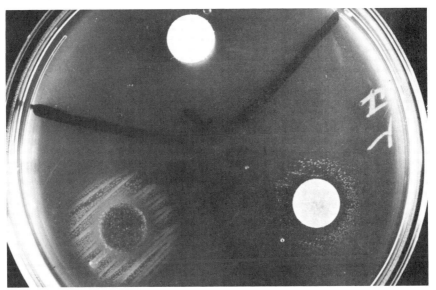

Table 26.1.   Pathogenic and Common *Haemophilus*-like Species

	X	V	Host	Clinical Significance
H. influenzae	+	+	Human	Meningitis, septicemia, otitis, epiglottitis, conjunctivitis, bronchopneumonia
H. suis	+	+	Swine	Doubtful
H. parasuis	−	+	Swine	Secondary pneumonia, Glässer's disease
H. gallinarum	+	+	Fowl	Original description of fowl coryza agent; may not exist
H. paragallinarum	−	+	Fowl	Infectious coryza of fowl
H. haemoglobinophilus	+	−	Dog	None (opportunistic)
H. somnus (*Histophilus ovis*, "*H. agni*")	−	−	Cattle* (sheep)	Septicemia, meningoencephalitis, pneumonia, abortion, epididymitis

* Require cyst(e)ine, are stimulated by thiamine pyrophosphate.

and meninges. Weaning, transport, and management stress are predisposing causes. The disease strikes sporadically within days of the stressing event. Morbidity and mortality are often low because of widespread acquired resistance but may be high in previously unexposed herds (e.g., specific pathogen-free herds). Disease manifestations include fever and general malaise, respiratory and abdominal distress, lameness, and paralytic or convulsive signs. Recovery begins in 1 to 2 weeks. Similar syndromes are due to *Mycoplasma hyorhinis*.

In chickens, infectious coryza (caused by *H. paragallinarum*) is an acute contagious upper-respiratory infection. It affects chickens of practically all ages. The signs include nasal discharge, swelling of sinuses, facial edema, and conjunctivitis. With air sac and lung involvement, rales may be detected. In the uncomplicated infection, mortality is low. Loss of productivity is the most damaging aspect. Superimposed infections with mycoplasmas and helminth parasites exacerbate and prolong outbreaks.

Of other species, only Japanese quail are highly susceptible.

In cattle, "*H. somnus*" causes a septicemia leading to thrombotic meningoencephalitis ("infectious thromboembolic meningoencephalitis," TEME) and infarcts in brain and cerebellum. The preencephalitic stage is marked by high fever.

With central nervous system (CNS) involvement, motor and behavioral abnormalities develop.

"*Haemophilus somnus*" occurs in pneumonic processes, usually with other agents, for example, *Pasteurella* spp. Isolations have been made from normal and inflamed female genitalia and from aborted fetuses. It is common in the genital tract of bulls.

In sheep, *Haemophilus*-like organisms ("*H. somnus*," "*Histophilus ovis*", "*H. agni*") cause respiratory and mammary infections, epididymitis of immature rams, and occasionally septicemias.

In dogs, *H. haemoglobinophilus*, a commensal of the canine lower genital tract, sometimes causes cystitis and neonatal infections. Its role in balanoposthitis and vaginitis, where it is frequently found, is uncertain.

In cats, a V factor-requiring *Haemophilus* sp. is associated with conjunctivitis (following *Chlamydia psittaci* and *Mycoplasma* spp. in prevalence).

Epidemiology

All the agents named, except for *H. paragallinarum*, inhabit normal mucous membranes of the respiratory or genital tract. Sources of infection are therefore often endogenous to herds or individuals. Colonization of pigs with *H. parasuis* probably occurs while animals are shielded by maternal immunity. Glässer's disease in pigs of all ages occurs in previously *H. parasuis*-free, stressed populations.

Respiratory and septicemic "*H. somnus*" infections are similarly related to stress factors, as their predilection for feed lots and the fall and winter months suggests.

Haemophilus spp. are generally host-specific.

IMMUNOLOGIC ASPECTS

Circulating antibody develops in infected individuals and has a protective function, at least in mammals. Presence of serum antibody correlates well with resistance to "*H. somnus*" infection. The role of cell-mediated immunity is unknown.

Immunity develops after infection. Following infectious coryza, it extends to heterologous serotypes.

Immunoprophylaxis is used to control infectious coryza, polyserositis, and TEME. Bacterins prevent serious disease but not infection owing to homologous serotypes.

LABORATORY DIAGNOSIS

Recovery of the organism from infected tissues or fluids is usually required to establish a diagnosis. Observation of gram-negative rods in these specimens prior to culture may suggest *Haemophilus* infection. Isolation of such an organism is followed by demonstration of a growth factor requirement.

Organisms requiring X factor cannot convert delta-aminolevulinic acid to urobilinogen and porphyrin. The porphyrin test determines this ability and X factor requirement most reliably. Definitive assignment to a species usually requires additional tests.

Fowl coryza can be diagnosed by agglutination, agar gel immunodiffusion, and hemagglutination-inhibition tests.

TREATMENT AND CONTROL

Most animal hemophili are susceptible to penicillin G, ceftiofur, and tetracyclines. Calves with shipping fever in which "*H. somnus*" was involved responded to tilmicosin.

For fowl coryza therapy, erythromycin or sulfonamides can be administered in feed or water.

"*Haemophilus somnus*" is susceptible to penicillin G and tetracycline. For the septicemic-meningoencephalitic form, timeliness and maintenance of treatment are critical.

Infectious coryza of fowl is controlled by elimination of carriers and immunization of individuals at risk. Bacterins are of value in prevention of TEME but are less effective in other "*H. somnus*" infections.

Poultry producers may depopulate infected flocks. When breeding stock must be preserved, flock additions are vaccinated at 16 weeks, four weeks before joining the infected flock.

SELECTED REFERENCES

Blackall PJ. The avian haemophili. Clin Microbiol Rev 1989; 2:270.

Corbeil LB, Bastida-Corcuera FD, Beveridge TJ. *Haemophilus somnus* immunoglobulin binding proteins and surface fibrils. Infect Immun 1997;65:4250.

Groom SC, Little RB. Effects of vaccination of calves against induced *Haemophilus somnus* pneumonia. Am J Vet Res 1988; 49:793.

Humphrey JD, Stephens LR. "*Haemophilus somnus*." A review. Vet Bull 1983;53:987.

Jamaluddin AA, Case JT, Hird DW, et al. Dairy cattle abortion in California: evaluation of diagnostic laboratory data. J Vet Diagn Infest 1996;8:210.

Kilian M. A rapid method for the differentiation of *Haemophilus* strains. The porphyrin test. Acta Path Microbiol Scand B 1974; 82:835.

Kilian M. A taxonomic study of the genus *Haemophilus*. J Gen Microbiol 1976;93:9.

King SJ. Porcine polyserositis and arthritis with particular references to mycoplasmosis and Glässer's disease. Aust Vet J 1968; 44:227.

Kirkham C, Biberstein EL, LeFebvre RB. Evidence of host specific subgroups among "*Histophilus ovis*" isolates. Int J Syst Bacteriol 1989;39:236.

Lederer JA, Brown JE, Czuprynski CJ. "*Haemophilus somnus*," a facultative intracellular pathogen of bovine mononuclear phagocytes. Infect Immun 1987;55:381.

Miller RB, Lein DH, McEntee KE, et al. *Haemophilus somnus* infection of the reproductive tract of cattle. A review. J Am Vet Med Assoc 1983;182:1390.

Moller K, Kilian M. V factor dependent members of the family Pasteurellaceae in the porcine upper respiratory tract. J Clin Microbiol 1990;28:2711.

Morozumi T, Nicolet J. Some antigenic properties of *Haemophilus parasuis* and a proposal for serological classification. J Clin Microbiol 1986;23:1022.

Musser J, Mechor GD, Grohn YT, et al. Comparison of tilmicosin with long-acting oxytetracycline for treatment of respiratory tract disease in calves. J Am Vet Med Assoc 1996;208: 102.

Riising HJ. Prevention of Glässer's disease (porcine polyserositis) through immunity to *Haemophilus parasuis*. Zbl Vet Med B 1981;28:630.

Rimler RB. Studies on the pathogenic avian haemophili. Avian Dis 1979;23:1006.

Sawata A, Kume K, Nukai T. Relationship between anticapsular antibody and protective activity of capsular antigen of *Haemophilus paragallinarum*. Jpn J Vet Sci 1984;46:475.

Vahle JL, Haynes JS, Andrews JJ. Experimental reproduction of *Haemophilus parasuis* infection in swine: clinical, bacteriologic, and morphologic findings. J Vet Diagn Invest 1995;7: 476.

Williams P, Griffiths E. Bacterial transferrin receptors-structure, function and contribution to virulence. Med Microbiol Immunol 1992;181:301.

27 Bordetella

Ernst L. Biberstein   Dwight C. Hirsh

The genus *Bordetella*, gram-negative coccobacilli belonging to the family *Alcaligenaceae*, contains several species, some of which are important pathogens of humans and other animals. Members of the genus *Bordetella* are aerobic gram-negative bacteria and are parasites of ciliated respiratory epithelium. *Bordetella pertussis* (and, rarely, *B. parapertussis*) causes whooping cough in humans. Of veterinary importance are *B. bronchiseptica*, which has been implicated in porcine atrophic rhinitis, canine kennel cough, and bronchopneumonia in many species; *B. avium*, which causes rhinotracheitis of turkeys; and rarely *B. parapertussis*, as a cause of pneumonia in sheep.

Descriptive Features

Morphology and Staining

Bordetellae are pleomorphic gram-negative coccobacilli, about 0.5 μm × up to 2 μm in size. *Bordetella bronchiseptica* has a capsule-like envelope and pili; *B. bronchiseptica* and *B. avium* are motile by peritrichous flagella.

Structure and Composition

Some colonial forms have a surface covering of fibrils. Otherwise, the cell structure is that of other gram-negative bacteria.

Some 20 heat-labile (K) and heat-stable (O; 120°C/60 min) antigens exist. Many are common to several species. Others are species- and type-specific.

Cellular Products of Medical Interest

A dermonecrotic toxin (sharing homology with CNF1 of *Escherichia coli* but different from the dermonecrotic toxin of *Pasteurella*), adenylate cyclase, proteases, hemolysin, hemagglutinins, and a tracheal cytotoxin (a muramyl peptide toxic to ciliated epithelium) are present in *B. bronchiseptica*. That agent also produces an adhesin that binds to sialic acid residues on ciliated epithelia. *Bordetella avium* produces a histamine-sensitizing factor resembling *B. pertussis* toxin, a cytotoxin, adhesin, and a dermonecrotic toxin. All members of the genus except *B. avium* contain the gene for pertussis toxin, but only *B. pertussis* possesses a functional promotor.

Bordetella bronchiseptica produces a hydroxymatic siderophore by which it acquires iron from iron-binding proteins of the host, even though it also produces a receptor for iron-transferrin complexes.

Growth Characteristics

Bordetella species are strict aerobes deriving energy from oxidation of amino acids. *Bordetella bronchiseptica* and *B. avium* grow on ordinary laboratory media, including MacConkey agar, under atmospheric conditions; the former is inconsistently hemolytic on blood agar.

Bordetella bronchiseptica is a facultative intracellular parasite able to exist within phagolysosomes of phagocytic cells.

Biochemical Activities

Bordetella avium and *B. bronchiseptica* are catalase and oxidase positive, ferment no carbohydrates, and utilize citrate as an organic carbon source, but only *B. bronchiseptica* reduces nitrate and splits urea.

Resistance

Bordetella spp. are killed by heat or disinfectants. They are susceptible to broad-spectrum antibiotics and polymyxin, but not to penicillin. Their environmental survival is epidemiologically significant.

Variability

Bordetella bronchiseptica dissociates into four phases varying in colonial characteristics, hemolytic activity, suspension stability in saline, ease of colonization, and toxicity. Some strains appear to be host-specific.

Three serotypes, based on surface agglutinogens, are recognized in *B. avium*.

Ecology

Reservoir

Bordetella spp. are parasites primarily of the ciliated respiratory tract tissue. *Bordetella bronchiseptica* occurs in wild and domestic carnivores, wild and laboratory rodents, swine, rabbits, and occasionally horses, other herbivores, primates, and turkeys. Although probably not part of the resident flora, it is found in the nasopharynx of healthy animals.

Bordetella avium inhabits the respiratory tract of infected fowl, principally turkeys.

Transmission

Mammalian infections are primarily airborne, while in turkeys indirect spread via water and litter is common.

Pathogenesis

Mechanisms.   Attachment of *B. bronchiseptica* to ciliated respiratory epithelium, preventable by neuraminidase treatment of host cells, is followed by bacterial proliferation, cilial paralysis, and inflammation. Adenylate cyclase may interfere with phagocytosis and intracellular killing. If phagocytosis occurs, *B. bronchiseptica* can survive within the phagolysosomes; it also has the ability to escape into an endocytic compartment that does not lead to fusion with lysosomes. In pigs, *B. bronchiseptica* provides nasal irritation, rendering the turbinates susceptible to the action of the dermonecrotic toxin (Pmt) of *Pasteurella multocida*, which has emerged as the primary agent of atrophic rhinitis (see Chapter 24).

Bordetella bronchiseptica from pigs appear different from the strains from dogs and horses (which are also different from each other).

Infectivity of *B. avium* is related to a plasmid. The agent depresses some cell-mediated immune reactions.

Bordetella infections depress respiratory clearance mechanisms, facilitating secondary complications.

Pathology.   The lesions of atrophic rhinitis have been described (Chapter 24). *Bordetella bronchiseptica* alone causes temporary turbinate atrophy by disturbing osteoblast physiology.

Canine infectious tracheobronchitis ("kennel cough") results in production of a tenacious mucoid to mucopurulent exudate and variable involvement of lungs and adjacent lymph structures. The exudate is predominately neutrophilic.

The organism produces a mild upper respiratory tract infection in cats, mainly those housed in colonies. Cats, like dogs, carry the organism asymptomatically (up to 19 weeks) following recovery.

Acute coryza of turkeys is characterized by catarrh of suppurative rhinitis, sinusitis, tracheitis, bronchopneumonia, and airsacculitis. Chronic lesions include tracheobronchitis, peribronchitis, and interstitial granulomatous.

Destruction of ciliated respiratory epithelium is common to *Bordetella* infections.

Disease Patterns.   Atrophic rhinitis of swine, due to combined infection with *P. multocida* and *B. bronchiseptica*, was considered under pasteurelloses (Chapter 24). Infection with *B. bronchiseptica* alone is transient and self-limiting but is believed to prepare the ground for establishment and activities of toxigenic *P. multocida*.

Canine infectious tracheobronchitis (kennel cough) is marked by hacking cough, high morbidity, and low mortality. Pneumonia is rare. The natural disease is often accompanied by mycoplasma and virus infections (canine parainfluenza virus, canine adenoviruses 1 and 2, and canine herpesvirus). While most dogs recover within a few weeks, the bacterium can persist for months.

Bordetella bronchiseptica causes respiratory tract infections in diverse domestic, wild, and laboratory mammals. It also causes rare human infections, which sometimes resemble whooping cough.

Turkey poults infected with *B. avium* develop tracheobronchitis, sinusitis, and airsacculitis. Signs include nasal exudate, conjunctivitis, tracheal rales, and dyspnea. Morbidity is high, but mortality, except by secondary infection, is generally low (<5%). Recovery may begin after 2 weeks, although some illnesses may last 6 weeks.

Epidemiology

Atrophic rhinitis affects pigs under 6 weeks old, when osteogenesis and bone remodeling are most active. *Bordetella bronchiseptica* is spread by affected pigs. The ultimate sources are carrier sows, in which carrier rates decline with age. Canine kennel cough usually affects young, nonimmune dogs.

Bordetella avium causes disease mainly in young poults. The contaminated environment is important in perpetuating the infection.

IMMUNOLOGIC ASPECTS

Pathogenic Factors

Depressed cell-mediated responses have been observed in experimental *B. avium* infections. Their relation to natural disease is undetermined. *Bordetella bronchiseptica* can parasitize dendritic cells, which results in a decrease in immune responses due to inefficient antigen processing.

Protective Role

Local antibody is believed to prevent *B. bronchiseptica* colonization in dogs. No other immune responses have been shown to be protective.

Bordetella avium antiserum was ineffective in protecting turkeys, but maternal immunization reduced losses in challenged progeny. Antibody to adhesin prevents adherence to tracheal epithelia.

Immunization Procedures

Bacterins used on pregnant sows provide some colostral immunity to piglets, especially when including toxigenic *P. multocida* strains. Bacterin-toxoid preparations protect piglets.

Intratracheal administered live attenuated vaccine has been beneficial in kennel cough control.

Of *B. avium* vaccines, those using attenuated live organisms intratracheally have been most effective.

LABORATORY DIAGNOSIS

Nasal swabs (atrophic rhinitis), sediment of transtracheal washes (canine tracheobronchitis), and tracheal swabs (coryza of turkeys) are cultured on blood and MacConkey agar.

Bordetella avium reacts like *Alcaligenes faecalis* in routine laboratory tests. Cellular fatty acid analysis differentiates the two. A microagglutination test is used for serodiagnosis.

TREATMENT AND CONTROL

Atrophic rhinitis is not treatable. Preventive measures include maintenance of an aged sow herd with a low carrier rate; thorough disinfection and cleanup of farrowing houses and nurseries after each use; vaccination (see p. 149); prophylactic use of sulfonamides in feed or water; and elimination of carrier sows based on nasal swab culture.

Canine tracheobronchitis responds poorly to injected antibiotics. Vaccination (see p. 149), fumigation of kennels, adequate ventilation, and isolation of affected dogs are useful preventive practices. Tetracycline remains the drug of choice.

Bordetella avium is susceptible to tetracycline, erythromycin, and nitrofurantoin, but resistant to penicillin, streptomycin, and sulfonamides. Mass medication and vaccination may prevent outbreaks without eliminating the infection.

SELECTED REFERENCES

Bemis DA, Wilson SA. Influence of potential virulence determinants on *Bordetella bronchiseptica*-induced ciliostasis. Infect Immun 1985;50:35.

Blackall PJ, Doheney CM. Isolation and characterization of *Bordetella avium* and an evaluation of their role in respiratory disease in poultry. Aust Vet J 1987;64:235.

Cimiotti W, Glunder G, Hinz KH. Survival of the bacterial turkey coryza agent. Vet Rec 1982;110:304.

Confer DL, Eaton JW. Phagocyte impotence caused by invasive bacterial adenylate cyclase. Science 1982;217:948.

Coutts AJ, Dawson S, Binns S, et al. Studies on natural transmission of *Bordetella brochiseptica* in cats. Vet Microbiol 1996; 48:19.

Giles CJ, Smith IM. Vaccination of pigs with *Bordetella bronchiseptica*. Vet Bull 1983;53:327.

Goodnow RA. Biology of *Bordetella bronchiseptica*. Microbiol Rev 1980;44:722.

Guzman CA, Rohde M, Bock M, Timmis KN. Invasion and intracellular survival of *Bordetella bronchiseptica* in mouse dendritic cells. Infect Immun 1994;62:5528.

Guzman CA, Rohde M, Timmis KN. Mechanisms involved in uptake of *Bordetella bronchiseptica* by mouse dendritic cells. Infect Immun 1994;62:5538.

Hausman SZ, Cherry JD, Heininger U, et al. Analysis of proteins encoded by the *ptx* and *ptl* genes of *Bordetella bronchiseptica* and *Bordetella parapertussis*. Infect Immun 1996;64:4020.

Ishikawa H, Sato W. Role of *Bordetella bronchiseptica* sialic acid-binding hemagglutinin as a putative colonization factor. J Vet Med Sci 1997;59:43.

Marcon MJ. Clinical and laboratory diagnostic features of *Bordetella* spp. — pertussis and beyond. Clin Microbiol News 1997; 19:185.

Pullinger GD, Adams TE, Mullan PB, et al. Cloning, expression, and molecular characterisation of the dermonecrotic toxin gene of *Bordetella* spp. Infect Immun 1996;64:4163.

Sakano T, Okada M, Taneda A, et al. Effect of *Bordetella bronchiseptica* and serotype D *Pasteurella multocida* bacterin-toxoid on the occurrence of atrophic rhinitis after experimental infection with *B. bronchiseptica* and toxigenic type A *P. multocida*. J Vet Med Sci 1997;59:55.

Speakman AJ, Binns SH, Dawson S, et al. Antimicrobial susceptibility of *Bordetella bronchiseptica* isolates from cats and a comparison of the agar dilution and E-test methods. Vet Microbiol 1997;54:63.

van der Zee A, Groenedijk H, Peeters M, Mooi FR. The differentiation of *Bordetella parapertussis* and *Bordetella bronchiseptica* from humans and animals as determined by DNA polymorphism mediated by two different insertion sequence elements suggests their phylogenetic relationship. Int J Syst Bacteriol 1996;46:640.

Walker KE, Weiss AA. Characterization of the dermonecrotic toxin in members of the genus *Bordetella*. Infect Immun 1994; 62:3817.

28 Moraxella

Ernst L. Biberstein   Dwight C. Hirsh

MORAXELLA

Moraxella spp. are aerobic, gram-negative, nonfermenting, nonflagellated coccobacilli. *M. bovis* causes infectious bovine keratoconjunctivitis (IBK), one of the most troubling diseases in beef herds.

DESCRIPTIVE FEATURES

Morphology and Staining

Moraxellae are short, plump gram-negative rods, 11.5 μm × 1.5 to 2.5 mm, and are often arranged in pairs ("diplobacilli") or short chains (Fig 28.1).

Structure and Composition

Pili (fimbriae) of *M. bovis* are virulence determinants and can be lost on subculture (see under *Variability* below). Capsules may be present in fresh isolates.

Cellular Products of Medical Interest

A soluble hemolysin (probably an RTX-like pore-forming toxin (see *Escherischia coli* haemolysin, Chapter 9) is correlated with virulence independently of pili. Enzymes active on lipids, peptides, and carbohydrates are produced. The pili are type 4 and similar to those of *Pseudomonas aeruginosa, Neisseria gonorrhoeae, Dicholobacter nodosus, Pasteurella multocida* and *Vibrio cholerae*. Pili appear responsible for adherence to corneal epithelial cells.

Growth Characteristics

Siderophores have not been demonstrated. Proteins that bind lactoferrin and transferrin have been found, however, and are probably involved with iron acquisition.

Moraxella bovis grows best at 35°C in the presence of serum and blood. No growth occurs on MacConkey agar or anaerobically. In 48 hours, fresh isolates produce flat, hemolytic, friable colonies, about 1 mm in size, that corrode the agar and autoagglutinate when suspended in saline. *Moraxella bovis* is oxidase positive, nonfermenting,

and catalase variable. Nitrates and urea are not attacked, but proteins are digested. Resistance to physical and chemical agents is not remarkable. It is susceptible to commonly used antibiotics.

Variability

In culture, *M. bovis* undergoes colonial dissociation producing smooth butyrous colonies, the cells of which lack pili (phase variation occurs due to inversion of the pilin-encoding gene) and infectivity and are less autoagglutinable. Nonhemolytic variants are nonpathogenic. Pili are immunogenically diverse and this trait is responsible for a classification scheme based on serological similarities.

ECOLOGY

Reservoir

Moraxella bovis occurs worldwide on the bovine conjunctiva and upper respiratory mucosa, often without clinical manifestations.

Transmission

Dissemination is by direct and indirect contact, including flying insects and possibly other airborne transmission.

Pathogenesis

Mechanisms. Pathogenicity is closely linked to hemolysin and pili, which mediate attachment to conjunctival epithelium. Leukotoxicity for macrophages has been described. Pathogenic contributions by lipopolysaccharides, collagenase, and hyaluronidase are likely.

Environmental factors implicated include ultraviolet irradiation, flies, dust, and woody pasture plants, all of which contribute to irritation of the target tissues. Concurrent infections with viruses, such as bovine herpesvirus I (IBR) and adenovirus, mycoplasma (*Mycoplasma bovoculi*), bacteria (*Listeria monocytogenes*), and nematodes (*Thelasia*), may complicate the disease.

Disease Pattern and Pathology. The disease begins with invasion of conjunctiva and cornea, producing edema and a

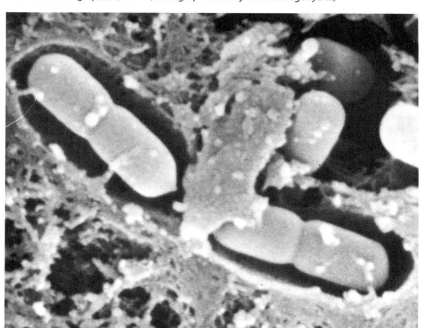

FIGURE 28.1. Moraxella bovis *in the cornea of an experimentally infected calf. There is evidence of digestion of corneal substance around the bacterial cells. Scanning electron micrograph, 22,000×. (Photograph courtesy of Dr. G. Kagonyera.)*

predominantly neutrophilic inflammatory response. It may progress from mild epiphora and corneal clouding to production of severe edema, corneal opacities, vascularization, ulceration, and rupture leading to uveal prolapse and panophthalmitis. Healing of the ulcers proceeds from the periphery and requires several weeks. Central scarring may persist for months. Though a self-limiting disease, losses occur because vision-impaired animals do not forage and loose condition. Deaths, which are due to ascending infection via the eye, are exceptional.

Epidemiology

Infectious bovine keratoconjunctivitis is a highly infectious disease, mostly of beef cattle. Young animals are preferentially affected, probably due to lack of acquired immunity. Lack of eyelid pigmentation and prominent placement of eyes are apparent predisposing factors, as is vitamin A deficiency.

Prevalence is greatest during summer and early fall, when environmental stresses are maximal.

IMMUNOLOGIC ASPECTS

Antibody of all isotypes is produced during infection, with secretory IgA predominating locally. Temporary resistance to reinfection follows recovery. The relative roles in immunity and recovery of general vs. local responses and humoral vs. cell-mediated responses are unsettled.

Experimental bacterins and fimbrial antigens stimulate resistance, optimally to homologous challenge. Apparently, fimbrial proteins, hemolysin, and proteolytic enzymes have protection-inducing activity. Fimbrial vaccines are commercially available.

LABORATORY DIAGNOSIS

The agent may be demonstrated in smears of exudate, most convincingly by immunofluorescence. Exudate is cultured on blood agar and *Moraxella* are identified by colonial characteristics, oxidase activity, hemolysis, proteolysis, and failure to ferment carbohydrates. Specific fluorescent antibody conjugates can be applied directly to suspect colonies on plates for identification even of dissociant colonies (epifluorescence).

TREATMENT AND CONTROL

Affected animals should be placed in a dark stall, free from dust and flies. Topical corticosteroids may relieve the inflammation, while antimicrobial drugs, given topically or systemically, may be beneficial. Long-acting tetracycline is considered the drug of choice.

Fimbrial vaccines are the most promising specific prophylactics.

RIEMERELLA (MORAXELLA) ANATIPESTIFER

The agent of "new duck disease," a severe polyserositic disease especially of ducklings (duck septicemia, infectious serositis of ducks), is unrelated to the genus *Moraxella* and has also been called *Pasteurella* and *Pfeifferella*.

DESCRIPTIVE FEATURES

Riemerella anatipestifer is a gram-negative, nonmotile, encapsulated, occasionally bipolar coccobacillus. It grows best under increased carbon dioxide tension on blood or chocolate agar. Colonies are nonhemolytic, transparent, and may exceed 1 mm in diameter after 24 hours of incubation. The organism is oxidase and catalase positive, proteolytic, ferments no carbohydrates, and survives for weeks in litter. Many serotypes exist.

ECOLOGY

Reservoir

The agent occurs in ducks and other fowl. Carrier birds constitute the reservoir.

Transmission

Infection occurs via respiratory, percutaneous, and possibly other routes.

Pathogenesis

Riemerella anatipestifer septicemia causes sudden mortality, or, less acutely, respiratory signs with sneezing, coughing, and discharges from nose and eyes. Central nervous involvement produces head tremors, torticollis, and ataxia. Diarrhea is also seen.

Fibrinous polyserositis is seen in the acute disease. The exudate is mostly mononuclear. In protracted cases, fibroblasts and giant cells are observed.

Mortality rates vary from 5% to 75%; duration is from one day to several weeks.

Epidemiology

Only ducks are consistently at risk. Stress factors play a significant predisposing role. Young birds are most susceptible.

IMMUNOLOGIC ASPECTS

Recovered birds are resistant to reexposure. Immunity is serotype-specific and may be induced by bacterins.

LABORATORY DIAGNOSIS

Isolation and identification of the agent are mandatory for diagnosis. Organisms may be demonstrated in organs and fluids by Gram stain or immunofluorescence.

Culture plates are incubated under increased carbon dioxide tension.

TREATMENT AND CONTROL

Sulfonamides (sulfamethazine, sulfadimethoxine, sulfaquinoxaline) may be given prophylactically in feed or water. Penicillin G, tetracycline, erythromycin, and novobiocin are used therapeutically. Corticosteroids administered along with antibiotics (penicillin G) do not influence resolution of lesions.

Vaccination with killed or live avirulent bacteria of appropriate serotypes is beneficial.

SELECTED REFERENCES

Allen LJ, George LW, Willits NH. Effect of penicillin or penicillin and dexamethasone in cattle with infectious bovine keratoconjunctivitis. J Am Vet Med Assoc 1995;206:1200.

Atwell JL, Tennent JM, Lepper AW, Elleman TC. Characterization of pilin genes from seven serologically defined prototype strains of *Moraxella bovis*. J Bacteriol 1994;76:4875.

Beard MK, Moore LJ. Reproduction of bovine keratoconjunctivitis with a purified hemolytic and cytotoxic fraction of *Moraxella bovis*. Vet Microbiol 1994;42:15.

Billson FM, Hodgson JL, Egerton JR, et al. A hemolytic cell-free preparation of *Moraxella bovis* confers protection against infectious bovine keratoconjunctivitis. FEMS Microbiol Lett 1994;124:69.

George LW. Antibiotic treatment of infectious bovine keratoconjunctivitis. Cornell Vet 1990;80:229.

Gerhardt RR, Allen JW, Greene WH, Smith RC. The role of face flies in an episode of infectious bovine keratoconjunctivitis. J Am Vet Med Assoc 1982;180:156.

Gray JT, Fedorka-Cray PJ, Rogers DG. Partial characterization of a *Moraxella bovis* cytolysin. Vet Microbiol 1995;43:183.

Lepper AW, Atwell JL, Lehrbach PR, et al. The protective efficacy of cloned *Moraxella bovis* pili in monovalent and multivalent vaccine formulations against experimentally induced infectious bovine keratoconjunctivitis (IBK). Vet Microbiol 1995; 45:129.

Marrs CF, Ruehl WW, Schoolnick G, Falkow S. Pilin-gene phase variation of *Moraxella bovis* is caused by an inversion of the pilin genes. J Bacteriol 1988;170:3032.

Moore LJ, Rutter MJ. Antigenic analysis of fimbrial proteins from *Moraxella bovis*. J Clin Microbiol 1987;25:2063.

Punch RI, Slatter DH. A review of infectious bovine keratoconjunctivitis. Vet Bull 1984;54:193.

Rosenbusch RE, Ostle AG. *Mycoplasma bovoculi* increases ocular colonization by *Moraxella bovis* in calves. Am J Vet Res 1986; 47:1214.

Ruehl WW, Marrs C, Beard MK, et al. Q pili enhance the attachment of *Moraxella bovis* to bovine corneas in vitro. Molec Microbiol 1993;7:285.

Ruehl WW, Marrs CF, George L, et al. Infection rates, disease frequency, pilin gene rearrangement, and pilin expression in calves inoculated with *Moraxella bovis* pilin-specific isogenic variants. Am J Vet Res 1993;54:248.

Sandhu TS, Rhoades KR, Rimler RB. *Pasteurella anatipestifer* infection. In: Calnek BW, ed. Diseases of poultry. 9th ed. Ames, IA: Iowa State University, 1991:66.

Segers P, Mannheim W, Vancanneyt M, et al. *Riemerella antipes-* *tifer* gen. nov., comb. nov., the causative agent of septicemia anserum exsudativa, and its phylogenetic affiliation within the *Flavobacterium-Cytophaga* rRNA homology group. Int J Syst Bacteriol 1993;43:768.

Yu R, Schryvers AB. Transferrin receptors on ruminant pathogens vary in their interaction with the C-lobe and N-lobe of ruminant transferrins. Can J Microbiol 1994;40: 532.

29

Burkholderia mallei *and* Burkholderia pseudomallei

Ernst L. Biberstein   Dwight C. Hirsh

Burkholderia mallei

Glanders, once a widespread infection of *Equidae*, remains important only in Asia (Mongolia and China) with pockets of activity in India, Iraq, Turkey, and the Philippines. It is a systemic pyogranulomatous infection varying in acuteness and severity. It also affects members of the cat family and occasionally dogs, goats, camels, sheep, and humans.

Descriptive Features

Burkholderia mallei (syn. *Pseudomonas, Malleomyces, Pfeifferella, Loefferella,* and *Actinobacillus*) is a gram-negative, acapsular, nonmotile rod 0.5 μm thick. It varies in length and morphology depending on conditions of growth. Endotoxins and exotoxins are reported but have not been characterized.

The organism grows best on media containing glycerol or blood. Nonhemolytic colonies develop in 48 hours or more at 20°C to 41°C. They range from mucoid to rough in five possible forms. Confluent growth is common.

The glanders bacillus is aerobic and oxidase and catalase positive; it reduces nitrates and hydrolyzes urea. Glucose is attacked oxidatively. Resistance is unremarkable, although in dark, damp, and cool environments the agent can survive for months. Sulfonamides, aminoglycosides, chloramphenicol, tetracyclines, and erythromycin inhibit *B. mallei*.

Of three serological types, one cross-reacts with *B. pseudomallei*.

Ecology

Reservoir

Infected *Equidae* are the reservoir.

Transmission

Exposure occurs via contaminated feed, water, and fomites, and sometimes through inhalation and wounds. Infectious material originates mostly in the respiratory tract or skin lesions.

Pathogenesis

Although toxins are suspected in pathogenesis, the mechanisms are uncertain. Primary lesions form at the point of entry — the pharynx, for example. Infection spreads along lymphatics, producing nodular lesions on the way to lymph nodes and the bloodstream, which disseminates the agent. Metastatic lesions form in the lungs or other organs, such as spleen, liver, and skin, producing cutaneous glanders ("farcy"). Frequent lesions in the nasal septum may be primary, hematogenous, or secondary to a pulmonary focus.

The basic nodular lesion is made up initially of neutrophils, fibrin, and red cells. The neutrophils degenerate and the central necrotic area becomes surrounded by epithelioid and giant cells and by lymphocytes embedded in granulation tissue. Near epithelial surfaces, ulceration is common. Strain variations determine the suppurative vs. granulomatous predominance in lesions.

Acute infections are characterized by fever, nasal discharge, and lymphadenitis of head and neck, with swelling along the upper respiratory tract. They tend to end fatally in about two weeks and predominate in donkeys and felids, less so in mules.

In horses, protracted chronic and subclinical infections are typical; signs, if present, include occasional fever, persistent respiratory problems, skin abscesses (farcy buds), and nodular induration of cranial lymph nodes.

Human exposures are traced to acutely ill horses and may lead to acute or chronic infections. All acute infections and 50% of chronic ones were fatal prior to the advent of effective antimicrobials.

Epidemiology

The persistence of glanders depends on an infected horse population. Susceptible nonequids acquire glanders from infected horses or horse meat, and appear to be dead-end hosts.

Immunologic Aspects

Humoral and cell-mediated responses occur.

Apparent recovery from glanders, including loss of dermal hypersensitivity, has been observed under natural conditions, but without increased resistance to reinfection.

No method of immunization is known.

LABORATORY DIAGNOSIS

Nodular contents are cultured on blood or glycerol agar. They may be examined for gram-negative rods and by immunofluorescence.

Guinea pigs and hamsters are highly susceptible to fatal infection with virulent strains.

Any suspect isolates should be submitted to a qualified reference laboratory. Differentiation from *B. pseudomallei* is important.

Serologically, glanders is diagnosed by complement fixation tests employing aqueous bacterial extracts as antigen. The intradermo-palpebral mallein test detects cell-mediated hypersensitivity, which indicates infection and has served as a basis for glanders eradication. Mallein is a heat extract of old *B. mallei* broth cultures.

TREATMENT AND CONTROL

Although glanders is treatable by many antimicrobics (see above), treatment is inappropriate in countries committed to glanders eradication. Equine imports from endemic areas are mallein-tested, and reactors are destroyed.

BURKHOLDERIA PSEUDOMALLEI

Burkholderia pseudomallei causes melioidosis, a disease superficially resembling glanders. Important distinctions are that 1) melioidosis affects a wide host range and 2) the agent is a saprophyte, whose prevalence is unaffected by elimination of infected animals.

DESCRIPTIVE FEATURES

Burkholderia pseudomallei is related to *B. mallei* but differs in being motile by means of polar flagella.

Unlike *B. mallei*, *B. pseudomallei* grows on MacConkey agar, in the presence of 2% sodium chloride, and at 42°C. The agents also differ in the utilization of carbon sources.

The relation of exotoxin-like substances (lethal, necrotizing) to virulence is uncertain.

Burkholderia pseudomallei appears to be a facultative intracellular pathogen. Within phagocytic cells it survives within phagolysosomes and is resistant to various defensins in vitro.

Burkholderia pseudomallei is killed by disinfectants and does not survive chilling and freezing in biologic specimens. It is generally susceptible to tetracyclines, chloramphenicol, trimethoprim-sulfamethoxazole, and novobiocin.

ECOLOGY

Reservoir

Burkholderia pseudomallei is considered a soil and water dweller. Although most prevalent between 20° northern and southern latitude, extratropical foci do exist, for example, in France, Iran, China, and the United States.

Transmission

Ingestion, wound infection, and possibly arthropod bites introduce infection. In humans, consumption of infected animal products and airborne infection may be significant.

Pathogenesis

Infections are typically systemic. Manifestations depend on the extent and distribution of lesions. Small abscesses may coalesce, developing into larger suppurative foci or granulomas. The equine disease may mimic glanders. In cattle, acute and chronic infections can localize in lung, joints, and uterus. Arthritis and lymphadenitis occur in sheep. Goats suffer loss of condition, respiratory and central nervous system disturbances, arthritis, and mastitis. Similar signs are seen in swine, along with abortions and diarrhea. Dogs develop a febrile disease with localizing suppurative foci.

Epidemiology

Clinical disease is usually sporadic. The host range in mammals is virtually unlimited, and avian cases are reported. Human infections range from the rapidly fatal to the subclinical. A wet environment, such as a swampy terrain or rice paddies, is related to exposure.

IMMUNOLOGIC ASPECTS

Complement-fixing and indirect hemagglutinating antibodies are produced during infections. Cell-mediated hypersensitivity has been demonstrated in infected goats. Successful vaccination of horses and zoo animals is reported.

LABORATORY DIAGNOSIS

The methods for isolating and identifying *B. mallei* apply to *B. pseudomallei*. Chilling and freezing of specimens should be avoided. Motility, growth on citrate, growth at 42°C, and reduction of nitrates to gaseous nitrogen distinguish *B. pseudomallei* from *B. mallei*.

Treatment and Control

Antimicrobial susceptibilities should be verified by laboratory tests. Vaccines are not commercially available.

Selected References

Farkas-Himsley H. Selection and rapid identification of *Pseudomonas pseudomallei* from other gram-negative bacteria. Am J Clin Pathol 1968;49:850.

Jones AL, Beveridge TJ, Woods DE. Intracellular survival of *Burkholderia pseudomallei*. Infect Immun 1996;64:782.

Ketterer RJ, Donald B, Rogers RJ. Bovine melioidosis in Southeastern Queensland. Aust Vet J 1975;51:395.

Laws L, Hall WTK. Melioidosis in animals in North Queensland. IV. Epidemiology. Aust Vet J 1964;40:309.

Minnett EC. Glanders (and melioidosis). In: Stableforth AW, Galloway LA, eds. Infectious diseases of animals. New York: Academic, 1959:296–318.

Redfearn MS, Palleroni NJ, Stanier RY. A comparative study of *Pseudomonas pseudomallei* and *Bacillus mallei*. J Gen Microbiol 1966;43:293.

Thomas AD. Prevalence of melioidosis in animals in Northern Queensland. Aust Vet J 1981;57:196.

Yabuuchi E. *Burkholderia pseudomallei* and melioidosis: be aware in temperate area. Microbiol Immunol 1993;37:823.

Yabuchi E, Kosako Y, Oyaizu H, et al. Proposal of *Burkholderia* gen. nov. and transfer of seven species of the genus *Pseudomonas* homology group II to the new genus, with the type species *Burkholderia cepacia* (Palleroni and Holmes 1981) comb. nov. Microbiol Immunol 1992;36:1251.

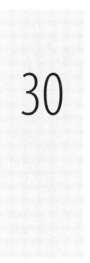

30 Mycobacterium *Species: The Agents of Animal Tuberculosis*

ERNST L. BIBERSTEIN   DWIGHT C. HIRSH

Tuberculosis is a chronic granulomatous disease caused by *Mycobacterium* spp. The tubercle bacilli are *M. tuberculosis*, the agent of the disease in primates, *M. bovis* in other mammals, and *M. avium* in birds. Host specificity is relative.

Of the 40-odd other *Mycobacterium* spp., some ("nontuberculous," "atypical," "anonymous," or saprophytic) cause tuberculosis-like infections. *Mycobacterium microti* causes tuberculosis of voles; *M. leprae* causes human leprosy; and *M. avium* ssp. *paratuberculosis* causes Johne's disease of ruminants (see Chapter 18). Other mycobacteria produce granulomatous skin diseases or bovine mastitis, while still others infect fish and other poikilotherms.

DESCRIPTIVE FEATURES

Morphology and Staining

Tubercle bacilli are predominantly rod-shaped, about 0.5 μm wide, and variable in length. Spores, flagella, and capsules are absent.

Mycobacteria, though cytochemically gram positive, often resist staining with Gram stain. Their most noted staining property is their acid fastness: once stained, they resist discoloration with 3% HCl in ethanol. Mycobacteria can be stained with fluorescent dyes (auramine-rhodamine).

Structure and Composition

Mycobacterial cells abound in lipids, especially in their walls. Lipids account for acid fastness and pathogenic and immunologic properties.

The surface mycosides (mostly glycolipids and peptidoglycolipids) determine colonial characteristics, serologic specificities, and bacteriophage susceptibilities. They are considered instrumental in ensuring bacterial survival within macrophages.

Subsurface layers of long-chain branched mycolic acids and their esters make up the bulk of cell wall lipids. Acid fastness somehow depends on these cell wall constituents. Mycolic acids are linked to the innermost peptidoglycan layer by way of arabinogalactans (see also Corynebacteria, Chapter 23; Nocardiae, Chapter 46).

"Wax D," an autolysate of *M. tuberculosis*, contains elements of all portions of the cell wall, has adjuvant activity, activates macrophages, stimulates particularly cell-mediated immune responses including delayed-type hypersensitivity, and induces granuloma formation. One of its constituents, cord factor (dimycolyl trehalose), among other effects, immobilizes neutrophils, acts as an adjuvant, evokes granulomatous responses, and causes mitochondrial disruption, which leads to disturbances in cellular respiration. Its relation to the "cord" pattern of mycobacterial growth is not proven.

Sulfolipids (or sulfatides) and a phospholipid, phosphatidyl inositol mannoside (PIM), may also aid in preventing the respiratory burst and phagolysosomal fusion, and may interfere with function of reactive oxygen intermediates following ingestion of tubercle bacilli by macrophages.

Mycobactins are cell wall amines involved in iron acquisition.

The presence of carotenoid pigments in some mycobacteria ("chromogens" vs. "nonchromogens") and their light dependence ("photochromogens" vs. "scotochromogens") is a basis for classifying nontuberculous mycobacteria.

Tuberculins are bacterial peptides liberated into culture media during growth. To some of them, or to their parent proteins, a delayed-type hypersensitivity develops during infection, making them useful diagnostic reagents (see *Immunologic Aspects* and *Laboratory Diagnosis*, p. 162).

No exotoxins are produced.

Growth Characteristics

Tubercle bacilli are strict aerobes that grow best on complex organic media such as Lowenstein-Jensen's, which contains, among other ingredients, whole eggs and potato flour. A dye, malachite green, inhibits contaminants. Oleic acid-albumin media, such as Middlebrook's 7H10 agar, are also used for isolation, often in combination with Lowenstein-Jensen's. Simple synthetic media containing ammonium salts, asparagine, citrate, glycerol, and minerals and vitamins are unsuitable for isolation but support growth from large inocula.

The presence of glycerol favors growth of *M. tuberculosis* (eugonic) and *M. avium*, but not *M. bovis* (dysgonic).

Nontuberculous mycobacteria often grow on routine laboratory media.

Generation times of tubercle bacilli range from 12 hours upward, and it may take weeks before colonies are visible. A wetting agent, tween 80, expedites growth in liquid media, and transparent oleic acid-albumin agar media permits early discernment of colonies. *Mycobacterium avium* grows more rapidly than mammalian types.

The mammalian species grow at 33°C to 39°C, while avian and related mycobacteria (see below) grow at 25°C to 45°C, with the optimum being near the top of that range.

Colonial growth of mammalian tubercle bacilli is dry and crumbly. Avian forms grow in dome-shaped colonies.

Resistance

Tubercle bacilli survive exposure to 1N NaOH or HCl for 15 to 30 minutes, a circumstance utilized in decontaminating diagnostic specimens. Mycobacteria are resistant to many antimicrobial drugs, bacteriostatic dyes, and disinfectants. Phenolic disinfectants are the most effective.

Tubercle bacilli resist drying and survive for long periods in soil. They are killed by sunlight, ultraviolet irradiation, and pasteurization.

Variability

Genetically, the mammalian tubercle bacilli are variants of one species, *M. tuberculosis*: human, bovine, and murine. The vaccine strain BCG (bacille de Calmette et Guérin) is a modified *M. bovis*.

The avian tubercle bacilli constitute one species within the *M. intracellulare* group of saprophytic mycobacteria. Of the approximately 20 numbered serotypes in the *M. avium-intracellulare* complex, 1 through 3 are avian tubercle bacilli.

ECOLOGY

Reservoir

The source of tubercle bacilli is tuberculous individuals. Humans perpetuate *M. tuberculosis*, cattle *M. bovis*, and chickens *M. avium*. The latter two can infect wild mammals and birds, respectively, which occasionally become sources of infection for domestic animals.

Most nontuberculous mycobacteria are saprophytes living in surface water and soil. Some are normal commensal bacteria of animals. Diseased individuals are not significant sources of infection.

Transmission

Tubercle bacilli are transmitted via the respiratory and alimentary routes through contaminated airborne droplet nuclei, feces, urine, genital discharges, milk from infected mammary glands, or contaminated feed and water. Percutaneous, transplacental, and transovarian (birds) infections are unusual. Intrauterine infection of calves occurred when bovine tuberculosis was common.

Pathogenesis

Mechanisms. The lipid components are implicated in pathogenesis. Mycosides and phospholipid and sulfolipid apparently protect tubercle bacilli against phagocytic killing. Other lipids can produce granulomas, and, with tuberculo-proteins, stimulate cell-mediated responses, a central feature of tuberculosis.

Pathology. Infection begins with deposition of tubercle bacilli in the lung or on pharyngeal or intestinal mucous membranes. In previously unexposed animals, local multiplication occurs as macrophages on the scene ingest the organisms. Resistance to phagocytic killing (cell wall chemistry and shunting to endosomal compartments rather than those that fuse with lysosomes) allows continued intracellular and extracellular multiplication. An inflammatory response (elicited by mycobacterial cell wall constituents) involving largely histiocytes and monocytes develops around the focus of proliferating organisms. Infected host cells and bacteria reach draining lymph nodes, where proliferation and inflammatory responses continue.

After the first week, cell-mediated immune reactions begin to modify the host response from essentially a foreign body reaction to a reaction characteristic of infectious granulomas. Infected macrophages secrete IL-12, a cytokine responsible for stimulating CD4$^+$ T$_{H1}$ lymphocytes to produce gamma interferon (INF), granulocyte monocyte colony stimulating factor (GM-CSF), and migration inhibition factor (MIF), which attract and activate macrophages. Activated macrophages acquire the capacity to kill mycobacteria. Their efficiency in doing so depends on the adequacy of the immune response and the virulence of bacteria. Stimulated CD4$^+$ T$_{H1}$ as well as gamma-delta T lymphocytes lyse mycobacteria-containing macrophages. Recognition of infected macrophages is probably due to increased expression of "stress" proteins by the infected macrophages.

Epithelioid cells appear among the macrophages. They have oblong vesicular nuclei and pale, poorly delineated cytoplasm; they often become the predominant cells. A third, rarer cell type is the Langhans giant cell, which is probably a cellular fusion product. It has a large amount of pale cytoplasm and, peripherally, many vesicular nuclei (Fig 30.1). Both cells are probably macrophage derivatives. They do not seem to be effective phagocytes. Their bacterial content presumably came from their macrophage precursors.

At the center of the lesion, caseation necrosis develops. A function of the allergic state, it may proceed to calcification or liquefaction.

At the periphery of the lesion are unaltered macrophages mixed with lymphocytes. Fibrocytes appear,

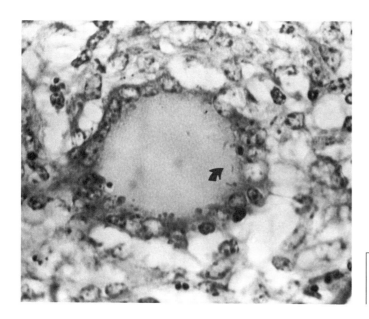

FIGURE 30.1. *Langhans giant cell with tubercle bacilli (arrow) among epithelioid cells in a bovine tuberculous lymph node. Ziehl-Neelsen stain, 1000×.*

FIGURE 30.2. *Sector of tubercle showing a central area of calcification (1), surrounded by caseation necrosis (2). Adjoining is a zone of epithelioid (3) and giant cells (arrow). The outermost zone (4) contains other mononuclear cells, particularly lymphocytes, among which tracts of fibrous tissue are discernible. Hematoxylin-eosin stain, 100×.*

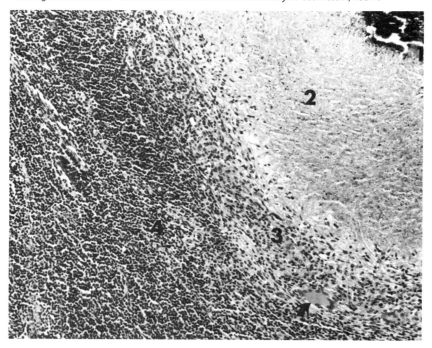

and a fibrous layer eventually invests the lesion, which is called a *tubercle* (Fig 30.2).

Tubercles may enlarge, coalesce, and eventually occupy sizable portions of organs. Such tubercles consist mostly of caseous material.

The process described is typical of human and ruminant tuberculosis caused by mammalian tubercle bacilli.

It is chronic; the lesion is called *productive* or *proliferative*. Occasionally an acute exudative process takes place, marked by predominantly neutrophilic responses and fluid effusion. It is thought to be favored by such factors as a large infecting dose, focally delivered; high virulence of the infecting strain; constitutional predisposition of the host; a loose tissue architecture as in the lung, serous membranes, or meninges; and a high degree of tuberculous hypersensitivity. One such acute process is *tuberculous pneumonia*, which may cause extensive necrosis and be rapidly fatal ("galloping consumption"), resolve almost completely, or subside into the chronic pattern.

Cell-mediated responses influence the course of the disease in several ways. Primary infection is disseminated via lymphatics to lymph nodes and beyond these through the bloodstream, seeding many reticuloendothelial tissues. Cell-mediated immunity and macrophage activation eliminate these foci, except where they have developed furthest — that is, the point of primary exposure and the adjacent lymph node. Here primary lesions (Ghon or Ghon-Ranke complexes) persist. Sometimes, especially with alimentary tract exposure, they are "incomplete" — that is, only the lymph node lesion is discernible.

Once cell-mediated reactivity is established, subsequent reinfection follows a different course: antigen-specific T lymphocytes and activated macrophages promptly converge on the site, contain the infection, and prevent lymphatic spread.

Antigen-specific T lymphocyte responses, however, also mediate allergic cytotoxic reactions and cause extensive tissue destruction, which is characteristic of progressive tuberculosis: while the lymphatic dissemination is limited by the immune response, tissue damage facilitates bacterial spread by contiguous extension, or erosion of bronchi, blood vessels, or viscera, introducing infection to new areas. Wherever microorganisms lodge, the allergic (as well as the immune) reaction will be repeated with cumulative consequences. Hematogenous dissemination may produce *miliary tuberculosis*: multifocal tubercle formation throughout an organ.

Reinfection tuberculosis is most often endogenous; that is, it results from reactivation of previously dormant foci.

Disease Patterns. Clinical tuberculosis is typically a debilitating illness characterized by progressive emaciation, erratic appetite, irregular low-grade fever, and occasionally by localizing signs such as enlarged lymph nodes, cough, and diarrhea.

Cattle are usually infected with *M. bovis* and the infection is centered on the respiratory tract and adjacent lymph nodes and serous cavities. The disease is commonly progressive via air spaces and passages. Hematogenous dissemination involving liver and kidney occurs. The uterus may serve as portal for fetal infection, a pattern virtually unknown in other domestic animals. Surviving calves commonly develop liver and spleen lesions. Udder infection is rare (<2% of cases) but has obvious public health implications.

Infection with *M. avium* is generally subclinical. Abortions resulting apparently from localization of *M. avium* in the uterine wall occur, in some instances repeatedly.

Mycobacterium tuberculosis causes minor, nonprogressive lesions in cattle.

The histopathology of bovine tuberculosis is as described under *Pathogenesis*, p. 159.

Horses are rarely infected, but relatively more often with *M. avium* than with *M. bovis*. Infection enters usually by the alimentary tract, with primary complexes related to pharynx and intestine and often incomplete. Secondary lesions may be in lung, liver, spleen, and serous membrane. Lesions in cervical vertebrae may be due to a secondary, nonspecific hypertrophic periostitis.

Gross lesions are tumor-like. They lack caseation and gross calcification and contain few lymphocytes. There is fibroblast proliferation but usually no firm encapsulation.

Swine can be infected by tubercle bacilli, usually via the alimentary route, but only *M. bovis* causes progressive disease with classical lesions. *Mycobacterium tuberculosis* infections do not advance past regional lymph nodes. *Mycobacterium avium* infection, the predominant form in many countries, may disseminate to viscera, bone, and meninges. The lesions lack the organization of tubercles, but contain granulomatous elements. Caseation, calcification, or liquefaction are negligible. Bacteria may be abundant.

Sheep and goats are susceptible to *M. bovis* and perhaps slightly less to *M. avium*, but they are resistant to progressive infection by *M. tuberculosis*. Disease patterns resemble those described in cattle.

Dogs and cats are readily infected with *M. bovis* but rarely with *M. avium*. Dogs are also susceptible to *M. tuberculosis*. Intestinal and abdominal localization of infection is more common in cats than in dogs, reflecting a likely alimentary route of exposure.

Hypertrophic pulmonary osteoarthropathy (Marie disease, acropachia), a nonspecific periostitis most noticeably affecting the long bones, sometimes affects tuberculous dogs (and horses). The etiology seems related to pulmonary incapacitation rather than to specific agents.

Ulcerative skin lesions are more common in cats than in other hosts, as is eye involvement, with tuberculous choroiditis leading to blindness.

Lesions, especially in dogs, often more closely resemble a foreign-body reaction than tubercles, since they may lack typical epithelioid and giant cells, and neither caseate, calcify, nor liquefy. The course is usually progressive.

Primates are susceptible to the two mammalian tubercle bacilli but resistant to *M. avium* unless severely compromised, as by AIDS or preexisting bronchopulmonary disease. Such individuals also become infected with nontuberculous mycobacteria.

In humans, infection is usually contracted by inhalation of droplet nuclei originating from "open" human cases (that is, respiratory shedders). When tuberculosis was widespread, most cases did not develop beyond the primary complex in the respiratory tract. A minority became progressive clinical tuberculosis, resembling the bovine disease described above.

Infection with *M. bovis* typically occurred following ingestion of unpasteurized milk from a tuberculous cow. Primary invasion, through pharynx or intestine, resulted in lymphadenitis of adjacent nodes. Hematogenous dissemination to vertebrae could result in a hunchback, a condition now rare thanks to pasteurization of milk and eradication of bovine tuberculosis.

Mycobacterium tuberculosis and *M. bovis* cause progressive disease in captive nonhuman primates, which are resistant to *M. avium*, although intestinal infections resembling Johne's disease of ruminants (Chapter 18) are associated with members of the *M. avium-intracellulare* complex.

Immunosuppressed humans, especially those with AIDS, appear susceptible to a variety of nontuberculous mycobacteria, for example, *M. genavense*, *M. avium-intracellulare* complex, *M. simiae*, *M. marinum*, and *M. haemophilum*.

Birds are naturally susceptible primarily to *M. avium*. Most poultry infections occur via the alimentary canal and disseminate to liver and spleen. Bone marrow, lung, and peritoneum are often affected. Although the agent has been isolated from eggs, transovarian infection of chicks is rare. *Mycobacterium genavense* affects canaries and parrots.

Tubercle formation stops short of calcification.

Although *M. avium* affects many species of birds, psittacines are resistant but are susceptible to *M. tuberculosis*. Canaries also are more susceptible to mammalian than to avian bacilli.

Epidemiology

With eradication of cattle tuberculosis in industrial countries, the traditional reservoir in domestic mammals has disappeared. Game farms, animal parks, and zoos remain foci of *M. bovis* in technically advanced countries. Sporadic cases of canine tuberculosis often prove to be *M. tuberculosis* infections traceable to human contacts — "reverse zoonoses" — which are also found in nonhuman primates in laboratory colonies and zoos.

In commercial poultry establishments, rapid population turnover (<1 year) eliminating transgenerational transmission has eradicated *M. avium*. It remains a problem in barnyard flocks, however, particularly since the agent can survive in soil for several years.

Tuberculosis is typically a disease of captivity and domestication. When wild and captive infected populations were compared, clinical improvement and lack of spread in free-living animals contrasted with deterioration and high communicability in confined groups. Tuberculosis in wild populations seems to be a relative rarity. Nevertheless, *M. bovis*, probably originating from cattle, is endemic in badgers of southern England and in brush-tailed opossums of New Zealand, both of which are considered sources of infection for livestock.

Immature individuals often develop more severe lesions than older ones. Breed susceptibilities differ: zebu cattle are more resistant than European breeds, and fox terriers and Irish setters are more often infected than dachshunds and Dobermans. The higher prevalence in dairy than beef cattle may reflect closer confinement, longer life spans, and greater productivity stress among dairy cows. Exemption from pregnancy and lactation may explain the lower disease prevalence in

bulls than cows, although in dogs the reverse sex ratio is observed.

IMMUNOLOGIC ASPECTS

Immune Mechanisms of Disease

The key role of cell-mediated immune responses in the pathogenesis of tuberculosis has been discussed. In their absence the disease may progress as a disseminating inflammatory disease (as it does in athymic mice) without the development of typical lesions.

Recovery and Resistance

Acquired resistance depends on cell-mediated responses. Under natural conditions this develops along with hypersensitivity, both of which are demonstrated in the *Koch phenomenon*: an already tuberculous guinea pig suffers a rapid, destructive, but limited reaction at the site of reexposure to tubercle bacilli, while a virgin animal develops persistent, progressive, disseminating, and eventually fatal disease when injected at the same anatomical site. Allergic reactivity and protective responses are separable: immunity can persist in experimentally desensitized animals and can be absent in sensitized subjects.

Antibody to tubercle bacilli does not protect against natural infection.

Artificial Immunization

Vaccination of humans with BCG (live attenuated *M. bovis*) produces temporary immunity and hypersensitivity. The benefits of vaccination have been greatest where exposure was most intense and negligible where prevalence was low. Vaccination in humans is focused on infants and tuberculin-negative individuals anticipating exposure.

BCG has been used in calves. This practice is inappropriate in countries attempting to eradicate tuberculosis because it interferes with the interpretation of the tuberculin test.

Mycobacterium microti, the vole bacillus, stimulates immunity to bovine and human tuberculosis. Its virulence is too variable to permit its use as a vaccine.

Among subcellular experimental immunogens, a ribosomal preparation is of interest because it produces protection without tuberculin allergy.

LABORATORY DIAGNOSIS

Sample Collection

Samples include tracheobronchial and gastric lavages; lymph node, thoracic, abdominal, and other aspirates; and urine, feces, and biopsy specimens. At necropsy, material is obtained from lesions.

Direct Examination

Fluids are concentrated by centrifugation in tightly capped containers. Samples intended for microscopy only are digested and disinfected with hypochlorite (bleach, Clorox). Smears of sediment or tissue are stained with an acid-fast stain, auramine-rhodamine where fluorescence microscopy is available. Histologic sections are stained with hematoxylin-eosin and acid-fast stains.

Positive results should be culturally confirmed.

Culture

Digestion and selective decontamination are advisable especially with specimens likely to contain a mixture of microorganisms.

Identification of mycobacteria is done almost exclusively in vitro.

Animal inoculations are sometimes used and DNA probes, specific for the main groups, are commercially available.

IMMUNODIAGNOSIS

Tuberculin Test

Cell-mediated hypersensitivity, acquired through infection, can be demonstrated systemically by fever, ophthalmically by conjunctivitis, or dermally by local swelling, when tuberculin or its purified protein derivative (PPD) is given by the subcutaneous, conjunctival, or intradermal route, respectively.

In cattle, tuberculin, the equivalent of a 0.2 to 0.3 mg/dose of bovine PPD, is injected intradermally in the caudal, vulvar, or anal skin or, in some situations, the neck region. In positive cases, a swelling (≥ 5 mm) develops within 72 hours. While tuberculin cannot induce the allergic state, it may desensitize animals for weeks or months.

A positive test implies past or present infection, requiring the reacting animal to be slaughtered and necropsied. Where tuberculosis is rare, no lesions are often found in reactors (NVL, for *nonvisible lesion* reactors). Such apparently false-positive reactions are explained by allergies to nontuberculous, related agents such as other mycobacteria, or nocardiae. Simultaneous use of avian tuberculin, which detects hypersensitivity to several nontuberculous mycobacteria, often helps to decide, by comparative size assessment of the two reactions, whether sensitivity is due primarily to mammalian or a heterologous tuberculin. Other explanatons for NVL are early states of infection, remote location of lesions, or microscopic sizes of lesions.

False-negatives occur in animals too recently infected and in advanced cases in which anergy develops due to antigen excess or immunosuppression. Nonspecific factors, such as malnutrition, stress, and impending or recent parturition, are alternative causes of anergy.

Rules governing the use of tuberculin tests in eradication programs vary from country to country.

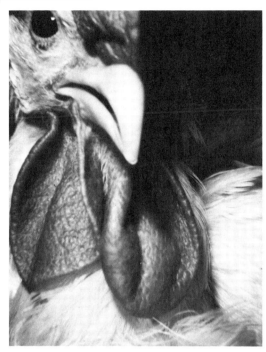

FIGURE 30.3. *Positive tuberculin reaction in the left wattle of a chicken experimentally infected three weeks earlier with Mycobacterium avium.*

Tuberculins of appropriate specificity are used on swine and poultry. In swine the ears are injected, in poultry the wattles (Fig 30.3). The reliability of tuberculin tests on horses, sheep, goats, dogs, and cats is not established.

Serology

Serologic tests have not been useful in diagnosis of mammalian tuberculosis. As a first step in poultry tuberculosis eradication, a whole-blood agglutination test is available. It is sensitive but lacks specificity.

TREATMENT AND CONTROL

First-line drugs for tuberculosis therapy are streptomycin, isoniazid (INH), ethambutol, and rifampin. Second-line drugs are pyrazinamide, para-aminosalicylic acid, kanamycin, cycloserine, capreomycin, and ethionamide. Because resistance often develops under a single-drug regimen, a combination is commonly used, the most favored one in human medicine being INH-ethambutol-rifampin. Treatment is 9 months with rifampin included, 18 to 24 months without it.

Because of the public health hazards inherent in the retention of tuberculous animals, antituberculous chemotherapy of animals is discouraged. Prophylactic treatment with INH may be considered for pets recently exposed to tuberculosis. Some experimental successes with INH for prophylaxis and treatment of calves have been reported. In countries with eradication programs, treatment is generally discouraged or illegal.

Bovine tuberculosis is controlled by identification and elimination of infected animals. This approach has resulted in near-eradication of the infection in many countries. Continued surveillance is required to prevent resurgence.

In poultry, tuberculosis in backyard flocks is perpetuated by retention of birds and persistence of soil contamination.

Eradication of bovine, human, and avian tuberculosis will diminish infection hazards for other species.

Treatment of atypical mycobacterial disease of the skin of cats involves surgery, a fluoroquinolone, or a macrolide (clarithromycin, azithromycin) antibiotic.

SELECTED REFERENCES

Bermudez LE, Wu M, Young LS. Interleukin-12 stimulated natural killer cells can activate human macrophages to inhibit growth of *Mycobacterium avium*. Infect Immun 1995;63:4099.

Brennan PJ. Structure of mycobacteria: recent developments in defining cell wall carbohydrates and proteins. Rev Infect Dis 1989;11(suppl. 2):S420.

Clemens DL, Horwitz MA. Characterization of the *Mycobacterium tuberculosis* phagosome and evidence that phagosomal maturation is inhibited. J Exp Med 1995;181:257.

Dannenberg AM. Immune mechanisms in the pathogenesis of pulmonary tuberculosis. Rev Infect Dis 1989;11(suppl. 2): S369.

Falkinham JO. Epidemiology of infection by nontuberculous mycobacteria. Clin Microbiol Rev 1996;9:177.

Farrar MA, Schreiber RD. The molecular cell biology of interferon gamma and its receptor. Annu Rev Immunol 1993;11:571.

Fenton MJ, Vermeulen MW. Immunopathology of tuberculosis: role of macrophages and monocytes. Infect Immun 1996;64: 683.

Fulton SA, Johnsen JM, Wolf SF, et al. Interleukin-12 production by human monocytes infected with *Mycobacterium tuberculosis*: role of phagocytosis. Infect Immun 1996;64:2523.

Grange JM, Yates MD, Boughton E. The avian tubercle bacillus and its relatives. J Appl Bacteriol 1990;68:411.

Hines ME, Kreeger JM, Herron AJ. Mycobacterial infections of animals: pathology and pathogenesis. Lab Anim Sci 1995;45: 334.

Hoop RK, Bottger EC, Pfyffer GE. Etiological agents of mycobacteriosis in pet birds between 1986 and 1995. J Clin Microbiol 1996;34:991.

Multhoff G, Hightower LE. Cell surface expression of heat shock proteins and the immune response. Cell Stress Chaperones 1996;1:167.

Orme IM, Andersen P, Boom WH. T cell response to *Mycobacterium tuberculosis*. J Infect Dis 1993;167:1481.

Ramis A, Ferrer L, Aranaz A, et al. *Mycobacterium genavense* infection in canaries. Avian Dis 1996;40:246.

Thoen CQ, Karlson AG. Tuberculosis. In: Calnek BW, ed. Diseases of poultry. 9th ed. Ames, IA: Iowa University, 1991:172–185.

Watt B. In-vitro sensitivities and treatment of less common mycobacteria. J Antimicrob Chemother 1997;39:567.

31 *Mollicutes*

Richard L. Walker

The mollicutes are members of the order *Mycoplasmatales* and class *Mollicutes* (soft skin). They are the smallest of the free-living prokaryotes and are devoid of cell walls. Six genera are recognized: *Acholeplasma, Anaeroplasma, Asteroplasma, Mycoplasma, Spiroplasma,* and *Ureaplasma.* Only members of the genera *Mycoplasma* and *Ureaplasma* are important in veterinary medicine. *Acholeplasma* are sometimes encountered, but usually as contaminants. *Mollicutes* is the correct term to use when collectively referring to members in this order; however, the trivial name *mycoplasma(s)* is also used for this purpose.

Members of the mollicutes infect a wide range of animal species. Infections range from subclinical to severely debilitating and sometimes fatal diseases. Clinical manifestations include respiratory and urogenital tract infections, arthritis, mastitis, and septicemia. Most pathogenic species exhibit a high degree of host specificity. Infections in humans usually present as respiratory or urogenital tract disease.

DESCRIPTIVE FEATURES

Morphology and Staining

The cell morphology of the mollicutes is extremely pleomorphic. Cell shapes include spherical, pear-shaped, spiral-shaped, and filamentous forms. Cells sometimes appear as chains of beads, the result of asynchronized genomic replication and cell division. The diameter of the spherical form ranges from 0.3 μm to 0.8 μm.

Although classified as gram negative, mollicutes stain poorly by the Gram method. Giemsa, Castañeda, Dienes and new methylene blue stains are preferred.

Structure and Composition

The mollicutes are not only devoid of cell walls but lack the genetic capacity to produce one. They are bound by single trilaminar membrane composed of proteins, glycoproteins, glycolipids, phospholipids, and sterols. Cholesterol in the membrane provides for osmotic stability. A polar bleb has been demonstrated in some species and has a role in adherence to host cell surfaces. Capsules have also been described for some species.

The mollicutes have a small genome (5×10^8 to 1×10^9 daltons) compared to other bacteria. The base composition is poor in guanine and cytosine with the mol% $G + C$ of DNA ranging from 23 to 40%. Sequence analysis of 16S rRNA indicates that mollicutes are most closely related to the genus *Clostridium*. Transposons, plasmids, and bacteriophages have been demonstrated in some species.

Cellular Products of Medical Interest

Various substances produced by the mollicutes are potentially important in disease pathogenesis. Peroxide and superoxide production may be important in disruption of host cell integrity. Urease, produced by *Ureaplasma* species, may be involved in injury to host tissue as a result of the production of ammonia by urea hydrolysis. Experimental inoculation of a 200 kDa protein from the supernatant of *M. neurolyticum* cultures causes neurologic signs in mice. Vascular damage in the brain is evident but the mechanism of action is unclear. Poorly defined products from some mollicutes induce interleukin-1, interleukin-6, and tumor necrosis factor production from activated macrophages. This accounts for the endotoxic-like activity observed with some infections. Bovine ureaplasmas produce IgA protease, which cleaves IgA_1 and may aid in avoiding the host immune response on mucosal surfaces. Other proteases, hemolysins, and nucleases are also produced.

Growth Characteristics

The mollicutes grow slowly and generally require 3 to 7 days' incubation before colonies are apparent. Growth is best at 37°C in an atmosphere of increased CO_2. Sterols are required by all genera except *Acholeplasma* and *Anaeroplasma*. Most genera are facultative anaerobes with the exception of *Anaeroplasma* and *Asteroplasma*, which are obligate anaerobes. Optimal pH for growth ranges from 6.0 for *Ureaplasma* up to 7.5 for other mollicutes.

Mollicute colonies are small and difficult to visualize with the unaided eye. Colony sizes vary from 0.01 mm to 1.0 mm. When observed with a dissecting microscope, many species exhibit a "fried egg" morphology. This umbonate appearance is the result of the central portion of the colony embedding into the agar with a peripheral zone of surface growth. Some species produce film spots, which are composed of cholesterol and phospholipids and which appear as a wrinkled film on the media surface.

Resistance

The lack of a cell wall renders mollicutes resistant to the action of antimicrobial agents that affect the cell wall or its synthesis. They are sensitive to compounds that interfere with protein and nucleic acid synthesis. *Acholeplasma* species are resistant to 1.5% digitonin, whereas the growth of other mollicutes is inhibited by this concentration. In general, mollicutes survive outside the host for substantial periods in moist, cool environments. They are very susceptible to heat and most detergents (tween) and disinfectants (quaternary ammonium, iodine, and phenol-based compounds).

Variability

Variations in nutritional and atmospheric requirements account for some of the diversity among genera and species within genera. Differences in colony morphology and size can be used to distinguish some of the mollicutes. *Ureaplasma* species produce substantially smaller colonies than other mollicutes and often lack the fried-egg colony morphology. The colony size of *M. mycoides* ssp. *mycoides* isolates from goats is consistently larger than those isolated from cattle. This size difference is used to distinguish between the two variants. While some antigens are shared among the mollicutes, antigenic differences are sufficiently specific to allow for species identification. Animal host specificity is strongly exhibited by the pathogenic mollicutes and may be explained by specific host receptors necessary for attachment or the failure of the host to recognize host-adapted species as nonself.

ECOLOGY

Reservoir

The major reservoir for mollicutes is the host they infect. Asymptomatically infected animals carry organisms on mucosal surfaces including nasal, conjunctival, oral, intestinal, and genital mucosa. The ear canal of goats has also been shown to be a reservoir for some of the pathogenic caprine mycoplasmas.

Transmission

Transmission occurs predominately by spread from animal to animal through direct contact and is mediated through aerosolization of respiratory secretions or through venereal transmission. Mechanical transmission is also important, especially with regard to bovine and caprine mycoplasma mastitis. In poultry, vertical transmission through hatching eggs is an important means of spread for many of the pathogenic avian species. Contaminated milk can be a source of infection for calves and goat kids. Little is known about the role of ectoparasites in transmission; however, pathogenic caprine species have been isolated from ear mites of goats.

Pathogenesis

Mechanisms.   Attachment to host cells is the first step in establishing infection and is mediated through the anionic surface layer on most mycoplasmas. In some species, special attachment structures have been demonstrated, which appear to be encoded by a common ancestral adhesin gene. Host receptors for attachment are glycoconjugates and allow for colonization of mucosal surfaces. The ciliostatic capability of some *Mycoplasma* species further promotes establishment of infection.

Latent infections are common. Factors that allow for persistence include mechanisms to avoid the immune system such as antigenic variability or biological mimicry. Underlying factors such as age, crowding, concurrent infections, and transportation stresses lead to overt disease. Breaks in integrity of the epithelial barrier probably account for the initial step in breaching host defenses.

Acute, septicemic forms of disease result in a coagulopathy and widespread vascular thrombosis, which resembles a gram-negative septicemia and is, at least in part, mediated through induction of cytokines.

The pathogenesis of chronic infections is directly related to persistence of the organisms in the face of an intense inflammatory response. Peroxidation causes host tissue damage. Activation of complement and cytotoxic T lymphocytes further contributes to host injury.

Virulence varies among species and strains within species and accounts for some of the variations in disease manifestation. In some species, virulence is correlated with presence of an outer surface layer. A galactan polymer in *M. mycoides* subsp. *mycoides* has been shown to modulate the immune response and promote dissemination. Virulence is rapidly lost by in vitro passage.

In addition to specific diseases, generalized effects on the immune system may increase susceptibility to secondary infections with other bacterial pathogens.

Pathology.   The lesions associated with mycoplasma infections vary from acute to chronic and are dependent on the agent involved and the site affected. In acute infections, there is an inflammatory reaction with an infiltration of neutrophils and fibrin accumulation. Generalized infections lead to a fibrinopurulent exudate on serosal surfaces and synovial membranes.

In persistent localized infections, tissue destruction can be substantial. Abscesses may develop at pressure sites in calves and are characterized by a eosinophilic coagulative necrosis with peripheral fibrosis. In cases of mycoplasma mastitis, pockets of purulent exudate may develop in affected mammary tissue. Eventually the affected gland becomes fibrosed. In the acute stage of mycoplasma infections of the joint, the joint becomes distended with fluid containing fibrin. As infections become chronic, there is villus hypertrophy of the synovia and a proliferative and erosive arthritis develops. A marked pleural effusion develops in respiratory tract infections due to *M. mycoides* ssp. *mycoides* in cattle and *M. capricolum* ssp. *capripneumoniae* in goats. The subpleural tissue and interlobular septa become thickened and fluid filled. Affected areas of lung become hepatized with resulting sequestration of necrotic tissue.

An infiltration of lymphocytes and plasma cells is often observed in mycoplasma infections, particularly around vessels and in the submucosa. Peribronchial and peribronchiolar lymphoplasmacytic cuffing is a characteristic finding in respiratory tract infection. The profound lymphoplasmacytic proliferation observed in many infections is due to nonspecific mitogenic effects as well as to a specific antimycoplasmal immune response.

Disease Patterns. Infections can manifest in a variety of ways. Common manifestations include septicemias, disseminated infections involving multiple sites, or localized infections. Common manifestations caused by the different pathogenic species in major animal species are listed in Table 31.1.

Avian. Mycoplasmosis in poultry has important economic consequences. *Mycoplasma gallisepticum* causes a chronic respiratory disease in chickens, turkeys, and a number of other domestic avian species. Clinical signs include coughing, nasal discharge, and tracheal rales. Turkeys can develop sinusitis with production of a thick,

Table 31.1. Animal Species, Agents, and Diseases Associated with Mycoplasma Infections

Animal Species	Agent	Common Clinical Manifestations
Cats	*M. felis*	Conjunctivitis
	M. gatae	Arthritis
Cattle	*M. alkalescens*	Arthritis, mastitis
	M. bovigenitalium	Infertility, mastitis, seminal vesiculitis
	M. bovis	Abscesses, arthritis, mastitis, otitis, pneumonia
	M. bovoculi	Keratoconjunctivitis
	M. californicum	Arthritis, mastitis
	M. canadense	Arthritis, mastitis
	M. dispar	Alveolitis, bronchiolitis
	M. mycoides subsp. *mycoides* (SC)	Arthritis, pleuropneumonia
	M. diversum	Infertility, pneumonia, vulvovaginitis
Chickens	*M. gallisepticum*	Respiratory disease
	M. synoviae	Airsacculitis, sternal bursitis, synovitis
Dogs	*M. canis*	Urogenital tract disease
	M. cynos	Pneumonia
	M. spumans	Arthritis
Goats	*M. agalactiae*	Agalactiae, arthritis, conjunctivitis
	M. capricolum subsp. *capricolum*	Arthritis, mastitis, pneumonia, septicemia
	M. capricolum subsp. *capripneumoniae*	Pleuropneumonia
	M. conjunctivae	Keratoconjunctivitis
	M. mycoides subsp. *mycoides* (LC)	Abscesses, arthritis, mastitis, septicemia
	M. mycoides subsp. *capri*	Pneumonia
	M. putrefaciens	Arthritis, mastitis
Horses	*M. felis*	Pleuritis
Mice	*M. neurolyticum*	Conjunctivitis, neurological disease
	M. pulmonis	Respiratory disease
Rats	*M. arthritidis*	Arthritis
	M. pulmonis	Respiratory disease, genital tract disease
Sheep	*M. agalactiae*	Agalactiae
	M. conjunctivae	Keratoconjunctivitis
	M. ovipneumoniae	Pneumonia
Swine	*M. hyopneumoniae*	Enzootic pneumonia
	M. hyorhinis	Arthritis, pneumonia, polyserositis
	M. hyosynoviae	Arthritis
Turkeys	*M. gallisepticum*	Sinusitis, respiratory disease
	M. iowae	Embryo mortality, leg deformities
	M. meleagridis	Airsacculitis, decreased egg hatchability, perosis
	M. synoviae	Sternal bursitis, synovitis

mucoid exudate that results in severe swelling of the paranasal sinuses. Occasionally, clinical signs related to brain and joint involvement are recognized. Decrease in egg production also occurs. *Mycoplasma synoviae* also infects a wide range of avian species. Synovitis resulting in lameness, swelling of joints and tendon sheaths, and retarded growth are common presentations. Sternal bursitis is also frequently observed. Airsacculitis, which is usually subclinical, is another manifestation. *Mycoplasma meleagridis* and *M. iowae* infections are mostly limited to turkeys. *Mycoplasma meleagridis* causes respiratory disease, predominately an airsacculitis, which is often clinically mild or inapparent. Skeletal deformities, including bowing or twisting of the tarsometatarsal bone and cervical vertebrae, are occasionally detected. Decreased egg hatchability is a serious consequence of *M. meleagridis* infections. Airsacculitis, leg deformities, and stunting in poults have been demonstrated experimentally with *M. iowae*. Decreased egg hatchability has also been noted with *M. iowae* infections.

Bovine. *Mycoplasma mycoides* subsp. *mycoides* (small-colony type) is considered the most virulent of the bovine mycoplasmas. It causes a respiratory disease, contagious bovine pleuropneumonia (CBPP), in cattle that ranges from a persistent, subclinical infection to an acute, sometimes fatal disease. Clinical signs include respiratory distress, coughing, nasal discharge, and reluctance to move. In severe cases, the animal will stand with its neck extended and mouth open to facilitate breathing. Subclinically affected animals serve as a source for maintaining and spreading infection in the herd. Most infections are limited to the respiratory tract, although arthritis occurs in calves.

Mycoplasma mastitis is caused by a number of species. *Mycoplasma bovis* is the most common cause and results in the most severe disease. *Mycoplasma californicum* and *M. canadense* are also frequently involved. *Mycoplasma alkalescens* and *M. bovigenitalium* have also been implicated as etiologic agents on occasion. Typically, there is a drop in milk production. The milk becomes thick and intermixed with a watery secretion and may progress to a purulent exudate (Fig 31.1). The udder is often swollen, although not painful. Sometimes all four quarters are involved. It is a destructive mastitis and often refractory to treatment. Most infections are limited to the mammary gland; however, arthritis subsequent to bacteremia occurs. Spread from cow to cow is directly related to inadequate management and sanitation practices.

Mycoplasma respiratory tract infections in calves often present as pneumonia in association with other bovine respiratory pathogens. *Mycoplasma bovis* is the predominant species recovered. *Mycoplasma dispar* causes a mild respiratory disease characterized by bronchiolitis and alveolitis and is usually precipitated by environmental stresses or a primary viral infection. Both *M. bovis* and *M. dispar* can be recovered as commensals from the upper respiratory tract.

Urogenital tract infections are caused by *M. bovigenitalium* and *Ureaplasma diversum*. Seminal vesiculitis in bulls and granular vulvitis, endometritis, and abortion in cows are associated with both of these organisms. Both are found as normal commensals in the lower urogenital tract.

Arthritis in calves occurs sporadically. While a number of different species can cause arthritis, *M. bovis* is most frequently recovered. Other less common presentations include otitis media and decubital abscesses. *Mycoplasma bovis*, again, is the usual agent.

Canine. A number of *Mycoplasma* species have been isolated from dogs; however, little is known about the role

FIGURE 31.1. *Milk from a cow with severe mycoplasma mastitis. The milk is thickened with a watery component containing small flakes of material.* Mycoplasma bovis *was isolated.*

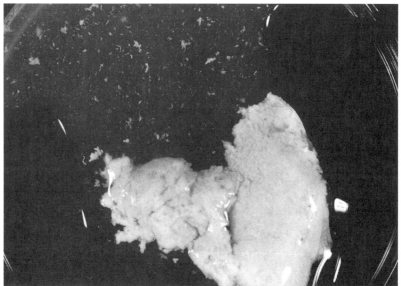

they play in disease. Experimental and clinical evidence suggests *M. canis* can cause urogenital tract disease including prostatitis, cystitis, endometritis, orchitis, and epididymitis. *Mycoplasma cynos* has been associated with pneumonia, usually as a secondary invader. *Mycoplasma spumans* has been reported to cause arthritis. The role of *Mycoplasma* in reproductive disorders of the bitch is uncertain.

Caprine. Mycoplasma infections in goats are economically important and can result in disease of epizootic proportion. *Mycoplasma mycoides* ssp. *mycoides* (large-colony type) infections present as a mastitis, pneumonia, or arthritis in adult animals. Some does develop a generalized toxic disease that can be fatal. A rapidly fatal septicemia is common in kids. Those that survive develop a chronic, destructive arthritis. *Mycoplasma mycoides* ssp. *capri* causes a pleuropneumonia similar to that of goat strains of *M. mycoides* ssp. *mycoides*. Septicemia, arthritis, and mastitis occur with *M. capricolum* ssp. *capricolum* infections. *Mycoplasma capricolum* ssp. *capripneumoniae* (formerly *Mycoplasma* sp. F-38) causes contagious caprine pleuropneumonia (CCPP), which is similar to CBPP in cattle. Both *M. agalactiae* and *M. putrefaciens* cause mastitis. The mastitis due to *M. putrefaciens* is purulent in nature, while infections with *M. agalactiae* result in a decrease or total cessation in milk production. Both species can cause arthritis. *Mycoplasma conjunctivae* causes a keratoconjunctivitis that presents with lacrimation, conjunctival hyperemia, and keratitis. Pannus is sometimes evident.

Equine. *Mycoplasma felis* is the only species that has been solidly associated with disease in the horse. It is recovered from the upper respiratory tract as a commensal but can cause a pleuritis, usually related to some exertional activity. The pleuritis is self-limiting and frequently resolves spontaneously.

Feline. A variety of commensal mycoplasmas have been recovered from mucosal surfaces of cats. Relatively few are associated with disease. *Mycoplasma gatae* has been recovered from cats with arthritis. *Mycoplasma felis* causes a serous to mucoid conjunctivitis. Typically the conjunctiva is edematous; however, the cornea is not involved. A mycoplasma-like organism has been associated with subcutaneous abscesses, but neither the disease nor the organism has been well characterized.

Murine. *Mycoplasma pulmonis* causes a low-grade respiratory disease in rats. Infections involve the nasal cavity, middle ear, larynx, trachea, and lungs. The most common clinical sign is a low-pitched wheezing or snuffling resulting from the purulent nasal exudate. In mice, clinical signs are often inapparent, although a chattering sound and continued rubbing of the eyes and nose may suggest infection in the colony. Mortality is low and when it occurs is related to pneumonia. Genital tract infections with *M. pulmonis* are also recognized in rats. *Mycoplasma arthritidis* causes a polyarthritis in rats and mice, although

many infections are subclinical. Experimental infections in mice result in joint swelling and, in some cases, posterior paralysis. Natural infections with *M. neurolyticum* generally do not cause disease, although conjunctivitis has been reported. Experimental inoculation with *M. neurolyticum* or cell-free filtrates causes a neurologic syndrome referred to as *rolling disease*.

Ovine. Compared to other ruminant species, mycoplasma infections in sheep are not as frequent or devastating. *Mycoplasma ovipneumoniae* is associated with pneumonia and usually in conjunction with other common bacterial pathogens of the ovine respiratory tract. Outbreaks of keratoconjunctivitis have been attributed to *M. conjunctivae*. Agalactic mastitis caused by *M. agalactiae* is similar to that observed in goats. Sheep can also be infected with many of the other species that affect goats.

Porcine. A number of important clinical entities are associated with mycoplasma infections in swine. Infections with *M. hyopneumoniae* present as a chronic respiratory disease, referred to as *enzootic pneumonia*. There is high morbidity but low mortality. The principal clinical sign is a chronic nonproductive cough. Affected pigs appear unthrifty and have retarded growth. *Mycoplasma hyorhinis* causes a systemic infection in pigs between 3 and 10 weeks of age. Initial signs include fever, inappetence, and listlessness. Swelling of the joints and lameness frequently follow. There is a characteristic polyserositis that involves pleural, peritoneal, and pericardial serosa. Synovial membranes are also affected. Chronic infections result in decreased weight gain. *Mycoplasma hyosynoviae* causes arthritis in growing pigs 12 to 24 weeks of age. Lameness and associated difficulty with mobility are the principal clinical signs.

Epidemiology

The primary source of most of the pathogenic mollicutes is the host that they infect. Introduction of an infected animal into an uninfected population accounts for dissemination of infection. Asymptomatic carriers, usually colonized on mucosal surfaces, serve as the source for maintaining organisms in the population. Young animals are very susceptible to infection and generally develop more severe disease than adult animals. Animal pathogens are not considered to have significant zoonotic potential.

IMMUNOLOGIC ASPECTS

Immune Mechanisms in Pathogenesis

The immune response of the host is intimately involved in the pathogenesis of disease. Consequences of both an active humoral and cellular immune response, as well as immunosuppressive effects of the pathogen itself, are involved in pathogenic process.

Some mollicutes have been shown to possess nonspecific mitogenic properties and are able to induce a polyclonal B-cell stimulation to a variety of antigens, including host antigens. *Mycoplasma arthriditis* possesses a small peptide that acts as a superantigen and stimulates a broad population of T-cells. The resulting production of various cytokines and inflammatory reaction are detrimental to the host. Shared host and mycoplasma antigens, such as the galactans found in the lungs of cattle and in *M. mycoides* ssp. *mycoides*, can result in auto-immune disease.

Mycoplasmas activate the complement cascade by the classical pathway, which contributes to the inflammatory response. While beneficial in controlling infections, the inflammatory response can result in damage to bystander host cells. Persistence of antigen in selected sites, such as joints, allows for further damage due to development of an immune-complex mediated inflammatory response. Induction of IL-1, IL-6, and TNF from activated macrophages by many mycoplasmas leads to activation of cytotoxic T lymphocytes and results in an endotoxin-like effect.

Suppression or lack of the host immune response is important in allowing for persistence and avoidance of recognition by the host. A number of *Mycoplasma* species have been shown to decrease phagocytic activity of neutrophils and macrophages. Proposed mechanisms include decreasing the respiratory burst (*M. bovis*) or decreasing phagocytosis as a result of capsule production (*M. dispar*). Antigens shared between *Mycoplasma* species and the host tissues may result in a biological mimicry, whereby the host recognizes the mycoplasma as self-leading to persistent infections. Antigenic variability is another mechanism employed to evade host defenses. Incorporation of host antigens by mycoplasmas, a condition referred to as *capping*, further aids some mollicutes in escaping detection by the immune system.

Mechanisms of Resistance and Recovery

Age, environmental conditions, genetic predisposition, crowding, and concurrent infections are all involved in contributing to resistance to infection or lack thereof. Minimizing predisposing stresses will minimize disease. Some of the innate host mechanisms for protection, such as the mucociliary escalator system in the respiratory tract, are important in preventing colonization.

The chronicity of mollicute infections suggests that the immune response is not very effective at controlling infection once established. Mycoplasmas stimulate a humoral response and specific antibodies can be demonstrated. Antibodies have been shown to enhance clearance. Cellular immunity is also recognized, although less is known about it. In the face of an intense inflammatory response, however, mycoplasmas generally appear able to avoid elimination.

Artificial Immunization

Vaccination is employed to control some mycoplasma diseases. An attenuated vaccine is used to protect cattle in areas where CBPP is enzootic. Protection lasts for approximately 18 months. Attenuated and killed, adju-

vanted vaccines have been used with variable success to control some caprine infections, specifically those caused by *M. agalactiae*, *M. mycoides* ssp. *capri*, and *M. capricolum* ssp. *capripneumoniae*. Inactivated vaccines afford some protection for swine against infection with *M. hyopneumoniae* and *M. hyorhinis*. In poultry, live and inactivated vaccines are employed to control egg production losses and respiratory disease associated with *M. gallisepticum* infections.

LABORATORY DIAGNOSIS

Sample Collection

The appropriate sample for isolation attempt is determined by the clinical presentation and includes exudates, swabs from affected sites, affected tissues, and milk. The ear canals of goats can be sampled to detect inapparent carriers. Because of the mollicutes' fastidious nature, samples should be submitted to the laboratory as soon as possible after collection. During transportation, samples should be kept cool and moist. Various commercially available media (Stuart's and Amies' without charcoal) are suitable for transporting swabs. If a prolonged transport time (greater than 24 hours) is expected, samples should be shipped frozen and preferably on dry ice or in liquid nitrogen.

Direct Examination

The variability in microscopic morphology and poor staining with the Gram method make direct examination for mollicutes unrewarding. Direct fluorescent antibody tests and DNA fluorochrome staining have been described, particularly for diagnosing conjunctivitis and mastitis, but they are not widely used.

Isolation

No one media formulation is suitable for growth of all of the mollicutes. The media selected should be based on the specific species or group of species of interest. In general, a fairly complex media is required. Serum is the usual source of sterols and is required by most species. Different species, however, grow better with different sources of serum. The exception is the *Acholeplasma*, which have the ability to synthesize their own fatty acids and therefore do not require exogenous sterols. Yeast extract is also included as a source of growth factors. Growth of some species is enhanced or requires incorporation of specific substances such as vaginal mucus (*M. agalactiae*) and nicotinamide adenine dinucleotide (*M. synoviae*). Penicillin, thallium acetate, and amphotericin B are commonly added to media to inhibit contaminating bacteria and fungi. Specific immune sera directed against commensal mycoplasmas can be incorporated in media to allow for selective isolation for pathogenic species. For optimal recovery, samples are inoculated into both a liquid and solid media and incubated at 37°C in 5% to 10% CO_2 for at least 7 days. Some species require longer incubation times. Semen and joint fluids may contain inhibitory factors and should be diluted prior to culture to enhance recovery. Blind passages from broth to broth may enhance the recovery of poultry pathogens. *Ureaplasma* species are susceptible to pH changes as a result of hydrolysis of urea included in the media and must be subcultured frequently to maintain their viability when isolation attempts are made.

Identification

Plate media is examined with the aid of a dissecting microscope. Colonies with the typical umbonate morphology are stained directly with the Dienes stain to differentiate them from other bacteria (Fig 31.2). The mollicutes stain blue because of their inability to reduce methylene blue in the stain. Other bacteria reduce methylene blue by using it as a hydrogen acceptor in maltose oxidation and therefore appear colorless with the Dienes stain. The exceptions are L-form bacteria, which exhibit a similar colony morphology and staining reaction as the mollicutes. L-forms must be differentiated from mollicutes by demonstrating reversion of the L-form bacteria back to a walled form.

Digitonin sensitivity is used to distinguish *Mycoplasma* and *Ureaplasma* from *Acholeplasma*. A zone of inhibition around paper disks saturated with 1.5% digitonin will be present with *Mycoplasma* and *Ureaplasma* but not *Acholeplasma*. Commonly used biochemical tests to further characterize isolates include detection of phosphatase activity, fermentation of glucose, and hydrolysis of arginine or urea.

Definitive identification is based on reactivity with specific antisera. A number of methods are employed based on either the ability of specific antisera to inhibit growth or metabolism or the demonstration of reactivity with a specific antisera using either a fluorescence or chromogen-based detection system. Growth inhibition tests employ antisera impregnated disks or antisera placed in wells in media and demonstrating a zone of inhibition. Metabolic inhibition tests use growth inhibition in liquid media and a color change based on pH as an indicator system. Other test procedures commonly used to demonstrate specific reactivity are direct or indirect immunofluorescence on colony impressions, colony epifluorescence, and immunoperoxidase staining of colonies on agar plates.

Nonserologic methods for species identification using polymerase chain reaction (PCR) have recently been described. Amplification of specific DNA sequences by PCR and restriction endonuclease analysis of PCR products have been used for identification and characterization of isolates. Randomly amplified polymorphic DNA analysis has been used for strain differentiation. Restriction endonuclease analysis, protein electrophoresis, and ribotyping have also been used to further characterize strains.

Antibiotics susceptibility testing of clinical isolates is not routinely performed.

Nonculture Detection Methods

Immunoperoxidase and immunofluorescent staining of histopathologic sections has been used successfully for identification of some species in tissues, including *M. bovis* in cattle tissues, *M. hyopneumoniae* in pig lungs, and some of the poultry mycoplasmas. A number of PCR methods have been described for identification of pathogenic species directly from clinical material. Polymerase chain reaction tests for direct detection of some of the pathogenic poultry mycoplasmas are commercially available.

FIGURE 31.2. *Dienes-stained mycoplasma colonies with densely staining centers and lighter staining peripheries (75×).*

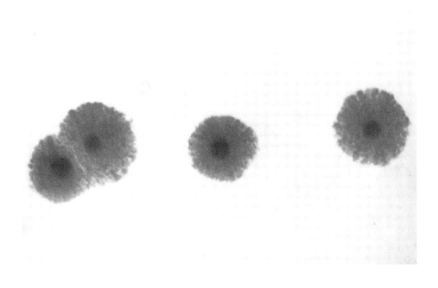

Immunodiagnosis

A number of immunodiagnostic tests have been developed for many of the important mycoplasma diseases. Many have not been standardized and are not in wide use. Problems with sensitivity, especially with asymptomatic carriers, are common. Lack of specificity as a result of cross-reacting antibodies is also a problem.

Enzyme-linked immunosorbent assays, plate agglutination, and hemagglutination inhibition tests are routinely used to detect flock infections with *M. gallisepticum*, *M. meleagridis*, and *M. synoviae* in poultry and are an important part of overall eradication programs used by commercial poultry operations.

TREATMENT, CONTROL, AND PREVENTION

Success of treatment varies depending on the species involved, the affected site, and time course of the disease. Although the mollicutes are susceptible to a number of antibiotics in vitro, treatment failures are common. Commonly used antibiotics include tetracyclines, tylosin, erythromycin, lincomycin, spectinomycin, and tilmicosin. Resistance to some of these antimicrobials has been noted. Animals that do respond to treatment often become carriers.

Control measures depend on the disease status of the country, specific disease, and animal species infected. Diseases such as CBPP and CCPP, which affect large populations of animals, are controlled by test and slaughter of affected herds in countries that are free of the disease. Vaccination, culling of infected animals, and management changes to prevent dissemination are employed in countries where the disease is enzootic. In general, because of the poor success in treating infected animals, culling of clinically ill animals is often employed as a control measure in infected populations where test and slaughter is not feasible. Industry-driven efforts, particularly in the poultry industry, have outlined measures to eliminate or prevent infection. Attempts to eradicate infections, particularly in breeding flocks, include serologic testing and elimination of positive flocks and antibiotic treatment of hatching eggs to produce mycoplasma-free chicks. Treatment of eggs involves immersing warmed eggs in a chilled antibiotic solution, which promotes antibiotic penetration into the egg. Routine culturing of bulk tanks is used to monitor for mammary infections in cow and goat herds. Animals identified as shedding organisms in the milk are usually culled.

Preventing infection should be based on following strict biosecurity practices to preclude introduction of infected animals into a mycoplasma-free herd. New animals should be quarantined and tested before being mixed with the herd. Taking animals to shows and fairs and returning them to the herd may also serve as a source for introducing infection. Good hygiene and management practices are important in preventing spread among animals where infections are enzootic. Because milk can be a source of infection, especially in goats, it should be pasteurized to prevent infecting young animals in the herd.

SELECTED REFERENCES

Almeida RA, Wannemuehler MJ, Rosenbusch RF. Interaction of *Mycoplasma dispar* with bovine alveolar macrophages. Infect Immun 1992;60:2914.

Bölske G, Mattsson JG, Bascuñana CR, et al. Diagnosis of contagious caprine pleuropneumoniae by detection and identification of *Mycoplasma capricolum* subsp. *capripneumoniae* by PCR and restriction enzyme analysis. J Clin Microbiol 1996;34:785.

DaMassa AJ, Wakenell PS, Brooks DL. Mycoplasmas of goats and sheep. J Vet Diagn Invest 1992;4:101.

Keeler CL, Hnatow LL, Whetzel PL, Dohms JE. Cloning and characterization of a putative cytadhesin gene (MGC1) from *Mycoplasma gallisepticum*. Infect Immun 1996;64:1541.

Kirk JH, Lauerman LH. Mycoplasma mastitis in dairy cows. Compend Cont Ed Pract Vet 1994;16:541.

Razin S, Jacobs E. Mycoplasma adhesion. J Gen Microbiol 1992;138:407.

Thomas CB, van Ess P, Wolfgram LJ, et al. Adherence to bovine neutrophils and suppression of neutrophil chemiluminescence by *Mycoplasma bovis*. Vet Immun Immunopathol 1991;27:365.

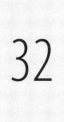

32

Chlamydiae

ERNST L. BIBERSTEIN   DWIGHT C. HIRSH

Chlamydiae are obligate intracellular gram-negative bacteria incapable of obtaining energy by metabolic activities. Their life cycle alternates between noninfectious proliferative stages and infectious nonproliferative stages. There are four species of *Chlamydia: C. trachomatis* causes human venereal, ocular, and respiratory infections; *C. psittaci* affects many mammals (including humans) and birds; *C. pneumoniae* causes human respiratory infections; *C. pecorum* causes encephalitis, polyarthritis, and enteritis in cattle, sheep, and pigs.

DESCRIPTIVE FEATURES

Morphology and Staining

Chlamydiae are coccobacilli 200 × up to 1500 nm in size. Though cytochemically gram-negative, they stain best with Gimenez, Macchiavello's, Castaneda, and Giemsa stains. *Chlamydia psittaci* and *C. pecorum* are indistinguishable phenotypically. Only genetically can the two species be resolved.

Life Cycle

Elementary bodies, 200 to 400 nm in size, enter susceptible cells by receptor-mediated endocytosis and the endosome "traffics" to pathways not involved with endosome-lysosome fusion. Elementary bodies change into noninfectious, metabolically active reticulate bodies, measuring 600 to 1500 nm, that generate, by binary fission, a new crop of elementary bodies that are released upon cell lysis (by lysosomal host enzymes). In vitro, the cycle requires 30 to 40 hours.

Elementary bodies appear red by Macchiavello's and Gimenez, blue by Castaneda, and reddish-purple by Giemsa stain, while reticulate bodies stain blue, green, reddish, and blue, respectively. Giemsa stain is best for the demonstration of both stages.

Structure and Composition

The cell envelope of elementary and reticulate bodies resembles a gram-negative cell wall but lacks peptidoglycan. A trilaminar outer membrane consists of protein and lipopolysaccharides. Proteins confer species and type-specificity, and may act as adhesins. Heparin-like derivates produced by chlamydiae are also proposed to act as adhesins by associating with heparin-binding receptors on host cells. The lipopolysaccharides, which have endotoxic properties, are genus-specific.

The genome size, 6.6×10^8 Da, is among the smallest in prokaryotes. There is much RNA in the reticulate but little in the elementary bodies. In the reticulate body, electron-dense material is fairly uniformly dispersed throughout the cell interior, while in the developing elementary body it becomes increasingly concentrated into a compact nucleoid, which, in the mature elementary body, occupies most of the cell (Fig 32.1).

Cellular Products of Medical Interest

A soluble hemagglutinin and cell-bound heat-labile toxic effect, demonstrable in mice and on macrophages and neutralizable by type-specific antibody, is associated with elementary but not reticulate bodies. Heparin-like derivates act as adhesins.

Growth Characteristics

Chlamydiae do not grow on cell-free media. They grow well in the yolk sac of embryonated chicken eggs and in tissue culture (e.g., L-cells, McCoy cells), where they form intracytoplasmic colonies.

Reticulate bodies transport adenosine triphosphate (ATP) into cells and adenosine diphosphate (ADP) out of cells. In the presence of ATP, peptides are synthesized. The agents are "energy parasites." Elementary bodies show little biochemical activity.

Resistance

There is little resistance to common disinfectants, heat, and sunlight. Elementary bodies survive in water for several days at ambient temperatures and apparently persist in dried animal excretions for long periods.

Variability

Chlamydia psittaci and *C. pecorum* include genetically and serologically distinct subgroups (immunotypes) related to host and disease specificities. Genital and intestinal isolates in cattle and sheep differ antigenically from encephalomyelitis-, polyarthritis-, and conjunctivitis-derived strains and may in fact reflect the distribution of *Chlamydia psittaci* and *C. pecorum* are indistinguishable

FIGURE 32.1. Chlamydia psittaci *inclusion containing reticulate bodies (RB), condensing forms (CF), and elementary bodies (EB). The nucleoid of the elementary body has a polar eccentric location but occupies most of the cell. Transmission electron micrograph, 15,000×. (Reproduced by permission of Storz J. Chlamydiales: properties, cycle of development and effect on eukaryotic host cells. Curr Topics Microbiol Immunol 1977;76:167.)*

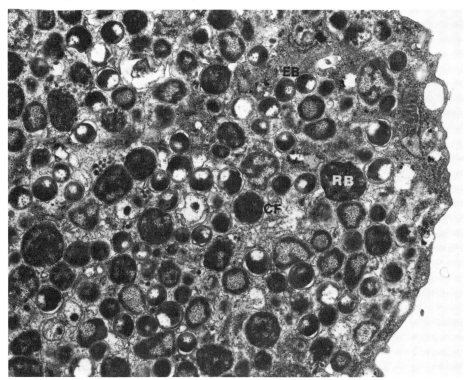

phenotypically. Both groups are distinct from strains affecting avian species.

ECOLOGY

Reservoir

The respiratory, intestinal, and genital tracts of mammals and birds constitute the reservoir.

Transmission

Exposure is through inhalation or ingestion of infectious material. The finding of *C. psittaci* in ectoparasites is of undetermined significance. Egg transmission occurs in some birds.

Pathogenesis

Mechanisms. Elementary bodies attach to and are endocytosed by epithelial cells, where they multiply, having somehow averted phagolysosomal fusion by trafficking to endosomes that do not readily fuse to lysosomes. Synthesis of host DNA, RNA, and protein ceases and cells eventually disintegrate through host enzyme action.

Microbial toxicity and tissue damage elicit inflammatory responses.

Pathology. Pathologic changes vary with localization of infection. In pulmonary chlamydiosis, an exudative bronchiolitis and bronchopneumonia develop mostly in the anterior lobes as reddish-gray areas of consolidation with purulent exudate in the bronchioles. Microscopically, the smallest bronchioles contain predominantly neutrophilic exudates. In the acini, alveolar macrophages predominate. Edema may be marked. Epithelial damage in the bronchioles is variable. Mononuclear cells gradually replace neutrophils, and lymphoreticular cuffing is common in ruminants.

Ocular infections take the form of a catarrhal conjunctivitis. Chlamydial arthritis involves all soft tissues near affected joints. Suppuration, edema, and hemorrhage are succeeded by granulomatous and fibrotic reactions.

In chlamydial abortion of ruminants, there is placentitis producing cotyledonary necrosis and edematous or leathery intercotyledonary thickening. Lesions in the male genital tract of ruminants (epididymis, testicle, deferent duct) are granulomatous.

In intestinal infections, there is granulomatous inflammation of the lamina propria and submucosa.

Chlamydiosis of birds is marked by fibrinous serositis of body cavities, air sacs, and organ surfaces. Lung, spleen, and liver are enlarged and congested. Microscopically, there is fibrinonecrotizing inflammation with mononuclear and heterophil leukocytes.

Chlamydial infections in ruminants appear to be manifest in two ways depending upon the microorganism: 1) abortion (almost always caused by *C. psittaci*) and 2) polyarthritis, polyserositis, encephalitis, and enteric infections (*C. pecorum*).

Avian chlamydiosis (ornithosis, psittacosis) is most significant economically in turkeys. Onset is insidious and may occur weeks after exposure. Early signs are inappetence, weight loss, and the voiding of greenish-yellow, gelatinous droppings. Egg production is reduced. Severity varies with strain virulence (toxicity); morbidity may range from 5% to 80%, mortality from 1% to 30%.

Geese and ducks are sometimes affected, chickens exceptionally so. Subclinical forms predominate in pigeons and psittacine birds.

Chlamydial abortion outbreaks occur among previously unexposed ewes (enzootic abortion of ewes) and goats. Abortion occurs sporadically in cattle and rarely in other species. Ewes abort typically late in pregnancy without premonitory signs or after effects, except for a vulvar discharge and occasionally a retained placenta. Bovine abortions follow similar patterns.

Chlamydial pneumonias, seen particularly in cats, sheep, goats, and cattle, are often subclinical or part of mixed infections (enzootic sheep pneumonia, shipping fever). The clinical importance of uncomplicated infections (e.g., "feline pneumonitis") is uncertain.

Chlamydial polyarthritis affects mainly lambs and calves. In "stiff lamb disease," morbidity may be 80%, but the mortality rate is <1%. In calves, there may be systemic complications and high mortality.

Chlamydial conjunctivitis, although reported in cattle, dogs, pigs, guinea pigs, and koalas, is most noted in cats and lambs. It may pass through acute and prolonged chronic phases. In lambs, where it accompanies polyarthritis, secondary complications, keratitis, and corneal ulcerations are seen.

Sporadic bovine encephalomyelitis (SBE) is a febrile disease predominantly of young cattle producing locomotor, postural, and behavioral disturbances. There may be mild cough, nasal discharge, and diarrhea. The disease lasts from days to weeks, and morbidity and case fatality rates may reach 50%. Some outbreaks may continue for months, with new cases appearing irregularly.

Clinical intestinal infections are seen in young animals, especially calves, and may be phases of systemic chlamydiosis (SBE, polyarthritis, ornithosis).

Chlamydiosis occurs in snowshoe hares, muskrats, ferrets, opossums, and guinea pig colonies.

Epidemiology

Chlamydia psittaci is recognized worldwide in most animal species that have been adequately studied. It should be pointed out, however, that many of the studies used to define the epidemiology of a chlamydial infection thought to be caused by *C. psittaci* may have been caused by *C. pecorum*.

Commensal intestinal carriage and latent infections are common. Infected individuals, regardless of clinical history, can excrete the organism in high concentration for indefinite periods and constitute significant reservoirs of infection.

Host-species predilection is related to immunotype and DNA endonuclease digestion patterns. The most noted zoonotic form, psittacosis (ornithosis), an often severe respiratory disease with systemic complications, is usually traced to birds.

IMMUNOLOGIC FACTORS

Recovery and Resistance

Ewes that have aborted rarely abort again, and calves recovered from SBE resist reinfection. In other chlamydial diseases, which are often chronic and marked by remissions and relapses, there is little evidence of heightened resistance.

Cell-mediated and humoral immune responses are demonstrable by skin tests, lymphocyte stimulation tests, and serological reactions. Protective responses appear to be cell-mediated.

Artificial Immunization

Vaccination of animals against chlamydial infections often produces only short-lived partial protection, except against enzootic abortion of ewes (see under *Treatment and Control,* p. 176).

LABORATORY DIAGNOSIS

Diagnosis requires laboratory confirmation. Chlamydial inclusions — that is, intracytoplasmic colonies of reticulate and elementary bodies — may often be demonstrated by appropriate stains (Fig 32.2) including immunofluorescence within infected epithelium and macrophages. An enzyme-linked immunoadsorbent assay (ELISA) technique detects chlamydial antigen in vaginal discharges.

Isolation

Chlamydiae are isolated on tissue culture line cells (L-cells) or in fertile chicken eggs. Decontamination of suspect feces, placentas, urine, semen, and conjunctival fluids can be accomplished by treatment with combinations of gentamicin (50 µg/ml), vancomycin (75 µg/ml), and nystatin (500 units/ml). With tissue culture, centrifugation of the inoculum onto the monolayer on a cover slip is beneficial, and addition of cycloheximide (2 µg/ml) provides an added boost to chlamydiae. Growth should occur within 2 to 3 days of incubation.

Eggs are inoculated into the yolk sac and candled daily thereafter. Yolk sacs of embryos dying 3 or more days after inoculation are examined for chlamydial inclusions.

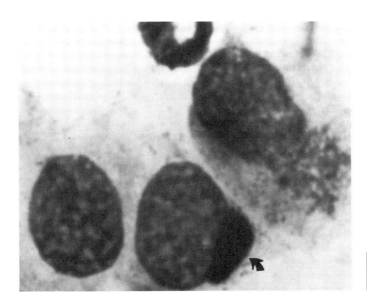

FIGURE 32.2.   *Chlamydial inclusion (arrow) in a conjunctival epithelial cell from a kitten. Wright stain, about 1000×.*

By either method serial subpasses are required to rule out chlamydiosis.

Presumptive isolates can be confirmed serologically by immunofluorescence or complement fixation tests.

In assessing the significance of chlamydial isolations, one must consider possible contamination by intestinal chlamydiae and rule out *Coxiella burnetti* (Chapter 53), which resembles chlamydiae.

Serologic Tests

Complement fixation and ELISA tests are not generally available to veterinarians, although genus-specific antigens are marketed. The presence of antibody confirms a diagnosis only if its titer increased fourfold during the course of illness.

TREATMENT AND CONTROL

Treatment

Tetracycline has been the drug of choice in the treatment of chlamydial infections. In birds, flock treatment involves incorporating the drug in feed. Moderate doses (200 g/ton) are adequate for disease control in turkeys. Higher doses (2800 g/ton) are needed for tissue clearance. To limit outbreaks of abortion in ewes, intramuscular injections (20 mg/kg) of long-acting forms are given at 2-week intervals. Tetracycline is given orally to lambs (150 to 200 mg/kg) to prevent arthritis. For pet birds, tetracycline-containing millet (0.5 mg/g) is available.

Prevention

Vaccination against *C. psittaci* infections has had variable success. Formalinized vaccines are beneficial in preventing enzootic ovine abortion. Feline chlamydial vaccines containing modified live or killed organisms attenuate clinical illness without curing or prevent-

ing infection. A vaccine for avian chlamydiosis is not available.

Prompt disposal of infected material and segregation of affected animals is helpful in control of ovine abortion. Young turkey poults should be placed in clean quarters, with no access to infected droppings and unexposed to potentially contaminated air currents.

Regulations governing import of exotic birds are designed to minimize introduction of psittacosis into household and resident bird populations.

SELECTED REFERENCES

Barron AL. Microbiology of *chlamydia*. Boca Raton, FL: CRC, 1988.

Beatty WL, Belanger TA, Desai AA, et al. Tryptophan depletion as a mechanism of gamma interferon-mediated chlamydial persistence. Infect Immun 1994;62:3705.

Beatty WL, Morrison RP, Byrne GI. Persistent chlamydiae: from cell culture to a paradigm for chlamydial pathogenesis. Microbiol Rev 1994;58:686.

Black CM. Current methods of laboratory diagnosis of *Chlamydia trachomatis* infections. Clin Microbiol Rev 1997; 10:160.

Buxton D. *Chlamydia psittaci* of ovine origin: an especial risk to pregnant women. In: Aitken ID, ed. Chlamydial diseases. Luxembourg: Office of Official Publications of the European Communities, 1986:121.

Cutlip RC, Smith RC, Page LA. Chlamydial polyarthritis of lambs. A review. J Am Vet Med Assoc 1972;161:1213.

Fukushi H, Hirai K. Proposal of *Chlamydia pecorum* sp. nov. for *Chlamydia* strains derived from ruminants. Int J Syst Bacteriol 1992;42:306.

Grayston JT, Kuo C-C, Campbell LA, Wang S-P. *Chlamydia pneumoniae* sp. nov. for *Chlamydia* sp. strain TWAR. Int J Syst Bacteriol 1989;39:88.

Grimes JE. Chlamydiosis in psittacine birds. J Am Vet Med Assoc 1987;190:394.

Harshfield GS. Sporadic bovine encephalomyelitis. J Am Vet Med Assoc 1970;156:466.

Isberg RR, Nhieu GTV. Two mammalian cell internalization strategies used by pathogenic bacteria. Annu Rev Genet 1994; 27:395.

Kaltenboeck B, Kousoulas KG, Storz J. Structures of and allelic diversity and relationships among the major outer membrane protein (*ompA*) genes of the four chlamydial species. J Bacteriol 1993;175:487.

Kirkbride CA. Diagnosis in 1,784 ovine abortions and stillbirths. J Vet Diagn Invest 1993;5:398.

Kuo C, Jackson LA, Campbell LA, Grayson JT. *Chlamydia pneumoniae* (TWAR). Clin Microbiol Rev 1995;8:451.

Moulder JW. Interaction of chlamydiae and host cells in vitro. Microbiol Rev 1991;55:143.

Nasisse MP, Guy JS, Stevens JB, et al. Clinical and laboratory findings in chronic conjunctivitis in cats: 91 cases (1983–1991). J Am Vet Med Assoc 1993;203:834.

Nietfeld JC, Leslie-Steen P, Zeman DH, Nelson D. Prevalence of intestinal chlamydial infection in pigs in the midwest, as determined by immunoperoxidase staining. Am J Vet Res 1997;58:260.

Peeling RW, Brunham RC. Chlamydiae as pathogens: new species and new issues. Emerg Infect Dis 1996;2:307.

Psittacosis Compendium Committee. Compendium of chlamydiosis (psittacosis) control, 1995. J Am Vet Med Assoc 1995; 206:1874.

Stephens RS. Molecular mimicry and *Chlamydia trachomatis* infection of eukaryotic cells. Trends Microbiol 1994;2:99.

Szeredi L, Schiller I, Sydler T, et al. Intestinal *Chlamydia* in finishing pigs. Vet Pathol 1996;33:369.

Vanrompay D, Ducatelle R, Haesebrouck F. *Chlamydia psittaci* infections: a review with emphasis on avian chlamydiosis. Vet Microbiol 1995;45:93.

Wills JM. Effect of vaccination on feline *Chlamydia psittaci* infection. Infect Immun 1987;55:2653.

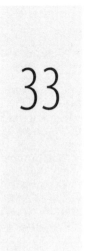

33

The Urinary Tract as a Microbial Habitat; Urinary Tract Infections

ERNST L. BIBERSTEIN   DWIGHT C. HIRSH

ANTIMICROBIAL DEFENSES OF THE URINARY TRACT

Because it is primarily an excretory system, the urinary tract is not subject to massive microbial exposure and has developed few specifically antimicrobial defenses. Protective features include the following:

1. The flow of urine, its direction, diluting effect, and frequent periodic removal, discourage the establishment of microorganisms in the normally sterile portions of the tract — that is, the kidneys, ureters, bladder, and proximal male urethra.
2. Bacterial interference may restrict colonization of the lower urinary tract by transient organisms.
3. The glycoprotein "slime" layer covering the epithelium may inhibit some bacterial adhesion.
4. Epithelial desquamation and a prompt, largely neutrophilic inflammatory response to bacterial colonization aid in clearing the bladder wall of invaders. In the lumen of the bladder, phagocytosis is less efficient.
5. Urine has certain antimicrobial properties.
   a. High osmolality (>1000 mOsm/kg) reduces growth, particularly of rod-shaped bacteria, in urine. It may, however, depress leukocyte activity and preserve bacteria with cell walls damaged by immune reactions or antibiotic therapy. Combined with high concentrations of ammonia, which is anticomplementary, it may contribute to the high susceptibility of the renal medulla to infection.
   b. While extremes in pH discourage multiplication of some bacteria, ranges bactericidal to common urinary tract pathogens are unlikely.
   c. Of urine constituents, urea imparts to urine an unexplained bacteriostatic effect, which is diminished by removal of urea from urine and enhanced by dietary supplementation. Methionine and hippuric and ascorbic acids produce an antibacterial effect largely by acidifying the urine. Urinary ammonium nitrogen is linked with antibacterial properties, as are prostatic secretion in humans.

All properties described above were observed in voided urine. All the same, most urines support in vitro growth of many microorganisms.

Immune responses to urinary tract infections have been studied mostly on humans or laboratory animals. Serum and urinary antibody titers tend to be low in cystitis and asymptomatic infections, high in pyelonephritis. Secretory IgA (sIgA) tends to be most prominent in urine, but IgG and IgM antibodies also occur regularly. Serum IgA, IgG, IgM, and sIgA antibodies are produced, particularly in kidney infection. The protective function of these antibodies is uncertain.

Cell-mediated responses are reportedly suppressed in pyelonephritis, less so in lower tract infection.

BACTERIA ENCOUNTERED IN THE URINARY TRACT

Small numbers of bacteria may enter the bladder via the urethra, especially in the female, but are normally removed during urination.

The canine distal urethra, external genitalia, and perineum are populated by resident and transient microorganisms. The resident flora of at least the external genitalia includes commensal anaerobes, which are largely gram-negative non-spore-formers; *Mycoplasma* spp.; alpha-hemolytic and beta-hemolytic streptococci; lactobacilli; *Haemophilus* spp. (particularly *H. haemoglobinophilus*); corynebacteria; propionibacteria; and coagulase-negative staphylococci. These, with the possible exception of mycoplasmas, rarely cause urinary tract infection.

Among the transients, which are derived from rectum and perineum, the most significant are *Escherichia coli*, coagulase-positive staphylococci, *Proteus* spp. (especially *P. mirabilis*), enterococci, *Klebsiella pneumoniae*, and *Pseudomonas aeruginosa*. These account for 85% to 90% of the bacteriuric episodes in dogs. The remainder involve mostly, in approximate order of prevalence, *Enterobacter* spp., beta-hemolytic streptococci (mainly Group G), *Mycoplasma* spp., *Providencia* spp., *P. vulgaris*, *Citrobacter* spp., *Pasteurella* spp., and *Candida albicans*.

URINARY TRACT INFECTIONS OF DOGS

Etiologic Agents

The prevalence of agents implicated in urinary tract infections (UTI) is shown in Table 33.1. Bacteria capable of initiating UTI require virulence determinants, the most firmly established of which are adhesins (e.g., the pyelonephritis-associated pilus, Pap). Other properties associated with UTI agents (*E. coli*) and rare in random *E. coli* strains, are resistant to serum bactericidal action, hemolytic activity, and possession of certain O-antigens and bacteriocins. These observations suggest that agents of urinary tract infections represent a select subpopulation within their species.

Host Factors

Interference with the free flow of urine and with complete emptying of the bladder predisposes to UTI. This can be due to tumors, polyps, calculi, anatomic anomalies, and neural defects. Vesico-ureteral reflux, the re-entry of urine into the ureters during urination, causes bladder urine to reach the renal pelvis, possibly carrying bacteria into a susceptible area. Reflux is aggravated (perhaps initiated) by infection and complicates existing infections by increasing the likelihood of renal involve-ment. It is a problem in humans and also occurs in dogs. Its significance in canine UTI is not known.

Other host factors include endocrine disturbances such as diabetes mellitus and hyperadrenocorticism (Cushing's disease). Long-term use of corticosteroids appears to predispose dogs to UTI. Canine UTI occurs at approximately equal frequencies in males and females.

Routes of Infection

There are three ways bacteria can reach the urinary tract:

1. The ascending route via the urethra is the most likely way. The abundance of the common agents near the urethral orifice and the usual localization of infection in the bladder point to this as a probable portal of entrance.
2. Hematogenous infection of the urinary tract occurs secondarily to bacteremia and primarily affects the kidneys. It is rare, due probably to the high resistance of the renal cortex, where it must start. It occurs naturally in septicemia, especially of young animals, resulting frequently in multiple cortical abscesses. Leptospirae (Chapter 34) infect kidneys by the hematogenous route.
3. UTI via lymphatic pathways from the gut is of undetermined importance.

The Infectious Process

Ability to adhere to epithelium is considered a prerequisite to establishment of UTI. Fimbrial attachment of *E. coli* to surface slime glycoproteins by Type I (mannose-

Table 33.1. Leading Bacterial Causes of Urinary Tract Infections (UTI) in Dogs

Species	Prevalence in UTI (%)	Typical Colonies on:		Confirmatory Tests		
		Blood Agar	MacConkey Agar	Gram Stain	Oxidase	Catalase
Escherichia coli	42–46	Smooth grey; often hemolytic	Red discrete, surrounded by red haze	Negative rods	Negative	NA
Enterococcus spp.	11–14	Very small (<1mm) α, β, or γ	No growth	Positive cocci	—	Negative
Coagulase positive *Staphylococcus*	12	White or off-white (often hemolytic)	No growth	Positive cocci	—	Positive
Proteus mirabilis	6–12	Swarms; no discrete colonies	Colorless	Negative rods	Negative	—
Klebsiella spp.	8–12	Large, wet mucoid, whitish-grey	Pink, slimy coalescing; not surrounded by red haze	Negative rods	Negative	—
Pseudomonas spp.	<5	Gray to greenish-gray; fruity or ammonia odor; often hemolytic	Colorless, surrounded by blue-green pigment	Negative rods	Positive	—

NA = not applicable.

sensitive) pili is probably of less significance than that mediated by several mannose-resistant adhesins, one of which is Pap, that attach to cell membrane glycolipids. Mannose-resistant adhesins occur commonly in uropathogenic *E. coli*, but irregularly in other strains.

The infection may begin with colonization of the urethral orifice by a potential pathogen that, through multiplication, extension along the epithelial surface, or migration through active motility or random movement, reaches the bladder. The resulting infection, after further multiplication, is marked by bacteriuria and usually pyuria and low-grade proteinuria. Inflammation is triggered by the interaction of lipopolysaccharide (gram negatives) or muramyl dipeptides (gram positives) with transitional cells of the bladder that then secrete IL-8 which attracts polymorphonuclear neutrophil leukocytes (PMNs). Often it is asymptomatic. Signs when present include dysuria or urinary frequency or urgency. There may be hematuria and incontinence.

The most serious complication of lower urinary tract infection is *pyelonephritis* caused by ascending infection via the ureters, which is aided often by vesicourethral and intrarenal bacterial reflux.

Signs of pyelonephritis are vague. Fever is transient even during the acute phase. Pain in the thoracolumbar area is not specific unless directly associated with kidney palpation. Urinalysis may reveal lowered specific gravity and casts. In advanced cases, blood urea nitrogen is elevated.

Uroliths of dogs are predominantly (70%) "infection stones" consisting of struvite or apatite, or various combinations, and are often called *triple phosphate* stones. Urease-producing bacteria are implicated — in dogs, chiefly coagulase-positive staphylococci, and to a lesser extent *Proteus mirabilis* (in humans, *P. mirabilis*). Inhibition of urease activity by urea analogues (e.g., acetohydroxamic acid) can suppress infection stone formation.

LABORATORY DIAGNOSIS OF URINARY TRACT INFECTIONS

Collection of Samples

Urine obtained by normal voiding ("clean midstream catch"), the usual collection method in humans, invariably contains some contaminants that must be taken into consideration in the interpretation of growth from such samples.

Catheterization yields less contaminated samples but cannot elude the normal flora of the distal urethra, which not only contaminates the sample but is introduced into a bladder that may have been sterile. Catheterization, especially if done repeatedly, may also cause irritation and trauma so that problems may be initiated where none existed before.

Antepubic cystocentesis (bladder tap) by needle and syringe is the most desirable for microbiological diagnosis. Any bacteria in samples properly collected by this technique have originated in the bladder. The procedure is performed under strict asepsis and only on a palpably filled bladder. A minimum of 5 ml should be submitted for culture.

Sample Processing

Transportation.   If culture has to be delayed for more than 2 hours after collection, the sample should be refrigerated. Relevant bacteria — except possibly *Mycoplasma* spp. — survive refrigeration for several hours.

Commercial urine transport media extend the permissible delay at ambient temperatures between collection and culture to 24 hours.

Direct Microscopic Examination

Unstained Urine.   The presence of inflammatory cells in unstained sediment from 5 ml of urine (>3/field at 400× magnification in urine obtained by cystocentesis; >8 otherwise) suggests infection. Bacteria, if present in appreciable numbers, can be detected at this magnification and their morphology (rods vs. cocci) can often be recognized, permitting prompt therapeutic decisions, especially with urine collected by bladder tap.

Stained Smear.   The observation of more than 1 organism in every 10 oil immersion fields of gram-stained films of uncentrifuged urine would suggest more than 10^5 bacteria per milliliter of the original urine, a level considered "significant" by traditional standards (see below) when observed in urine obtained by midstream catch or by catheterization.

Isolation of UTI Agents

Quantitative Considerations.   By comparisons between midstream urine samples from pyelonephritic and normal women, the threshold of "significant bacteria" was determined to be more than 10^5 organisms per milliliter. This criterion has also been found useful in canine urology. Accordingly, urine culture procedures are designed to permit rough quantitation of bacteriuria. The threshold 10^5 of bacteria per milliliter cannot be applied without reference to clinical and clinicopathological considerations. In dogs and humans, serious infections can exist at bacteriuria levels well below this threshold. Conversely, "significant bacteriuria" is seen in the absence of illness. Asymptomatic bacteriuria in human adults has not been proven to be a forerunner of kidney disease, and its treatment as an illness has been questioned. Although a majority of canine bacteriuria episodes are asymptomatic, their relation to pyelonephritis is undetermined. They are treated as clinical cases.

Standard Culture.   Within its interpretive limitations, quantitative culture remains a standard procedure for culturing urine obtained by midstream catch or by catheterization and is carried out by the surface plating of 1 μl and/or 10 μl amounts of fresh, well-mixed urine on blood agar and a selective enteric medium, such as MacConkey agar. Special media for the recovery of *Mycoplasma* spp.

and *Ureaplasma* spp. can be included. Inocula are applied by calibrated loops. Some laboratories culture only one amount. Culture of sediment is advisable for monitoring patients under treatment or detecting specific organisms of interest (e.g., *Salmonella*).

Culture of urine obtained by bladder tap is performed by inoculating a portion of sediment to blood agar and a selective medium (MacConkey agar). Recovery of bacteria in any number is considered significant.

Identification. Recovered bacteria can be identified by the characteristics described in relevant chapters. The six bacterial agents accounting for nearly 90% of canine UTI (see above) can usually be identified by their growth patterns on blood and MacConkey agars as shown in Table 33.1.

A pour-plate method employing a nonselective, bloodless medium is optimal for quantitative accuracy but must be used in conjunction with surface plating for prompt characterization of isolates.

Recovery of more than one species in significant numbers from cystocentesis is common in dogs (15% to 20% of UTI).

Alternative Tests. A variety of usually miniaturized devices — paddles, cups, strips, slides — are available for semiquantitative culture of UTI agents and their presumptive identifications. Most are satisfactory for screening purposes and for monitoring effects of therapy, but they are designed for detecting more than 10^5 organisms per milliliter and are thus only useful for urine obtained by midstream catch or by catheterization.

Some test systems are based on instantaneous chemical reactions. One of these systems tests for nitrite, a product of bacterial reduction of urinary nitrate. It works only when bacteria have been in contact with urine in the bladder for extended periods (overnight), a condition rarely satisfied by dogs visiting veterinary clinics. Another detects the presence of leukocytic enzymes, thereby indirectly reflecting a likely state of infection. This test is not an adequate indicator of "significant" bacteriuria in dogs.

Localization of Urinary Tract Infection. Available methods for distinguishing cystitis from pyelonephritis are bladder washout, demonstration of antibody-coated bacteria, ureteral catheterization, and use of isotopes with affinity for inflammatory tissue. The first two have been used in veterinary medicine.

In bladder washout following the demonstration of bacteriuria, the bladder is drained and flushed with an antimicrobial solution. A sample drawn from the bladder immediately afterward is usually sterile. A subsequent urine sample is collected 15 minutes later. If the infection was confined to the bladder, this will be sterile. If the source of the bacteriuria was the kidney, the follow-up samples will have bacterial contents similar to those obtained before washout.

Antibody-coated bacteria in urine, demonstrable by fluorescent anti-immunoglobulin, have been described as indicative of renal infection. Tests employing the procedure on dogs of known infected status yielded many false results.

THERAPY

Susceptibility tests are recommended. The interpretive standards used must be based on antimicrobic concentrations in urine. Disc diffusion (Kirby-Bauer) tests are irrelevant. Antimicrobial susceptibilities of common urinary isolates are shown in Tables 33.2 through 33.7.

Therapy should be continued for 2 weeks for cystitis. For pyelonephritis, longer treatment may be required.

Table 33.2. Susceptibility of Canine Urinary Isolates of *Escherichia coli* to Antimicrobial Agents

Antibiotic	% Susceptible
Ampicillin	77
Amoxicillin-clavulanate	96
Cephalosporin	77
Chloramphenicol	76
Enrofloxacin	85
Tetracycline	52
Trimethoprim sulfanate	68

From the Veterinary Medical Teaching Hospital, University of California, Davis.

Table 33.3. Susceptibility of Canine Urinary Isolates of *Enterococcus* to Antimicrobial Agents

Antibiotic	% Susceptible
Ampicillin	72
Amoxicillin-clavulanate	97
Cephalosporin	54
Chloramphenicol	100
Enrofloxacin	79
Tetracycline	95
Trimethoprim sulfanate	92

From the Veterinary Medical Teaching Hospital, University of California, Davis.

Table 33.4. Susceptibility of Canine Urinary Isolates of Coagulase Positive *Staphylococcus* to Antimicrobial Agents

Antibiotic	% Susceptible
Ampicillin	100
Amoxicillin-clavulanate	100
Cephalosporin	100
Chloramphenicol	100
Enrofloxacin	100
Tetracycline	100
Trimethoprim sulfanate	87

From the Veterinary Medical Teaching Hospital, University of California, Davis.

Table 33.5.   Susceptibility of Canine Urinary Isolates of *Klebsiella* to Antimicrobial Agents

Antibiotic	% Susceptible
Ampicillin	94
Amoxicillin-clavulanate	100
Cephalosporin	94
Chloramphenicol	94
Enrofloxacin	100
Tetracycline	100
Trimethoprim sulfanate	100

From the Veterinary Medical Teaching Hospital, University of California, Davis.

Table 33.6.   Susceptibility of Canine Urinary Isolates of *Proteus mirabilis* to Antimicrobial Agents

Antibiotic	% Susceptible
Ampicillin	97
Amoxicillin-clavulanate	100
Cephalosporin	97
Chloramphenicol	100
Enrofloxacin	100
Tetracycline	94
Trimethoprim sulfanate	90

From the Veterinary Medical Teaching Hospital, University of California, Davis.

Table 33.7.   Susceptibility of Canine Urinary Isolates of *Pseudomonas aeruginosa* to Antimicrobial Agents

Antibiotic	% Susceptible
Ampicillin	0
Amoxicillin-clavulanate	0
Cephalosporin	0
Chloramphenicol	56
Enrofloxacin	100
Tetracycline	94
Trimethoprim sulfanate	100

From the Veterinary Medical Teaching Hospital, University of California, Davis.

URINARY TRACT INFECTIONS OF CATS

Urinary tract disorders of cats are collectively called *feline urological syndrome (FUS)*. Viral, nutritional, and metabolic factors have been implicated in the etiology, particularly of obstructive forms. When bacteria are recognized as causes of feline UTI, it is usually in association with systemic disturbances, including immunosuppressive drug therapy. Feline urine is more inhibitory to bacterial

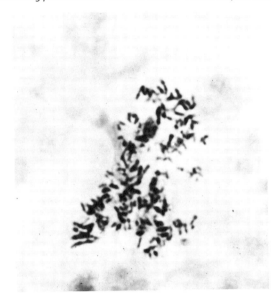

FIGURE 33.1.   Corynebacterium renale *in urinary sediment of a cow with pyelonephritis. Note "diphtheroid" configurations, including palisades and "Chinese letters." Gram stain, 3000×.*

growth than human or canine urine, perhaps owing to its higher osmolality. The agents found in the relatively rare instances of high-level bacteriuria are most frequently coliforms and coagulase-positive staphylococci.

CORYNEBACTERIUM RENALE GROUP

Diphtheroid bacteria, traditionally called *Corynebacterium renale* but actually constituting three species (see below), colonize the lower genital tract of cattle and sometimes sheep. Associated diseases are bovine pyelonephritis and ovine posthitis (pizzle rot).

DESCRIPTIVE FEATURES

These bacteria are diphtheroids in staining properties, cell wall composition, and cellular configurations (see Fig 33.1). Metachromatic granules may be present. No capsules are formed. Fibrillar surface structures (pili, fimbriae) are present. Renalin, a CAMP-like protein (Chapter 22), is produced.

Members of the *C. renale* group are facultative anaerobes capable of growing on most common laboratory media.

Pyelonephritis in cattle is more frequently caused by *E. coli.*

Nonhemolytic, opaque, off-white colonies develop within 48 hours at 37°C on blood agar.

Members of the *C. renale* group have impressive urease activity, which is demonstrable in most strains within minutes of contact with its substrate. Glucose is slowly acidified, other carbohydrates variably so. All strains are catalase positive. The agents are not particularly resistant to heat or disinfectants.

Three serotypes were found, by DNA homology studies, to constitute separate species: *C. renale* (Type I), *C. cystidis* (Type II), and *C. pilosum* (Type III). Type III strains are the most and Type II the least virulent in bovine UTI.

Ecology

Reservoir

Members of the *C. renale* group inhabit the lower genital tract of cattle and sometimes other ruminants. Occasionally they are implicated in urinary tract disease of sheep, horses, dogs, and nonhuman primates. No human infections are known. Distribution is global.

Transmission

Organisms pass between animals by direct and indirect contact. Many clinical cases are probably endogenous.

Pathogenesis

Pili-mediated attachment to urothelium and urea hydrolysis are considered critical in pathogenesis. Urea breakdown with production of ammonia initiates an inflammatory process, high alkalinity in urine (pH > 9.0), and suppression of antibacterial defenses, possibly through complement inactivation by ammonia.

Pathology. A chronic pyelonecrotic process attacks successively the bladder, ureter(s), renal pelvis, and renal parenchyma.

Disease Patterns. In cattle, the process is an ascending urinary tract infection, beginning with cystitis, which proceeds to ureteritis and pyelonephritis. Rectal palpation reveals thickened bladder and ureteral walls, distended ureters, and enlarged kidneys with obscured lobulations. Early cases show pollakiuria, hematuria, and increasing degrees of abdominal pain. Chronic infections progress to debilitation and death due to uremia.

The more common form of infection in sheep is posthitis or "pizzle rot," a necrotizing inflammation of the prepuce and adjacent tissues in wethers or rams. Disease develops in the presence of the urealytic agent in an area constantly irrigated with urine. Ammonia is thought to initiate the inflammatory process. A similar condition occurs in goats. Only *C. renale* and *C. pilosum* have been found in ovine posthitis.

Epidemiology

Bovine pyelonephritis is found mostly in cows near parturition, appearing as an opportunistic infection by a commensal organism. Bulls are rarely affected, but are commensal hosts of all three types and the sole commensal source of Type III (*C. cystitidis*).

Pizzle rot occurs typically in animals on rich legume pasture that is high in proteins, which increase urea excretion, and estrogens, which cause preputial swelling and urine retention in the sheath.

Immunologic Aspects

No useful immunity develops in the course of the infection. Serum antibody is present and antibody coating (mostly IgG) of bacteria in urine occurs in bovine pyelonephritis (not cystitis).

No immunizing agents exist.

Laboratory Diagnosis

Gross examination of urine may reveal the presence of red blood cells and high alkalinity (pH 9.0). Microscopically, packets of pleomorphic gram-positive diphtheroid rods are seen (see Fig 33.1). The agent is readily cultured from sediment. A generous inoculum of colonial growth planted in one spot on a Christensen's urea agar slant will produce an alkaline shift, indicating urea hydrolysis, within minutes of inoculation. A diphtheroid isolate from urine capable of producing this reaction and fermenting glucose probably belongs to the *C. renale* group.

Treatment and Control

Members of the *C. renale* group are susceptible to penicillin, but antimicrobic therapy is successful only in the early stage of the infection.

Ovine posthitis is treated by surgical care of lesions, local antiseptic applications, dietary restriction, and testosterone administration.

Eubacterium suis

An anaerobic diphtheroid, first described as *Corynebacterium suis*, causes urinary tract infection of sows. Like bovine pyelonephritis, the disease is an apparently ascending infection by a urealytic diphtheroid agent, limited to females and often related to breeding operations, pregnancy, and parturition. Boars are frequent carriers. The infection is recognized primarily in Britain and continental Europe but also in North America, Australia, and Hong Kong. Treatment is rarely successful.

Selected References

Urinary Tract Infections of Dogs (and Cats)

Clarridge JE, Pezzio MT, Vosti KL. Laboratory diagnosis of urinary tract infections. CUIMITECH 2A. Washington: American Society for Microbiology, 1987.

Ihrke PJ, Norton AL, Ling GV, Stannard AA. Urinary tract infection associated with long-term corticosteroid administration in dogs with chronic skin diseases. J Am Vet Med Assoc 1985;186:43.

Johnson JR. Virulence factors in *Escherichia coli* urinary tract infections. Clin Microbiol Rev 1991;4:80.

Ko Y, Mukaida N, Ishiyama S, et al. Elevated interleukin-8 levels in the urine of patients with urinary tract infections. Infect Immun 1993;61:1307.

Ling GV. Lower urinary tract diseases of dogs and cats: diagnosis, medical management, prevention. St. Louis: Mosby-Year Book, 1995.

Low DA, Braaten BA, Ling GV, et al. Isolation and comparison of *Escherichia coli* strains from canine and human patients with urinary tract infections. Infect Immun 1988;56:2601.

Roberts JA. Pathogenesis of pyelonephritis. J Urol 1983;129:1102.

Roberts JA. Tropism in bacterial infections: urinary tract infections. J Urol 1996;156:1552.

Corynebacterium renale

Barajas-Rojas JA, Biberstein EL. The diphtheroid agent of ovine posthitis: its relationship to *Corynebacterium renale*. J Comp Pathol 1974;84:301.

Brown MA, Kadis S, Chapman WL. Evaluation of penicillin in conjunction with acetohydroxamic acid in treatment of experimental *Corynebacterium renale* pyelonephritis. Can J Microbiol 1981;27:1306.

Coyle MB, Lipsky BA. Coryneform bacteria in infectious diseases: clinical and laboratory aspects. Clin Microbiol Rev 1990; 3:227.

Hayashi A. Adhesion of bovine urinary corynebacteria to the epithelial cells of various parts of the bovine urinary tract, and survival of the bacteria in soil. Jpn J Vet Res 1984;32:90.

Nicolet J, Fey H. Antibody-coated bacteria in urine sediment from cattle infected with *Corynebacterium renale*. Vet Rec 1979;105:301.

Patti JM, Allen BL, McGavin MJ, Hook M. MSCRAMM-mediated adherence of microorganisms to host tissues. Annu Rev Microbiol 1994;48:585.

Rebhun WC, Dill SG, Peerdrizet JA, Hatfield CE. Pyelonephritis in cows: 15 cases (1982–1986). J Am Vet Med Assoc 1989; 194:953.

Shelton M, Livingstone CW. Posthitis in angora wether goats. J Am Vet Med Assoc 1975;167:154.

Yanagawa R, Honda E. *Corynebacterium pilosum* and *Corynebacterium cystitidis*, two new species from cows. Int J Syst Bacteriol 1978;28:209.

Eubacterium (Corynebacterium) suis

Jones JET, Daynall GJR. The carriage of *Corynebacterium suis* in male pigs. J Hyg 1984;93:381.

Narucka V, Westendorp JE. *Corynebacterium suis* in swine II. Netherlands J Vet Sci 1975;5:116.

Soltys MA. *Corynebacterium suis* associated with a specific cystitis and pyelonephritis. J Pathol Bacteriol 1961;81:441.

Weigienek J, Reddy A. Taxonomic study of "*Corynebacterium suis*" Soltys and Spratling: proposal of *Eubacterium suis* (nom. rev.) comb. nov. Int J Syst Bact 1982;32:218.

34 *Leptospirae*

Rance B. LeFebvre

Leptospirae are spirochetes that are morphologically and physiologically uniform but serologically and epidemiologically diverse. Domestic animals most commonly affected are dogs, cattle, swine, and horses. Canine leptospirosis manifestations are septicemic, hepatic, and renal disease. In cattle and swine, septic illness is largely confined to the young, while abortion is the principal manifestation in adults. Abortion and recurrent uveitis (moon blindness, or periodic ophthalmia) are the most common manifestations in horses. California sea lions are also susceptible to acute, septicemic leptospiral infections. Other host species, though susceptible to infection, develop clinical signs less frequently. Leptospirosis in humans is typically an acute febrile disease.

Taxonomy studies, based on DNA analyses, have led to the description of eight pathogenic species: *Leptospira borgpetersenii, L. inadae, L. interrogans sensu stricto, L. kirschneri, L. meyeri, L. noguchii, L. santarosae,* and *L. weilee.* Leptospires have historically been classified by antigenic composition divided into 23 serogroups and greater than 200 serovars. Reference to serovars is more common in clinical settings. Serovars important in North America and their principal hosts and clinical hosts (in parentheses) are:

> *L. icterohaemorrhagiae:* rodents (dogs, horses, cattle, swine)
> *L. grippotyphosa:* rodents (dogs, cattle, swine)
> *L. canicola:* dogs (swine, cattle)
> *L. pomona:* cattle, swine (horses, sheep, sea lions)
> *L. hardjo:* cattle
> *L. bratislava:* swine (horses, sea lions)

DESCRIPTIVE FEATURES

Morphology and Staining

Leptospirae (from the Greek *leptos,* meaning "thin") are thin spiral organisms $0.1\,\mu m \times 6\,\mu m$ to $20\,\mu m$. Because they stain poorly, they require darkfield or phase contrast microscopy for visualization. The spirals are best demonstrated by electron microscopy. Typical cells have a hook at each end making them S- or C-shaped. Wet mounts reveal them to be motile.

Leptospirae are gram negative but unrecognizable in routinely fixed stained smears. They can be demonstrated by fluorescent antibody or silver impregnation (Fig 34.1).

Cellular Anatomy and Composition

Leptospiral cells consist of an outer sheath, axial fibrils ("endoflagella"), and a cytoplasmic cylinder. The outer sheath combines features of a capsule and outer membrane. The cytoplasmic cylinder is covered by a cell membrane and the peptidoglycan layer of the cell wall.

Endotoxin is present in the cell wall. A hemolysin, sphingomyelinase C, is associated with some serovars and cytotoxicity has been demonstrated in vivo.

Growth Characteristics

Leptospirae are obligate aerobes, which grow optimally at 29°C to 30°C. Generation time averages about 12 hours. No growth occurs on blood agar or other routine media. Traditional media are essentially rabbit serum (<10%) in solutions ranging from normal saline to mixtures of peptones, vitamins, electrolytes, and buffers. Some newer media have substituted polysorbates and bovine albumin for rabbit serum. Protein is not required. Unlike most prokaryotes, leptospirae do not incorporate exogenous pyrimidines like the toxic 5-fluorouracil, which is used in leptospiral selective media.

Most media are fluid or semisolid (0.1% agar). In fluid media, little turbidity develops. In semisolid media, growth is concentrated in a disc — called a *dinger zone* — about 0.5 cm below the surface.

Biochemical Reactions

Leptospirae are oxidase and catalase positive; many have lipase activity. Some produce urease. Identification beyond genus is based on serology. However, the development of species specific DNA primers in conjunction with the polymerase chain reaction (PCR) is a promising new development for a more accurate characterization of pathogenic leptospirae.

Resistance

Leptospirae are killed by drying, freezing, heat (50°C for 10 minutes), soap, bile salts, detergents, acidic environments, and putrefaction. They persist in a moist, temperate environment at neutral to slightly alkaline pH (see *Epidemiology,* p. 187).

FIGURE 34.1.   Leptospira (interrogans serovar) pomona *in the renal tubules of a pig. Levaditi stain, 1000×.*

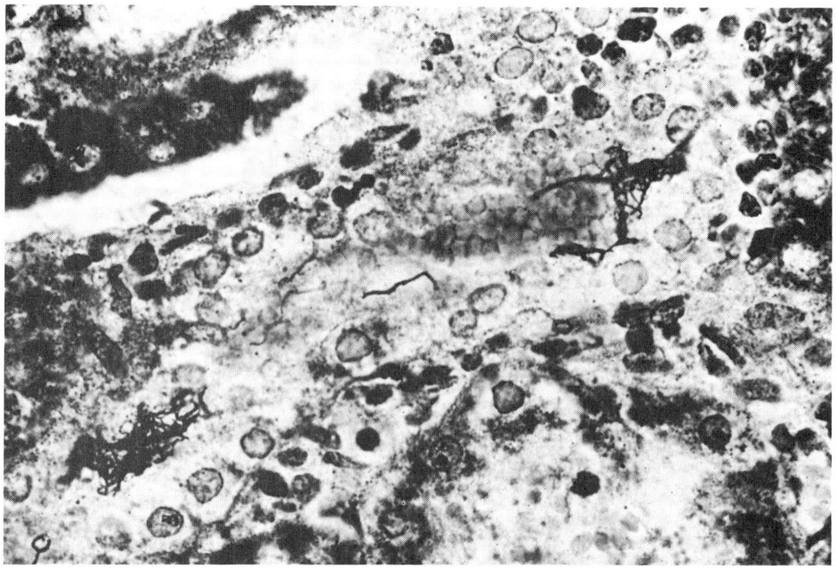

Variability

Greater than 200 serovars of parasitic leptospirae exist. They vary in host and geographic distribution and in pathogenicity.

ECOLOGY

Reservoir

Leptospira interrogans inhabits the tubules of mammalian kidneys. Leptospirae have been isolated from birds, reptiles, amphibians, and invertebrates, but the epidemiologic significance of such associations is not established.

Rodents are the most frequent leptospiral carriers, with wild carnivores ranking second. No mammal can be excluded as a possible host. Typically reservoir hosts show minimal, if any, signs of disease. Leptospirae and serovars *L. icterohaemorrhagiae, L. canicola, L. pomona, L. hardjo,* and *L. grippotyphosa* occur on all continents.

Transmission

Exposure is through contact of mucous membranes or skin with urine-contaminated water, fomites, or feed. Other sources are milk from acutely infected cows and genital excretions from cattle and swine of either sex.

Pathogenesis

Clinical and pathological manifestations suggest toxic mechanisms. Filtrates of tissue fluids from experimentally infected animals contain cytotoxic factors producing vascular lesions like leptospirosis.

The spirochetes enter the bloodstream subsequent to mucous membrane or reproductive inoculation, colonizing particularly liver and kidney, where they produce degenerative changes. Other affected organs may be muscles, eyes, and meninges, where a nonsuppurative meningitis may develop. Leptospirae damage vascular endothelium, resulting in hemorrhages. All serovars produce these changes to varying degrees. *Leptospira pomona* in cattle causes intravascular hemolysis due to a hemolytic exotoxin. Autoimmune phenomena may also contribute to this condition. Secondary changes include icterus due to liver damage and blood destruction, and acute, subacute, or subchronic nephritis due to renal tubular injury. The cellular exudates contain predominantly lymphocytes and plasma cells. In surviving animals, leptospirae disappear from circulation with the appearance of serum antibody but persist in the kidneys for many weeks (see Fig 34.1).

Disease Patterns. Most leptospiral infections run an inapparent course probably due to infection of the animal by a host-adapted serovar. Clinical infections manifesting overt signs are primarily due to non-host-adapted serovar infections. These occur mainly in dogs, cattle, and swine; increasingly in sea lions; occasionally in horses, goats, and sheep; and exceptionally in cats.

Dogs. Leading serovars involved are *L. icterohaemorrhagiae* and *L. canicola*, with the latter the more common. Increasing numbers of acute renal failure due to *L. grippotyphosa, L. pomona,* and *L. bratislava* infections are being reported. (Currently available vaccines for canine leptospirosis contain bacterins of *L. icterohaemorrhagiae* and *L. canicola* only).

The most acute form affects young pups preferentially, produces fever without localizing signs, and is commonly fatal within days. Hemorrhages are often apparent antemortem on mucous membranes and skin, or manifested by epistaxis or by blood-stained feces and vomitus. Icterus is absent.

The icteric type runs a slower course, and hemorrhages are less conspicuous. Icterus is prominent. Renal localization causes nitrogen retention, while renal casts and leukocytes appear in the urine.

The uremic type, centered in the kidneys, results subsequent to either of the types of infections described above or may develop in their absence. It may be acute and rapidly fatal with signs of gastrointestinal upsets, uremic breath, and ulcerations in the anterior alimentary tract; or it may run a slow course with delayed onset. The relationship of leptospirosis to chronic interstitial nephritis leading to uremic death is controversial.

Cattle. The predominant manifestation of bovine leptospirosis is abortion, usually late term, but may occur at any time following infection. Abortion is due to primary fetal death rather than placental infection. Fetal retention with progressive autolysis is common. Abortions due to *L. hardjo*, the host-adapted serogroup for cattle, is primarily a problem of heifers in dairies due to management practices that differ between beef cattle and dairy operations. *Leptospira hardjo* infections affect calves in utero, leading either to abortion or "weak-calf syndrome." These infections are often subclinical or may be marked by "milk-drop syndrome," reproductive failure, and infertility. Chronic infection of the kidneys and the shedding of leptospirae in urine are common.

Acute leptospirosis due to *L. pomona* affects mostly calves and sometimes adult cattle. It is marked by fever, hemoglobinuria, icterus, anemia, and a fatality rate of 5% to 15%.

In some parts of the world, *L. grippotyphosa*, *L. icterohaemorrhagiae*, and *L. canicola* cause bovine leptospirosis.

Swine. The serovars implicated in porcine leptospirosis include *L. pomona*, *L. icterohaemorrhagiae*, *L. canicola*, *L. tarassovi*, *L. bratislava*, and *L. muenchen*. As in bovine leptospirosis, septicemia with icterus and hemorrhages occurs, especially in piglets, while abortion and infertility are the manifestations in sows.

Horses. Equine leptospirosis is due most often to serovars *L. pomona*, *L. grippotyphosa*, and *L. icterohaemorrhagiae*. Signs in natural infections have been fever, mild icterus, and abortion. Leptospirosis is probably involved in equine recurrent iridocyclitis (periodic ophthalmia; see under *Immunologic Factors*, below).

Other Animals. In small ruminants, leptospirosis, usually due to *L. pomona*, resembles that seen in cattle. Infections with *L. hardjo* and *L. grippotyphosa* also occur. Epidemics due to *L. pomona* have caused high mortality among California sea lions periodically since the 1940s.

Humans. Humans are susceptible to all serovars with no host-adapted strains identified. Infections cause fever, icterus, muscular pains, rashes, and nonsuppurative meningitis, manifestations varying somewhat with the serovars involved. A malignant form, most often associated with *L. icterohaemorrhagiae*, can cause fatal liver or renal disease.

Epidemiology

Leptospirosis is perpetuated by the many tolerant hosts and the protracted shedder state. Indirect exposure depends on mild and wet conditions, which favor environmental survival of leptospirae. More direct transfer occurs by urine aerosols in milking barns and cattle sheds or by canine courting habits, which may explain the male bias of canine leptospirosis.

Contaminated bodies of water are important sources of infection to livestock, aquatic mammals, and humans. Animal handlers, sewer workers, field hands, miners, and veterinarians are at increased risk of exposure.

IMMUNOLOGIC FACTORS

Immune Mechanisms of Disease

Immunologic mechanisms may relate to some features of leptospiral disease:

1. The hemolytic anemia characteristic of septicemic leptospirosis due to *L. pomona* in ruminants is associated with the presence of cold hemagglutinins, suggesting an autoimmune process. The relative roles of this and the bacterial hemolysin are uncertain.
2. Canine chronic interstitial nephritis is considered by many a postleptospiral lesion. A leptospiral etiology is suggested by a frequent history of leptospirosis and the presence of leptospiral antibody, particularly in urine. An allergic theory is attractive as antirenal antibody has been demonstrated in infected dogs.
3. Evidence of a leptospiral basis for equine recurrent iridocyclitis (uveitis, periodic ophthalmia, moon blindness) rests in part on leptospiral antibody and its relative titers in serum and aqueous humor. The condition has been reproduced in horses by experimental leptospirosis and in dogs by leptospiral antigens.

Mechanisms of Resistance and Recovery

Recovery from acute leptospirosis coincides with the cessation of septicemia and the appearance of circulating antibody, usually during the second week of infection. Protective antibodies are of IgM and IgG isotypes and are directed mainly at the outer sheath antigens.

Agglutinating antibody (mostly IgM), which may persist for years after recovery, is no indication of immunity nor of the shedder state, which may exist in the absence of antibody or have terminated before its disappearance.

Immunity following recovery is generally solid and serovar-specific, but repeated abortions due to *L. hardjo* have been seen in cows.

Artificial Immunization

Vaccination by bacterins is used on dogs (bivalent containing *L. icterohaemorrhagiae* and *L. canicola*), cattle, swine (at least a pentavalent bacterin with the addition of serovar *L. bratislava* and a second *L. hardjo* component in some vaccines), and occasionally humans. Protection is serovar-specific and temporary, requiring at least annual boosters. Vaccination prevents disease but not necessarily infection.

LABORATORY DIAGNOSIS

Diagnosis of leptospirosis must be established by laboratory confirmation.

Sample Collection

From living subjects, blood, urine, cerebrospinal fluid, uterine fluids, and placental cotyledons are examined. Blood is usually negative after the first febrile phase. Milk is destructive to leptospirae and not a promising source of cultures. Urine should always be tested.

From cadavers, including aborted fetuses, kidneys are most likely to harbor leptospirae. In septic fatalities (including abortions) many organs, especially the liver, spleen, lung, brain, and eye, may contain the agent.

Culturing is done promptly after sample collection, although leptospirae can survive in oxalated human blood for 11 days.

Direct Examination

Methods of direct visual demonstration are wet mounts, examined by darkfield (or phase) microscopy; immunofluorescent stains; and silver impregnation of fixed tissue.

Routine darkfield microscopy should be limited to urine. Other body fluids contain artifacts similar to leptospirae. Brief, low-speed centrifugation clears the specimen of interfering particles but will not sediment leptospirae. Methods using formalinized urine have been described, but they destroy motility, and motility aids in the identification of leptospira. Negative results of direct examinations do not rule out leptospirosis.

Fluorescent antibody has been used on fluids, tissue sections, homogenates, organ impressions, and, most effectively, on aborted bovine fetuses, where examination of kidney was most rewarding. Silver-impregnated sections must be interpreted with caution, because argyrophilic tissue fibrils can mimic leptospirae.

DNA amplification using PCR and specific DNA primers has become an excellent diagnostic tool for detecting the presence of leptospirae in animal tissues and fluids.

Isolation and Identification

The medium of Ellinghausen, McCullough, Johnson, and Harris (EMJH medium) is a good isolation medium, especially for *L. hardjo*, the slowest growing of the common serovars. Replicate inoculations are made into EMJH medium with and without selective inhibitors (5-fluorouracil, neomycin, cycloheximide). Cultures are examined microscopically at intervals during incubation for up to several months.

Animal inoculation (hamsters or guinea pigs) eliminates minor contaminants from the primary inoculum, which is injected intraperitoneally. Blood is drawn periodically for culture starting a few days after inoculation. After 3 to 4 weeks, the animals are sacrificed and their kidneys examined and cultured for leptospirae. If infected with leptospirae, they will have developed antibody. Any isolate recovered by these methods can be identified morphologically as *Leptospira* sp. Definitive identification is carried out by reference laboratories (Centers for Disease Control, Atlanta, GA; National Animal Disease Center, Ames, IA).

Serology

Because direct examination is often unreliable and culture laborious, expensive, and slow, serology is the most common diagnostic method. The microscopic agglutination test employing live antigen is most widely used. Others include macroscopic plate and tube agglutination tests, complement fixation tests, and enzyme-linked antibody assays. Paired samples are preferred: one collected at first presentation and one 2 weeks later. If leptospirosis was the problem, a fourfold or greater rise in titer should have occurred in the interval. In bovine abortion, these relations may not hold. This is due to the fact that *L. hardjo* infections of cattle elicit a very poor immune response that is probably due to their adaptation to this animal species.

Antibody persists for extended periods postinfection. Postvaccination titers are lower and decline well before the vaccination immunity. Agglutination titers are type-specific. Diagnostic laboratories generally maintain all common serovars for serologic testing.

TREATMENT AND CONTROL

Leptospirae are susceptible to penicillin, fluoroquinolones, tetracycline, chloramphenicol, streptomycin, and erythromycin. Treatment, to be of benefit, must be instituted early, possibly even prophylactically in cases of known exposure. Doxycycline is used to treat humans prophylactically. However, evidence of leptospiral infection in the kidneys and reproductive tracts of cattle subsequent to antibiotic treatment is not uncommon.

Vaccination generally prevents disease. It does not prevent infection nor shedding, although it does reduce its extent.

SELECTED REFERENCES

Bolin CA, Zuerner RL, Trueba G. Effect of vaccination with a pentavalent leptospiral vaccine on *Leptospira interrogans* serovar *hardjo* type hardjo-bovis infection of pregnant cattle. Am J Vet Res 1989;50:161.

Brown CA, Roberts AW, Miller MA, et al. *Leptospira interrogans* serovar *grippotyphosa* infection in dogs. J Am Vet Med Assoc 1996;209:1265.

Cousins DV, Ellis TM, Parkinson J, McGlashan CH. Evidence for sheep as a maintenance host for *Leptospira interrogans* serovar *hardjo*. Vet Rec 1989;124:123.

Dhaliwal GS, Murray RD, Dobson H, et al. Effect of *Leptospira interrogans* serovar *hardjo* infection on milk yield in endemically infected dairy herds. Vet Rec 1996;139:319.

Dierauf LA, Vandenbroek DJ, Roletto J, et al. An epizootic of leptospirosis in California sea lions. J Am Vet Med Assoc 1985;187:1145.

Ellis WA. Recent developments in bovine leptospirosis. Vet Annual 1983;23:91.

Ellis WA, Bryson DG, O'Brien JJ, Neill SD. Leptospiral infection in aborted equine fetuses. Equine Vet J 1983;15:321.

Ellis WA, Little TWA. The present state of leptospirosis: diagnosis and control. Amsterdam: Nijhoff, 1986.

Harwood CS, Canale-Perola E. Ecology of spirochetes. Annu Rev Microbiol 1984;38:161.

Holt SL. Anatomy and chemistry of spirochetes. Microbiol Rev 1978;42:114.

Isogai RB, Isogai H, Kurebayashi Y, Ito N. Biological activities of leptospiral lipopolysaccharide. Zbl Bakt Hyg A 1986;261:53.

LeFebvre RB, Thiermann AB, Foley J. Genetic and antigenic differences of serologically indistinguishable leptospires of serovar hardjo. J Clin Microbiol 1987;25:2094.

Little TWA, Hathaway SC. Leptospirosis in pigs. Vet Annual 1983;23:116.

Merien F, Amouriaux P, Perolat P, et al. Polymerase chain reaction for detection of *Leptospira* spp. in clinical samples. J Clin Microbiol 1992;30:2219.

Miller BD, Chappell RJ, Adler B. Detection of leptospires in biological fluids using DNA hybridization. Vet Microbiol 1987;15:71.

Ramadass P, Jarvis BD, Corner RJ, et al. Genetic characterization of pathogenic *Leptospira* species by DNA hybridization. Int J Syst Bacteriol 1992;42:215.

Stalheim OHV. Leptospira. In: Blobel H, Schliesser T, eds. Handbuch der bakteriellen Infektionen bei Tieren. Stuttgart, Germany: Gustav Fischer, 1985:90–154.

Takafuji ET, Kirkpatrick JN, Miller RN, et al. An efficacy trial of doxycycline chemoprophylaxis against leptospirosis. N Engl J Med 1984;310:497.

Taylor RL, Hanson LE, Simon J. Serologic, pathologic, and immunologic features of experimentally induced leptospiral nephritis in dogs. Am J Vet Res 1970;31:1033.

Torten M. Leptospirosis. In: Steele JE, ed. Handbook series in zoonoses. A1. Boca Raton, FL: CRC, 1979:363–421.

Yasuda PH, Steigerwalt AG, Haufman AF, et al. Deoxyribonucleic acid relatedness between serogroups and serovars in the family *Leptospiraceae* with proposals for seven new leptospiral species. Int J Syst Bacteriol 1987;37:407.

35

The Genital Tract as a Microbial Habitat

Dwight C. Hirsh

The female genital tract possesses a resident microbial flora caudal to the external cervical os. The uterus is normally devoid or transiently contaminated with small numbers of microorganisms. The vagina contains a flora that is mainly composed of species of obligate anaerobic bacteria, including both gram-negative and gram-positive species. The aerobic and facultative organisms, about one-tenth the number of obligate anaerobes, include gram-positive and gram-negative species as well as *Mycoplasma*.

The role played by the normal flora of the vagina is uncertain. However, as is the case with other mucosal surfaces, the flora should be thought of as protective insofar as other, perhaps more pathogenic strains, are excluded (colonization resistance, see Chapters 2 and 7). In a more practical sense, the normal flora contains those species that will contaminate the uterus should it become compromised. Some examples include *Streptococcus zooepidemicus* in mares with endometritis; *Arcanobacterium* (*Actinomyces*) *pyogenes* along with *Fusobacterium necrophorum* in cows with pyometra; and *Escherichia coli* in bitches with pyometra. All of the organisms mentioned above are part of the normal vaginal flora of the affected species. If the normal flora is disturbed, as during antibiotic treatment of bacterial endometritis in the mare, the vagina will be repopulated with other, more resistant strains, which will ultimately infect the uterus if the underlying compromise goes uncorrected.

The prepuce and the distal urethra of the male genital tract possesses a resident flora. The role played by these organisms is probably similar to that played by the flora in the vagina. The origin of organisms responsible for bacterial disease of this area is almost always endogenous.

Hormones play a part in protecting the genital tract from disease. Estrogens, which increase during estrus, increase the blood supply to the vagina and uterus, the number of polymorphonuclear neutrophil leukocytes (PMNs) in the cervix and uterus, and the myeloperoxidase activity of phagocytic cells in the tract. These activities are important because the vagina and perhaps the uterus may become contaminated with potentially harmful agents during coitus.

Hormones also play a role in making the genital tract more susceptible to disease. At least in bitches, during the luteal phase, receptors for *E. coli* are expressed. Colonization by *E. coli* expressing appropriate adhesins results in

cystic endometrial hyperplasia and ultimately pyometra. Whether the same occurs in other species is unknown.

The immune system of the genital tract appears to be similar in structure and function to other mucosal surfaces. There are lymphoid follicles in the submucosa from the cervix caudally. These follicles supply the cells that will ultimately secrete IgA. IgG and IgM will be found in this area as well, but these isotypes probably arrive through transudation. In the uterus, IgG and IgM (it is uncertain whether these are locally synthesized) and some sIgA are found. In the prepuce, mainly sIgA is found; it is probably secreted by the accessory glands or locally from cells arising from the lymphoid follicles in this area.

The defensive potential of these antibodies depends upon the isotype. Antibodies of the IgA isotype make particles more hydrophilic, thereby negating any surface attraction an organism might have for usually hydrophobic host cell surfaces as well as sterically hindering attachment. IgG and IgM, on the other hand, will opsonize, trigger the complement cascade, and sterically hinder attachment. All immunoglobulins, if specific for epitopes comprising flagella, immobilize bacteria that use motility as a way to ascend the tract from the more caudal regions.

SELECTED REFERENCES

Bara MR, McGowan MR, O'Boyle D, Cameron RDA. A study of the microbial flora of the anterior vagina of normal sows during different stages of the reproductive cycle. Aust Vet J 1993;70:256.

Clemetson LL, Ward ACS. Bacterial flora of the vagina and uterus of healthy cats. J Am Vet Med Assoc 1990;196:902.

Hinrichs K, Cummings MR, Sertich PL, Kenney RM. Clinical significance of aerobic bacterial flora of the uterus, vagina, vestibule, and clitoral fossa of clinically normal mares. J Am Vet Med Assoc 1988;193:72.

Hirsh DC, Wiger N. The bacterial flora of the normal canine vagina compared with that of vaginal exudates. J Small Anim Pract 1977;18:25.

Kenney KJ, Matthiesen DT, Brown NO, Bradley RL. Pyometra in cats: 193 cases (1979–1984). J Am Vet Med Assoc 1987;191:1130.

Nomura K, Kawasoe KL, Shimada Y. Histological observations of canine cystic endometrial hyperplasia induced by intra-uterine scratching. Jpn J Vet Sci 1990;523:979.

Potter K, Hancock DH, Gallina AM. Clinical and pathologic features of endometrial hyperplasia, pyometra and endometritis in cats: 79 cases (1980–1985). J Am Vet Med Assoc 1991; 198:1427.

Rosendal S. Canine mycoplasmas: their ecologic niche and role in disease. J Am Vet Med Assoc 1982;180:1212.

Sanholdm M, Vasenius H, Kivisto A. Pathogenesis of canine pyometra. J Am Vet Med Assoc 1975;167:1006.

Winter AJ. Microbial immunity in the reproductive tract. J Am Vet Med Assoc 1982;181:1069.

36 Campylobacter — Arcobacter (Reproductive Tract)

Dwight C. Hirsh

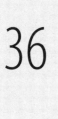

Members of the genus *Campylobacter* are responsible for economically important diseases of the reproductive system of food-producing animals. The disease produced by these organisms is sometimes referred to as *vibriosis* because the agents were once classified as members of the genus *Vibrio*. They are not actually members of this genus, however, because members of the genus *Vibrio* are facultatively anaerobic, ferment carbohydrates, and have a moles % G + C of 40 to 50. Members of the genus *Campylobacter*, on the other hand, are microaerophilic, nonfermentative, and have a moles % G + C of 30 to 35.

Two species of *Campylobacter* are important in regard to the genital tract and reproductive performance: *C. fetus* and *C. jejuni*. *Campylobacter fetus* has two subspecies, *venerealis* and *fetus*.

The genus *Arcobacter* (at one time designated as *Campylobacter*-like organisms) contains four species: *A. cryaerophilus*, *A. butzleri*, *A. skirrowii*, and *A. nitrofigilis*. The first three species are associated with diarrheal conditions (Chapter 14) and reproductive disease of livestock, especially swine.

DESCRIPTIVE FEATURES

Cell Morphology, Anatomy, and Composition

Cell morphology is described in Chapter 14. *Campylobacter* spp. possess a glycoprotein microcapsule (designated a or K), somatic antigens typical of gram negatives (O), and flagella (H). *Campylobacter fetus* ssp. *fetus* contains two serovars, A-2 and B, based on heat-stable surface antigens. Strains with both antigens occur. *Campylobacter fetus* ssp. *venerealis* has two serovars, A-1 and A-sub 1. The serovars differ not only with respect to heat-stable surface antigen (A) but also culturally and biochemically. *Campylobacter jejuni* possesses one serovar C, based on heat-stable surface antigen. A number of other serovars are determined by extractable heat-labile (22) or extractable heat-stable antigens (23).

Cellular Products of Medical Interest

The glycoprotein capsule has been shown to be antiphagocytic, and to protect the outer membrane from deposition of membrane attack complexes of the complement system. The role of toxins, either endotoxin or exotoxin, of *C. jejuni* (Chapter 14) in producing disease of the reproductive tract is unknown.

Physiologic Characteristics

The physiologic properties of *Campylobacter* spp. and *Arcobacter* spp. are described in Chapter 14.

Campylobacter sputorum biovar *fecalis* ("*C. fecalis*") is sometimes isolated from the prepuce of bulls or vagina of cattle, but are not considered significant.

ECOLOGY

Reservoir

The reservoir of *C. fetus* ssp. *venerealis* is the preputial crypts of the bull (main) and the vagina of carrier animals (rare after one to two breeding seasons without exposure). The reservoir for *C. fetus* ssp. *fetus* is the intestinal tract of infected (recovered) sheep (perhaps through contamination from a colonized gallbladder). The reservoir for *C. jejuni* is the intestinal tract of normal animals (especially young ruminants, various birds) or animals that have had the disease.

The reservoir for *Arcobacter* spp. appears to be normal animals (at least in swine) and diseased individuals.

Transmission

Animals acquire campylobacters venereally (*C. fetus* ssp. *venerealis* [cattle]) or by ingestion (*C. fetus* ssp. *fetus* and *C. jejuni* [sheep and goats, rarely cattle]).

It is unknown how animals acquire arcobacters. Ingestion and entry through other mucosal surfaces are likely possibilities.

Pathogenesis

Cattle. The agent *C. fetus* ssp. *venerealis* is introduced into a susceptible female by an infected bull at coitus. The organisms remain at the cervicovaginal junction until the end of estrus. This is probably a consequence of the increased blood supply and active polymorphonuclear neutrophil leukocytes (PMNs) seen in the reproductive tract during this time (see Chapter 35). The organisms multiply at this site and, when conditions are suitable, move into the uterus. Further multiplication and perhaps active invasion result in inflammation of the uterus with resultant endometritis and cessation of pregnancy. The animal will return to estrus. This process continues until the female makes an immune response sufficient to eliminate the agent from the uterus. Subsequently, the endometritis subsides, and the animal conceives and pregnancy goes to term. Sporadic abortions sometimes occur.

Clinically, there are signs of repeat breeding and extended cycles (10-to-60-day cycles; 21 days is normal), which are usually manifested by prolonged calving interval and extended calving periods. In addition, the herd bull will show loss of condition. The herd, if it remains closed, develops an immunity, and calving intervals gradually return toward normal. This process takes years, however, and the economic consequences of the disease are disastrous.

Sheep and Goats. These species are infected following ingestion of *C. fetus* ssp. *fetus* or *C. jejuni*. The organism somehow gains entry into the bloodstream and localizes in the pregnant uterus, especially in the latter stages of pregnancy. Incubation may be as long as 2 months. A placentitis develops along with infection of the fetus (amniotic fluid) and abortion results. The placenta, fluids, and fetus contain large numbers of the organism and act as a source of infection for susceptible animals. Abortions, when they occur, are usually in "storms" occurring in great numbers relatively suddenly following a few scattered abortions. Cattle are rarely infected with *C. fetus* ssp. *fetus* and, when they are, sporadic abortions are observed.

Swine. Arcobacters (*A. cryaerophilus* is most common) are associated with a variety of reproductive abnormalities of swine — for example, late-term abortion and infertility.

Epidemiology

The disease is seen mainly in beef cattle, since the agent is effectively killed by techniques used to prepare and store semen for insemination in the dairy industry.

The gallbladder of sheep, and presumably goats, may become colonized with *Campylobacter*. If this occurs, these animals become a source of infectious organisms for susceptible stock.

In addition to producing disease of the reproductive tract of animals, members of the genus *Campylobacter* are a significant cause of human disease. *Campylobacter jejuni* is one of the leading causes of gastroenteritis in human beings. Both subspecies of *C. fetus* have been isolated from the blood of septic human beings.

IMMUNOLOGIC ASPECTS

Cattle

Development of an active immune response results in the uterus being cleared of the organism. Specific serum IgG

and IgM function by initiating the complement cascade (IgG and IgM) and by acting as opsonizing agents (IgG). In the latter case, these antibodies bind to the antigenic determinants composing the capsular antigens, resulting in the phagocytosis and subsequent destruction of the agent. Secretory IgA, IgG, and IgM specific for surface structures bind and prevent the adherence of the organism to the surface of the epithelium. All isotypes, if specific for the flagellar antigens, prevent movement of more organisms from the vagina. Animals clear the entire tract of the agent if they are not reinfected. Clearance rarely takes more than one year. The mechanism responsible for clearing is unknown but is probably due to the fact that the campylobacters have to deal with an immune response as well as the normal flora of the vagina.

The disease can be controlled by vaccinating heifers or cows with bacterins or by eliminating carrier animals, including the bull. Bulls do not carry the organism efficiently until they are older than about five years. The most commonly held explanation is that the preputial crypts of older bulls are deeper and more hospitable than the shallower crypts found in younger bulls.

Sheep and Goats

Sheep and goats are immune following abortion. The basis for this immunity is mainly antibody of the IgM and IgG types. These antibodies bind to the surface of the agent while it is in the bloodstream, resulting in removal by liver and spleen. Antibody bound to the surface also initiates the complement cascade leading to lysis of the agent. The immune response would also be effective in killing organisms that had reached the placenta but had not yet produced enough damage to terminate pregnancy.

Swine

Little is known concerning the immunological consequences of the interaction of *Arcobacter* spp. and host. There is, however, a report of an effective autologous bacterin.

LABORATORY DIAGNOSIS

Sample Collection

Cattle. Samples for culture or observation are best taken from the prepuce of the bull. Smegma is collected by aspiration into the tip of an insemination pipette. If the female is to be cultured, samples are collected from the anterior vagina. With either sex, 10% of the herd or 20 animals (whichever is greater) are sampled for diagnostic testing.

Sheep and Goats. Samples from the liver and the abomasum of the aborted fetus are most rewarding. The placenta and fluids of the abortus are usually too contaminated.

Swine.   Arcobacters have been isolated from stomach contents, kidney, and placenta of aborted fetuses.

Direct Examination

Cattle.   The low numbers of campylobacters together with the high numbers of organisms of the normal flora make it very difficult to observe the campylobacters in stained smears (Gram or Romanovsky). Fluorescent antibody-stained preparations have proven useful in detection. Campylobacters exhibit a characteristic "tumbling" motility when observed in wet mounts of affected material.

Sheep and Goats.   Gram (carbol fuchsin as counterstain) or Romanovsky stained preparations of stomach contents from aborted fetuses often demonstrate the agent (Fig 36.1). Such findings, in conjunction with doughnut-shaped necrotic foci sometimes found on the liver, help support the diagnosis. Examination of wet mounts of affected material is sometimes useful.

Swine.   Arcobacters and campylobacters are indistinguishable in direct smear, both in fixed preparations and wet mounts.

Isolation

Smegma, vaginal fluid, or stomach contents are plated onto media that contain antimicrobial agents (vancomycin, polymyxin B or C, and trimethoprim are commonly added to decrease the growth of noncampylobacters; amphotericin B is included in some formulations to inhibit growth of fungi). The plate is incubated at 37°C in an atmosphere containing 6% oxygen and 5% to 10% carbon dioxide. Plates are examined in 48 hours.

Arcobacters are aerotolerant (the main trait that distinguishes them from members of the genus *Campylobacter*).

Identification

Isolation of a gram-negative, curved rod that is oxidase positive is presumptive evidence that a member of the genus *Campylobacter* has been isolated. Methods based on detection of specific DNA sequences have proven useful for identification. Likewise, analyses of cell wall fatty acids have been useful.

DIAGNOSIS

The disease can be diagnosed by tests of cervicovaginal mucus for antibody to campylobacter antigens. For collection, a tampon is placed in the vagina near the cervix. Following removal, the mucus is collected and diluted serially. Agglutinins appear in the cervicovaginal mucus in 3 to 80 days of infection and persist for approximately 7 months. Samples are collected 4 to 5 days after estrus or 1 to 2 days before. Samples taken at estrus are too dilute due to the excess mucus. The presence of blood invalidates the test. Antibody to *C. fetus* can also be detected by using an enzyme-linked immunosorbent assay (ELISA). Reportedly, this test can be run on samples collected during estrus and will be positive within 18 to 40 days after infection.

DNA probes and other molecular procedures have been useful in identifying members of the genus *Arcobacter* from *Campylobacter*. In addition, the various species of *Arcobacter* can be identified by molecular approaches.

TREATMENT, CONTROL, AND PREVENTION

Cattle

Bulls can be treated parenterally with streptomycin. For topical treatment, an aqueous solution of penicillin and streptomycin may be instilled into the prepuce. Vaccination of bulls has been reported to clear the carrier state.

The disease is best controlled by prevention. Sound husbandry practices reduce the chances of introducing the organism into the herd. The use of young bulls that have tested negative when bred to a virgin heifer, and barring of replacement heifers or cows originating from herds with unknown history, are means to keep out campylobacters. Once the agent is in the herd, a number of alternatives are available. The least acceptable to the producer is to rest the herd for one breeding season and eliminate the bulls. This eliminates the organism from the females and removes a source of the organism when breeding resumes. Artificial insemination is a very effective way to control and eliminate the disease from a herd.

FIGURE 36.1.   Campylobacter fetus *ssp. fetus in the stomach fluid of an aborted lamb. Gram stain, 1000×.*

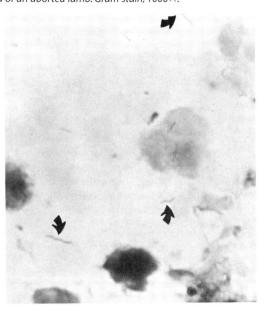

Antibiotic treatment of females is unrewarding, but bacterins are used to prevent the disease in herds in which it is endemic. Vaccination is performed yearly.

Sheep and Goats

Abortion storms can be stopped by administering antibiotics. The most effective is penicillin. Aborting ewes should be isolated from those that are apparently unaffected.

The disease can be prevented by administering a bacterin prior to breeding.

Swine

Treatment of arcobacter-associated conditions in swine is poorly documented.

SELECTED REFERENCES

Allos BM, Blaser MJ. *Campylobacter jejuni* and the expanding spectrum of related infections. Clin Infect Dis 1995;20:1092.

Blaser MJ, Pei Z. Pathogenesis of *Campylobacter fetus* infections: critical role of high-molecular-weight S-layer proteins in virulence. J Infect Dis 1993;167:372.

Blaser MJ, Smith PF, Repine JE, Joiner KA. Pathogenesis of *Campylobacter fetus* infections. Failure of encapsulated *Campylobacter fetus* to bind C3b explains serum and phagocytosis resistance. J Clin Invest 1988;81:1434.

Blom K, Patton CM, Nicholson MA, Swaminathan B. Identification of *Campylobacter fetus* by PCR-DNA probe method. J Clin Microbiol 1995;33:1360.

Borden MM, Firehammer BD. Antigens of *Campylobacter fetus* subsp. *fetus* eliciting vaccinal immunity in heifers. Am J Vet Res 1980;41:746.

Carroll EJ, Hoerlein AB. Diagnosis and control of bovine genital vibriosis. J Am Vet Med Assoc 1972;161:1359.

Corbeil LB, Corbeil RR, Winter AJ. Bovine venereal vibriosis: activity of inflammatory cells in protective immunity. Am J Vet Res 1975;36:403.

Fliegelman RM, Petrak RM, Goodman LJ, et al. Comparative in vitro activities of twelve antimicrobial agents against *Campylobacter* species. Antimicrob Agents Chemother 1985; 27:429.

Frank MM. The mechanism by which microorganisms avoid complement attack. Curr Opin Immunol 1992;4:14.

Hewson PI, Lander KR, Gill KRN. Enzyme-linked immunosorbent assay for antibodies to *Campylobacter fetus* in bovine vaginal mucus. Res Vet Sci 1985;38:41.

Horstmann RD. Target recognition failure by the nonspecific defense system: surface constituents of pathogens interfere with alternative pathway of complement activation. Infect Immun 1992;60:721.

Kirkbride CA. Diagnosis in 1784 ovine abortions and stillbirths. J Vet Diagn Invest 1993;5:398.

Pickett CL, Auffenberg T, Pesci EC, et al. Iron acquisition and hemolysin production by *Campylobacter jejuni*. Infect Immun 1992;60:3872.

Schroeder-Tucker L, Wesley IV, Kiehlbauch JA, et al. Phenotypic and ribosomal RNA characterization of *Arcobacter* species isolated from porcine aborted fetuses. J Vet Diagn Invest 1996; 8:186.

Smibert RM. The genus *Campylobacter*. Annu Rev Microbiol 1978;32:673.

Taylor DE, deGrandis SA, Karmali MA, Fleming PC. Transmissible plasmids from *Campylobacter jejuni*. Antimicrob Agents Chemother 1981;19:831.

Vandamme P, Vancanneyt M, Pot B, et al. Polyphasic taxonomic study of the emended genus *Arcobacter* with *Arcobacter butzleri* comb. nov. and *Arcobacter skirrowii* sp. nov., an aerotolerant bacterium isolated from veterinary specimens. Int J Syst Bacteriol 1992;42:344.

Wesley IV, Baetz AL, Larson DJ. Infection of cesarean-derived colostrum-deprived 1-day-old piglets with *Arcobacter butzleri*, *Arcobacter cryaerophilus*, and *Arcobacter skirrowii*. Infect Immun 1996;64:2295.

Wesley IV, Schroeder-Tucker L, Baetz AL, et al. *Arcobacter*-specific and *Arcobacter butzleri*-specific 16S rRNA-based DNA probes. J Clin Microbiol 1995;33:1691.

Winter AJ. Vibriosis: toward an understanding of immunity in genital infections. Cornell Vet 1973;63:5.

37 Brucella

Richard L. Walker

Brucellosis is an infectious bacterial disease caused by members of the genus *Brucella*. It is a disease of worldwide importance and affects a number of animal species. *Brucella* are obligate parasites, requiring an animal host for maintenance. Infections tend to localize to the reticuloendothelial system and genital tract with abortions in females and epididymitis and orchitis in males the most common clinical manifestations. Chronic infections are common.

Although DNA-DNA hybridization studies indicate all *Brucella* belong to a single genospecies, traditional species designations are used in this chapter. The different *Brucella* species exhibit host preferences and vary in severity of the disease caused. Dye and phage susceptibility along with biochemical, cultural, and serologic characteristics are used to distinguish among species. The six *Brucella* species are *B. abortus*, *B. canis*, *B. melitensis*, *B. neotomae*, *B. ovis*, and *B. suis*.

Many species of *Brucella* are capable of causing disease in humans. Infections are chronic and debilitating. The signs of brucellosis in humans are relatively nonspecific and individuals with brucellosis are sometimes labeled hypochondriacs because of the vague presenting clinical signs.

DESCRIPTIVE FEATURES

Morphology and Staining

Brucella are small, gram-negative coccobacilli measuring 0.6 to 1.5 μm × 0.5 to 0.7 μm in size. Cells are fairly uniform and can easily be mistaken for cocci. They are typically arranged singly but also occur in pairs or clusters. No capsules, flagella, or spores are produced; however, an external envelope has been demonstrated by electron microscopy around *B. abortus*, *B. melitensis*, and *B. suis*. *Brucella* stain red with Macchiavello and modified Ziehl-Neelsen stains.

Cellular Structure and Composition

Brucella possess a typical gram-negative cell wall. Dominant surface antigens are located on the lipopolysaccharide. Specifically, the A and M antigens are found in varying concentrations among the different smooth *Brucella* species. The outer membrane contains other major surface antigens. Porin proteins in the outer membrane are thought to stimulate delayed-type hypersensitivity and account for the varying susceptibility to dyes observed for the different species. The peptidoglycan layer (3 nm to 5 nm) is more prominent than that of *Escherichia coli*. The periplasmic space varies from 3 nm to 30 nm. The cytoplasmic membrane is a typical three-layered lipoprotein membrane. L-form variants are recognized and may play a role in persistence of infections in the host.

The mol% G + C of DNA is 57. Plasmid DNA has not been demonstrated. The overall fatty acid composition is sufficiently unique to be useful for identification and taxonomic purposes.

Growth Characteristics

On initial isolation, colonies are not apparent until 3 to 5 days' incubation. Most colonies are detected by 10 to 14 days, but in some cases incubation for up to 21 days is required. Growth is best in an aerobic environment at 37°C but occurs between 20°C and 40°C. Optimal pH is 6.6 to 7.4. *Brucella ovis* and some biovars of *B. abortus* require an increased concentration of CO_2. Enriched media with 5% serum is required by *B. abortus* biovar 2 and *B. ovis*.

Brucella colonies have a characteristic bluish color when examined with obliquely transmitted light. Colonies have smooth or nonsmooth morphologies that are determined by the presence or absence, respectively, of the polysaccharide side chain in the lipopolysaccharide. These morphologic variations are the result of spontaneous mutation and are influenced by specific growth factors. Smooth colonies are white, convex with an entire edge and have a creamy consistency. Nonsmooth colonies have intermediate, rough, or mucoid forms. Rough colonies are dull yellow, opaque, and friable. They are difficult to suspend in solution and agglutinate spontaneously. The mucoid colonies are similar to the rough colonies except for having a glutinous texture.

Resistance

Brucella survive freezing and thawing. Under proper environmental conditions, they survive for up to 4 months in milk, urine, water, and damp soil. Most disinfectants active against other gram-negative bacteria kill *Brucella*. Pasteurization effectively kills *Brucella* in milk.

Diversity

The colony morphology of *Brucella* varies from rough to smooth forms (see *Growth Characteristics*, p. 196). *Brucella abortus*, *B. melitensis*, *B. suis*, and *B. neotomae* are typically isolated in the smooth form but can develop rough forms on subsequent laboratory passage. *Brucella ovis* is always in a rough form. Isolates of *B. canis* have a mucoid appearance. In general, smooth strains of *Brucella* are more virulent than rough strains.

Variation in CO_2 requirement, H_2S production, urease production, susceptibility to varying concentration of certain dyes (thionin and basic fuchsin), and susceptibility to naturally or mutagen-derived bacteriophages account for diversity among species and biovars within species. The different species of *Brucella* vary in host preference and degree of virulence within and among animal species.

ECOLOGY

Zoologic and Geographic Reservoirs

As obligate parasites, *Brucella* require an animal reservoir. Host preference is exhibited by the different *Brucella* species; however, a broad host range has been demonstrated for some species. Survival time outside the host is variable and depends on temperature and moisture. Colder weather extends survival time.

Cattle are the preferential host for *B. abortus*. Other animals, including bison, camels, and yaks, are commonly infected. The different biovars of *B. abortus* have different geographic distributions. Biovars 1 and 2 have a worldwide distribution, while biovar 3 is predominantly found in India, Egypt, and Africa. Biovar 5 is most commonly encountered in Germany and the United Kingdom.

Swine are the preferential host for *B. suis* biovar 1. This biovar is widely distributed. Biovar 2 is found in swine and wild hares (*Lepus timidus*), predominately in western and central Europe. *Brucella suis* biovar 3 is predominately recovered from the midwestern United States. Biovar 4 affects reindeer and caribou in Alaska, Canada, and Siberia.

Brucella melitensis infects goats and sheep worldwide except for North America, Australia, and New Zealand. Camels, alpacas, and llamas are also infected.

Brucella ovis infections are limited to sheep and *B. canis* infections are limited to dogs. Both have a worldwide distribution. *Brucella neotomae* has only been found in the wood rat (*Neotoma lepida*) with geographic distribution limited to the Salt Lake Desert of Utah.

Transmission

Brucella are disseminated by direct or indirect contact with infected animals. Ingestion is the most common route of entry, although exposure through the conjunctival and genital mucosa, skin, and respiratory routes occurs. The major source for exposure to *B. abortus* in cattle and *B. melitensis* in sheep and goats is through aborted fetuses, the placenta, and postabortion uterine fluids. Aborted tissue and fluids are also a common means for transmission of *B. suis* and *B. canis*. Genital infections in cattle routinely clear within 30 days after calving and cows are not considered infectious for other cattle after that time. Genital infections in swine, in some cases, persist longer than those in cattle.

Ingestion of milk from infected cattle and goats is another source for infection of calves and kids. Direct transfer in utero has also been documented.

Infections of the accessory sex glands of males allows for dissemination of organisms through the semen. Infections can occur in the accessory sex organs without testicular or epididymal lesions being present. Venereal transmission of *B. suis* in swine, *B. ovis* in sheep, and *B. canis* in dogs is common. Urine is another vehicle for disseminating *B. canis* to other dogs.

Insects may play a minor role in transmission and maintenance of infection in a herd. Face flies have been shown to take up and excrete *Brucella* in feces.

Pathogenesis

Mechanisms. Following exposure, *Brucella* penetrate intact mucosal surfaces. In the alimentary tract, the epithelium covering the ileal Peyer's patches are a preferred site for entry. After penetrating mucosal barriers, organisms may be engulfed by phagocytic cells. Specific receptors on macrophages appear to mediate attachment and uptake of *Brucella*. Various mechanisms are employed by *Brucella* to allow for survival inside phagocytic cells. They are capable of surviving and multiplying inside macrophages by inhibiting phagolysosome fusion. Adenine and 5'-guanosine monophosphate in crude supernatants from *Brucella* suspensions have been shown to inhibit phagolysosome fusion in neutrophils. Intracellular survival in macrophages and, to a lesser extent, neutrophils is enhanced by suppressing the myeloperoxidase-H_2O_2-halide system. Superoxide dismutase and catalase production may play a role in defense against oxidative killing. Stress proteins have been demonstrated in *Brucella* and could be a factor in intracellular survival in the host. These proteins are thought to play a role in protecting organisms from hydrolytic enzymes, oxygen radicals, and myeloperoxidase killing systems in the phagolysosome. The lipopolysaccharide of *Brucella* is directly associated with virulence and is thought to play a role in enhancing intracellular survival. It is believed that the variations in virulence observed among the *Brucella* species may, in part, be related to the greater ability of some species to avoid host defenses.

Following entry into the host, *Brucella* organisms, either free in the extracellular environment or in phagocytic cells, localize to regional lymph nodes. There they proliferate and infect other cells or are killed and the infection is terminated. Some cattle appear to be innately resistant to infection. This resistance is related to the macrophages' ability to contain the organisms. From the regional lymph nodes, *Brucella* disseminate hematogenously and localize in the reticuloendothelial system and reproductive tract.

There is preferential localization to the reproductive tract of the pregnant animals. Unknown factors in the gravid uterus, collectively referred to as *allantoic fluid factors*, stimulate the growth of *Brucella*. Erythritol, a four-carbon alcohol, is considered to be one of these factors.

Experimental infection studies have demonstrated that, at the cellular level, *Brucella* localizes into the cisternae of the rough endoplasmic reticulum of trophoblasts of the placentome. Infection subsequently spreads to the fetus. The exact mechanism of abortion is unclear; however, likely possibilities are that abortion results from 1) interference with fetal circulation due to the existing placentitis, 2) the direct effect of endotoxin, and/or 3) fetal stress resulting from the inflammatory response in fetal tissue.

Although less is known about the factors involved in localization of *Brucella* in the reproductive tract of males, the presence of growth stimulating compounds may be a factor. The prolonged bacteremia observed with some of the *Brucella* species may account for the greater likelihood for extragenital manifestations to occur in those species.

Pathology. There are grossly visible lesions in the placenta associated with *Brucella* abortions. Intercotyledonary thickening with a yellow gelatinous fluid is present. The cotyledons are frequently necrotic, yellow-gray in color, and covered with a thick brown exudate. The degree of necrosis varies among the *Brucella* species with *B. melitensis* infections in goats being most severe. The aborted fetus is frequently edematous. Abomasal contents may be turbid and have a lemon-yellow color. The most common histologic findings in the fetus are bronchitis and bronchopneumonia with a predominately mononuclear cell infiltrate. In general, *Brucella* induce a granulomatous-type inflammatory reaction.

In males palpable enlargement of the epididymis, especially involving the tail portion, is common. Epididymal lesions are characterized by hyperplasia and hydropic degeneration of tubular epithelium. Resulting extravasation of sperm leads to the formation of a spermatic granuloma (Fig 37.1). In bulls with orchitis the scrotum is swollen, largely due to an inflammation of the tunica and fibrinopurulent exudate in the tunica vaginalis. The testicular parenchyma becomes necrotic and is sometimes replaced by pus. Pathology of the accessory sex organs includes prostatitis in dogs and fibrinopurulent seminal vesiculitis in bulls.

Extragenital tract pathology includes lymphocytic endophthalmitis in dogs (*B. canis*), purulent or fibrino-purulent synovitis in swine (*B. suis*), osteomyelitis in dogs and swine (*B. canis* and *B. suis*), necrotizing and purulent bursitis in horses (*B. abortus*), and hygroma development in cattle (*B. abortus*).

Disease Patterns. The primary clinical manifestations of brucellosis are related to the reproductive tract. In general, animals do not exhibit overt systemic illness. In females, abortion is the most common presentation. No premonitory signs are usually apparent. Abortion in cattle commonly occurs in the fifth month of gestation or later. Retained placenta is a possible sequela. Females usually abort only once, presumably due to acquired immunity. *Brucella melitensis* infections in goats and sheep are similar to *B. abortus* in cattle except that acute mastitis develops

FIGURE 37.1.   *Swelling and irregular conformation of the tail of the epididymis of a ram infected with* Brucella ovis *(left). Cross-section of the tail of the epididymis revealed a pocket of inspissated material resulting from extravasation of sperm (right).*

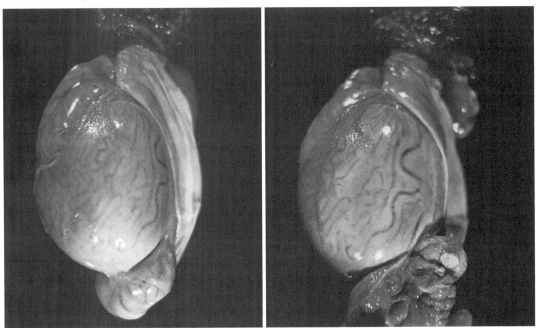

in goats infected with *B. melitensis*. The mastitis in goats presents with palpable nodules in the udder and milk that is clotted and watery. Abortions in swine can occur at any time in gestation and are related to time of exposure. Abortions in dogs due to *B. canis* occur around 50 days of gestation. *Brucella ovis* infections in sheep only rarely result in abortions in ewes.

In males, epididymitis and orchitis are the most common presenting signs. Lesions are usually unilateral but may be bilateral. Semen examination reveals increased numbers of neutrophils in acute cases. Neutrophils are few in number in more chronic infections. *Brucella ovis* infections in rams predominately affect the epididymis with testicular lesions being uncommon. Palpable lesions in the epididymis of mature rams are frequently the result of infection with *B. ovis*, whereas epididymitis in yearlings and ram lambs are invariably caused by a variety of other organisms. In bulls, infection with *B. abortus* frequently involves the testicle. Dogs infected with *B. canis* develop scrotal swelling as a result of fluid accumulation in the tunica. Scrotal dermatitis may develop because of constant licking of the scrotum. Infections of the male genital tract result in decreased fertility and, in some cases, sterility.

Extragenital manifestations develop in many animal species. Swine infected with *B. suis* may develop arthritis, especially in the large joints of the limbs, or lumbar spondylitis. Lesions in the lumbar vertebrae result in tissue necrosis that puts pressure on the spinal cord and can lead to posterior paralysis. Dogs infected with *B. canis* can develop meningoencephalitis, osteomyelitis, discospondylitis, and anterior uveitis. Ocular manifestations in dogs may be the initial presenting sign for canine brucellosis. Chronic infections with *B. abortus* in cattle can result in hygromas. Horses infected with *B. abortus* develop "poll evil" or "fistulous withers" and present with fistulous tracts originating from the atlantal or supraspinous bursas, respectively. Infections in horses usually result from contact with infected cattle.

Brucellosis in humans is primarily a disease of the reticuloendothelial system. A mild lymphadenopathy, splenomegaly, and hepatomegaly may be detected. Onset of signs occurs within 2 to 3 weeks of exposure. Clinical signs are nonspecific and include alternating fever and chills with night sweats, fatigue, muscle and joint pains, and backaches. Depression and insomnia are common.

Epidemiology

Humans acquire infections by handling tissues containing *Brucella* organisms. *Brucella melitensis* is considered the most virulent species for humans followed by *B. suis*, *B. abortus*, and *B. canis*. *Brucella ovis* and *B. neotomae* do not infect humans. Common sources for infection are aborted fetuses, placentas, and postabortion uterine fluids, all of which contain large numbers of organisms. Veterinarians, ranchers, and slaughterhouse workers are particularly at risk for acquiring infections.

The prolonged bacteremic phase of *B. suis* infections in swine poses a special risk for slaughterhouse workers handling infected tissues. Individuals who participate in the hunting of feral swine are also at risk for contracting *B. suis* infections. Relatively few cases of infections in humans due to *B. canis* have been reported. Individuals at risk are kennel workers and breeders coming in contact with contaminated fluids from infected dogs.

Infected animals also shed organisms in the milk. Raw milk or raw milk products of bovine or caprine origin are ready sources for infections in humans.

Accidental self-inoculation with live *Brucella* vaccine strains can result in disease. Human-to-human transmission is rare.

Characteristics of the Animals and Herd. Susceptibility to infection depends on age, sex, breed, and pregnancy status. Younger animals tend to be more resistant to infection and frequently clear infections, although latent infections do occur. Only 2.6% of animals infected at birth remain infected as adults. Sexually mature animals are much more susceptible to infection, regardless of gender. Most animals infected as adults remain infected for life.

Herd size and animal density are directly related to prevalence of disease and difficulty in controlling infection in a population. Calving practices also play a major role in the spread of brucellosis. Separate calving pens allow for minimizing exposure of uninfected animals. Whether a herd raises its own replacement animals or purchases replacement animals affects the potential for introduction into the herd.

In contrast to cattle, where bulls play a relatively minor role, boars are more likely to be a source for introducing *Brucella* into a swine herd. Both venereal transmission or exposure to aborted fetuses and fetal membranes are important for maintaining infections in a herd. Confinement of breeding swine in common pens or lots provides the ideal setting for spreading infection. Management practices directed at eliminating infected boars and minimizing exposure to aborted tissue greatly reduce the incidence of disease in commercial swine operations. Feral swine serve as a reservoir for *B. suis* and are more commonly infected than commercial swine in some countries. In some European countries where *B. suis* biovar 2 is found, the European hare acts as a source for infection in swine.

Dissemination of *B. ovis* in sheep occurs during the breeding season. Older rams are more likely to be infected than yearlings. Introduction of an infected ram during the breeding season can lead to rapid spread of infection within the flock. Transmission occurs when an uninfected ram breeds a ewe recently bred by an infected ram. The ewe acts mainly as a mechanical vector for transmitting infection. Homosexual activity of rams is another means of spreading infection among rams.

Dogs in suburban areas are least likely to be infected with *B. canis*. Prevalence of infection is greatest in economically depressed areas. Close confinement settings such as kennels increase the likelihood for transmitting infections.

IMMUNOLOGIC ASPECTS

Immune Mechanisms in Pathogenesis

Evidence indicates that antibodies against *Brucella* play both a protective and detrimental role. IgM antibodies, which appear initially after infection, and low levels of IgG will cause complement-mediated lysis of *Brucella*. Elevated levels of IgG antibodies, however, appear to act as blocking antibodies that modulate the ability of the complement membrane attack complex to lyse cells. This may account for resistance to complement-mediated lysis in the face of high specific antibody levels and the lack of correlation between protection and high antibody titers. The blocking antibodies are opsonizing and promote uptake by phagocytes where *Brucella* have developed mechanisms for survival and proliferation.

Phagocytic cells unable to eliminate *Brucella* play a role in dissemination of organisms to other parts of the body and in persistence of infection.

IgA autoantibody has been demonstrated in dogs infected with *B. canis* and may explain some of the observed effect on fertility.

Mechanisms of Resistance and Recovery

Effective immunity is primarily cellular in nature. Specifically sensitized T-lymphocytes release cytokines that activate macrophages, which in turn control *Brucella* by reactive oxygen intermediates. A more effective immunity develops when animals are infected prior to sexual maturity.

Artificial Immunization

Cattle are immunized with either nonviable (*B. abortus* 45/20) or attenuated live (*B. abortus* strains 19 and RB51) vaccines. These products provide protection from abortion, the major mode of dissemination, but not from infection. A single dose at 3 to 7 and 3 to 10 months of age is required with *B. abortus* strain 19 and strain RB51, respectively. Two doses 6 weeks apart in animals over 6 months of age are required with *B. abortus* 45/20. Adult cow vaccination is sometimes performed as a regulatory effort to control infection in a herd. Strain 19 is occasionally shed in the milk and can cause abortions in cattle. Adult vaccination with *B. abortus* strain RB51 only rarely causes abortion. Bulls should not be vaccinated because orchitis can develop. The type of vaccine used is generally established by the particular country's regulatory agency in charge of brucellosis control. Recently, in a number of regulatory programs *B. abortus* strain RB51 has replaced strain 19 as the approved calfhood vaccine because it does not interfere with serologic evaluation.

Brucella melitensis Rev 1, a partially attenuated vaccine, is used to control brucellosis in goats and sheep caused by *B. melitensis*. A killed product, *Brucella melitensis* H38, is also available.

Bacterins for control of *B. ovis* are available, but their efficacy is limited. *Brucella melitensis* Rev 1 has been used to protect against *B. ovis* infections in sheep; however, it cannot be used in countries free of *B. melitensis* because the antibody titers interfere with serologic evaluations for *B. melitensis* infection.

Vaccination is not practiced for control of disease caused by *B. suis* or *B. canis*.

LABORATORY DIAGNOSIS

Specimens

Great care should be employed when working with infected tissues and cultures in the laboratory. All *Brucella* cultures should be handled following biosafety level 3 practices because of the potential for laboratory infection. All laboratory procedures should be performed in a manner that prevents aerosolization.

Appropriate samples for diagnosis of brucellosis depend on the animal species affected, species of *Brucella* involved, and clinical presentation. Abscess material, semen, and vaginal fluids associated with recent abortions are useful for recovering organisms antemortem. Milk samples from cattle and goats are used in antemortem isolation attempts and for immunodiagnostic evaluation. In dogs, blood cultures are useful for isolation of *B. canis* because of the prolonged bacteremia that occurs. Serum is used for serologic evaluation.

Samples collected at necropsy should include spleen, liver, udder, and multiple lymph nodes, including the supramammary, retropharyngeal, internal iliac, lumbar, and mesenteric lymph nodes. The supramammary lymph node is superior to other lymph nodes for isolating *Brucella* from dairy cattle. Abomasal fluid and lungs of the aborted fetus and the placenta are the preferred specimens in the case of abortion. In males the epididymis, testicle, and accessory sex organs are examined.

Direct Examination

Gram stains of fetal stomach contents from an aborted fetus and the placenta reveal large numbers of gram-negative coccobacilli. Modified Ziehl-Neelsen and Macchiavello stains are also used to demonstrate *Brucella*. Organisms can be detected in semen but are usually in low numbers. *Brucella* is difficult to detect by direct examination in other samples, especially from chronically infected animals.

Isolation

Tissues are cultured directly on solid media. Milk cultures are performed by centrifuging milk at 5900 to 7700 × g for 15 minutes or by allowing for gravity cream separation to occur overnight. Both the cream layer and sediment, if the centrifugation technique is used, should be plated on solid media. Commonly used media include serum dextrose, tryptose, and brucella (Albimi) agars. If contamination is likely to be a problem, isolation attempts should be made using media containing actidione (30 mg/L), bacitracin (7500 U/L), and polymyxin B (1800 U/L). Selective media are used both with and without the incorporation of ethyl violet (1 : 800,000). Cultures should be incubated at 37°C in 10% CO_2 for a minimum of 10 days and up to 21 days in highly suspicious cases.

Animal inoculation is the most sensitive method for detection of *Brucella* and is sometimes necessary when very low numbers of organisms are present. Guinea pigs are the most sensitive laboratory animals for this purpose. Two guinea pigs are inoculated and at 3 and 6 weeks postinoculation an animal is sacrificed. Serum is examined for antibodies and tissues are cultured for organisms.

Identification

Preliminary identification of *Brucella* species requires demonstrating colonies of gram-negative coccobacilli that are nonhemolytic, catalase positive, and oxidase positive (except for *B. ovis* and some strains of *B. abortus*). Most species, except *B. ovis*, are strongly urease positive. Glucose and lactose are not fermented by any of the species. Agglutination in unadsorbed antismooth *Brucella* serum helps in preliminary identification of smooth strains.

Definitive identification is usually performed by a *Brucella* reference laboratory. A fluorescent antibody test is used for rapid identification. Urease production, CO_2 requirement, H_2S production, oxidation of metabolic substrates, agglutination in monospecific antisera, growth in the presence of varying concentration of thionin, and basic fuchsin and phage typing are used to determine species and biovars within species. *Brucella abortus* strain 19 can be differentiated from field strains of *B. abortus* by its lack of requirement for CO_2 for growth and inhibition by 5 mg/ml penicillin or 1 mg/ml of erythritol. Strain RB51 can be differentiated from field strains and strain 19 by demonstrating its resistance to rifampin (200 μg/ml), staining with crystal violet, and agglutination with acriflavin.

Polymerase chain reaction (PCR) methods have been described for differentiation of *Brucella* species.

Immunodiagnosis

Antibody detection is commonly used for diagnosing brucellosis and in control programs. Samples tested include blood, milk, and occasionally semen. A number of immunodiagnostic tests have been developed for cattle. These tests detect different classes and types of antibodies and vary in their sensitivity and specificity. Individual blood samples can be tested by tube agglutination, plate agglutination, rose bengal plate, or card tests. Other tests include the buffered plate agglutination assay, rivanol agglutination, complement fixation, and enzyme-linked immunosorbent assay (ELISA).

Frequently, highly sensitive but less specific tests are used for screening purposes and are followed by more specific tests for confirmation purposes. A similar approach to that used in cattle is employed when testing goats and sheep for *B. melitensis*. Sera are screened with a test such as the rose bengal test and results confirmed with a more specific test.

Milk is screened with the *Brucella* milk ring test, which identifies specific antibodies in milk. The test is performed on bulk tank milk samples as a means of screening dairy herds. Stained *Brucella* antigen is added to milk. If antibodies are present, agglutinated antigen is buoyed to the top by the rising cream and a purple ring develops at the top of the tube (Fig 37.2).

Serologic tests are commonly used to identify infected swine herds and monitor herd status. These tests are less accurate when testing individual pigs because some infected swine do not have detectable antibody titers. Herds can be screened by the brucellosis card test. Tests such as rivanol agglutination and 2-mercaptoethanol agglutination are used for confirmation.

Rams are tested for antibodies to *B. ovis* using either a complement fixation test or ELISA.

For canine brucellosis, screening is performed with a rapid slide agglutination test (RSAT). The RSAT is sensitive but not very specific, therefore positive results should be confirmed with additional tests that are more specific. An agar gel immunodiffusion test using cytoplasmic antigen is more specific but not as sensitive as the RSAT and is used as a confirmatory test.

Nonculture Detection Methods

A number of nonculture methods, including PCR, immunoperoxidase staining, DNA probes, and coagglutination, have been described for detection of *Brucella* in tissues and fluids.

FIGURE 37.2. Brucella *milk ring test for detection of antibodies in milk. In a negative sample, the added, stained* Brucella *antigen remains dispersed in the milk portion and the cream layer is white (left). In a positive sample, the antibodies react with stained antigen and the complex rises to the top in the cream layer. The cream layer appears purple (right).*

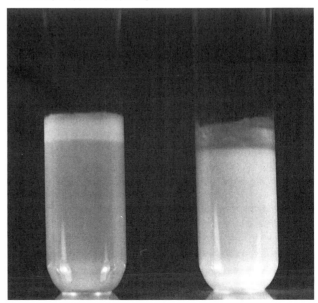

TREATMENT

As a general rule, treatment of infected livestock is not attempted because of the high treatment failure rate, cost, and potential problems related to maintaining infected animals in the face of ongoing eradication programs. Tetracycline and dihydrostreptomycin have been used to treat *B. ovis* infections in rams with variable results. Once a palpable epididymal lesion is present, antibiotic treatment will not be beneficial because the lesion is the result of extravasation of sperm. The presence of abscesses and fibrosis in tissues of the accessory sex organs makes penetration with antibiotics to these areas difficult.

Treatment of dogs with brucellosis requires a prolonged course of antibiotic therapy. The combination of dihydrostreptomycin and tetracycline or minocycline for a 2-to-4-week period is commonly used. Quinolones may also be useful; however, only limited information about their effectiveness is available. Treatment failures are common. Treatment should also consist of neutering affected animals. Treatment is not recommended in canine breeding colonies. In this case, infected dogs should be culled.

CONTROL AND PREVENTION

Approaches at control and prevention of brucellosis depend on the animal species involved, *Brucella* species, management practices, and availability and efficacy of vaccines. Approaches used to control brucellosis include 1) immunization alone, 2) testing and removal of infected animals in conjunction with an immunization program, and 3) testing and removal of infected animals without immunization.

Control by Immunization Alone

Immunization by itself reduces the number of abortions and, thereby, reduces potential for exposure. By itself, immunization will not result in eradication of the infection in a herd. Immunization alone should be considered as a means of controlling the level of disease only.

Immunization Followed by Test and Slaughter

Control of bovine brucellosis routinely employs a combination of vaccination of females and a test and slaughter program. Cattle are vaccinated at a young age and tested by immunodiagnostic tests when they reach sexual maturity and vaccination titers have diminished. Vaccination with strain 19 is approximately 70% effective on an individual basis but more effective when evaluated on a herd basis. In experimental challenge, vaccination with strain RB51 provided protection similar to vaccination with strain 19. Any animals identified as infected are culled from the herd and slaughtered. Routine testing is done by the milk ring test in dairy cattle or blood tests from beef cattle at slaughter. A similar program is followed with *B. melitensis* infections in sheep and goats.

Test and Slaughter Without Immunization

Immunization control programs are not used for swine brucellosis. The most successful method of control is depopulation of the entire herd and restocking with uninfected replacement animals. Methods other than depopulation, such as removing only adult animals and retaining weanlings, are less successful. Removal of only the serological reactors will not control infection in the herd. Confinement operations and closed herds make establishing and maintaining a swine herd free of brucellosis readily achievable. In some instances, depopulation is practiced with *B. melitensis* infections in sheep and goats.

Control of *Brucella ovis*

Removing infected rams and preventing new infections in rams are the main means of controlling *B. ovis* infection in a flock. Practices that allow for introduction of infected rams into a flock, such as loaning of rams, should be avoided. Yearling rams should be maintained separately from mature rams. All rams should be palpated for epididymal lesions at least twice a year before breeding season and rams with palpable lesions culled. Serologic tests (ELISA, CF) are used to identify infected rams without lesions. Serologic testing should be performed a minimum of two times before rams are turned in to breed ewes. Vaccination can be employed but its efficacy is limited and it interferes with serologic interpretation. No effort is made to control infections in ewes. Ewes, although playing a role in transmission of infection at breeding, are only transiently infected and naturally eliminate the infection by the next breeding season.

Control of *Brucella canis*

Efforts to prevent canine brucellosis involve serologic testing of dogs prior to breeding. Males are also evaluated by palpating for epididymal and testicular lesions. In breeding colonies with brucellosis, infected animals identified by serologic tests are removed. Repeat serologic testing is performed to identify previously undetected infected animals. Until at least three negative test results are obtained, a kennel should not be considered free of brucellosis. Kennel areas should be thoroughly disinfected with quaternary ammonium compounds or iodophors.

SELECTED REFERENCES

Alton GG, Jones LM, Angus RD, Verger JM. Techniques for the brucellosis laboratory. Institut National de la Recherche Agronomique. INRA, Paris, 1988, pp 24–61.

Anderson TD, Cheville NF. Ultrastructural morphometric analysis of *Brucella abortus*-infected trophoblasts in experimental placentitis. Am J Pathol 1986;124:226.

Campbell GA, Adams LG, Sowa BA. Mechanisms of binding of *Brucella abortus* to mononuclear phagocytes from cows naturally resistant or susceptible to brucellosis. Vet Immunol Immunopathol 1994;41:295.

Hoffman EM, Houle JJ. Contradictory roles for antibody and complement in the interaction of *Brucella abortus* with its host. Crit Rev Microbiol 1995;21:153.

Jiang X, Leonard B, Benson R, Baldwin C. Macrophage control of *Brucella abortus*: role of reactive oxygen intermediates and nitric oxide. Cell Immunol 1993;151:309.

Laboratory procedures for isolating, identifying and typing of *Brucella*. US Dept of Agriculture, Animal and Plant Inspection Services, Veterinary Services, National Veterinary Services Laboratories, 1985.

Smith LD, Ficht TA. Pathogenesis of *Brucella*. Crit Rev Microbiol 1990;17:209.

Young EJ. An overview of human brucellosis. Clin Infect Dis 1995;21:283.

38 Taylorella equigenitalis

ERNST L. BIBERSTEIN

Contagious equine metritis (CEM) is an acute, suppurative, self-limiting infection of the uterus of mares. It causes temporary sterility, is highly communicable, and is followed by long-term asymptomatic carriage of the agent *Taylorella equigenitalis* (syn. contagious equine metritis organism [CEMO], *Haemophilus equigenitalis*).

Stallions develop no signs of illness but may remain carriers of the agent indefinitely. The disease is geographically limited at present.

DESCRIPTIVE FEATURES

Morphology and Composition

Taylorella equigenitalis is a gram-negative, nonmotile, inconsistently piliated, and encapsulated coccobacillus, about $0.8\,\mu m \times 5$ to $6\,\mu m$ in size.

Some antigens are shared by *Haemophilus*, *Pasteurella*, and *Brucella* spp.

Growth Characteristics

Taylorella equigenitalis is a facultative anaerobe that grows optimally at 37°C under 5% to 10% carbon dioxide on chocolate agar in a rich base (Columbia, Eugon). After 48 hours of incubation, colonies have a diameter of 1 mm and may enlarge further upon longer incubation. They are shiny, smooth, grayish-white, waxy, and sometimes pleomorphic.

The organism is oxidase, catalase, and phosphatase positive and produces no acid from carbohydrates.

The resistance of *T. equigenitalis* is not remarkable. Samples on swabs are shipped in transport medium under refrigeration and cultured within 48 hours of collection. This requirement adds a safety margin to survival times observed in the laboratory.

Most antibiotics except streptomycin inhibit *T. equigenitalis*, although they are strain-susceptible to this antibiotic. Trimethoprim-sulfamethoxazole, lincomycin, and clindamycin are sufficiently well tolerated to have been included in selective isolation media.

The agent is unrelated to other gram-negative genera, including *Alcaligenes* and *Bordetella*.

Apart from harboring streptomycin-susceptible variants, the species appears to be homogeneous, though some strains appear more virulent than others as measured by entry into cells in vitro.

ECOLOGY

Reservoir

Taylorella equigenitalis is a parasite exclusively of the equine genital tract. Antibodies to the agent but no infections have been found in cattle and humans. Donkeys appear to harbor a CEM-like organism whose significance is unclear at this writing.

The reservoir is in Europe, but the agent has been recovered from CEM in Japan, Australia, and the United States.

Transmission

CEM is sexually transmitted, although its occurrence in newborn and virgin animals suggests alternative means of exposure.

Pathogenesis

Within a few days of exposure, a purulent endometritis develops with variable amounts of exudate. The main damage is to uterine epithelium (exclusive of glands), which becomes covered by neutrophilic exudate. The cellular infiltrate in the endometrial stroma is predominantly mononuclear. Epithelium is eroded or undergoes severe degenerative changes. The uterine infection usually subsides spontaneously within several weeks. Endometrial repair is complete and there is no lasting impairment of breeding performance. Infection has been demonstrated in placentas and newborn foals, but abortions have been few.

There is no fever or other sign of illness. The only effect may be failure of conception. Alternatively, there may be a mucoid to mucopurulent vulvar discharge of variable abundance some days after service; internal examination reveals a cervicovaginal exudate of uterine origin. External signs of disease disappear within 2 weeks, although the uterine infection may persist longer.

Epidemiology

Inapparent persistence of *T. equigenitalis* is frequent in recovered mares and in stallions in endemic areas. The foci of carriage in mares are the clitoridal fossa and sinuses; in stallions, the foci are the prepuce, urethra, and the urethral fossa and sinus.

Dissemination of infection is tied to breeding operations and the movement and use of infected animals.

IMMUNOLOGIC ASPECTS

Recovered animals show increased resistance for several months, manifested by milder signs and lower numbers of bacteria when reinfected. The mechanism of resistance is uncertain.

Complement-fixing serum antibody appears late in the first week and rises for 3 weeks after experimental exposure. Duration of titers in mares varies, but tests are consistently positive during the third to the seventh week postinfection. Titers are apparently unrelated to the carrier status. Antibody is present in vaginal mucus, but its relation to infection is unknown.

Bacterins did not prevent infection, but they did reduce its severity.

LABORATORY DIAGNOSIS

Diagnosis of CEM and carrier identification require demonstration of *T. equigenitalis* in the genital tract. In clinical cases, the agent can be demonstrated in the uterine exudate by Gram stain.

Definitive identification of an infected animal requires replicate cultures of appropriate specimens (see under *Treatment and Control,* below) on chocolate Eugon agar (prepared with horse blood) with and without added streptomycin. A third medium incorporating clindamycin and trimethoprim permits growth of all strains. Plates are examined daily from the second to the seventh days of incubation (see under *Growth Characteristics,* p. 204). Gram-negative, oxidase positive, and catalase positive organisms from suspect colonies must be confirmed serologically. Any identification of *T. equigenitalis* should be considered tentative until confirmed by a competent reference laboratory.

A polymerase chain reaction (PCR) based assay has been developed and found to be more sensitive than traditional culture techniques.

Serological testing (CF) may be done on suspect mares between the fifteenth and fortieth day postbreeding.

TREATMENT AND CONTROL

Uterine infusions of disinfectants or antimicrobics and systemic antibiotic treatment are used in attempts to reduce the severity and duration of illness and perhaps abort the carrier state. Their benefit has been questioned.

Topical treatment of affected mares consists of a cleansing of the clitoridal fossa with 2% chlorhexidine followed by liberal application of nitrofurazone ointment (0.2%). The prepuce, urethral sinus, and fossa glandis of stallions imported into the United States from countries in which CEM is known to exist are cultured. The stallions are then bred to two uninfected mares, which subsequently are sampled three times for culture of clitoridal fossa and clitoridal sinuses. In mares to be imported, each of these sites is cultured repeatedly throughout one estrus.

Some countries require surgical obliteration of the clitoridal sinuses in imported mares.

In CEM-endemic countries, attempts at control have included mandatory veterinary examinations, negative cultures of all animals intended for breeding, and supervision of the movement of horses.

SELECTED REFERENCES

Atherton JC. Evaluation of selective supplements used in media for the isolation of sensitive organisms of contagious equine metritis. Vet Rec 1983;43:299.

Bleumink-Pluym NM, Ter Laak EA, van der Zeijst BA. Differences between *Taylorella equigenitalis* strains in their invasion of and replication in cultured cells. Clin Diagn Lab Immunol 1996;3:47.

Bleumink-Pluym NM, van Dijk L, van Vliet AH, et al. Phylogenetic position of *Taylorella equigenitalis* determined by analysis of amplified 16S ribosomal DNA sequences. Int J Syst Bacteriol 1993;43:618.

Bleumink-Pluym NM, Werdler ME, Houwers DJ, et al. Development and evaluation of PCR test for detection of *Taylorella equigenitalis*. J Clin Microbiol 1994;32:893.

Bryans JT, Darlington RW, Smith B, Brooks RR. Development of a complement fixation test and its application to diagnosis of contagious equine metritis. J Eq Med Surg 1979;3:467.

Ensink JM, van Klingeren B, Houwers DJ, et al. In-vitro susceptibility to antimicrobial drugs of bacterial isolates from horses in the Netherlands. Eq Vet J 1993;25:309.

Kanemaru T, Kamada M, Wada R, et al. Electron microscopic observation of *Taylorella equigenitalis* with pili in vivo. J Vet Med Sci 1992;54:345.

Sahu SP, Rommel FA, Fales WH, et al. Evaluation of various serotests to detect antibodies in ponies and horses infected with contagious equine metritis bacteria. Am J Vet Res 1983;44:1405.

Swerczek TW. Elimination of CEM organisms from mares by excision of clitoral sinuses. Vet Rec 1979;105:131.

Timoney PJ, Shin SJ, Jacobson RH. Improved selective medium for isolation of the contagious equine metritis organism. Vet Rec 1982;111:107.

Timoney PJ. Contagious equine metritis. Comp Immunol Microbiol Infect Dis 1996;19:199.

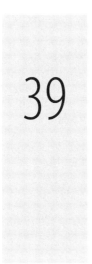

39

The Skin as a Microbial Habitat: Bacterial Skin Infections

ERNST L. BIBERSTEIN

ANTIMICROBIAL PROPERTIES OF THE SKIN

The skin is less favorable to microbial growth than mucous membranes owing to the following properties:

1. *Dryness.* Conditions interfering with evaporation from the skin cause proliferation of resident and transient skin flora through increased moisture retention, temperature, pH, and CO_2 tension.
2. *pH.* Skin pH varies over the surface of the animal body. Growth of many bacteria is discouraged at pH less than 6.0.
3. *Desquamation.* Continuous shedding of superficial skin layers eliminates transient organisms. Resident flora are promptly replenished from the residual population.
4. *Secretions and excretions.* Holocrine sebaceous glands secrete lipids, including long-chain fatty acids, many of which inhibit bacteria. They and the apocrine sweat glands contribute to an intercellular seal in superficial epidermal layers, limiting microbial access. Apocrine and eccrine sweat glands excrete lactate, propionate, acetate, caprylate, and high concentrations of sodium chloride. Interferon, lysozyme, transferrin, and all classes of immunoglobulins are also present. All these substances may contribute to the "self-sterilizing" action of the skin — that is, its resistance to colonization by transient microorganisms.
5. *Microbial interactions.* Resident bacteria exclude intruders by excreting inhibitory metabolites (volatile fatty acids, antibiotics), bacteriocins, and occupying available niches.
6. A skin immune system (SIS) responds to local antigenic stimuli, including microbial ones, and comprises cell types corresponding functionally to those operating on mucosal surfaces (see Chapter 2). A nonphagocytic, antigen-presenting Langerhans cell is a prominent constituent of the system.

MICROBIAL SKIN FLORA

Microorganisms are limited to the superficial epidermal layers, where intercellular cohesion is relaxed prior to desquamation, and to the distal portions of gland ducts and hair follicles. Their density varies but is heaviest in moist, protected areas such as the axilla, inguinal region, interdigital spaces, and skin folds of certain breeds or obese individuals. Their concentration is lower than on colonized mucous membranes, rarely exceeding $10^5/cm^2$ and, in some areas, $10^2/cm^2$.

Gram-positive organisms predominate among the resident flora. Coagulase-negative staphylococci make up the leading component. Facultative (*Corynebacterium* spp.) and anaerobic (*Propionibacterium* spp.) diphtheroids are consistently present. *Micrococcus* spp. and "viridans" streptococci are likely residents. Of gram negatives, only *Acinetobacter* spp. are considered part of the resident flora. Lipophilic yeasts (*Malassezia*) may be found in small numbers.

The most important transients are coagulase-positive staphylococci, probably derived from the distal nares and gastrointestinal tract. Beta-hemolytic streptococci (generally Group G) on cat or dog skin are usually associated with abnormal conditions. Members of the family *Enterobacteriaceae*, particularly *Escherichia coli* and *Proteus mirabilis*, and enterococci are common transients. *Pseudomonas aeruginosa* is sometimes found in cutaneous lesions. The feet of farm animals carry fecal bacteria, some of which participate in foot infections, most notably *Fusobacterium necrophorum* and *Prevotella melaninogenica*. The agent of ovine footrot, *Dichelobacter (Bacteroides) nodosus* (see below), although hardly a normal commensal, is limited to epidermal tissues.

SKIN STERILIZATION

Sterilization of the skin is impossible due to the physical inaccessibility of much of the skin flora. Thorough cleansing of the shaved skin with soap and water, followed by soaking with 70% alcohol, will remove 95%. More than 99% removal of skin flora is claimed for repeated povidone iodine (alcoholic) applications and rinses with chlorhexidine (0.5%) in alcohol.

Following such treatment there is rapid repopulation, usually by the same organisms.

BACTERIAL SKIN INFECTIONS

Only infections whose agents are primarily or exclusively skin inhabitants and pathogens are considered here. The many agents causing skin lesions, along with other disease manifestations, are discussed under their chief habitat or theater of pathogenic activity.

FOOTROT OF SMALL RUMINANTS

Footrot is a contagious infection affecting the epidermal portions of the foot of sheep and goats. The fully developed lesions cause a crippling lameness. Two gram-negative non-spore-forming anaerobes are primarily implicated: *Dichelobacter (Bacteroides) nodosus* and *Fusobacterium necrophorum*. Numerous other bacteria common in the ruminant environment (*Arcanobacterium [Actinomyces] pyogenes*, *Treponema* spp.) are secondarily involved.

DICHELOBACTER (BACTEROIDES) NODOSUS

DESCRIPTIVE FEATURES

Structure

Dichelobacter nodosus, the specific cause, is a nonmotile rod measuring 2 to 10 μm × 0.5 to 1.0 μm. In smears from

lesions, its ends are commonly swollen (Fig 39.1). Pili (Type 4, as are those of *Moraxella bovis*, *Neisseria gonorrheae*, *Pasteurella multocida*, and *Pseudomonas aeruginosa*) act as adhesins and confer twitching motility.

Cellular Products of Medical Interest

Pili and proteolytic enzymes (serine and basic proteases) are the major traits associated with virulence. Less clear are the proteins encoded in two pathogenicity islands: virulence-associated proteins (Vap) and the gene product of virulence-related locus (*vrl*).

Growth Characteristics

Dichelobacter nodosus is a strict anaerobe requiring added carbon dioxide and a rich medium, preferably containing protein. After several days, smooth colonies about 1 mm in diameter are produced.

Resistance

Dichelobacter nodosus survives in the environment 2 to 3 days and is killed by disinfectants and many antibiotics.

Variability

Colonial variation and virulence are related to abundance of piliation. Virulence also varies with proteolytic activities of strains. Nine major immunotypes (A–I) are recognized.

ECOLOGY

Reservoir

The significant reservoir is the infected foot of sheep or goats. Cattle and swine strains are of low virulence.

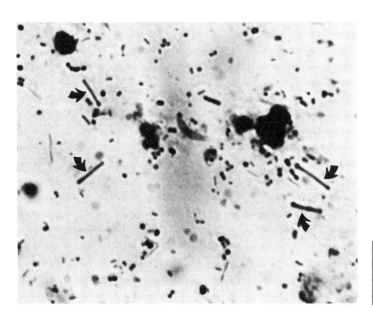

FIGURE 39.1. *Exudate from ovine footrot. Mixture of bacterial species, with* Dichelobacter nodosus *recognizable as large rods with swollen ends: "dumbbells" (arrows). Gram stain, 1000×.*

Transmission

Transmission is by direct or indirect contact. The brief environmental survival time of the agent requires prompt colonization of new hosts.

Pathogenesis

Pathogenic mechanisms include the pili-mediated attachment to host cells, proteolytic activity, and synergy with *F. necrophorum*, to which *D. nodosus* supplies growth factors.

Disease Patterns

The sequence of events is typically as follows:

1. The interdigital epidermis is damaged, most commonly by maceration due to persistent soaking.
2. *Fusobacterium necrophorum*, a constituent of the fecal flora, infects the macerated skin and produces superficial inflammation, hyperkeratosis, parakeratosis, and necrosis (ovine interdigital dermatitis [OID]).
3. *Dichelobacter nodosus* from a footrot lesion colonizes (with the aid of its pili) and proliferates in the lesion initiated by *F. necrophorum*, producing interdigital swelling. Invasion of epidermal structures begins at the medial aspect of the claw and, probably with the help of bacterial proteases, advances to the epidermal matrix of the hoof, eventually separating it from the underlying dermal tissues ("underrunning").

Secondary invaders help maintain or aggravate the process. The result is extreme lameness, which becomes paralyzing when two or more feet are involved. Affected animals may starve.

Epidemiology

Footrot occurs on all continents. It is most serious in regions with a mild climate and periods of abundant rainfall (>20 inches [500 mm]). Dissemination of *D. nodosus* essentially ceases at ambient mean temperatures of less than 50°F (10°C), and footrot does not occur in arid regions and improves during dry periods in endemic areas. All ages of animals beyond nursing stages are susceptible, but genetic differences in susceptibility exist. Fine wool breeds are most severely affected. The agent is eliminated from contaminated pastures within 2 weeks.

IMMUNOLOGIC ASPECTS

Resistance is related to circulating antifimbrial antibody; it is serogroup-specific. Natural infection produces no immunity, but oil-adjuvant vaccines of appropriate specificity induce temporary protection and improve existing cases.

LABORATORY DIAGNOSIS

Diagnosis is usually clinical. Direct smears from the lesion reveal stout rods with terminal swellings (see Fig 39.1). Other microorganisms are usually also present, some of which — small gram-negative rods — often coaggregate around *D. nodosus*. Immunofluorescence confirms identification.

Culture (on selective media) is not routinely done.

TREATMENT AND CONTROL

Treatment begins with removal and exposure of diseased tissue by hoof trimming, followed by topical application of disinfectants or antibiotics, such as repeated treatment with 5% to 10% formalin, 5% copper sulfate, 10% to 20% zinc sulfate, or 5% tetracycline tincture. Use of chloramphenicol (10%) is not permissible in the United States. Formalin and copper and zinc sulfate are used in foot baths. Three 1-hour 20% zinc sulfate soaks at weekly intervals have proven effective without foot paring.

Systemic treatment with large doses of penicillin and streptomycin has been successful in the absence of topical therapy.

Control is achieved by a combination of repeated examination, vaccination, treatment of active cases, and segregation of active cases from the healthy flock. Care must be taken not to add infected animals to the flock. Contaminated lots should not be restocked for 2 weeks. Control programs should be instituted during dry weather.

FOOTROT OF CATTLE (INFECTIOUS PODODERMATITIS: FOULS)

Dichelobacter nodosus combined with *Fusobacterium necrophorum* can cause a coronary and interdigital dermatitis in cattle.

What is often called *bovine footrot* is etiologically and pathologically distinct from the ovine disease. The chief agent is *F. necrophorum*. Other bacteria, particularly pigmented anaerobic rods (*Prevotella*) are implicated. The process involves the dermis and subcutis, and produces a diffuse, often febrile necrotizing cellulitis, which may extend to joints or spread hematogenously. Sinus tracts develop in the foot region.

Injury, irritation, and maceration are likely predisposing factors. Their presence, rather than transmissibility, probably determines disease prevalence.

Cases are treated topically and by hoof trimming. Uncomplicated cases respond to systemic sulfonamides or tetracycline.

Cat Leprosy and Other Feline Cutaneous Mycobacterioses

There is no true leprosy in domestic animals. Since a disease of cats is called *feline leprosy*, key features of the prototype condition are summarized.

1. *Mycobacterium leprae*, the acid-fast causative bacterium of human leprosy, has not been propagated in vitro. Limited infections can be produced in rodents. The nine-banded armadillo is susceptible to natural and experimental infection.
2. Leprosy affects superficial tissues, mainly skin and upper respiratory tract. Only in advanced cases are internal organs colonized.
3. Particular targets of infection are peripheral nerves.
4. The disease picture ranges between two extremes.
    a. In lepromatous leprosy, bacterial proliferation is profuse. Poorly circumscribed nondestructive lesions develop, dominated by a histiocytic response but little other inflammatory reactivity. Cell-mediated immunity is suppressed, but circulating immunoglobulins are high.
    b. In tuberculosis leprosy, bacteria are scarce. Lesions are granulomatous and cell-mediated inflammatory responses are well developed. They cause neural damage, leading to anesthesia, paralysis, dystrophy, disfigurement, and mutilation.
5. The course extends over years and decades. Affected individuals die of complications traceable directly or indirectly to immune disorders or neural destruction.

Feline leprosy is a chronic noduloulcerative, nontuberculous mycobacterial infection of the skin, reported from New Zealand, Australia, Great Britain, the Netherlands, and western North America.

Its acid-fast agent is believed by many to be *Mycobacterium lepraemurium*, a cause of leprosy-like disease in rodents. It is cultivable on a special medium, which also supports growth of the feline isolate. Known *M. lepraemurium* has failed to infect cats. However, sequence comparisons of DNA obtained from tissues of cats with feline leprosy show significant identity with *M. lepraemurium*.

Ecology

Reservoir and Transmission

Sources, mode of spread, and pathogenic mechanisms are unknown. Transmission by rodent bite or arthropod is suspected.

Disease Pattern

Judged from experimental infections, lesions of feline leprosy develop in 2 to 6 months. They occur in cutis or subcutis in many sites. They are freely movable and painless. Ulceration and lymph node involvement are frequent. The general health is unaffected. Microscopically, the lesions are granulomas consisting largely of histiocytes with variable neutrophilic, lymphocytic, plasma, and giant cell admixtures. Caseation necrosis and irregular neural involvement occur. Acid-fast bacteria abound within histiocytes.

Immunologic Aspects

Limited observations suggest the existence of lepromatous and tuberculoid forms.

Laboratory Diagnosis

Diagnosis depends on demonstration of a noduloulcerative granulomatosis associated with mycobacteria not cultivable on routine mycobacterial media.

Treatment and Control

Discrete lesions are excised. Antimicrobic therapy (topical injection of streptomycin, systemic administration of dapsone and rifampin) is not dependably effective, and dapsone is potentially hemotoxic. Clofazamine is reportedly effective in some cases.

Postsurgical relapses are common.

Mycobacterial ulcerative dermatitis of cats (occasionally dogs) can be associated with opportunistic mycobacteria (Runyon's Group IV, rapid growers, see Chapter 30), most frequently *M. fortuitum*, sporadically *M. phlei, M. smegmatis, M. xenopi, M. ulcerans, M. thermoresistible*, and unspeciable mycobacteria of this group. Percutaneous wound infection is the likely portal of entry.

The division between these mycobacterioses and cat leprosy is tenuous and possibly invalid. Distinctive features of nonfeline leprosy mycobacterioses are the following:

1. Lesions tend to be restricted to the ventral part of the trunk, particularly the abdomen.
2. Lesions tend to be more suppurative than granulomatous.
3. Sinus tracts are frequent.
4. Nodular features are less conspicuous.
5. Lymph node involvement is less consistent.

Most of the agents grow readily on lifeless media, usually blood agar, within 48 hours to 1 week. Identification should be left to a mycobacterial reference laboratory.

As some cases regress spontaneously, the benefits of treatment are uncertain. The agents often test susceptible to azithromycin, clarithromycin, aminoglycosides, tetracycline, fluoroquinolones, and chloramphenicol, and are usually resistant to first-line antituberculous drugs, except ethambutol. Surgery is sometimes palliative.

BOVINE MYCOBACTERIAL ULCERATIVE LYMPHANGITIS

Noduloulcerative skin lesions occur in cattle, particularly on the lower extremities and ventral trunk. They resemble tubercles and typically contain noncultivable acid-fast bacteria. They are of interest mainly because of their association with false-positive tuberculin reactivity.

CANINE OTITIS EXTERNA

The agents associated with canine otitis externa are *Pseudomonas aeruginosa*, *Staphylococcus intermedius*, *Streptococcus canis*, *Proteus mirabilis*, *Escherichia coli*, *Klebsiella pneumoniae*, *Enterobacter* spp., *Enterococcus* spp., and the yeast *Malassezia pachydermatis*, a skin commensal that is oval in shape and produces single buds attached by a broad base (Fig 39.2). *Candida* spp. and *Aspergillus* spp. are rarely encountered.

A primary role of any microorganism in otitis externa is doubtful.

ECOLOGY

Reservoir and Transmission

Infection is probably endogenous. There is no evidence of communicability.

Pathogenesis

A predisposing factor is the configuration of the canine ear. The external meatus is roughly L-shaped, with the vertical leg leading to the outside. This arrangement interferes with aeration and drainage, especially in dogs with floppy ears and abundant secretions and meatal hair, which are particularly otitis-prone. Infection, once begun, initiates cycles of further accumulation of exudate and aggravated infection. It is common to recover three or four isolates in large numbers from these processes, which may be acute or chronic, purulent, and become ulcerative or eventually verrucous. There is usually abundant malodorous discharge and evidence of pain and pruritus.

Epidemiology

Predisposing conditions, which are influenced by breed, climate, season, life-style, and management, include floppy ears, pilose ear canals, foreign bodies, parasites, seborrhea, and hot, humid weather.

IMMUNOLOGIC ASPECTS

Allergic dermatitis may be one possible initiator. No immunologic mechanisms are recognized in the recovery from otitis.

LABORATORY DIAGNOSIS

Swabs are satisfactory for microbial culture. Gram-stained smears often reveal the presence of yeasts (see Fig 39.2), gram-positive cocci, and gram-negative rods along with neutrophils and epithelial debris. All bacteria commonly involved grow on blood agar. *Malassezia pachydermatis*

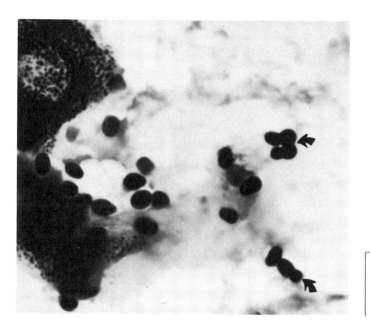

FIGURE 39.2.   *Exudate of canine otitis externa containing* Malassezia pachydermatis. *Note characteristic "shoe print" pattern of budding yeasts (arrows). Gram stain, 1000×.*

grows sparingly as small, dry colonies (<1 mm) on blood agar and on fungal media with or without antibiotics. Some strains of *M. pachydermatis* require a medium rich in lipid for isolation.

TREATMENT AND CONTROL

The objectives of treatment are symptomatic relief and

1. Establishment of aeration and drainage (surgically if necessary).
2. Control of infection (which step 1 will greatly aid).
3. Alleviation of the underlying condition.

Topical medications contain 1) local analgesics or anesthetics, 2) anti-inflammatory drugs (usually corticosteroids), and (3) antimicrobials, including a broad spectrum antibacterial (enrofloxacin, neomycin, gentamicin, chloramphenicol) and often an antimycotic (nystatin, thiabendazole).

DERMATOPHILOSIS

Streptothricosis (cattle and other species), rain scald or rain rot (horses), grease heal (horses), lumpy wool (sheep), and strawberry footrot (sheep) are infections due to *Dermatophilus congolensis*, a gram-positive bacterium. In temperate climates, dermatophilosis is often a cosmetic problem controllable by management practices. In sheep and cattle, especially in tropical areas, it can severely affect productivity.

DESCRIPTIVE FEATURES

Morphology and Composition

Dermatophilus congolensis is an actinomycete, as indicated by its staining characteristics, filamentous growth, and branching patterns. Its reproductive unit is the motile coccoid "zoospore," about 2 μm in diameter. Upon germinating the spore sprouts a germ tube, about 1 μm thick, which elongates and thickens, dividing both transversely and longitudinally and forming a strand several cell layers thick. Enclosed in a gelatinous sheath, constituent cells become coccoid as they differentiate into multiflagellated zoospores, which are liberated as the strand disintegrates, completing the life cycle.

Like some other actinomycetes, *Dermatophilus* has a cell wall containing mesodiaminopimelic acid, but lacking glycine and arabinogalactan.

Growth Characteristics

Dermatophilus congolensis grows on blood and infusion media, but not on Sabouraud agar. It is aerobic and capnophilic. Hemolytic colonies, which develop in 48 hours, vary from mucoid to viscous and waxy, whitish-gray to yellow, and smooth to wrinkled. Glucose and some other carbohydrates are attacked nonfermentatively. Catalase, urease, and proteases are produced. The agent survives well in soil and on fomites.

There is colonial and antigenic variability, but all strains appear to share antigens.

ECOLOGY

Reservoir

Dermatophilus congolensis does not multiply saprophytically. Its reservoir is infected animals. Cattle, sheep, goats, and horses are common hosts. It has been diagnosed in swine, dogs and cats, turkeys, primates (including humans), and wild mammals, including marine mammals. The distribution of *D. congolensis* is worldwide, but its greatest economic significance is in tropical Africa.

Transmission

Spread is by direct and indirect contact. Transmission occurs through flying and nonflying, biting and nonbiting arthropods. Injury by thorny range plants and shearing cuts may create portals of infection or inoculate the agent.

Pathogenesis

The disease is an exudative epidermitis. Its primary activity is confined to the living epidermis. As access to this is limited by hair, wool, sebaceous secretions, and the stratum corneum, infection depends on their disruption by soaking or trauma. Deposited zoospores, responding to a CO_2 gradient, "home" into deeper cell layers. Upon germination, germ tubes and filaments arborize within the epidermis and colonize hair follicles. A layer of inflammatory cells (largely neutrophils) forms under the infected epidermis, which keratinizes. Beneath the neutrophils new epidermis forms, which in turn is invaded. The eventual result is a scab consisting of layers of neutrophilic exudate and infected keratinizing epidermis. The scabs are easily lifted by the hair, which protrudes from both surfaces.

The primary lesions are painless and nonpruritic. Wetting favors their expansion. Biting arthropods can infect areas protected from soaking rain (axilla, flank, ventral trunk). Soaking provides the preparatory step for lesions on the back (equine "rain scald"), feet, and legs (ovine "strawberry footrot," equine "grease heel"). The extent varies from a few scabby areas of roughened hair or "lumpy wool" to widespread loss of epidermis, causing secondary parasitisms or infections and eventual loss of the animal. This progressive form affects African cattle. Neglected cases of "lumpy wool" may lead to complete solidification of the fleece.

Dermatophilosis in nonepidermal tissue — tongue, the urinary bladder, lymph nodes, and subcutis — is reported in cats.

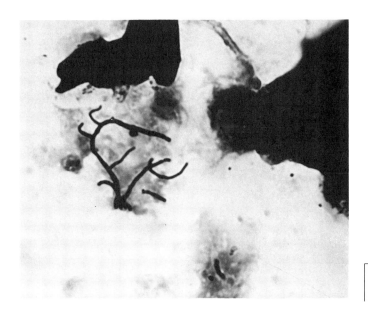

FIGURE 39.3.   Dermatophilus congolensis *in smear from a lesion of "rain scald" in a horse. Gram stain, 1000×.*

Epidemiology

The prevalence of dermatophilosis depends on 1) infected animals, 2) dissemination, for example, by arthropods or thorny plants, and 3) susceptible hosts' epidermis rendered accessible by trauma or wetting.

IMMUNOLOGIC ASPECTS

Antibody is widespread among cattle in endemic areas. Its protective role, relative to that of cell-mediated resistance, is at present unsettled.

Attempts at artificial immunization have been inconclusive.

LABORATORY DIAGNOSIS

Gram or Giemsa stains of ground-up scabs usually show typical phases of the life cycle described (see Fig 39.3). In subacute and chronic cases, bacterial elements may be rare and lack, for example, multicellular branching filaments. Zoospores resemble large cocci. They and other *Dermatophilus* fragments in skin debris may be identified by fluorescent antibody.

Dermatophilus congolensis is cultured on blood agar under 5% to 10% carbon dioxide. Colonies appear within 48 hours and when gram-stained are seen to consist of branching filaments and zoospores. A wet mount reveals motile zoospores.

TREATMENT AND CONTROL

Acute cases are often self-limited. Mild cases respond to grooming and removal to shelter. Severe cases can be treated parenterally with penicillin G, tetracycline, chloramphenicol, or spiramycin.

Control should be aimed at minimizing skin trauma and exposure to rain and arthropods.

SELECTED REFERENCES

Cutaneous Microbiology

Ayliffe GAJ. Surgical scrub and skin disinfection. Infect Control 1984;5:23.

Bos JD, Kapsenberg ML. The skin immune system. Immunol Today 1986;7:235.

Garthwaite G, Lloyd DH, Thomsett LR. Location of immunoglobulins and complement at the surface and within the skin of dogs. J Comp Pathol 1983;93:185.

Ihrke P. An overview of bacterial skin disease in the dog. Br Vet J 1987;143:112.

Ihrke P, Schwartzman RM, McGinley K, et al. Microbiology of normal and seborrheic skin. Am J Vet Res 1978;39:1487.

Krogh HV, Kristensen S. A study of skin diseases in dogs and cats. II. Microflora of the normal skin of cats and dogs. Nord Vet Med 1976;28:459.

Muller GH, Kirk RW, Scott DW. Bacterial skin diseases. In: Small animal dermatology. 4th ed. Philadelphia: W.B. Saunders, 1989:244–287.

Noble WC. Skin microbiology: coming of age. J Med Microbiol 1984;17:1.

Scott DW. Large animal dermatology. Philadelphia: W.B. Saunders, 1988.

Wagner DK, Sohnle PG. Cutaneous defenses against dermatophytes and yeasts. Clin Microbiol Rev 1995;8:317.

Footrot

Bagley CV, Healey MC, Hurst RL. Comparison of treatments for ovine footrot. J Am Vet Med Assoc 1987;191:541.

Berg JN, Loan RW. *Fusobacterium necrophorum* and *Bacteroides melaninogenicus* as etiologic agents of foot rot in cattle. Am J Vet Res 1975;36:1115.

Billington SJ, Johnston JL, Rood JI. Virulence regions and virulence factors of the ovine footrot pathogen, *Dichelobacter nodosus*. FEMS Microbiol Lett 1996;145:147.

Dewhirst FE, Paster BJ, LaFontaine S, Rood JI. Transfer of *Kingella indologenes* (Snell and Lapage 1976) to the genus *Suttonella* gen. nov. as *Suttonella indologenes* comb. nov., transfer of *Bacteroides nodosus* (Beveridge 1941) to the genus *Dichelobacter* gen. nov. as *Dichelobacter nodosus* comb. nov., and assignment of the genera *Cardiobacterium*, *Dichelobacter*, and *Suttonella* to *Cardiobacteriaceae* fam. nov. in the gamma division of *Proteobacteria* on the basis of 16S rRNA sequence comparisons. Int J Syst Bacteriol 1990;40:426.

Egerton JR, Cox PT, Anderson BJ, et al. Protection of sheep against footrot with recombinant DNA-based fimbrial vaccine. Vet Microbiol 1997;14:393.

Every D, Skerman TM. Surface structure of *B. nodosus* in relation to virulence and immunoprotection in sheep. J Gen Microbiol 1983;129:255.

Gradin JL, Schmitz JA. Selective medium for isolation of *Bacteriodes nodosus*. J Clin Microbiol 1977;6:298.

Knott AA, Burns JE, Stewart DJ. Detection of the extracellular proteases of *Bacteroides nodosus* in polyacrylamide gels: a rapid method of distinguishing virulent and benign ovine isolates. Res Vet Sci 1983;35:171.

Lee CA. Pathogenicity islands and the evolution of bacterial pathogens. Infect Agents Dis 1996;5:1.

Patel P, Marrs CF, Mattick JS, et al. Shared antigenicity and immunogenicity of type 4 pilins expressed by *Pseudomonas aeruginosa*, *Moraxella bovis*, *Neisseria gonorrheae*, *Dichelobacter nodosus*, and *Vibrio cholerae*. Infect Immun 1991;59:4674.

Feline Mycobacterioses

Hughes MS, Ball NW, Beck L-A, et al. Determination of the etiology of presumptive feline leprosy by 16S rRNA gene analysis. J Clin Microbiol 1997;35:2464.

McIntosh DW. Feline leprosy: a review of forty-four cases from western Canada. Can Vet J 1982;23:291.

Pattyn SR, Portaels F. In vitro cultivation and characterization of *Mycobacterium lepraemurium*. Int J Leprosy 1980;48:7.

Schiefer HB, Middleton DM. Experimental transmission of a feline mycobacterial skin disease (feline leprosy). Vet Pathol 1983;20:460.

White SD, Ihrke PJ, Stannard AA, et al. Cutaneous atypical mycobacteriosis in cats. J Am Vet Med Assoc 1983;82:1218.

Canine Otitis Externa

Bond R, Anthony RM. Characterization of markedly lipid-dependent *Malassezia pachydermatis* isolates from healthy dogs. J Appl Bacteriol 1995;78:537.

Bond R, Anthony RM, Dodd M, Lloyd DH. Isolation of *Malassezia sympodialis* from feline skin. J Med Vet Mycol 1996;34:145.

Hayes HM, Pickle LW, Wilson GP. Effects of ear type and weather on the hospital prevalence of canine otitis externa. Res Vet Sci 1987;42:294.

Kennis RA, Rosser EJ, Olivier NB, Walker RW. Quantity and distribution of *Malassezia* organisms on the skin of clinically normal dogs. J Am Vet Med Assoc 1996;208:1048.

Uchida Y, Nakade T, Kitazawa K. Clinico-microbiological study of the normal and otitic external ear canals in dogs and cats. Jpn J Vet Sci 1990;52:415.

Uchida Y, Nakade T, Kitazawa K. In vitro activity of five antifungal agents against *Malassezia pachydermatis*. Jpn J Vet Sci 1990;52:851.

van der Gaag I. The pathology of the external ear canal in dogs and cats. Vet Qtly 1986;8:307.

Dermatophilus

Aronolo ROA, Arnakiri SF, Nwufoh KJ. Chemotherapeutic agents used in the treatment of dermatophilosis: a review. Bull An Hlth Prod Africa 1987;35:5.

Chastain CB, Corithers RW, Hogle RM, et al. Dermatophilosis in two dogs. J Am Vet Med Assoc 1976;169:1079.

How SJ, Lloyd DH. Use of a monoclonal antibody in the diagnosis of infection by *Dermatophilus congolensis*. Res Vet Sci 1988;45:416.

Jones RT. Subcutaneous infection with *Dermatophilus congolensis* in a cat. J Comp Pathol 1976;86:415.

Lloyd DH. Immunology of dermatophilus. Recent developments and prospects for control. Prev Vet Med 1984;2:93.

McNeil MM, Brown JM. The medically important aerobic actinomycetes: epidemiology and microbiology. Clin Microbiol Rev 1994;7:357.

Sellers L, ed. Dermatophilus infection in animals and man. New York: Academic, 1976.

40 *Dermatophytes*

ERNST L. BIBERSTEIN

Dermatophytes are molds capable of parasitizing only keratinized epidermal structures: superficial skin, hair, feathers, horn, hooves, claws, and nails. Those that have a sexual reproductive phase belong to the ascomycetes. Dermatophyte infections are called *ringworm (tinea)*.

DESCRIPTIVE FEATURES

Morphology

In their nonparasitic state, including culture, dermatophytes produce septate, branching hyphae collectively called *mycelium*. The asexual reproductive units (conidia) are found in the aerial mycelium. These units may be either *macroconidia:* pluricellular, podlike structures up to 100μm long; or *microconidia:* unicellular spheres or rods less than 10μm in any dimension. Shape, size, structure, arrangement, and abundance of conidia are diagnostic criteria. Hyphal peculiarities — spirals, nodules, "rackets," "chandeliers," and chlamydoconidia — are more common in some species than others, but they are rarely diagnostic. Pigmentation is useful in dermatophyte differentiation.

In the parasitic state, only hyphae and arthroconidia, another asexual reproductive unit, are seen. Except in size ranges, which overlap among dermatophyte species, arthroconidia are indistinguishable from species to species.

Sexual spores (ascospores) are absent in the parasitic phase.

The distinguishing features of the three genera of dermatophytes — *Microsporum*, *Trichophyton*, and *Epidermophyton* — are shown in Table 40.1. Only the first two affect animals consistently.

Growth Characteristics

The traditional medium for propagating dermatophytes (and other pathogenic fungi) is Sabouraud's dextrose agar, a 2% agar containing 1% peptone and 4% glucose. Its acidity (pH 5.6) renders it mildly bacteriostatic and selective. The selectivity is enhanced by addition of cycloheximide (500μg/ml), which inhibits other fungi, and gentamicin and tetracycline (100μg/ml of each), or chloramphenicol (50μg/ml). Dermatophytes are aerobes and nonfermenters. Some attack proteins and deaminate amino acids. They grow optimally at 25°C to 30°C and require several days to weeks of incubation.

Some dermatophytes in skin and hair (but not in culture) produce a green fluorescence due to a tryptophan metabolite that is visible under a Wood's light (λ = 366 nm). Of animal dermatophytes, only *Microsporum canis* produces this reaction.

Resistance

Dermatophytes are susceptible to common disinfectants, particularly those containing cresol, iodine, or chlorine. They survive for years in the inanimate environment.

ECOLOGY

Reservoir

One speaks of geophilic, zoophilic, and anthropophilic dermatophytes when discussing dermatophytes having a soil, animal, or human reservoir, respectively. Table 40.2 shows the important dermatophytes affecting animals, with reservoirs and clinical hosts.

Rare causes of animal dermatophytosis are the anthropophilic, globally prevalent *M. audouinii, T. rubrum, T. tonsurans*, and *E. floccosum*, and the zoophilic *M. distortum*, which has been recovered from lesions of dogs, cats, horses, monkeys, and humans and appears to be restricted to Australia, New Zealand, and the Americas.

Transmission

Dermatophytes are disseminated by direct and, owing to their persistence on fomites and premises, indirect contact.

Pathogenesis

Mechanisms. Proteolytic enzymes (elastase, collagenase, keratinase) may determine virulence, particularly in severe inflammatory disease. Localization in the keratinized epidermis has been attributed to the lack of sufficient available iron elsewhere. This may account for the frequent arrest of dermatophytoses by inflammatory responses (through the influx of iron-binding proteins) and by enzyme inhibitors.

The infectious unit — a conidium — enters via a defect in the stratum corneum. Germination is triggered by chemical stimuli. The germ tube develops into mycelium branching among cornified epithelium. Portions of mycelium differentiate into arthroconidia. This growth pattern in the hairless skin predominates with some dermatophytes (*M. nanum, T. rubrum*). Hair invasion, which is prominent in most animal ringworm, begins with germination of a spore near a follicular orifice. Hyphal strands grow into hair follicles along outer root sheaths and invade growing hairs near the living root cells. Hyphae grow within the hair cortex, in the outer parts of which arthroconidia form and accumulate on the surface of the hair. This pattern, called *ectothrix*, is characteristic of all significant animal dermatophytes. (*Endothrix* describes arthroconidial accumulation within hair).

Pathology. The pathogenic process begins with colonization, during which the events just described occur but evoke little host response. There may be hypertrophy of the stratum corneum with accelerated keratinization and exfoliation, producing a scurfy appearance and hair loss. In dogs with *M. canis* infections, this is often the main effect. In adult cats there may be no signs.

The second phase begins at about the second week with inflammation at the margin of the parasitized area. Manifestations range from erythema to vesiculopustular reactions and suppuration. Mild forms are seen in *T. verrucosum* infection of calves. Severe reactions are typical in *T. mentagrophytes* infection of dogs and *M. gypseum* infection of horses. Local plaques ("kerion") may resemble certain skin tumors, especially in dogs. The inflammatory reaction may arrest the mycotic infection but become the primary problem through secondary suppurative bacterial infection.

The roughly circular pattern of the lesions and their inflamed margins suggested the terms *ringworm* and *tinea* (Latin for worm). Occasional cases of myetoma are linked to dermatophyte infection.

Disease Patterns. The patterns of dermatophytosis in domestic animals are summarized in Table 40.3.

Ringworm generally regresses spontaneously within a few weeks or months, unless complicated by secondary infections or constitutional factors. The agents may persist after clinical cure.

Epidemiology

Dermatophytoses often affect the young. Extent and severity are influenced by environmental factors. Crowding of animals or assembling of large numbers is often associated with increased prevalence. Improvement in calves often follows their release from damp, dark, crowded winter quarters to the outdoors.

The important dermatophytoses of animals are perpetuated by infected individuals of the same species. Rodent sources of sporadic *T. mentagrophytes* infections in dogs and cats seem likely. Sporadic occurrence of the soil-derived *M. gypseum* infections contrasts with endemic to epidemic but bland infections of swine with geophilic *M. nanum*.

The major agents of animal ringworm are globally distributed.

Table 40.1. Features of Dermatophyte Genera

	Microsporum	*Trichophyton*	*Epidermophyton*
Macroconidia	Usually present	Variable; often absent	Present
Walls	Thick	Thin	Thick
Surface	Rough	Smooth	Smooth
Shape	Spindle, cigar	Club (slender)	Club (broad)
Microconidia	Variable, often absent	Usual	Absent
Sexual form	*Nannizzia*	*Arthroderma*	None known

Table 40.2. Important Dermatophytes of Animals and their Reservoirs

Dermatophyte Species	Reservoir	Affected Animal Hosts	Humans Affected	Geographic Distribution
Microsporum canis	Cat	Cat, dog, horse[a] (goat, cattle, swine, others)[b]	+ +[c]	Worldwide
M. gallinae	Chicken, turkey	Poultry (cat, dog)	+[d]	Worldwide
M. gypseum	Soil	Dog, horse (cattle, cat, swine, others)	+	Worldwide
M. nanum	Soil	Swine	+	Africa, Australia, N. America
Trichophyton equinum	Horse	Horse	+	Worldwide
T. mentagrophytes	Rodent	Dog, horse, cattle, cat, swine, others	+ +	Worldwide
T. verrucosum	Cattle	Cattle	+ +	Worldwide
T. simii	Monkey	Monkey, poultry	+	India

[a] Equine isolates are usually sufficiently distinct to qualify for the recently validated species of *M. equinum*.
[b] ( ) = uncommon host.
[c] Important pathogen.
[d] Occurrence noted.

Table 40.3. Important Dermatophyte Infections in Domestic Animals

Host	Agent	Nature of Lesions
Horse	*T. equinum*	Dry, scaly usually noninflammatory (unless secondarily infected)
	M. gypseum	Often suppurative under alopecic thickened areas
	M. equinum	Not more than mildly inflammatory, resembling *T. equinum* lesions
Cattle	*T. verrucosum*	Painless, thick, white, "asbestos" plaques, local alopecia
Swine	*M. nanum*	Tannish, crusty, spreading centrifugally on trunk; painless, margins slightly inflamed. No hair loss.
Dog	*M. canis*	Typically noninflammatory, scaly, alopecic patches, occasional kerion
	T. mentagrophytes	Often spreading, extensively scaling to inflammatory lesions, secondary suppuration
	M. gypseum	As *T. mentagrophytes*
Cat	*M. canis*	Often subclinical in adults. Generally noninflammatory except in young kittens; may become generalized in debilitated kittens. Occasional mycetoma (Persian cats).
	T. mentagrophytes	As in dogs
Chicken	*M. gallinae*	Generally affects unfeathered portions. Whitish chalky scaling on comb and wattles, noninflammatory
	T. simii	Superficially similar to *M. gallinae* but often inflammatory and even necrotizing. A poultry problem only in India.

Ringworm is rare in sheep. Agents are *T. verrucosum, T. mentagrophytes,* and *M. canis.* The same species affect goats.

IMMUNOLOGIC ASPECTS

Immune Mechanisms of Disease

The major antigens associated with dermatophyte infections are the keratinases (elicit cell-mediated responses) and glycoproteins (carbohydrate moieties stimulate antibody; protein moieties stimulate cell-mediated responses).

Antibody-mediated and cell-mediated hypersensitivities occur in the course of dermatophytoses. Their onset generally coincides with that of the inflammatory phase of infection and may contribute to its manifestations.

Sterile inflammatory skin lesions (phytids) occur in human ringworm infections. They are allergic reactions to circulating fungal antigens.

Recovery and Resistance

Antibodies play at best a limited role in resistance. Evidence favors cell-mediated mechanisms as decisive in protection and recovery.

Recovered individuals resist reinfection, although local reactions may be more acute and intense than on primary exposure. Acquired resistance varies in degree and duration with host, dermatophyte species, and possibly anatomical area.

Artificial Immunization

Mycelial *T. verrucosum* vaccines, inactivated and live avirulent, are used in Europe. They are credited with reducing the number of infected herds and new infections. Commercially available adjuvant vaccines have been shown to be effective in cats.

LABORATORY DIAGNOSIS

Direct Examination

In 50% to 70% of cases, hairs and skin scales infected with *M. canis* or *M. audouinii* may emit a bright greenish-yellow fluorescence under ultraviolet light ($\lambda = 366$ nm).

Microscopic Examination

Skin scrapings and hair are examined microscopically for the presence of hyphae and arthroconidia. The scraping should include material from the margins of any lesion and the full thickness of the keratinized epidermis. The hair is plucked, so as to include the intrafollicular portion. The sample is placed on a slide, flooded with 10% to 20% potassium hydroxide, covered with a cover slip, and heated *gently*. The treatment clears the sample (makes it "transparent") while leaving fungal structures and enough of the hair and epidermis intact to reveal the agent in its relation to the parasitized structures.

Microscopic examination should begin under low power (100×) and subdued light. Infected hairs are encased in an irregular sheath of arthrospores that may double their normal thickness (Fig 40.1). At higher magnification (400×) of such hairs, individual, spherical arthroconidia are recognizable (Fig 40.2). In hairless skin, branching hyphae and chains of arthroconidia occur (Fig 40.3).

Stains and penetrating and wetting agents (permanent ink, lactophenol cotton blue, dimethylsulfoxide) improve visualization. Calcofluor white reagent imparts fluorescence to fungal structures and facilitates diagnosis where appropriate equipment is available.

Culture

Scrapings are planted onto and into the surface of selective media (Sabouraud's agar with chloramphenicol and cycloheximide, Dermatophyte Test Medium [DTM], Rapid Sporulation Medium [RSM]), which are incubated at 25°C for up to 3 weeks. Samples suspected of containing *T. verrucosum* are incubated at 37°C. On DTM and

FIGURE 40.1. *Cat hairs infected (center left) and uninfected (center right) with* Microsporum canis. *15% KOH mount. 100×.*

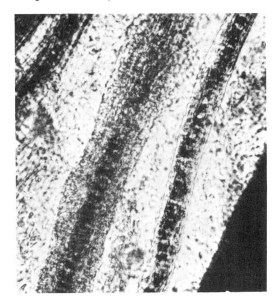

FIGURE 40.2. *Cat hair infected with* Microsporum canis. *Focus is on arthroconidia surrounding the hair (ectothrix). 15% KOH mount. 400×.*

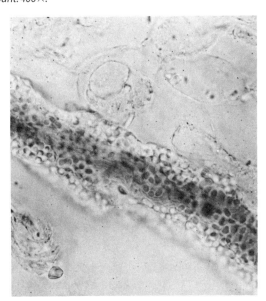

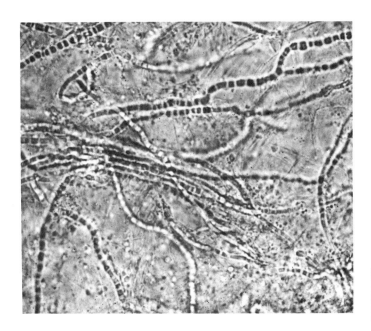

FIGURE 40.3. *Dog skin scraping infected with* Tricophyton mentagrophytes *showing septate hyphae and chains of arthroconidia. 15% KOH mount. 400×.*

RSM, an alkaline reaction suggests presence of a dermatophyte.

Suspicious growth is examined microscopically. The adhesive side of a clear cellophane tape strip is pressed gently on the suspect colony (from RSM; dermatophytes do not sporulate well on DTM) and mounted in a drop of lactophenol cotton blue on a slide to be examined for diagnostic characteristics (see Table 40.1, Figs 40.4–40.6). With *Trichophyton* spp., in the absence of diagnostic conidia, auxotrophic tests are used for speciation.

Knowledge of source (host species, type of lesion) aids significantly in provisional identification of animal dermatophytes.

TREATMENT AND CONTROL

Combined topical and systemic treatment is often preferable. Of two systemic agents available, griseofulvin and ketoconazole, the latter is more costly and less proven.

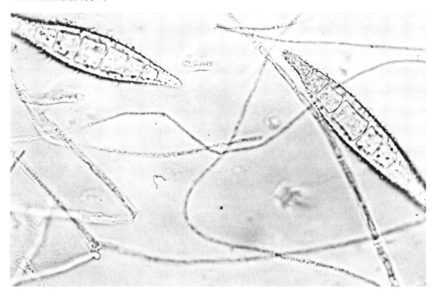

FIGURE 40.4. Microsporum canis. *Lactophenol cotton blue mount from potato flake glucose agar. Note thick- and rough-walled spindle-shaped macroconidia, absence of microconidia. 400×.*

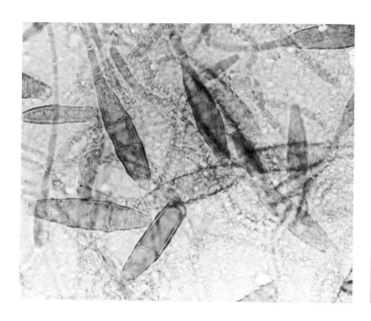

FIGURE 40.5. Microsporum gypseum. *Lactophenol cotton blue mount from Sabouraud's agar culture. Macroconidia are cigar-shaped and thin-walled; microconidia are absent. 400×.*

Both drugs are given orally and are relatively well tolerated. Griseofulvin in small carnivores is given for at least a month, or 2 weeks beyond clinical recovery. Use in large animals is inadequately documented. It is not approved for use in food animals. It is teratogenic in pregnant cats.

Antifungal orchard spray is effective on ringworm of large and small animals (Captan 45% powder, 2 tablespoons/gal). Affected areas are first clipped. In large animals, two applications at biweekly intervals are recommended. With dogs, weekly dips can be repeated to effect. Contact with human skin should be avoided. Thi-

abendazole (Tresaderm, Merek) is used on small and large animals.

Povidone-iodine (Betadine, Purdue Frederick) and chlorhexidine (Nolvasan, Fort Dodge), available as lotions and ointments, are general antiseptics with antifungal action.

A thorough cleanup of premises involving use of an iodine, chlorine, or phenol-containing disinfectant is essential. Utensils and equipment are disinfected with Captan or Bordeaux orchard spray.

Identification of carriers in kennels and catteries can be attempted by culture of brushings. The Wood's light is

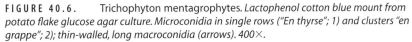

FIGURE 40.6. Trichophyton mentagrophytes. *Lactophenol cotton blue mount from potato flake glucose agar culture. Microconidia in single rows ("En thyrse"; 1) and clusters "en grappe"; 2); thin-walled, long macroconidia (arrows). 400×.*

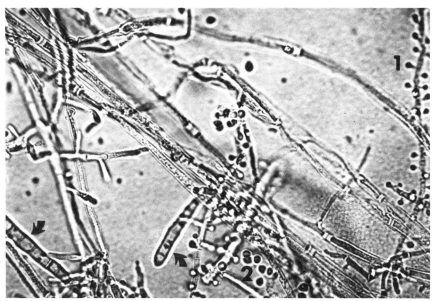

useful in population screening of cat colonies where *M. canis* is the only concern. Infected individuals should be isolated and treated. Exposed animals are treated prophylactically.

Successful vaccination is widely practiced on European cattle. A live attenuated strain (*T. verrucosum*) appears to be most immunogenic.

Selected References

Angarano DW, Scott DW. Use of ketoconazole in treatment of dermatophytosis in dogs. J Am Vet Med Assoc 1987; 190:1433.

Gudding R, Naess B. Vaccination of cattle against ringworm caused by *Trichophoton verrucosum*. Am J Vet Res 1986; 47:2415.

Hageage GJ, Harrington BJ. Use of calcofluor white in clinical mycology. Lab Med 1984;15:109.

Medleau L, Chalmers SA. Resolution of generalized dermatophytosis without treatment in dogs. J Am Vet Med Assoc 1992;201:1891.

Miller WH, Goldschmidt MH. Mycetomas in the cat caused by a dermatophyte. J Am Anim Hosp Assoc 1986;22:255.

Moriello KA, DeBoer DJ. Fungal flora of the coat of pet cats. Am J Vet Res 1991;52:602.

Moriello KA, DeBoer DJ. Fungal flora of the haircoat of cats with and without dermatophytosis. J Med Vet Mycol 1991;29:285.

Pier AC, Hodges AB, Lauze JM, Raisbeck M. Experimental immunity to *Microsporum canis* and cross reactions with other dermatophytes of veterinary importance. J Med Vet Mycol 1995;33:93.

Rebell G, Taplin D. Dermatophytes — their recognition and identification. Rev. ed. Miami: University of Miami, 1970.

Richard JL, Debey MC, Chermette R, et al. Advances in veterinary mycology. J Med Vet Mycol 1994;32:169.

Rippon JW. The changing epidemiology and emerging patterns of dermatophyte species. Curr Topics Med Mycol 1985;1:208.

Scott DW. Large animal dermatology. Philadelphia: W.B. Saunders, 1988.

Scott DW, Horn RT. Zoonotic dermatoses of dogs and cats. Vet Clin N Am Small Anim Pract 1987;17:117.

Wagner DK, Sohnle PG. Cutaneous defenses against dermatophytes and yeasts. Clin Microbiol Rev 1995;8:317.

Weitzman IR, Summerbell C. The dermatophytes. Clin Microbiol Rev 1995;8:240.

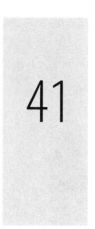

41

Agents of Subcutaneous Mycoses

ERNST L. BIBERSTEIN

This chapter deals with fungi affecting mostly skin and subcutis. Systemic mycoses, of which skin lesions may be one manifestation, are described in Chapter 47.

SPOROTHRIX SCHENCKII

Infections caused by *Sporothrix schenckii*, a dimorphic saprophyte, are usually chronic ulcerative lymphangitides of skin and subcutis.

DESCRIPTIVE FEATURES

Cellular Characteristics

The saprophytic, mold phase of *S. schenckii*, consisting of septate mycelium, produces oval or tear-shaped conidia (2 to 3 μm × 3 to 6 μm) in clusters on conidiophores and along hyphae (Fig 41.1), or it produces thick-walled, pigmented conidia. Mycelial growth occurs on Sabouraud's agar at room temperature. In tissue or rich media at 37°C, budding pleomorphic yeast cells measuring up to 10 μm in the longest dimension (Fig 41.2) are produced. These can be Gram stained. Either phase accepts Giemsa or fungal stains (periodic acid–Schiff, Grocott methenamine silver, Gridley).

Growth Characteristics

After several days on Sabouraud's agar at room temperature, initially moist, off-white to black colonies develop that become wrinkled and fuzzy. On blood agar at 37°C, whitish, smooth yeast colonies appear within a few days.

ECOLOGY

Reservoir

Sporothrix schenckii is associated with plant material and soil worldwide. Occasionally it is isolated from mucous membranes of normal animals and animal products.

The disease occurs — rarely — in humans, horses, dogs, and cats and has been reported in mice, pigs, rats, camels, dolphins, foxes, mules, goats, and chickens.

Transmission

The agent enters through skin contact, usually trauma. Rare cases of internal infection are due to inhalation or ingestion. Discharging lesions may be contagious.

Pathogenesis

Proteases are possible virulence factors and protease inhibitors have been shown to suppress nodule formation. Typically the first lesion is an ulcerating cutaneous nodule. Infection follows subcutaneous lymph channels, producing suppurating ulcers at intervals. These heal slowly but often re-erupt. Lymphatics become thickened. In dogs and cats, dissemination to viscera, joints, bones, and central nervous system is common.

Lesions are pyogranulomatous, having a purulent center surrounded by epithelioid cells, giant cells, and, peripherally, lymphocytes and plasma cells.

The course is protracted. Observations on humans suggest possible spontaneous recoveries.

Epidemiology

Sporotrichosis is acquired from the nonliving environment ("sapronosis"), but transmission from suppurating lesions is possible, particularly from cats. In humans, disseminated disease is seen in the immunosuppressed.

IMMUNOLOGIC ASPECTS

Observations on human infections suggest that cell-mediated reactivity is significantly related to resistance. No artificial immunization procedures exist.

LABORATORY DIAGNOSIS

Direct examination of exudates is often unrewarding except in cases of feline specimens, which generally

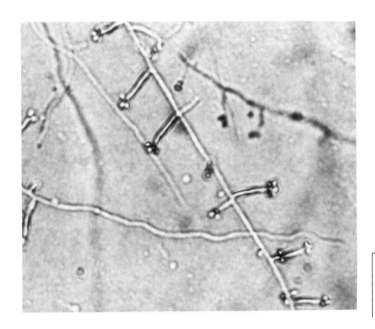

FIGURE 41.1.   Sporothrix schenckii. *Hyphal strands on a plate of Sabouraud's agar incubated at 25°C. Hyphae bear conidiophores with daisylike clusters of ovate conidia. About 400×.*

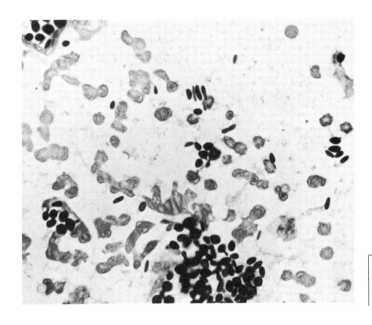

FIGURE 41.2.   *Exudate from sporotrichosis lesion in a cat. Wright-Giemsa stain. Note pleomorphism of dark-staining yeast cells, some of which are budding. 1000×.*

contain abundant yeast cells (see Fig 41.2). With other hosts, fungal stains (see above) and immunofluorescence may help detect yeast cells.

The agent grows readily in culture. Identification requires demonstration of both phases.

Serologic tests (yeast cell and latex agglutination, agar gel diffusion) have had limited use in animals.

TREATMENT AND CONTROL

The cutaneous form responds generally to the oral administration of inorganic iodides. Sodium iodide is given until signs of iodism appear (hypersalivation, anorexia,

vomiting). Doses are then reduced, but treatment is continued for a month beyond clinical cure. The azole drugs, especially itraconazole, are effective. Amphotericin B and flucytosine are used on human deep and disseminated forms.

HISTOPLASMA CAPSULATUM VAR. FARCIMINOSUM

Epizootic lymphangitis (pseudoglanders) is a chronic pyogranulomatous infection of equine skin and lymphatics caused by *Histoplasma capsulatum* var. *farciminosum*. Adjacent tissues, regional lymph nodes, and, rarely, internal organs may be involved.

DESCRIPTIVE FEATURES

Morphology

Histoplasma capsulatum var. *farciminosum*, a dimorphic fungus, produces a budding yeast in tissue and usually sterile hyphae in its mycelial form. Exceptionally, arthroconidia, chlamydoconidia, and spherical, thick-walled macroconidia are seen.

Growth Characteristics

The organism grows slowly on Sabouraud's glucose, infusion, and blood-supplemented media with cycloheximide and antibacterial agents. At room temperature, mycelial colonies form within several weeks. Conversion to yeast on blood agar requires incubation at 37°C under 15% to 20% CO_2.

ECOLOGY

Reservoir

The reservoir is unknown. Endemic areas include parts of Africa, much of Asia, and the Mediterranean littoral.

Transmission

Infection is thought to occur through skin wounds. Arthropods may play a part. Respiratory, conjunctival, and gastrointestinal infections are also reported.

Pathogenesis

A local skin nodule is found, which becomes abscessed and ulcerated. The ulcer may recur, enlarging each time, and ultimately heal by scarring. Typically, adjacent lymphatics develop nodules along their course, showing the same alternating activity. Adjacent lymph nodes develop abscesses draining by sinus tracts to the outside. Hematogenous spread and visceral involvement is possible. Histologically, the process evolves from suppurative to granulomatous, marked by lymphocytes, macrophages, and giant cells, to eventual fibrosis. Yeast cells occur extracellularly and intracellularly, especially in macrophages.

Skin lesions, chiefly on head, neck, and limbs, are the predominant signs. The general condition is usually unaffected except in primary respiratory tract or disseminated infections. Some mild cases do not progress beyond the local stage.

Epidemiology

The epidemiology of *H. capsulatum* var. *farciminosum* infection is unclear. Manifestations vary with geographic area. Seasonal peaks suggest arthropod transmission. The agent may colonize unrelated lesions on the body surface or in the gastrointestinal tract.

IMMUNOLOGIC FACTORS

The role of immune mechanisms in pathogenesis or resistance is not known. Skin sensitivity develops following exposure, even in the absence of disease. Circulating antibodies, demonstrable by indirect fluorescent antibody tests, are indicative of infection.

LABORATORY DIAGNOSIS

Differential diagnosis includes sporotrichosis and corynebacterial ulcerative lymphangitis. The agent must be demonstrated. Direct examination of stained exudates (Giemsa) or biopsy material (hematoxylin-eosin, periodic acid–Schiff, Grocott methenamine silver) may reveal intracellular or extracellular yeasts.

Histoplasma capsulatum var. *farciminosum* grows on Sabouraud's glucose agar with inhibitors. Mycelial extracts contain genus-specific antigens demonstrable by agar gel diffusion. Growth patterns and microscopic morphology differentiate *H. capsulatum* var. *farciminosum* from *H. capsulatum* var. *capsulatum* (Chapter 47).

TREATMENT AND CONTROL

Treatment of epizootic lymphangitis is poorly documented. In nonendemic areas, destruction of infected animals is advisable.

CHROMOBLASTOMYCOSIS AND PHAEOHYPHOMYCOSIS

These infections are due to dark-pigmented (dematiaceous) fungi. Most of the roughly 70 species implicated belong to the genera *Alternaria*, *Cladosporium*, *Cladophialophora*, *Curvularia*, *Exserohilum*, *Exophiala*, *Fonsecaea*, and *Phialophora*. In chromoblastomycosis, the fungal elements in tissue are large ($\leq 12\,\mu m$), pigmented, "sclerotic bodies" (Fig 41.3). Infections in which mycelium is present are called *phaeohyphomycoses*.

Chromoblastomycosis is rare in nonhuman mammals, but occurs in frogs and toads. Phaeohyphomycosis is seen sporadically in cats, dogs, horses, cattle, and goats and may be systemic.

The agents, soil- and plant-associated saprophytes, enter through skin and multiply subcutaneously, causing pyogranulomatous reactions. No tissue colonies or granules are seen. Nodular or larger swellings develop, which may ulcerate and discharge pus.

Diagnosis is by biopsy and culture. Sclerotic bodies and hyphae are seen in stained biopsy sections. Culture, on Sabouraud's agar without inhibitors, often requires lengthy incubation. The resulting colonies range from olive to brown to black.

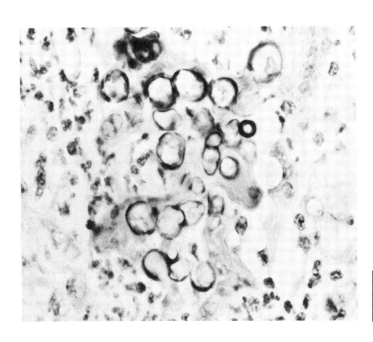

FIGURE 41.3.   *Chromoblastomycosis in the skin of a horse. Pigmented bodies suggestive of blastoconidia are surrounded by inflammatory reaction. Hematoxylin-eosin stain, 400×.*

Lesions are excised, but may recur. Medical treatment (flucytosine, itraconazole, amphotericin B, ketoconazole) has not been adequately tested in animals.

MYCETOMAS

Mycetoma, or "fungal tumor," is characterized by swelling, granule formation, and discharging sinus tracts. They may be associated with bacteria, most notably an actinomycete (actinomycotic) or fungi (eumycotic) and are rarely reported in cattle, horses, dogs, and cats. The cutaneous form is often nodular and is associated with similar nasal lesions.

Causative fungi include *Pseudollescheria boydii*, *Cochliobolus spicifer* (the sexual forms of *Scedosporium apiospermum* and *Bipolaris spicifera*, respectively), and *Curvularia geniculata*. All are saprophytes that presumably enter via a wound. It is not clear what triggers this course of pathogenesis, because the same agents can cause other pathologic patterns.

Fungal colonies are surrounded by suppuration bordered by granulomatous reactions. Sinus tracts carry pus and granules, consisting of microorganisms and inflammatory components, to the surface. The processes are slowly progressive, involving adjacent tissues.

Treatment is excision.

CUTANEOUS PYTHIOSIS ("SWAMP CANCER," "FLORIDA HORSE LEECHES")

Pythium insidiosum ("*Hyphomyces destruens*") causes ulcerative pyogranulomatous or fibrogranulomatous skin infections in horses, cattle, and dogs mainly in tropical or subtropical areas. The agent is an aquatic fungus with wide (4 μm), sparsely septate hyphae. Lesions in horses are large (≤45 cm) discharging swellings, usually on extremities, ventral trunk, or head. The nasal mucosa may be involved. Hyphae are demonstrable within granulomatous coagula ("leeches") consisting of necrotic macrophages, epithelioid cells, and giant cells, with eosinophilic admixtures. Identification requires isolation and demonstration of zoospores. An immunodiffusion test exists.

Treatment is surgery and antifungal therapy (amphotericin B). Benefits are claimed for immunotherapy.

SELECTED REFERENCES

General

Hogan LH, Klein BS, Levitz SM. Virulence factors of medically important fungi. Clin Microbiol Rev 1996;9:469.

McGinnis MR, Rinaldi MG. Selected medically important fungi and some common synonyms and obsolete names. Clin Infect Dis 1995;21:277.

Sporothrix schenckii

Dunstan RW, Langham RF, Reimann KA, Wakenell PS. Feline sporotrichosis: a report of 5 cases with transmission to humans. J Am Acad Dermatol 1996;15:37.

Dunstan RW, Reimann KA, Langham RF. Feline sporotrichosis. J Am Vet Med Assoc 1986;189:880.

Kauffman CA. Old and new therapies for sporotrichosis. Clin Infect Dis 1995;21:981.

Winn RE, Anderson J, Piper J, et al. Systemic sporotrichosis treated with itraconazole. Clin Infect Dis 1993;17:210.

Histoplasma capsulatum var. *farciminosum*

Gabal MA, Hassan FS, Siad AA, Karim KA. Study of equine histoplasmosis farciminosi and characterization of *Histoplasma farciminosum*. Saboraudia 1983;21:121.

Singh T. Studies on epizootic lymphangitis. Study of clinical cases and experimental transmission. Ind J Vet Sci 1966;36:45.

Singh T, Varmani BML, Bhalla NP. Studies on epizootic lymphangitis. II. Pathogenesis and histopathology of equine histoplasmosis. Ind J Vet Sci 1965;35:111.

Standard PC, Kaufman L. Specific immunological test for the rapid identification of members of the genus *Histoplasma*. J Clin Microbiol 1976;3:191.

Chromoblastomycosis and Phaeohyphomycosis

Abid HN, Walter PA, Litchfield H. Chromomycosis in a horse. J Am Vet Med Assoc 1987;191:711.

Dhein CR, Leathers CD, Padhye AA, Ajello L. Phaeohyphomycosis caused by *Aternaria alternata* in a cat. J Am Vet Med Assoc 1988;193:1101.

Dillehay DL, Ribas JL, Newton JC, Kwapien RP. Cerebral phaeohyphomycosis in two dogs and a cat. Vet Pathol 1987;24:192.

Kaplan W, Chandler FW, Ajello L, et al. Equine phaeohyphomycosis caused by *Drechslera spicifera*. Can Vet J 1975;16:205.

Lomax LG, Cole JR, Padhye AA, et al. Osteolytic phaeohyphomycosis in a German shepherd caused by *Phialemonium obovatum*. J Clin Microbiol 1986;23:987.

McKeever PJ, Caywood DD, Perman V. Chromycosis in a cat: successful medical therapy. J Am Anim Hosp Assoc 1983;19:533.

Simpson JG. A case of chromoblastomycosis in a horse. Vet Med 1966;61:1207.

Mycetoma

McEntee M. Eumycotic mycetoma: review and report of a cutaneous lesion caused by *Pseudollescheria boydii* in a horse. J Am Vet Med Assoc 1987;191:1459.

van den Brock AHM, Thoday KL. Eumycetoma in a British cat. J Small Anim Pract 1987;28:827.

Cutaneous Pythiosis

Berrocal A, van den Ingh TSGAM. Pathology of equine phycomycosis. Vet Qtly 1987;9:180.

de Cock AW, Mendoza L, Padhye AA, et al. *Pythium insidiosum*, the etiologic agent of pythiosis. J Clin Microbiol 1987;25:344.

Miller RI. Equine phycomycosis. Comp Cont Ed Pract Vet 1983;5:472.

Miller RI. Cutaneous pythiosis in beef cattle. J Am Vet Med Assoc 1985;186:984.

O'Neill CS, Foil CS, Short BG, et al. A report of subcutaneous pythiosis in five dogs and a review of the etiologic agent *Pythium* spp. J Am Anim Hosp Assoc 1984;20:959.

42 Listeria

Richard L. Walker

Listeriosis is an infectious disease affecting humans and many species of animals and birds. Of six recognized species of *Listeria* — *L. monocytogenes*, *L. innocua*, *L. welshimeri*, *L. seeligeri*, *L. ivanovii*, and *L. grayi* — *L. monocytogenes* and *L. ivanovii* are important pathogens.

Ruminants are the most frequently affected domestic animals. Principal forms of listeriosis include septicemia, meningoencephalitis, and abortion. In sheep and cattle, abortion is the usual manifestation of *L. ivanovii* infections. Listeriosis occurs worldwide, especially in temperate climates.

DESCRIPTIVE FEATURES

Morphology and Staining

Listeria are gram-positive, non-acid-fast, non-spore-forming, acapsular coccobacilli, which measure 0.5 to 2 μm × 0.4 to 0.5 μm.

Structure and Composition

Listeria has a typical gram-positive cell wall. Meso-diaminopimelic acid is the major diamino acid. Cell wall polysaccharides determine O-antigen. Peritrichous flagella and motility are present at 22°C. Motility is poor at 37°C.

Cellular Products of Medical Interest

A hemolysin of *L. monocytogenes*, listeriolysin O, which resembles streptolysin O, aids in the survival of *Listeria* in cells by lysing phagosome and ferritin vesicles. Its loss through transposon mutagenesis abolishes the ability of the agent to grow in mouse tissue. Its recovery restores virulence. Ivanolysin, another thiol-activated cytolysin, is the counterpart in *L. ivanovii*. Production of a phosphatidylinositol-specific phospholipase C and lecithinase also appears to be important in mediating membrane lysis.

Growth Characteristics

Listeria are facultative anaerobes that grow best under reduced oxygen and increased carbon dioxide concentration. Growth occurs at 4°C to 45°C, with an optimum at 30°C to 37°C. Simple laboratory media support growth, preferably at an alkaline or neutral pH. On sheep blood agar, most strains of *L. monocytogenes* produce a narrow zone of hemolysis. Colonies are usually 1 to 2 mm in diameter and appear blue-green in obliquely transmitted light on solid media such as tryptose agar. Colonies of *L. ivanovii* typically produce a larger and more intense zone of hemolysis.

Listeria tolerates 0.04% potassium tellurite, 0.025% thallium acetate, 3.75% potassium thiocyanate, 10% NaCl, and 40% bile in media. Most strains grow over a pH range of 5.5 to 9.6. It has greater heat tolerance than other non-spore-forming bacteria; however, short-time high-temperature pasteurization is effective at killing *Listeria*.

Variability

There are 16 recognized serovars in the genus *Listeria* based on somatic (O) and flagellar (H) antigens. There is no correlation between serovars and species, except that strains of serovar 5 are *L. ivanovii*. No relationship between serovars and host specificity has been recognized. Various nucleic acid-based methods have been used to further discriminate between *Listeria* strains for epidemiologic analysis and strain tracking purposes.

Smooth and rough colonial variants occur. In rough colonies, filaments 20 μm or more in length may be observed. L-forms develop on media containing penicillin and have been isolated from clinical cases in humans.

ECOLOGY

Reservoir

Listeria have a worldwide distribution and have been isolated from soil, silage, sewage effluent, stream water, and over 50 species of animals, including ruminants, swine, horses, dogs, cats, and various species of birds. In some areas, up to 70% of humans are reported to be asymptomatic fecal carriers. Many isolates from environmental samples, previously called *L. monocytogenes*, would now be identified as one of the nonpathogenic species based on current taxonomic criteria.

Transmission

Soil contamination and ingestion of contaminated feed are the primary modes of transmission of *Listeria*. Poor quality silage, with a pH greater than 5.5, is commonly implicated and accounts for listeriosis often being referred to as "silage disease." An asymptomatic carrier can be a source for further contamination of the environment and therefore an indirect source of infection.

Pathogenesis

Mechanisms. Exposure to *Listeria* occurs via the oral route. Entry into intestinal epithelial cells or M cells is mediated by internalin, a surface protein, and its interaction with host cell receptors. After passage through the intestinal barrier, *Listeria* can be observed in phagocytic cells within the lamina propria. Further dissemination occurs via the bloodstream. *Listeria* can be internalized by phagocytic cells or by nonphagocytic cells through induced phagocytosis. After internalization, it escapes from the phagosome, becomes associated with actin filaments in the cytoplasm, and propels itself to the cell's plasma membrane via actin polymerization. In this way, it is able to pass to neighboring cells in plasma membrane protrusions and thus avoid host defense mechanisms.

An alternative proposed route of entry has been through damaged oral, nasal, or ocular mucosal surfaces via the neural sheath of peripheral nerve endings, particularly the trigeminal nerve, into the central nervous system. Organisms have been demonstrated in the myelinated axons of the trigeminal nerve and cytoplasm of medullary neurons.

Pathology. With central nervous system involvement, the cerebrospinal fluid may be cloudy and the meningeal vessels congested. Occasionally, areas of softening in the medulla are observed. Histologically, perivascular cuffing predominated by lymphocytes and histiocytes is commonly observed. Focal necrosis and microglial and neutrophilic infiltrates are seen in parenchymal tissue. Resulting microabscesses are characterized by liquefaction of the neuropil. The medulla and pons are most commonly involved.

In the septicemic form, multiple foci of necrosis in the liver and, less frequently, the spleen may be noted.

In the aborted fetus of ruminants, gross lesions are minimal. Autolysis is usually present as a result of the dead fetus being retained for a period before being expelled.

Disease Patterns. Septicemia, meningoencephalitis, and abortion are the major disease forms. The septicemic form marked by depression, inappetence, fever, and death is the most common in monogastric animals and in neonates. Septicemia in neonates is the most common presentation in horses. Chinchillas are particularly susceptible to listerial septicemia.

The encephalitic form, sometimes called "circling disease," is the most common form in ruminants. In cattle, it is subacute to chronic. Signs include depression, anorexia, tendency to circle in one direction, head pressing or turning of the head to one side, unilateral facial paralysis, and bilateral keratoconjunctivitis. Similar signs

are seen in sheep and goats, but the course is more acute and frequently fatal.

Abortion is common in ruminants, but also occurs in other species. Abortion is usually late term — after 7 months in cattle and 12 weeks in sheep. The fetus may be macerated or delivered weak and moribund. Retained placenta and metritis may result. Systemic signs are rare in the cow unless the fetus is retained and triggers a fatal septicemia. Although abortion is usually sporadic, abortion rates of up to 10% have been noted. It is uncommon to find the encephalitic form and abortions occurring in a single outbreak.

In humans, meningitis is the most common of the three forms of listeriosis. Still other disease manifestations include infective endocarditis, oculoglandular disease, and dermatitis.

Epidemiology

The widespread distribution of environmental and animal-associated occurrence of *Listeria* makes localizing the source of a particular outbreak difficult. Contaminated silage is a classic source of infection. Other sources include particularly organic refuse (e.g., poultry litter). Stress factors predisposing to clinical disease include nutritional deficiencies, environmental conditions (including iron concentrations), underlying disease, and pregnancy. Cases are usually sporadic and may involve up to 5% of cattle herds or 10% of sheep flocks over a two-month period of time. Listeriosis in animals usually occurs in the winter and spring.

Most human cases occur in urban environments in the summer. There are occasional reports of listerial dermatitis in veterinarians and others after handling tissues from listerial abortions. Otherwise, animals are unlikely direct sources of human infections. Human epidemics have been traced to food sources of animal origin, including milk, Latin-style cheeses, and liver pâté. Coleslaw made from cabbage originating on a farm with recent history of ovine listeriosis was the source in one outbreak. In many instances, postprocessing contamination is found to be the source for *Listeria* contamination. Frequently there is also opportunity for selective growth of *L. monocytogenes* to occur during long periods of refrigeration.

IMMUNOLOGIC ASPECTS

The majority of human cases of listeriosis are associated with immunosuppressed individuals, the elderly, the very young, and pregnant women.

As a facultatively intracellular parasite, *Listeria* is primarily contained by cell-mediated responses. Humoral factors may play some limited role in host defense.

No immunizing preparations have met with significant success. Killed preparations have been ineffective, while live attenuated vaccines afforded some protection in sheep.

LABORATORY DIAGNOSIS

Specimens

Laboratory diagnosis is based upon isolation of the organism. Spinal fluid, blood, brain tissue, spleen, liver, abomasal fluid, and/or meconium are cultured, depending on signs, lesions, and tissues available.

Direct Examination

A direct smear of infected tissue may reveal numerous gram-positive rods in septicemias and abortions; however, only few numbers of organisms are observed in the encephalitic form. Negative findings are inconclusive. Immunohistochemical staining with specific antisera is useful in diagnosing encephalitic listeriosis.

Isolation

Samples are plated on sheep blood agar and incubated at 35°C in 10% CO_2. Isolation of *L. monocytogenes* from brain tissue may be enhanced by pour plate methods. After the initial isolation attempts, remaining tissue is stored at 4°C for "cold enrichment." Such tissue is subcultured weekly for up to 12 weeks. Cold enrichment is not necessary for isolation from listerial abortions or septicemias. For samples where contamination is likely, enrichment and the use of selective media (lithium chloride-phenylethanol-moxalactam medium, Oxford medium, or PALCAM *Listeria* selective medium) are advisable. Various DNA-based methods for detection of *Listeria* have been described.

Identification

Typical colonies consisting of gram-positive, diphtheroid rods are suggestive. *Listeria* is catalase positive, motile at 25°C, and hydrolyses esculin. *Listeria monocytogenes* is CAMP positive when cross-streaked with a beta-toxin producing *Staphylococcus aureus* on 5% washed sheep blood agar. A similar phenomenon is observed when *L. ivanovii* is cross-streaked with *Rhodococcus equi* (Fig 42.1). In semisolid motility media incubated at room temperature, a characteristic umbrella pattern of motility develops 3 mm to 4 mm below the surface, due to the microaerophilic nature of *Listeria*. An end-over-end tumbling type of motility with intermittent periods of quiescence is seen in hanging drop preparations. Acid is produced from glucose and L-rhamnose but not D-mannitol or D-xylose by *L. monocytogenes*. *Listeria ivanovii* differs by fermenting D-xylose but not L-rhamnose. Fluorescent antibody staining or agglutination with specific antiserum is helpful.

Mouse inoculation causes death within 5 days, with necrotic foci present in the liver. This procedure differentiates *L. monocytogenes* from nonpathogenic species of *Listeria*; however, it is rarely necessary for definitive identification.

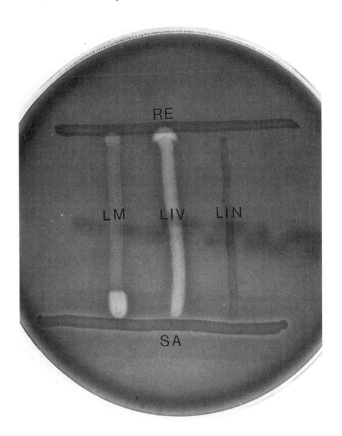

FIGURE 42.1. *Positive CAMP reactions of* Listeria monocytogenes *(LM) with* Staphylococcus aureus *(SA) and* L. ivanovii *(LIV) with* Rhodococcus equi *(RE). No reaction is detected with* L. innocua *(LIN). The variation in the degree of intensity of hemolysis of* L. monocytogenes *compared to* L. ivanovii *is apparent.* Listeria innocua *is not hemolytic.*

Immunodiagnosis

Serology has not been useful for diagnosis due to the prevalence of positive titers in apparently normal animals and cross-reactions with *S. aureus*, *Enterococcus faecalis*, and *Arcanobacterium pyogenes*.

TREATMENT, CONTROL, AND PREVENTION

Listeria monocytogenes is sensitive in vitro to penicillin, ampicillin, erythromycin, tetracycline, and rifampin. Chlortetracycline and penicillin may be effective in timely treatment of cattle with meningoencephalitis. Treatment of sheep has been less successful.

Control measures include reduction or elimination of feeding of silage, particularly poor-quality silage. All forms of stress should be minimized. Affected animals should be isolated and infected material disposed of properly.

Vaccination has not proven to be highly successful and may not be warranted due to the sporadic nature of the disease.

SELECTED REFERENCES

Blenden DC, Kampelmacher EH, Torres-Anjel MJ. Listeriosis. J Am Vet Med Assoc 1987;191:1546.

Czuprynski CJ. Host defense against *Listeria monocytogenes* — implications for food safety. Food Microbiol 1994;11:131.

Doyle MR. Survival of *Listeria monocytogenes* in milk during high temperature, short-time pasteurization. Appl Environ Microbiol 1987;53:1433.

Dramsi S, Biswas I, Maguin E, et al. Entry of *Listeria monocytogenes* into hepatocytes requires expression of inlB, a surface protein of the internalin multigene family. Molec Microbiol 1995;16:251.

Fiedler F. Biochemistry of the cell surface of *Listeria* strains: a locating general view. Infection 1988;16(suppl. 2):S92.

Geoffroy C, Gaillard JL, Alouf JE, Berche P. Purification, characterization, and toxicity of the sulfhydryl-activated hemolysin listeriolysin O from *Listeria monocytogenes*. Infect Immun 1987;55:1641.

Goldfine H, Knob C, Allford D, Bentz J. Membrane permeabilization by *Listeria monocytogenes* phosphatidylinositol-specific phospholipase C is independent of phospholipid hydrolysis and cooperative with listeriolysin O. Proc Nat Acad Sci USA 1995;92:2979.

Schwan WR, Demuth A, Kuth M, Goebel W. Phosphatidylinositol-specific phospholipase C from *Listeria monocytogenes* contributes to intracellular survival and growth of *Listeria innocua*. Infect Immun 1994;62:4795.

Sheehan B, Kocks C, Dramsi S, et al. Molecular and genetic determinants of the *Listeria monocytogenes* infectious process. Curr Top Microbiol 1994;192:187.

Van Netten P, Perales I, van de Moosdijk A, et al. Liquid and solid selective differential media for the detection and enumeration of *Listeria monocytogenes* and other *Listeria* spp. Int J Food Microbiol 1989;8:299.

Wiedmann M, Czajka J, Bsat N, et al. Diagnosis and epidemiological association of *Listeria monocytogenes* strains in two outbreaks of listerial encephalitis in small ruminants. J Clin Microbiol 1994;32:991.

World Health Organization Working Group. Foodborne listeriosis. Bull WHO 1988;66:421.

43 Erysipelothrix

Richard L. Walker

Erysipelothrix rhusiopathiae is the type species of the genus and is the species of primary importance. A second species, *E. tonsillarum*, has been described for some strains previously designated as serotypes of *E. rhusiopathiae*. *Erysipelothrix tonsillarum* is biochemically and morphologically similar to *E. rhusiopathiae* but is genetically distinct by DNA-DNA homology. *Erysipelothrix tonsillarum* is only occasionally involved in clinical disease and is nonpathogenic for swine.

Erysipelothrix can be isolated from a wide variety of environmental settings as well as from the alimentary tract and lymphoid tissue of healthy animals. The disease, erysipelas, occurs in various animal species, with swine the most frequently and severely affected. Other susceptible animals include turkeys and sheep. Clinical presentations include septicemia, a generalized skin form, arthritis, and vegetative endocarditis. In humans, the most commonly recognized form of infection is *erysipeloid*, a self-limiting infection of the skin, usually involving the hand.

DESCRIPTIVE FEATURES

Morphology and Staining

Erysipelothrix is a gram-positive, nonmotile, non-acid-fast, non-spore-forming bacillus, which measures 0.2 to 0.4 μm × 0.8 to 2.5 μm in size. On subculture, rough colonies may develop and produce filamentous forms 60 μm or more in length.

Structure and Composition

Erysipelothrix exhibits a cell wall typical of gram-positive organisms. The diamino acid of cell wall peptidoglycan is lysine. The DNA base composition is 36–40 mol% G + C. A capsule has been described for *E. rhusiopathiae* and related to virulence.

Cellular Products of Medical Interest

Most strains produce hyaluronidase, coagulase, and neuraminidase. Although neuraminidase production varies directly with virulence of strains, there does not appear to be a relationship between virulence and hyaluronidase or coagulase production.

Growth Characteristics

Growth is best on media supplemented with glucose. *Erysipelothrix* is a facultative anaerobe preferring an environment containing 5% to 10% CO_2. Optimal growth occurs at 30°C to 37°C and at a pH of 7.2 to 7.6; however, it is capable of growing over a temperature range of 5°C to 42°C and a pH range of 6.7 to 9.2.

Resistance

Erysipelothrix is resistant to drying and withstands salting, pickling, and smoking. It survives for up to 6 months in swine feces and fish slime at cool temperatures. It is killed by moist heat (55°C) in 15 minutes, but grows in the presence of potassium tellurite (0.05%), crystal violet (0.001%), phenol (0.2%), and sodium azide (0.1%).

Erysipelothrix rhusiopathiae is susceptible to penicillin, cephalosporin, clindamycin, and fluoroquinolones but is resistant to novobiocin, sulfonamides, and aminoglycosides. Resistance to erythromycin, oleandomycin, oxytetracycline, and dihydrostreptomycin has been observed. Resistance was apparently not plasmid-mediated.

Variability

Common heat-labile antigens account for cross-reactions between strains. Heat-stable, somatic antigens account for the existence of at least 23 serotypes. No relationship between host species and serotype has been recognized. Serotypes 3, 7, 10, 14, 20, 22, and 23 exhibited a higher degree of DNA-DNA homology with the type strain of *E. tonsillarum* than with the type strain of *E. rhusiopathiae*. Cultures dissociate on passage from convex, circular, smooth colonies with entire edges to rough colonies with undulate edges. L-forms have been reported.

ECOLOGY

Reservoir

Erysipelothrix is often recovered from sewage effluent, abattoirs, surface slime of fresh and saltwater fish, and soil, but its saprophytic character is in question. It has been recovered from over 50 species of mammals and 30 species of wild birds, and it can be isolated from the tonsils of apparently healthy swine, the most prominent reservoir.

Transmission

Transmission among animals is mostly by ingestion of contaminated material (surface water, fish meal). Wound infections and arthropod bites are other possible routes.

Pathogenesis

Mechanisms.   Strains of *E. rhusiopathiae* vary in virulence. Virulent strains produce high levels of neuraminidase, which is considered an important virulence factor in acute septicemic infections. Neuraminidase cleaves sialic acid present on cell surfaces, leading to vascular damage and hyaline thrombus formation. Antibodies to neuraminidase are protective against experimental infections in mice. The presence of capsules has been described and appears to play a role in resistance to phagocytosis.

Partial immunity of the host and low virulence of strains are felt to account for the localized skin form in swine.

Localization of *E. rhusiopathiae* in joints of swine leads to fibrinous exudation and pannus formation. Subsequent damage to the articular cartilage and an immunologic response to persistent bacterial antigens in synovial tissue and chondrocytes are responsible for the chronic articular changes.

Valvular endocarditis, presumably initiated by bacterial emboli and vascular inflammation, results in chronic changes and damage to the heart valves.

Pathology.   Pigs dying from acute erysipelas infections exhibit hemorrhages of the gastric serosa, skeletal and cardiac muscles, and renal cortex. Congestion of lungs, liver, spleen, skin, and urinary bladder is frequent. Vascular damage with microthrombi is observed microscopically. A mononuclear infiltrate predominates in most cases.

In joints, acute synovitis often proceeds to more chronic articular changes. Synovial membranes become hyperplastic and villous and are infiltrated with mononuclear cells. Spreading of granulation tissue over articular surfaces and erosion of articular cartilage may occur. Ankylosis of the joint may be the ultimate outcome.

In valvular endocarditis, the mitral valve is most commonly involved with development of large, valvular vegetations due to fibrin deposition and connective tissue proliferation. Emboli may produce infarcts in the spleen and kidney.

In turkeys, the pathology associated with erysipelas infections is generally marked by congestion and intramuscular and subpleural hemorrhages. The liver and spleen are often swollen and the abdominal fat is petechiated. A swollen, cyanotic snood and diffuse reddening of the skin are frequent.

Disease Patterns.   Swine with the septicemic form present with fever, anorexia, depression, vomition, stiff gait, and

reluctance to walk. Urticarial lesions in the skin may be palpable before becoming visible. They may be pink or, in severe cases, purplish, especially on the abdomen, thighs, ears, and tail. In severe cases, the skin becomes necrotic and is sloughed. If untreated, this form has a high mortality rate.

In a less severe form of erysipelas in swine, lesions are limited to the skin but may be accompanied by a mild fever. Skin lesions are red to purple rhomboidals — "diamond skin disease." Lesions may progress to necrosis or resolve, leaving a mild scruffiness to the skin. Mortality is seldom associated with this form.

Localization to certain tissues leads to chronic forms, which may occur as sequelae to the acute stages or without previous illness. A vegetative endocarditis is manifested by signs of cardiac insufficiency or sudden death. Arthritis is the other chronic form seen in swine. Signs include limping, stiff gait, and enlargement of the affected joints. Infrequently, sows abort due to *Erysipelothrix* infection.

Erysipelas in birds, especially turkeys, is usually a septicemia. Turkeys develop a cyanotic skin, become droopy, and may subsequently die. A swollen cyanotic snood, if present, is considered almost pathognomonic. Mortality rates range from 2% to 25%. Chronic manifestations include vegetative endocarditis and arthritis. Turkeys with endocarditis appear weak and emaciated or die suddenly without prior signs. Other affected avian species include chickens, chukars, ducks, emus, parrots, peacocks, and pheasants.

Polyarthritis is the most common presentation of *Erysipelothrix* infection in sheep. Entry is thought to be through the umbilicus or wounds associated with castration, docking, or shearing. Affected animals have a stiff gait and, often, swollen joints. They may have trouble getting up and down. A cutaneous infection following dipping also occurs in sheep. Pneumonia has been described in ewes. *Erysipelothrix rhusiopathiae* causes arthritis and endocarditis in dogs. *Erysipelothrix tonsillarum* can also be a canine pathogen and has been isolated from dogs with endocarditis. Septicemia and urticaria due to *E. rhusiopathiae* have been reported in dolphins.

Human infections of skin and subcutis are called *erysipeloid* and are seen mostly in animal and fish handlers. Septicemia, endocarditis, and polyarthritis are rare. Human "erysipelas" is a streptococcal infection.

Epidemiology

Pigs less than 3 months and over 3 years of age are least susceptible. Variable passive and active immunity probably accounts for age-related susceptibility. Predisposing factors include environmental stress, dietary change, fatigue, and subclinical aflatoxicosis.

In turkeys, the male is most frequently infected, possibly through fight wounds. Insemination of hens with contaminated semen is thought to be an important source of infection.

IMMUNOLOGIC ASPECTS

Immune Mechanisms in Pathogenesis

Persistence of antigen in the joint tissue is thought to act as a chronic stimulus for immune reaction and development of arthritis. In addition, an autoimmune process secondary to the erysipelas infection may be responsible for some of the chronic joint changes.

Mechanisms of Resistance and Recovery

Cell-mediated and humoral responses occur, directed at neuraminidase and cell wall components. Serum opsonins apparently play a decisive role. Phagocytosis is carried out primarily by mononuclear phagocytes.

Artificial Immunization

Attenuated vaccines and bacterins have been used for vaccination in swine. While effective against the acute forms, neither type appears to be highly protective against chronic erysipelas. Attenuated vaccines are given orally, parenterally, or, in some countries, by aerosol. Whole-cell bacterins and soluble antigen are given subcutaneously or intramuscularly. Most commercial vaccines are prepared from serotype 2. Certain strains have been refractory to vaccine-induced immunity. Formalin-inactivated, aluminum-hydroxide-absorbed bacterins appear to be effective in turkeys.

LABORATORY DIAGNOSIS

Specimens

Specimens are collected from appropriate sites according to signs. Blood cultures from several affected animals are useful in diagnosing septicemia. Necropsy specimens include liver, spleen, kidney, heart, and synovial tissue. Recovery of the organisms from skin lesions is also possible. In the more chronic forms, cultures from joints or heart valves are less successful.

Direct Examination

Specimens are examined by Gram stain for the presence of gram-positive rods. A negative result does not preclude infection.

Culture

Samples are plated on blood agar and incubated at 37°C in 10% CO_2. Colonies are often nonhemolytic and pinpoint after 24 hours' incubation. At 48 hours, a greenish hemolysis may be apparent. *Erysipelothrix* is catalase and oxidase negative and nonmotile. Inoculation of triple sugar iron agar slants will show an acid reaction and H_2S production along the stab line. A "pipe cleaner" type of growth occurs in gelatin stab cultures of rough colonies held at room temperature for 3 to 5 days. *Erysipelothrix* does not hydrolyze esculin or urea, reduce nitrates, or produce indole. Fermentative activity is weak. Fermentable carbohydrates include glucose, lactose, levulose, and dextrin. *Erysipelothrix tonsillarum* usually ferments saccharose while *E. rhusiopathiae* does not.

Selective media containing various aminoglycosides and vancomycin may be used to isolate *Erysipelothrix* from contaminated tissue. Other selective media contain sodium azide (0.1%) and crystal violet (0.001%).

Serology is of little value in diagnosing erysipelas infections.

TREATMENT, CONTROL, AND PREVENTION

Treatment with penicillin for at least 5 days is effective against the acute forms of erysipelas in swine. Tetracycline and tylosin are alternatives, although resistance to oxytetracycline and some macrolides has been reported. Antiserum (equine origin) is sometimes used in conjunction with antibiotic therapy. Treatment of chronic forms is less successful.

Good sanitation and nutrition are beneficial in preventing outbreaks. Infected carcasses should be disposed of in a proper manner and replacement animals isolated for at least 30 days before introduction into the herd. Vaccination is recommended in areas with previous history of erysipelas.

In turkeys, penicillin is the drug of choice. Subcutaneous injection of penicillin and vaccination with erysipelas bacterin are recommended, if practicable. Penicillin in the drinking water for 4 to 5 days has been effective in controlling some outbreaks. Injectable erythromycin is a recommended alternative treatment.

Good management practices including preventing fighting among toms, ensuring proper insemination practices of turkey hens, rotating turkey ranges away from contaminated areas, and using vaccination in areas with a history of erysipelas are useful preventive and control measures.

SELECTED REFERENCES

Franz B, Davies ME, Horner A. Localization of viable bacteria and bacterial antigens in arthritic joints of *Erysipelothrix rhusiopathiae*-infected pigs. FEMS Immunol Med Microbiol 1995;12:137.

Griffiths IB, Done SH, Readman S. *Erysipelothrix* pneumonia in sheep. Vet Rec 1991;128:382.

Müller HE. Neuraminidase and other enzymes of *Erysipelothrix rhusiopathiae* as possible pathogenic factors. In: Deicher H, Schulz LC, eds. Arthritis: models and mechanisms. New York: Springer-Verlag, 1980:58–67.

Müller HE, Böhm KH. In vitro studies of *Erysipelothrix rhusiopathiae* neuraminidase. Zentralbl Bakteriol (Orig A) 1973; 223:220.

Shimoji Y, Yokomizo Y, Mori Y, et al. Presence of a capsule in *Erysipelothrix rhusiopathiae* and its relationship to virulence for mice. Infect Immun 1994;62:2806.

Takahashi T, Fujisawa T, Tamura Y, et al. DNA relatedness among *Erysipelothrix rhusiopathiae* strains representing all 23 serovars and *Erysipelothrix tonsillarum*. Int J Syst Bacteriol 1992;42:469.

Takahashi T, Sawada T, Ohmae K, et al. Antibiotic resistance of *Erysipelothrix rhusiopathiae* isolated from pigs with chronic swine erysipelas. Antimicrob Agents Chemother 1983;25:385.

Venditti M. Antimicrobial susceptibilities of *Erysipelothrix rhusiopathiae*. Antimicrob Agents Chemother 1990;34:2038.

Wood RL. Swine erysipelas — a review of prevalence and research. J Am Vet Med Assoc 1984;184:944.

44 The Clostridia

ERNST L. BIBERSTEIN   DWIGHT C. HIRSH

Clostridia are gram-positive, spore-forming, usually motile anaerobic rods. Pathogenic species produce one or more exotoxins, which accounts for their pathogenicity. Two groups are recognized. One, which includes *C. botulinum* and *C. tetani*, is noninvasive and colonizes affected individuals to a very limited extent, if at all. These species cause identical diseases in humans and animals. The members of the other group, the "gas gangrene" clostridia, spread from the portal of infection causing local and systemic manifestations. Important animal diseases attributable to this group are enterotoxemias, which with few exceptions are of minor prominence in human medicine. Clostridial wound infections, resembling human gas gangrene, occur in animals.

Of some 80 species of *Clostridium*, perhaps 10 are of veterinary importance.

DESCRIPTIVE FEATURES

Morphology and Staining

Clostridia measure 0.2 to 4 μm × up to 20 μm. Location and shape of endospores are consistent within species. Clostridial spores distend their sporangia (spore-containing bacteria).

Not all clostridia are strongly gram positive. Those that are motile have peritrichous flagella. Of pathogenic species, only *C. perfringens* is encapsulated.

Structure and Composition

Little of medical relevance is known of the ultrastructure and composition of clostridia. Considerable cellular intraspecific antigenic diversity and interspecific cross-reactivity exist but are of less interest than the serologic properties of toxins (see under respective species).

Growth Characteristics

Strictness of anaerobic requirements varies among clostridial species and can be expressed as oxidation reduction (redox) potential (Eh) in millivolts. For practical purposes, redox indicators (e.g., methylene blue, resazurin) are adequate measures of conditions for cultivation of pathogenic anaerobes. Clostridia prefer 2% to 10% CO_2 in their environment. These conditions can be produced in a jar in which the oxygen is reduced catalytically by hydrogen, generated along with carbon dioxide from a commercially available packet.

Most pathogenic clostridia require complex media including amino acids, carbohydrates, and vitamins. Blood or serum is beneficial. A near-neutral pH and temperature of 37°C are optimal.

Growth is usually visible within 1 or 2 days. Colonies are often irregular in shape and contour. Several clostridia swarm across moist agar media without forming colonies. Most clostridia produce hemolysis.

In liquid media, clostridia often grow in air provided a reducing agent is present (cooked meat pieces, thioglycolate). Growth occurs only in reduced portions of the medium.

Biochemical Activities

Clostridial cultures typically emit putrid odors due to products of peptide catabolism, which is a common mode of energy production.

Most clostridia attack carbohydrates, proteins, lipids, or nucleic acids. Biochemical reactions and their end products furnish a basis for species identification.

Resistance

Vegetative clostridia are as susceptible to environmental stresses and disinfectants as other bacteria. Endospores impart resistance to drying, heat, irradiation, and disinfectants.

THE INVASIVE CLOSTRIDIA

CLOSTRIDIUM PERFRINGENS (SYN. WELCHII)

DESCRIPTIVE FEATURES

Clostridium perfringens is relatively aerotolerant. It is non-motile and has a polysaccharide capsule in tissue. Spores are rarely demonstrable in exudates obtained from normally sterile sites.

Diagnostic features include 1) phospholipase C hemolytic activity (hot-cold lysis), 2) the clotting of milk followed by gaseous disruption ("stormy fermentation"), and 3) neutralization of phospholipase C (a toxin) activity (on egg yolk agar) by specific antibody (Nagler reaction).

Table 44.1. *Clostridium perfringens* Types in Animal Disease

Type	Major Toxin Present			
	Alpha	Beta	Epsilon	Iota
A	+	−	−	−
B	+	+	+	−
C	+	+	−	−
D	+	−	+	−
E	+	−	−	+

Type E strains often present in cattle and sheep intestines, but are rarely implicated in enterotoxemia.

There are five types (A to E), based on toxin production. Each type produces a different combination of toxins designated by Greek letters alpha, beta, epsilon, and iota (Table 44.1). The genes encoding some of the toxins (beta and epsilon) are located on plasmids.

ECOLOGY

Clostridium perfringens, Type A, occurs in intestinal tracts of humans and animals and in most soils. Types B to E are found mostly in the intestinal tracts of animals, and their survival in soil is variable.

Transmission is by ingestion and wound infection.

Pathogenesis

1. Wound Infections. Type A *C. perfringens*, alone or with other bacteria, causes anaerobic cellulitis and gas gangrene in humans. Alpha toxin (phospholipase C, lecithinase C) attacks cell membranes, causing cell and tissue destruction. Other toxins, such as theta (hemolytic), kappa (collagenase), mu (hyaluronidase), and nu (DNAse), may contribute to the damage. Infection produces a necrotizing cellulitis or myonecrosis with edema, hemorrhage, emphysema, and a febrile, often fatal, toxemia. This type of *C. perfringens* infection in animals is rare, but when it occurs it is associated most often with injection sites deep in muscle (mainly horses).

2. Enterotoxemias. Most animal diseases due to *C. perfringens* are intestinal and involve Types A, B, C, or D. Type A has been implicated in outbreaks of gastritis and hemolytic disease of ruminants (enterotoxemic jaundice, the "yellows," "yellow lamb disease"), and in hemorrhagic enteritis in cattle, horses, and infant alpacas. *Clostridium perfringens*, Type A, causes necrotic enteritis in poultry and a mild form of food poisoning in humans and is associated with diarrhea in dogs and cats (see below).

In the Old World, *C. perfringens*, Type B, causes "lamb dysentery" in newborn lambs. Occasionally foals, calves, and mature sheep and goats are affected. Beta toxin is considered the principal factor producing hemorrhagic enteritis affecting the small intestine. Its trypsin suscep-tibility explains in part the predilection of the disease for the newborn (colostrum contains antitrypsin substances). The signs are depression, anorexia, abdominal pain, and diarrhea. The course is rapid, with mortality rates near 100%. A chronic form occurs in older animals. Extraintestinal lesions include congestion, edema, serosal effusions, and hemorrhages in various organs.

Clostridium perfringens, Type C, causes hemorrhagic enterotoxemia in neonatal calves, foals, piglets, and lambs worldwide. This type is associated with necrotic enteritides in humans and birds and an often rapidly fatal toxemia-bacteremia of older sheep called *struck*.

Beta toxin, and perhaps others, is the pathogenic factor. Clostridial attachment to intestinal villi precedes toxemia. Lesions and clinical features resemble those seen in Type B enterotoxemias.

Clostridium perfringens, Type D, produces an enterotoxemia ("overeating disease," "pulpy kidney disease") in older lambs (<1year) and occasionally in goats and calves. The key epsilon toxin is secreted as protoxin activated by intestinal proteases. It increases intestinal permeability, ensuring its absorption into the circulation where it damages vascular endothelium, leading to fluid loss and edema. Stress responses to cerebral edema trigger catecholamine release, resulting in adenylate cyclase activation, adenosine 3′,5′-monophosphate (cAMP)-related hyperglycemia, and glycosuria, a frequent finding in enterotoxemia.

Gross lesions may be absent. Postmortem autolysis is rapid. Subserous and subendocardial hemorrhages and excess fluid in the body cavities are sometimes seen. Cerebral hemorrhage and degenerative lesions are common in less acute cases. Histopathology may reveal enteritis.

Lambs may die without premonitory signs. Convulsions occur in agonal stages and diarrhea in protracted cases. Cattle and older sheep show neural manifestations. In goats, diarrhea is common.

Death rates are high in lambs. In calves and goats, nonfatal subacute and chronic cases occur.

3. Type A *C. perfringens* is commonly associated with diarrhea in dogs and sometimes in cats. Whether the microorganism is a contagious entity, as suggested by reports of hospital-associated outbreaks of diarrhea, or an endogenous disease is unknown. Strains of *C. perfringens* possessing the gene encoding *C. perfringens* enterotoxin (CPE) secrete the toxin when triggered to sporulate. CPE is a 35.3kDa protein that binds to a receptor on the surface of intestinal epithelial cells resulting in the insertion of an enterotoxin–host cell membrane complex into the host cell membrane, increasing the permeability of the cell, and ultimately cytolysis. Intestinal secretion (diarrhea) notably occurs as a consequence of epithelial cell damage leading to inflammatory events, and/or by way of the enteric nervous system.

Epidemiology

The agents are commonly carried by some normal animals, especially adults. During outbreaks of diarrheal disease, pathogenic strains survive in soil long enough to infect other animals.

The determinant of enterotoxemic disease is the intestinal environment, which is influenced by diet and age. Overeating, especially on protein and energy-rich food (milk, legume forage, grain) is almost a prerequisite. In young animals, the excess feed is often passed, inadequately digested, into the intestine, where it provides a rich medium for proliferation and toxigenesis by ingested or resident bacteria. Overloading slows intestinal motility, thereby favoring retention of bacteria and absorption of their toxins.

The age predilection of these diseases is due to the diet and the infantile digestive tract, which often lacks enzymes to inactivate the toxins. Colostral antitrypsin activity exacerbates this aspect. *Clostridium perfringens* spores are destroyed in the functional rumen, an organ that is rudimentary at birth. Type D proliferation in older lambs appears to be favored by high-carbohydrate intake.

Seasonal prevalence relates to the seasonal abundance of susceptible populations and rich forage.

Type B lamb dysentery occurs in Europe and South Africa, while Type B enteritis of sheep or goats is reported from Iran. Type C occurs worldwide and also causes overeating-type enterotoxemia in humans ("pig bel"). Type D is prevalent wherever sheep are raised. Type E is found in Britain, the United States, and Australia, and has been implicated in enterotoxemia. A toxin similar to its iota toxin is also produced by *C. spiroforme* and *C. difficile* (see below).

IMMUNOLOGIC ASPECTS

Immunity is antibody mediated and correlates with antitoxin levels. Immunizing preparations often include bacterial components as well.

Passive and active immunization are important in the control of the diseases (see under *Treatment and Control*, below).

LABORATORY DIAGNOSIS

In enterotoxemia, gram-stained contents of the small intestine often contain large numbers of gram-positive rods resembling *C. perfringens*. This test is of limited value due to rapid postmortem bacterial overgrowth in all parts of the gut.

Demonstration of toxin in the contents of the small intestine is definitive. Small amounts (<0.5 ml) of clarified fluid are injected into the tail vein of mice. Death after more than a few minutes postinjection constitutes presumptive evidence of enterotoxemia. A preferable procedure utilizes injections of mixtures of three parts test fluid to one part known antitoxin to the various *C. perfringens* types.

An intradermal test for necrotizing activity in guinea pigs is more specific. If used on broth cultures, tests must be performed on both trypsinized and untrypsinized supernatants, since some toxins are destroyed (B, C) while others are activated (E, D) by trypsin. Samples must be fresh or kept frozen until tested.

Antemortem tissue invasion occurs consistently only with struck, the Type C enterotoxemia of mature sheep. In other forms, isolation and typing may furnish supportive but rarely definitive evidence.

Lambs with Type D enterotoxemia usually test positively for glycosuria.

DNA primers specific for the various genes encoding the toxins have been developed for detection in feces or cultures by using the polymerase chain reaction (so-called multiplex PCR).

CPE is detected immunologically by an enzyme-linked immunosorbent assay (ELISA) in feces of affected dogs or cats. Although sporulation and CPE production are co-regulated, there is disagreement regarding the usefulness of determining the presence of spores in stained smears of feces as a method of diagnosis.

TREATMENT AND CONTROL

Most cases of enterotoxemia are too acute for successful treatment. Antitoxin of appropriate type may be given to sick animals and those at risk. Protection lasts 2 to 3 weeks. Prophylactic dosages, given subcutaneously, can be doubled and given intravenously for therapy.

Active immunization of dams with two injections of (bacterin) toxoid prior to parturition ensures nurslings passive protection for the first weeks of life.

During outbreaks, antitoxin and toxoid are often given and a second dose of toxoid is administered some weeks later. Protection of lambs against Type D enterotoxemia requires two vaccinations at monthly intervals. The course should be completed 2 weeks before the lambs are placed on full feed.

Commercial immunizing products usually cover Types C and D.

Ensuring against overeating is a worthwhile preventive measure where practicable. Feeding broad-spectrum antibiotics reduces the prevalence of enterotoxemia of lambs, but creates other problems (see Chapters 4 and 5). Feeding antibiotic to poultry reduces mortality in chickens due to necrotizing enteritis caused by *C. perfringens*, Type A.

Diarrhea in dogs and cats associated with *C. perfringens*, Type A, responds to metronidazole, macrolides (tylosin), or ampicillin.

CLOSTRIDIUM NOVYI

DESCRIPTIVE FEATURES

Clostridium novyi is a noncapsulated, motile, strict anaerobe, producing large, oval, highly heat-resistant spores. To three types (A to C), which differ biochemically, epidemiologically, and pathogenically, some would add *C. haemolyticum* as Type D.

ECOLOGY

Reservoir and Transmission

Type A is common in soil. Types A and B occur in normal intestine and liver of herbivores. All enter their hosts by ingestion or wound infection.

Pathogenesis

Of several toxins (alpha through eta) produced by Types A and B, alpha, which is lethal and necrotizing, is of established pathogenic significance. The pathogenic roles of the other toxins — hemolysins, a lipase, and myosinase — are uncertain.

Type A is implicated in gas gangrene of humans and wound infections in animals. One of these, "bighead" of rams, starts as a fight injury at the top of the head. Toxic endothelial damage produces edema involving head, neck, and cranial thorax. Death occurs in 2 days. The yellow tinge of the edema fluid, which is clear and gelatinous with little hemorrhage, is a postmortem change.

Clostridium novyi Type B causes infectious necrotic hepatitis ("black disease") of sheep and cattle, rarely horses and swine. Spores originating in the intestine reach the liver and remain there dormant within Kupffer cells. When liver cells are injured, as by fluke migration, resulting anaerobic conditions cause the spores to germinate. Vegetative growth causes toxin production and dissemination. Death may be sudden or within 2 days of clinical onset. Signs include depression, anorexia, and hypothermia. Necropsy reveals edema, serosal effusion, and one or more areas of liver necrosis, containing bacteria. Subcutaneous venous congestion secondary to pericardial edema darkens the underside of the skin, suggesting the name "black disease."

Type C, the reported cause of osteomyelitis of water buffalo in Southeast Asia, produces no toxins or experimental disease.

Epidemiology

The agent occurs worldwide. "Bighead" is recognized in Australia, South Africa, and North America. Distribution of "black disease" largely coincides with that of *Fasciola hepatica*. Both diseases occur mostly in adult sheep, during summer and fall. "Black disease" affects preferably well-nourished animals.

IMMUNOLOGIC ASPECTS

Circulating antitoxin (alpha) and antibody to cellular components of the organism presumably are the basis of immunity to *C. novyi* infections. Whole culture bacterins and toxoid have prophylactic value.

LABORATORY DIAGNOSIS

Liver lesions contain large gram-positive to gram-variable rods with oval subterminal large spores, identifiable by fluorescent anti-*C. novyi* conjugate.

Culture requires the strictest anaerobic conditions, especially for Type B, which is also nutritionally fastidious. *Clostridium novyi* may be demonstrable in normal livers of herbivores within hours after death.

Toxin, in serosal effusions, can be demonstrated by animal tests (see under *C. perfringens*, above), but antitoxins are not as readily available.

TREATMENT AND CONTROL

There is no effective treatment.

Control is directed at eliminating flukes and other hepatopathic agents. Prophylactic vaccination (two injections a month apart) with a bacterin-toxoid is generally effective.

CLOSTRIDIUM HAEMOLYTICUM

Clostridium haemolyticum (*C. novyi*, Type D) resembles *C. novyi* Type B in practically all phenotypic traits. Its toxin, lecithinase C, though identical to *C. novyi* Type B beta toxin, is produced in much larger amounts.

Serologic and toxigenic variants of *C. haemolyticum* have been noted.

The agent causes bacillary hemoglobinuria ("redwater") of cattle and sheep.

ECOLOGY

Reservoir and Transmission

Clostridium haemolyticum exists in the ruminant digestive tract and liver and in soil. Appearance of the disease in new, widely separated regions suggests that movement of cattle plays a part in its dissemination. Transmission is by ingestion.

Pathogenesis

The pathogenesis of bacillary hemoglobinuria involves ingestion of spores, colonization of the liver, liver injury, spore germination, and toxigenesis (cf. "black disease"). The toxin is a phospholipase C (beta toxin), which produces a hemolytic crisis and death within hours or days. Other effects include serosal effusions and widespread hemorrhages. The diagnostic lesions are circumscribed areas of liver necrosis ("infarcts"), which are the effects of the necrotizing toxin. Clinically there are fever, pale, icteric mucous membranes, anorexia, agalactia, abdominal pain, hemoglobinuria ("redwater"), and hyperpnea. Pregnant cows may abort.

Epidemiology

"Redwater" disease occurs in North America in the Rocky Mountain and Pacific Coast states and along the Gulf of Mexico, and in Latin America, parts of Europe, and New Zealand. Although swampy lowlands are associated with endemic disease and flooding with the spread of infection, little is known of the agent's persistence in soil. Shedder animals may have a role in dissemination.

Cases are clustered in the second half of the year, typically among well-nourished animals a year or more of age. Correlation with fluke infection is less consistent than in "black disease."

IMMUNOLOGIC ASPECTS

Immunity is antitoxic. Animals in endemic areas develop some immunity. Whole culture bacterin-toxoids are effective prophylactically.

LABORATORY DIAGNOSIS

Liver lesions are the best source of positive smears for Gram stains and immunofluorescence tests. Cultivation requires freshly poured blood agar and strict anaerobic conditions.

TREATMENT AND CONTROL

Early treatment of sick animals with a broad spectrum antibiotic (e.g., tetracycline), antitoxin, and blood transfusion produces good results. Animals in endemic areas are vaccinated minimally every 6 months and preferably 3 to 4 weeks before anticipated exposure.

CLOSTRIDIUM SEPTICUM

The leading *Clostridium* in wound infections of farm animals is *C. septicum*. Cells are short, stout, and pleomorphic. In some exudates, long filaments are found. *Clostridium septicum* produces DNAse, hyaluronidase, neuraminidase, hemagglutinin, and two hemolytic toxins, one of which, alpha, is also leukotoxic, necrotizing, and lethal. *Clostridium septicum* grows on ruminant blood agar under reasonably good anaerobic conditions, producing within 48 hours hemolytic colonies up to 5 mm in diameter, with rhizoid contours and a frequent tendency to swarm.

ECOLOGY

Reservoir and Transmission

Clostridium septicum occurs in soils worldwide and in the animal and human intestine. It is acquired by wound infection and ingestion.

Pathogenesis

Pathogenesis is presumably related to toxin production. Wound infections, called "malignant edema," radiate from the point of infection within hours to days of exposure. A hemorrhagic, edematous, necrotizing process frequently follows fascial planes as adjacent muscle is darkened.

With muscular involvement and emphysema, there may be close resemblance to "blackleg" (see below) and "gas gangrene."

Crepitant swellings change from painful and hot to anesthetic and cold. Signs include fever, tachycardia, anorexia, and depression. The course may be rapid and fatal within a day.

"Braxy" (Scots) or "bradsot" (Danish) is a fatal *C. septicum* cold-weather disease of sheep. It produces a lesion in the abomasal wall comparable to the subcutaneous one described. Clinical signs are mostly toxemia and gastrointestinal distress.

Human wound infections due to *C. septicum* can develop into cellulitis or "gas gangrene."

Epidemiology

"Malignant edema" may follow such procedures as castration, docking, shearing, tagging, and injections. Postparturient genital infections are sometimes linked to dystocia and unskilled obstetrical assistance.

"Braxy" or "bradsot" is seen mostly in Scotland and Scandinavia.

IMMUNOLOGIC ASPECTS

Immunity is probably antitoxin-dependent.

LABORATORY DIAGNOSIS

Sporulated rods may be demonstrable in exudates by Gram stain or immunofluorescence.

Recovery and identification of this agent by culture are not difficult. Positive results should be interpreted with some caution. *Clostridium septicum* is an aggressive postmortem invader. Its presence may be unrelated to the problem at hand and may obscure that of more significant pathogens, such as *C. haemolyticum* and *C. chauvoei*.

TREATMENT AND CONTROL

Prognosis should be guarded.

Possible therapy includes penicillin or tetracycline given systemically and topically, incision, drainage, and irrigation of lesions with antiseptics.

Calves are vaccinated at 3 to 4 months of age, sheep and goats at weaning. Annual revaccination is advisable. Hygienic precautions at times of likely exposure are helpful.

CLOSTRIDIUM CHAUVOEI

STRUCTURAL AND FUNCTIONAL ASPECTS

Cattle, sheep, and, rarely, other ungulates are subject to "blackleg," an emphysematous necrotizing myositis. Its agent, C. chauvoei, is a typical clostridium bearing subterminal or subcentral spores.

Its spore antigen cross-reacts with that of C. septicum.

Four toxins related to those of C. septicum, an edema factor, and, often, a neuraminidase are produced.

Clostridium chauvoei requires strict anaerobic condition and media rich in cysteine and water-soluble vitamins. Colonies are round with smooth contours, attaining sizes up to 4 mm in 2 days. Hemolysis is variable. The agent resembles C. septicum and is frequently recovered with it. (Unlike C. septicum it ferments sucrose but not salicin and will not grow at 44°C).

Spores last for years when dried, are killed by boiling 2 to 5 minutes, and resist phenol, alcohol, and quaternary ammonium disinfectants. Lye and formalin are reasonably sporicidal.

ECOLOGY

Reservoir and Transmission

Clostridium chauvoei inhabits the intestine, liver, and other tissues of susceptible and resistant species. Evidence that soil transmits "blackleg" is circumstantial (see under Epidemiology, below).

Routes of infection are not known. Endogenous and soil-acquired infection via ingestion or injury is assumed.

Pathogenesis

Toxin(s), particularly the necrotizing alpha toxin, but possibly also edema factor, hyaluronidase (gamma), DNAse (beta), oxygen-labile hemolysin (delta), and neuraminidase, are believed to be responsible for the initial lesions. Bacterial metabolism, producing gas from fermentation, may be contributory.

Disease in cattle is presumably preceded by seeding of tissues, especially skeletal muscle, with spores from the intestine. Conditions favoring spore germination, bacterial growth, and toxin production cause formation of local lesions marked by edema, hemorrhage, and myofibrillar necrosis. The centers of lesions become dry, dark, and emphysematous due to bacterial fermentation, while the periphery is edematous and hemorrhagic. A rancid-butter odor is typical.

Microscopically, one finds degenerative changes in muscle fibers disrupted by edema, emphysema, and hemorrhage. Leukocytic infiltration is minor.

Clinically, there is high fever, anorexia, and depression. Lameness is common. Superficial lesions cause visible swellings, which crepitate on being handled. Often lesions are entirely internal (diaphragm, myocardium, tongue). Some animals die suddenly, others within 1 or 2 days.

Epidemiology

"Blackleg" occurs worldwide at rates that differ between and within geographic areas, which suggests a soil reservoir or climatic or seasonal factors yet to be defined. Young, well-fed cattle (<3 years) are preferentially attacked.

Exertion, bruising, or acute indigestion are suspected triggering events.

In sheep and some other species, C. chauvoei typically causes wound infections resembling malignant edema or gas gangrene. Other clostridia (C. septicum, C. novyi, and C. sordelli) may be present.

IMMUNOLOGIC ASPECTS

Circulating antibody to toxins and cellular components apparently determines resistance to C. chauvoei. Commercial formalinized adjuvant vaccines include up to six other clostridial components.

LABORATORY DIAGNOSIS

Sporulated gram-positive rods can be demonstrated in smears of infected tissues and identified with immunofluorescent reagents.

Ground muscle in saline is cultured on blood agar plates, which are incubated anaerobically. Because of the possible presence of swarming C. septicum, early subcultures should be attempted from some plates, with others left for 48 hours. Identification is by immunofluorescence or biochemical tests.

TREATMENT AND CONTROL

Treatment is often disappointing. Penicillin should be given intravenously at first, followed by repository forms intramuscularly, if possible into the affected muscle.

Cattle are vaccinated at 3 to 6 months of age and annually thereafter. Vaccination should precede exposure by at least 2 weeks. During an outbreak, all cattle are vaccinated and given long-acting penicillin.

Pregnant ewes are vaccinated 3 weeks prior to parturition, when infection often occurs. Lambs may require vaccination during their first year.

Change of pasture is advisable when cases are first observed.

CLOSTRIDIUM DIFFICILE

This agent is a significant cause of diarrheal disease in human beings, but its significance in other animals is less clear. The microorganism has been isolated from symptomatic as well as asymptomatic dogs and cats. Association with a "trigger event," such as use of antimicrobial agents, has been suggested but not proven. *Clostridium difficile* has also been isolated from normal horses; however, it is more frequently isolated from horses with diarrhea and associated protein-losing enteropathy, suggesting a causal relationship. Pathological findings in horses from which *C. difficile* has been isolated include hemorrhagic necrotizing enterocolitis, typhlocolitis, and pseudomembranous colitis. As with dogs and cats, there is some suggestion of association with antimicrobial agents, though *C. difficile*-associated disease has been reported in previously normal, unmedicated foals.

ECOLOGY

Reservoir and Transmission

Clostridium difficile is found in the intestinal canal of normal as well as clinically affected animals. The spores are resistant to most environmental stresses, which results in its widespread distribution in locations where animals are housed. There does not seem to be an overlap between those strains that produce disease in human patients and those that are associated with animals.

Pathogenesis

Clostridium difficile probably associates normally by adhering to mucus or epithelial cells of the large intestine. Adhesins have not been characterized, but surface proteins are probably involved. Disease most often follows a "trigger" event (e.g., antibiotics, nonsteroidal drugs, chemotherapeutic agents) that results in relaxation of the tight control the normal flora has on the numbers of *C. difficile*. The agent produces two large toxins — toxin A and toxin B — both of which are approximately 300 kDa and are very similar in amino acid sequence. Almost all clinical isolates produce both toxins, which are responsible for disruption of the actin cytoskeleton of the large intestine epithelial cell leading to cytolysis. In addition, the toxins elicit an intense inflammatory response inducing the formation of proinflammatory cytokines IL-1, IL-6, IL-8, and tumor necrosis factor. Moreover, the toxins are lethal to macrophages. Thus, following a

"trigger" event, *C. difficile* multiplies and secretes the two toxins. Diarrhea (with or without blood) results.

Epidemiology

Clostridium difficile-associated diarrhea appears to be linked to administration of antibiotics, stress, chemotherapeutic agents, or nonsteroidal anti-inflammatory drugs, although newborn foals have been shown to develop disease without a recognizable "trigger" event. Whether this organism moves among hospitalized patients, as with human patients in human hospitals, is unknown.

IMMUNOLOGIC ASPECTS

Immunity is probably antitoxic, although the role of antibodies to *C. difficile* is unknown. Orally administered antitoxin (made in bovines) is protective for human patients.

LABORATORY DIAGNOSIS

The genes encoding the toxin(s) can be detected in feces by assays based on polymerase chain reaction (PCR). Immunologically based tests are available for the detection of the toxin (toxin A) in fecal specimens. *Clostridium difficile* can be isolated from feces by using a selective medium, CCFA (cycloserine, cefoxitin, and fructose agar).

TREATMENT AND CONTROL

Diarrhea associated *C. difficile* responds rapidly to metronidazole. Unfortunately, metronidazole-resistant strains exist. The alternative antibiotic is vancomycin. There are no vaccines available. However, the use of an orally administered yeast, *Streptomyces boulardii*, has been shown to be useful in preventing the disease in human patients. In human hospitals, handwashing by health care personnel is a very efficient mechanism for curtailing spread. Disinfectants are not effective against the spores.

CLOSTRIDIUM PILIFORME ("BACILLUS PILIFORMIS")

An acute fatal diarrheal disease of laboratory mice with focal liver necrosis (Tyzzer's disease) is associated with a spore-forming organism, *Clostridium piliforme*, that occurs in bundles within hepatocytes. It is unable to grow on cell-free media. It is linked to identical diseases in rabbits, hares, gerbils, rats, hamsters, muskrats, dogs, cats, snow leopards, foals, and rhesus monkeys. Tyzzer's disease has been reported in a human patient infected with the human immunodeficiency virus, but not in immunocompetent persons.

DESCRIPTIVE FEATURES

Clostridium piliforme is a large, gram-negative, spore-forming rod that is motile by peritrichous flagella. Giemsa and silver stains are preferable to hematoxylin-eosin and Gram stains.

Growth has been obtained in embryonated hen's eggs and on cultured mouse hepatocytes.

Vegetative cells die even when deep frozen or freeze-dried. Spores survive moderate heating, freezing, and thawing. Litter remains infective for months. Strains are pathogenically and morphologically uniform.

ECOLOGY

Reservoir and Transmission

The source of the agent is the infected animal. The agent spreads by the ano-oral route and transplacentally. Many infections are believed to be endogenous and stress-triggered.

Pathogenesis

Lesions suggest hepatic invasion from the intestine via lymphatics and blood vessels. Foci of coagulation necrosis are periportal. There may be dissemination to the myocardium. Parasitized cells include hepatocytes, myocardial cells, and smooth muscle and epithelial cells of the intestine, in which a dysentery-like condition may develop. Lymphadenitis, especially of hepatic nodes, is seen in foals.

The course is usually under 3 days.

Epidemiology

Outbreaks are often stress-related (crowding, irradiation, steroid administration). Morbidity is high in laboratory animal colonies. Case fatality rates reach 50% to 100%, especially among young stock. In many colonies, subclinically infected individuals are evidently present; these are often identifiable serologically by a complement-fixation test utilizing an infected mouse liver extract as antigen.

LABORATORY DIAGNOSIS

Laboratory diagnosis rests on the demonstration of typical bundles of intracellular bacilli (0.5 μm × 8.0 to 10.0 μm), especially in hepatocytes surrounding lesions. Fluorescent antibody aids diagnosis.

TREATMENT AND CONTROL

Treatment of clinical cases is usually unsuccessful. Prophylactically effective antimicrobic drugs include erythromycin and tetracycline.

OTHER SPECIES OF VETERINARY INTEREST

Clostridium sordellii is linked to fatal myositis and hepatic disease in ruminants and horses, although the precise pathogenic process is not known. The agent produces numerous toxins and is experimentally pathogenic for many species of animals. Mixed clostridial bacterin-toxoids usually contain *C. sordellii*.

Clostridium colinum causes quail disease, an ulcerative enteritis and necrotizing hepatitis of several species of fowl. The agent is fastidious nutritionally and forms spores sparingly. Its life cycle is unknown, and a toxin has not been identified. The untreated disease is usually fatal. Streptomycin has been effective in the field.

Clostridium spiroforme is isolated frequently from rabbits with juvenile enteritis ("mucoid enteritis"). It may be one of several microorganisms implicated. Its exotoxin is identical to the iota toxin of *C. perfringens* Type E and the toxins of *C. difficile*, and acts by ADP-ribosylating cellular actin.

THE NONINVASIVE CLOSTRIDIA

CLOSTRIDIUM BOTULINUM

Botulism, a neuroparalytic intoxication, is caused by any of seven protein neurotoxins (A to G) that are identical in action but differ in potency, antigenic properties, and distribution. They are produced by a heterogeneous group of clostridia, called *C. botulinum* (*C. botulinum* Group G has been renamed *C. argentinense*) on the basis of the toxins, which in some types (C and D) are bacteriophage-encoded.

Botulinum toxin paralyzes skeletal muscle. Animal botulism is seen mainly in ruminants, horses, mink, and fowl, particularly water fowl. Swine, carnivores, and fish are rarely affected.

DESCRIPTIVE FEATURES

Morphology

The agent is unremarkable morphologically. At a pH near and above neutrality, it produces subterminal oval spores.

Cellular Products of Medical Interest

Vegetative cells, at 12°C to 35°C, produce neurotoxin and other diffusible proteins, including hemagglutinin, some of which protect the neurotoxin against inactivation. Neurotoxin released after lysis of the bacterial cell is produced as protoxin activated by proteases (bacterial or tissue). At peripheral cholinergic nerve junctions, it inhibits acetylcholine release, thereby blocking transmis-

Table 44.2.   Botulinum Toxin Types: Distribution, Origin, Pathogenicity

Type	Cultural Types	Geographic Occurrence	Source	Affected Species	Toxins Present
A	I	Western U.S., Canada, ex-U.S.S.R.	Vegetables, fruits (meats, fish)[a]	Humans (chickens, mink)	A
B	I, II	Eastern U.S., Canada, Europe, ex-U.S.S.R.	Meat, pork products (vegetables, fish)	Humans (horses, cattle)	B
Cα	III	Western U.S., Canada, S. America, Australia, New Zealand, Japan, Europe	Vegetation, invertebrates, carrion	Waterfowl	C_1 (C_2)
Cβ	III	Australia, S. Africa, Europe, U.S.	Spoiled feed, carrion	Horses, cattle, mink, dogs (humans)	C_2, D (C_1)
D	III	S. Africa, ex-U.S.S.R., Southwest U.S., France	Carrion	Cattle, sheep (horses, humans)	C_2, D
E	II	N. America, N. Europe, Japan, ex-U.S.S.R.	Raw fish, marine mammals	Humans (fish)	E
F	I, II	U.S., N. Europe, ex-U.S.S.R.	Meat, fish	Humans	F
G[b]	IV	Argentina	Soil	Humans	G

[a] Parentheses indicate infrequency or variability.
[b] Strains producing this toxin are part of the species *C. argentinense* (Int J Syst Bacteriol 1988;38:375).

sion of neural impulses.[1] The toxin is acid- and pepsin-resistant, but inactivated by protein denaturing agents, including heat, especially at alkaline pH.

Botulinum toxins and tetanus toxin work in the same fashion. Both are zinc endopeptidases that interfere with "docking" of vesicles containing neurotransmitter with the membrane lining the presynaptic cleft. Interference is due to hydrolysis of the proteins (synaptobrevins) involved with "docking." Hydrolysis of these proteins leads to degeneration of the synapse. Regeneration takes several months.

The differences in activity of botulinum toxins (hydrolysis of the "docking" proteins at the neuromuscular junction) and tetanus toxin (hydrolysis of the "docking" proteins at the inhibitory interneurons of the ventral horn of the spinal cord) are related to toxin trafficking after internalization. It is important to note that the receptors on the surface of the motor neuron are different for the different botulinum toxins as well as for tetanus toxin, which helps explain the different susceptibilities of the various animal species to the different types of botulinum toxin. After binding, the toxin is internalized within a vesicle. The vesicles containing botulinum toxin remain at the neuromuscular junction, while the vesicles containing tetanus toxin travel retrograde up the neuron to the ventral horn. Following another cleaving event, a fragment of the toxin (either botulinum or tetanus toxin) translocates across the vesicle membrane into the cytosol where it acts on the synaptobrevins.

Physiologic Characteristics

Clostridium botulinum is a strict anaerobe. Culture groups (see below) vary in colonial characteristics. Some fail to grow on agar surfaces. Most are hemolytic.

Resistance

Although heat resistance of spores varies between culture groups, toxin types, and strains, moist heat at 120°C for 5 minutes is generally lethal. Exceptions exist. Low pH and high salinity enhance heat sterilization. The toxin is inactivated by heating to 80°C for 20 min.

Salt, nitrates, and nitrites suppress germination of spores in foods.

Variability

There are seven types of toxins; they differ in antigenicity, heat resistance, and lethality for different animal species (probably related to receptor density on the surface of the motor neuron). Four culture groups are also recognized (Table 44.2).

ECOLOGY

Reservoir

Reservoirs of *C. botulinum* are soil and aquatic sediments. Vehicles of intoxication are animal and plant material contaminated from these sources. When animals die, *C. botulinum* spores, which are common in gut and tissues, germinate and generate toxin. This may be ingested by carrion eaters or contaminate the environment. In rotting vegetation, a similar process occurs.

Transmission

Apart from toxin ingestion, spore ingestion and wound contamination may lead to botulism.

Spore ingestion is important in human infant botulism. Wound-infection botulism is seen occasionally in humans and horses.

Pathogenesis

Ingested toxin is absorbed from the glandular stomach and anterior small intestine and distributed via the blood-

---

1. Type C2 is not a neurotoxin but an ADP-ribosylating toxin affecting fluid movement across membranes. Its effects are cardiopulmonary-enteric and its role in animal botulism is poorly defined.

stream. It binds to receptors and enters the nerve cell after receptor-mediated endocytosis. Vesicles containing toxin remain at the myoneural junction. A fragment of the toxin translocates across the vesicle membrane and subsequently hydrolyzes a "docking" protein (which protein depends upon which botulinum toxin). The synapse degenerates and flaccid paralysis results. When this affects muscles of respiration, death due to respiratory failure occurs. No primary lesions are produced.

Clinical signs include muscular incoordination leading to recumbency, extrusion of the tongue, and disturbances in food prehension, chewing, and swallowing. No changes in consciousness occur. The temperature remains normal unless secondary infections such as aspiration pneumonia supervene. In nonfatal cases, recovery is slow and residual signs may persist for months.

In birds the disease has been named "limberneck," after the drooping head posture, which often causes waterfowl to drown.

Epidemiology

Types A and B are found in all soils, including virgin soils; C, D, E, and F are linked with wet environments — that is, muddy soils or aquatic sediment. In animals, Types C and D predominate.

Dead cats or rodents in feed can be sources of outbreaks, as can chicken manure when used as a cattle feed supplement. Outbreaks on mink ranches are usually due to tainted meat, and those in fish hatcheries to fish food containing Type E spores that germinate in bottom sludge. Decaying vegetation triggers outbreaks in waterfowl. As lakes recede in summer leaving muddy shores or shallow pools, rotting plant material becomes accessible. *Clostridium botulinum* and its toxin are ingested and after death permeate the carcass, which is fed upon by blowfly larvae. These absorb toxin and bacteria, becoming the source of further cases.

Type D botulism is classically linked to phosphorus-deficient ranges, where grazing animals feed on carcasses and bones that often contain botulinum toxin. In South African cattle, the condition is called *lamziekte* ("lame disease").

Type B botulism has been seen in cattle and mules. In "toxo-infectious botulism" of foals ("shaker foal syndrome") and adult horses, no toxin has been demonstrated, but the agent was isolated consistently from tissue.

Human botulism is usually traced to improperly processed meat, seafood, or canned vegetables. Infant botulism involves clostridial growth and toxinogenesis in the intestinal tract, producing the "floppy baby syndrome." Wound-infection botulism results from contaminated external injuries.

Immunologic Aspects

Resistance to botulism depends on circulating antitoxin. Some animals, such as turkey vultures, apparently acquire immunity through repeated sublethal exposure.

Laboratory Diagnosis

Diagnosis of botulism requires demonstration of toxin in plasma or tissue before death or from a fresh carcass. Isolation of the organism, especially from intestinal contents, or postmortem demonstration of toxin is not definitive. Demonstration of toxin in feedstuffs, fresh stomach contents, or vomitus supports a diagnosis of botulism.

Toxin is extracted from suspect material (unless fluids) overnight with saline. The mixture is centrifuged and the clear portion filter-sterilized and trypsinized (1% at 37°C for 45 minutes). Guinea pigs or mice are injected intraperitoneally with the extract, mixtures of extract and antitoxins, and extract heated to 100°C for 10 minutes. Death due to botulism will occur within 10 hours to 3 weeks (average is 4 days) preceded by muscular weakness, limb paralysis, and respiratory difficulties. Any toxin must be neutralizable by one of the *C. botulinum* antitoxins.

Isolation of *C. botulinum* from suspect feeds or tissue begins with heating suspect material for 30 minutes at 65°C to 80°C to induce germination. Type E spores require, in addition, treatment with lysozyme (5 mg/ml of medium). Culture anaerobically on blood agar plates. Identification is by biochemical reactions and toxin production. Immunofluorescence is used to identify some cultural groups.

Treatment and Control

If recent ingestion is suspected, evacuation of the stomach and purging are helpful. Antitoxin treatment following onset of signs is sometimes beneficial, especially for mink and ducks. Mink and other animals at risk should be vaccinated with toxoid (Types A, B, C, D).

Removal of affected waterfowl to dry land saves many from exposure and drowning. Placing feed on dry ground lures birds from contaminated areas.

Guanidine and aminopyridine stimulate acetylcholine release, and germine intensifies neural impulses. Clinical reports on their use are few and mixed.

Clostridium tetani

Tetanus is caused by an exotoxin of *C. tetani* and manifested by tonic-clonic convulsions. The organism is introduced traumatically and produces its toxin in a nidus often undetectable at the time of illness. All mammals are susceptible to varying degrees, with horses, ruminants, and swine more susceptible than carnivores and poultry. In all animals, the mortality rate is high.

DESCRIPTIVE FEATURES

Morphology

A distinguishing morphologic feature of *C. tetani* is the spherical shape and terminal position of its spores ("drumstick," "racket," Fig 44.1).

Cellular Products of Medical Interest

Of two exotoxins, tetanolysin, an oxygen-labile hemolysin, has no known pathogenic significance. Tetanospasmin is the plasmid-coded neurotoxin responsible for disease. Like botulinum toxin, it acts presynaptically on motor neurons, blocking release of neurotransmitters by hydrolysis of "docking" proteins (see under *C. botulinum*, above). The significant activity is on afferent inhibitory fibers in the ventral horn of the spinal cord. The toxin is destroyed by heat and proteases.

Growth Characteristics

Clostridium tetani grows on blood agar under routine anaerobic conditions. There may be swarming.

Its differential reactions (carbohydrate fermentation, proteolysis, indol production) vary with the medium used.

Spores resist boiling up to 1.5 hours, but not autoclaving (121°C/10 min.). Disinfection by some halogen compounds (3% iodine) can be effective within several hours, but phenol, lysol, and formalin in the usual concentrations are ineffective.

Variability

Ten serologic types, based on flagellar antigens, are somewhat related to geographic strain origin. The neurotoxin is antigenically uniform.

ECOLOGY

Reservoir and Transmission

Clostridium tetani is widely distributed in soil and is often a transient in the intestine. Spores are introduced into wounds.

Pathogenesis

Spore germination requires an anaerobic environment as found in tissues devitalized by crushing, burning, laceration, breakdown of blood supply (umbilical stump or placental remnants), or bacterial infection. Under these circumstances, *C. tetani* will proliferate and its toxin diffuse via vascular channels or peripheral nerve trunks. The toxin attaches to receptors of the nearest motor nerve terminals and is internalized within a vesicle, which travels inside the axons to the cell bodies in the ventral horns of the spinal cord. A fragment of the toxin translocates across the vesicle membrane into the cytosol where it hydrolyzes "docking" proteins and suppresses release of afferent inhibitory messenger substances (glycine, gamma-aminobutyric acid) causing the innervated muscles to remain in sustained clonic or tonic spasms. The toxin also travels within the cord to other levels affecting additional muscle groups. Synapses degenerate following hydrolysis of the "docking" proteins, taking several weeks to regenerate.

The process described ("ascending tetanus") is typical of animals not highly susceptible to tetanus toxin (e.g., dogs and cats). Only nerve trunks near the toxigenic site absorb sufficient toxin to produce overt signs.

"Descending tetanus" is typical of highly susceptible species (horses, humans) in which effective toxin quantities are disseminated via vascular channels to nerve endings in areas remote from the toxigenic site. Toxin enters the central nervous system at many levels

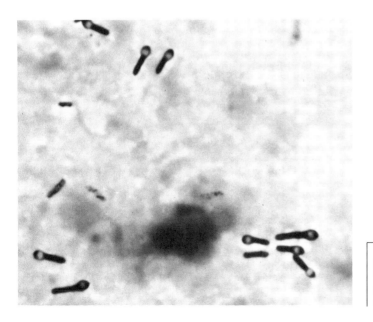

FIGURE 44.1. *Tetanus in a lamb recently castrated by the "elastrator" (rubber band) method. Scrotal impression showing terminally sporulated rods consistent with* Clostridium tetani. *Gram stain, 1000×.*

producing generalized tetanus, frequently beginning cranially. The sequence reflects susceptibility of various neurons.

No primary lesions are attributable to tetanus. Secondary lesions include fractures, hemorrhages, and hypostatic and aspiration pneumonias.

Disease Patterns.   Early signs, following an incubation period of a few days to several weeks, are stiffness, muscular tremor, and increased responsiveness to stimuli. In horses and food animals, which usually develop descending tetanus, retraction of the third eyelid, erectness of ears, grinding of teeth, and stiffness of the tail are observed. Bloat is common in ruminants. Feeding becomes impossible ("lockjaw"). Rigidity of extremities causes "sawhorse" attitudes and, eventually, recumbency. Tetanic spasms occur first in response to stimuli, but later become permanent. There is fecal and urinary retention, sweating, and high fever. Consciousness persists. Death, due to respiratory arrest, occurs in lambs and piglets within the first week, in adult animals in 1 to 2 weeks. Full recovery requires weeks to months.

In carnivores, the incubation period tends to be longer, and local (ascending) tetanus (stiffness, tremors) is frequently seen near the original wound. Progression may be slower than in ungulates, but signs and course are comparable.

Mortality is at least 50% and highest in the young.

Epidemiology

Occurrence of tetanus is linked to the introduction of *C. tetani* spores into traumatized tissue (see under *Pathogenesis*, above): penetrating nail wounds of the foot, barnyard surgery, the use of rubber bands for castrating and docking sheep, ear tagging, injections, shearing wounds, postpartum uterine infections, perinatal umbilical infections, and small animal fights and leghold traps.

IMMUNOLOGIC ASPECTS

Acquired resistance to tetanus depends on circulating antitoxin. Small amounts have been demonstrated in normal ruminants. Survivors of tetanus with the possible exception of dogs and cats are susceptible to reinfection. The amount of toxin needed to result in tetanus in dogs and cats is sometimes enough to elicit an antitoxin response.

Passive and active protection are provided by administration of antitoxin or immunization with toxoid, respectively (see under *Treatment and Control*, below).

LABORATORY DIAGNOSIS

A gram-stained smear from a suspect wound may reveal the typical "drumstick" type of bacteria (see Fig 44.1). Their absence does not exclude tetanus, and their presence is merely suggestive as the morphology is not unique.

Wound exudate is plated on blood agar for anaerobic culture. Increased agar content (up to 4%) inhibits swarming, and a drop of antitoxin will inhibit hemolysis on that portion of the plate.

Replicate cooked meat broth cultures are incubated and some are heated at 80°C for varying periods (up to 20 minutes). All are incubated at 37°C for 4 days, and subcultured to blood agar periodically during that time. Previously unheated ones are heated before subculture. Suspect isolates are identified by differential tests and confirmed as tetanus toxin producers by intramuscular injection of a 48-hour broth culture into two mice, one of which has received antitoxin.

TREATMENT AND CONTROL

Therapy aims at 1) neutralization of circulating toxin, 2) suppression of toxin production, and 3) life support and symptomatic relief to the patient.

The first objective is pursued by injection of adequate doses of antitoxin: 10,000 to 300,000 units for horses. Some suggest intrathecal administration.

Wound care and large doses of parenteral penicillin or metronidazole are aimed at stopping toxin production. Supportive treatment includes use of sedatives and muscle relaxants and exclusion of external stimuli. Artificial feeding by stomach tube or intravenously may be necessary after the hyperesthetic phase. Nursing care is most important.

PREVENTION

Wounds should be properly cleaned and dressed. During surgical procedures, especially on a mass scale under farm conditions, appropriate hygienic precautions should be observed. Horses, unless actively immunized, are given antitoxin after injury or surgery, and depot penicillin.

Active immunization employs formalinized toxoid, given twice at 1-to-2-month intervals and annually thereafter.

Passive immunity passes from immunized mare to nursing foals and appears to provide protection for about 10 weeks, when toxoid can be given.

SELECTED REFERENCES

Baker JL, Waters DJ, DeLahunta A. Tetanus in two cats. J Am Anim Hosp Assoc 1987;24:159.

Bartlett JG. *Clostridium difficile*: history of its role as an enteric pathogen and the current state of knowledge about the organism. Clin Infect Dis 1994;18:S265.

Dillon ST, Rubin EJ, Yakubovich M, et al. Involvement of Ras-related Rho proteins in the mechanisms of action of *Clostridium difficile* toxin A and toxin B. Infect Immun 1995;63:1421.

Gumerlock PH, Tang YJ, Weiss JB, Silva J Jr. Specific detection of toxigenic strains of *Clostridium difficile* in stool specimens. J Clin Microbiol 1993;31:507.

Jang SS, Hansen LM, Breher JE, et al. Antimicrobial susceptibility of equine isolates of *Clostridium difficile* and molecular characterization of metronidazole resistant strains. Clin Infect Dis 1997;25(suppl):S266.

Jang SS, Hirsh DC. Broth-disk elution determination of antimicrobial susceptibility of selected anaerobes isolated from animals. J Vet Diagn Invest 1991;3:82.

Jones RL, Adney WS, Alexander AF, et al. Hemorrhagic necrotizing enterocolitis associated with *Clostridium difficile* in four foals. J Am Vet Med Assoc 1988;193:76.

Kruth SA, Prescott JF, Welch MK, Brodsky MH. Nosocomial diarrhea associated with enterotoxigenic *Clostridium perfringens* infection in dogs. J Am Vet Med Assoc 1989;195:331.

Madewell BR, Tang YJ, Jang S, et al. Apparent outbreak of *Clostridium difficile*-associated diarrhea in horses in a veterinary medical teaching hospital. J Vet Diagn Invest 1995;7:343.

Malik R, Church DB, Maddison JE, Farrow BR. Three cases of local tetanus. J Small Anim Pract 1989;30:469.

Mastrantonio P, Pantosti A, Cerquetti M, et al. *Clostridium difficile:* an update on virulence mechanisms. Anaerobe 1996;2:337.

Meer RR, Songer JG. Multiplex polymerase chain reaction assay for genotyping *Clostridium perfringens*. Am J Vet Res 1997;58:702.

Midura TF. Update: infant botulism. Clin Microbiol Rev 1996;9:119.

Montecucco C, Schiavo G. Mechanism of action of tetanus and botulinum neurotoxins. Molec Microbiol 1994;13:1.

O'Neill G, Adams JE, Bowman RA, Riley TV. A molecular characterization of *Clostridium difficile* isolates from humans, animals and their environments. Epidemiol Infect 1993;111:257.

Schiavo G, Benfanati F, Poulain B, et al. Tetanus and botulinum-B neurotoxins block neurotransmitter release by proteolytic cleavage of synaptobrevin. Nature 1992;359:832.

Sears CL, Kaper JB. Enteric bacterial toxins: mechanisms of action and linkage to intestinal secretion. Microbiol Rev 1996;60:167.

Songer JG. Clostridial enteric diseases of domestic animals. Clin Microbiol Rev 1996;9:216.

Struble AL, Tang YJ, Kass PH, et al. Fecal shedding of *Clostridium difficile* in dogs: a period prevalence survey in a veterinary medical teaching hospital. J Vet Diagn Invest 1994;6:342.

Summanen P. Microbiology terminology update: clinically significant anaerobic gram-positive and gram-negative bacteria. Clin Infect Dis 1995;21:273.

Twedt DC. *Clostridium perfringens* associated diarrhea in dogs. Presented at the Eleventh Annual ACVIM Forum, 1993.

Wilcox MH. Cleaning up *Clostridium difficile* infection. Lancet 1996;348:767.

Clostridium piliformis ("Bacillus piliformis")

Bennett AM, Huxtable CR, Love DN. Tyzzer's disease in cats experimentally infected with feline leukemia virus. Vet Microbiol 1977;2:49.

Boschert KR, Allison N, Allen TLO, Griffen RB. *Bacillus piliformis* infection in an adult dog. J Am Vet Med Assoc 1988;192:791.

Duncan AJ, Carman RJ, Olsen GJ, Wilson KH. Assignment of the agent of Tyzzer's disease to *Clostridium piliforme* comb. nov. on the basis of 16S rRNA sequence analysis. Int J Syst Bacteriol 1993;43:314.

Fries AS. Studies on Tyzzer's disease: transplacental transmission of *Bacillus piliformis* in rats. Lab Anim 1979;13:43.

Ganaway JR, Allan AM, Moore TO. Tyzzer's disease. Am J Pathol 1971;64:717.

Ganaway JR, Spencer TH, Waggie KS. Propagation of the etiologic agent of Tyzzer's disease (*Bacillus piliformis*) in cell culture. In: Archibald J, Ditchfield J, Rowsell HC, eds. The contributions of laboratory animal science to the welfare of man and animals: past, present and future. Eighth ICLAS/CALAS Symposium, 1983. Vancouver: G. Fisher, 1985:59–70.

Smith KJ, Skelton HG, Hilyard EJ, et al. *Bacillus piliformis* infection (Tyzzer's disease) in a patient infected with HIV-1: confirmation with 16S ribosomal RNA sequence analysis. J Am Acad Dermatol 1996;34:343.

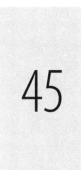

45 *The Genus* Bacillus

ERNST L. BIBERSTEIN   DWIGHT C. HIRSH

Bacillus spp. are spore-forming, aerobic, gram-positive rods that typically inhabit soil and water. Some species cause diseases of insects. The only consistent pathogen of vertebrates, including humans, is *B. anthracis*, a close relative of *B. cereus* that causes canine and human food poisoning.

BACILLUS ANTHRACIS

DESCRIPTIVE FEATURES

Morphology and Staining

Cells of *B. anthracis* are gram-positive, nonmotile, roughly rectangular rods with square ends (about $1\,\mu m \times 3$ to $5\,\mu m$). Chains are common. Spores within the cell cause no swelling. A capsule is formed in vivo.

Cellular Composition

The plasmid-encoded capsule (pXO2) consists of D-glutamyl polypeptide. The cell wall is largely polysaccharide.

Cellular Products of Medical Interest

A 110 mDa plasmid (pXO1) encodes a protein toxin with three components: protective, lethal, and edema factors. The host-cell-activated edema factor (I) is a calmodulin-dependent adenylate cyclase, which raises cellular cAMP levels, causing electrolyte and fluid loss. Lethal factor not only causes release of large amounts of IL-1 from macrophages, it is cytotoxic and also triggers apoptosis of this cell type. The protective fraction (II), the apparent equivalent of the B fragment of other exotoxins, is required for activity of the other factors.

Toxigenicity is lost ("cured") subsequent to loss of pXO1 when the agent multiplies at 42°C.

A feeble hemolysin affects goat, sheep, and rabbit erythrocytes.

Growth Characteristics

Bacillus anthracis, a facultative anaerobe, grows on common media between 15°C and 40°C. Colonies reach a diameter of 2 mm or greater in 24 hours at 37°C. Colonies grown in air have a dull surface and wavy margin formed by strands of bacterial chains ("medusa-

head"). Cells are nonencapsulated. Colonies grown in greater than 20% carbon dioxide on serum agar containing 0.7% bicarbonate are mucoid and consist of encapsulated bacteria (Fig 45.1).

Sporulation occurs under abundant oxygen and never in vivo. Organisms in infected tissue exposed to air sporulate after several hours.

Biochemical Activities

Reactions differentiating *B. anthracis* from *B. cereus*, its nearest relative and a frequent contaminant, are summarized in Table 45.1.

Resistance

Vegetative cells in unopened carcasses may survive for up to 1 to 2 weeks, but spores can persist for decades in a stable, dry environment. Spores are killed by autoclaving (121°C/15 min) and dry heat (150°C/60 min), but not by boiling (100°C) for under 10 minutes. They are not highly susceptible to phenolic, alcoholic, and quarternary ammonium disinfectants. Aldehydes, oxidizing and chlorinating disinfectants, beta-propiolactone, and ethylene oxide are more useful. Heat fixation of smears does not kill spores.

Variability

Colonial and pathogenic variability may be caused by environmental manipulation or spontaneous mutations. Under natural conditions the bacterium is antigenically uniform.

ECOLOGY

Reservoir

The soil is the source of anthrax infection for herbivores. Other species, including humans, are exposed via infected animals and animal products.

Transmission

Infection takes place by ingestion of contaminated feed or water or via wound infection and arthropod bites.

Human infections occur via skin wounds (malignant carbuncle), inhalation ("wool-sorter's disease") and, exceptionally, ingestion, which is also the likely exposure for predators.

Pathogenesis

Mechanisms. Under temperature and bicarbonate concentrations found in vivo, the genes encoding capsule and toxins are turned on. Known virulence factors include the antiphagocytic polypeptide capsule and the "tripartite toxin" (see under *Cellular Products of Medical Interest*, above). The toxin is leukocidal, but the increase in vascular permeability and capillary thrombosis leading to shock is related to the generalized release of IL-1.

Pathology. In tissue, spores germinate and proliferate, producing gelatinous edema. Inflammatory reactions are minimal. Infection disseminates to reticuloendothelial sites. When these are saturated, a terminal bacteremia

occurs, with enormous numbers of organisms in circulation. Postmortem findings are widespread hemorrhages; a black, engorged, friable spleen; tarry, nonclotting blood; and absence of rigor mortis. Bleeding at body orifices is common.

Disease Pattern. The process described is typical for the most susceptible species — cattle and sheep. The course, following an incubation period of 1 to 5 days, ranges from a few hours to 2 days. Some animals die without preceding illness. Others develop high fever, chills, and agalactia, and they may abort. There is congestion of mucous membranes, hematuria, hemorrhagic diarrhea, and often regional edema. These forms are regularly fatal. Occasional animals show just localized edema or an ulcerative skin lesion and recover.

Horses develop colic and diarrhea; edema also occurs, particularly of dependent parts and at the point of infection (e.g., the intestine or the throat) where it may cause death by asphyxiation. Alternatively, the course may be septicemic, as in ruminants.

In swine, localization in pharyngeal tissues is typical. An ulcerative lesion at the portal of entry is associated with regional lymphadenitis. Obstructive edema may cause death. Ulcerative hemorrhagic enteritis and mesenteric lymphadenitis sometimes occur.

Carnivores (including mink) are rarely affected; when they are, the disease pattern is similar to that in swine, although massive exposure through tainted meat may trigger septicemia.

In humans, percutaneous introduction of spores causes "malignant carbuncle" (pustule), a local ulcerative inflammatory lesion covered by a black scab (eschar). Possible complications are subcutaneous edema and septicemia. The case fatality rate is 10% to 20%. A shock-like state precedes death. Inhalation anthrax produces pulmonary edema, hemorrhagic pneumonia, and sometimes meningitis. Mortality rates approach 100%.

Table 45.1. Differentiation of *Bacillus anthracis* from *Bacillus cereus**

	B. anthracis	B. cereus
Motility	−	d+
Hemolysis (sheep blood agar)	±	+++
Reduction of methylene blue	±	+++
Fermentation of salicin	−	+
Growth at 45℃	−	+
Mucoid colonies on bicarbonate agar under 20% CO₂	+	−
Susceptible to gamma phage	+	−

* Modified after Burdon KL. Rapid isolation and identification of *Bacillus anthracis*. Presented at the Symposium on anthrax in man, Philadelphia, October 1954.

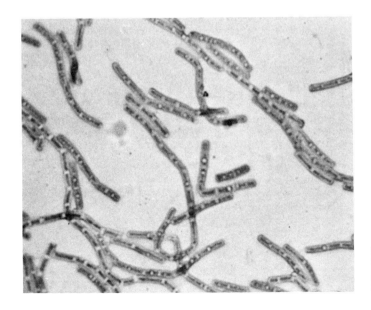

FIGURE 45.1. Bacillus anthracis *grown on calcium carbonate agar under 20% carbon dioxide for capsule production. McFadyean capsule stain, 1000×.*

Epidemiology

A soil rich in calcium and nitrate, with a pH range of 5.0 to 8.0, favors sporulation and bacterial proliferation at temperatures above 15.5°C (60°F), especially after flooding. The geography and seasonality of outbreaks reflect such circumstances. In cattle, sheep, and possibly horses, outbreaks begin with a few cases contracted from the soil. After excretions and postmortem discharges seed the area, secondary cases occur. Areas may be contaminated by floods and industrial effluents from rendering works, tanneries, carpet mills, brush factories, or wherever else carcasses are salvaged. Bone meal, an animal feed supplement, is a common vehicle in nonendemic areas. Carnivores (mink) are usually exposed via infected meat.

Human exposures are contracted in occupations dealing with animals and animal-derived material such as imported hides, wool, and bone. Anthrax occurring under industrial conditions is often the lethal airborne version.

IMMUNOLOGIC ASPECTS

Hyperimmune sera can prevent and alleviate disease. Antibacterial and antitoxic factors are thought to be involved. In most species, immunity is directed against the leukotoxic activity of the toxin, especially the protective antigen. Capsular polypeptide fails to stimulate protective antibody.

Artificial immunization of livestock has utilized mostly modified live spore vaccines. Currently these are derived from avirulent (noncapsulated) mutants. The most widely used is the Sterne vaccine. A cell-free vaccine consisting of concentrated culture filtrate has been used on humans exposed to industrial anthrax. It produces temporary protection against cutaneous infection. Protective antigen, produced by microorganisms into which the encoding gene has been placed, shows promise.

LABORATORY DIAGNOSIS

Sample Collection

During sample collection, precautions against contamination of the environment are important. Blood may be aspirated from a superficial vessel. Aqueous humor has the added advantage of remoteness from sources of early postmortem contamination. For direct examination, bloody discharges from orifices are sampled.

If the carcass has been opened, spleen material may be collected.

Direct Examination

Blood and organ smears are stained by Gram stain and a capsule stain such as McFadyean's methylene blue. Chains of encapsulated, gram-positive, non-spore-forming rods (see Fig 45.1) suggest *B. anthracis*. Contaminant *Bacillus* spp. are usually not encapsulated and lack the clipped, squared-off appearance of anthrax bacilli. Fluorescent antibody helps in the differentiation.

Isolation and Identification

Bacillus anthracis grows on all common media. Definitive identification is by specific bacteriophage (gamma phage). Fluorescent antibody and lectins of appropriate specificities are helpful. Experimental animals (mice, guinea pigs) are injected subcutaneously with suspect material.

Death from anthrax occurs after 24 hours. Lesions include hemorrhages, gelatinous exudate near the inoculation site, and an engorged spleen. The encapsulated agent is demonstrable in blood and tissue.

Immunodiagnosis

Bacillus anthracis antigens can be demonstrated in extracts of contaminated products by a precipitation test using high-titered antiserum (Ascoli test).

Molecular biological methods (DNA probes, polymerase chain reaction [PCR]) have been designed to detect specific sequences on DNA found in pXO1, pXO2, and the chromosome of *B. anthracis*.

TREATMENT, PREVENTION, AND CONTROL

Bacillus anthracis is susceptible to penicillins, chloramphenicol, streptomycin, tetracycline, fluoroquinolones, and erythromycin. Treatment should continue for at least 5 days. In some areas, antiserum is given simultaneously. Antiserum is not available in the United States. In acute anthrax, antimicrobial treatment is often unsuccessful.

Populations at risk are vaccinated annually.

When an outbreak or a case of anthrax has occurred, animal health authorities are notified to supervise control measures. Carcass disposal involves incineration or deep burial (>6.5 ft) under a layer of unslaked lime. Surviving sick animals are isolated and treated. Susceptible stock are vaccinated. The premises are quarantined for 3 weeks subsequent to the last established case. Milk from infected animals is discarded under appropriate precautions. Barns and fences are disinfected with lye (10% sodium hydroxide). Boiling for 30 minutes will kill spores on utensils. Surface soil is cleared of spores by treatment with 3% peracetic acid solution at the rate of 8 liters (2 gal) per square meter. Some other material can be gas-sterilized with ethylene oxide.

Prevention of anthrax exposure through animal products imported from endemic areas requires disinfection of such material as hair and wool by formaldehyde. Bone meal is sterilized by dry heat (150°C/3 h) or steam (115°C/15 min).

Bacillus cereus

Bacillus cereus can cause opportunistic infections, most notably abortions and bovine mastitis. This is often acutely gangrenous and rapidly fatal or destructive to entire quarters. Frequent initiators are udder surgery and intramammary medications.

Bacillus cereus is responsible for several forms of human food poisoning manifested by diarrhea or vomiting, the former being associated with various foods, the latter mostly with rice. Toxins are involved: an emetic toxin (cereulide) and three secretory enterotoxins (HBL, NHE, T).

Selected References

Bacillus anthracis

Abramova FA, Grinberg LM, Yapolskaya OV, Walker DH. Pathology of inhalational anthrax in 42 cases from the Sverdlovsk outbreak of 1979. Proc Nat Acad Sci USA 1993;90:2291.

Beyer W, Glockner P, Otto J, Bohm R. A nested PCR method for the detection of *Bacillus anthracis* in environmental samples collected from former tannery sites. Microbiol Res 1995;150:179.

Cole HB, Ezzell JW, Keller KF, Doyle RJ. Differentiation of *Bacillus anthracis* and other *Bacillus* species by lectins. J Clin Microbiol 1984;19:48.

Dai Z, Sirard JC, Mock M, Koehler TM. The *atxA* gene product activates transcription of the anthrax toxin genes and is essential for virulence. Molec Microbiol 1995;16:1171.

Dragon DC, Rennie RP. The ecology of anthrax spores: tough but not invincible. Can Vet J 1995;36:295.

Etienne-Toumelin I, Sirard JC, Duflot E, et al. Characterization of the *Bacillus anthracis* S-layer: cloning and sequencing of the structural gene. J Bacteriol 1995;177:614.

Fouet A, Mock M. Differential influence of the two *Bacillus anthracis* plasmids on regulation of virulence gene expression. Infect Immun 1996;64:4928.

Gordon VM, Leppla SH. Proteolytic activation of bacterial toxins: role of bacterial and host cell proteases. Infect Immun 1994;62:333.

Hanna PC, Acosta D, Collier RJ. On the role of macrophages in anthrax. Proc Nat Acad Sci USA 1993;90:10198.

Hunter L, Corbett W, Grinolem C. Anthrax. J Am Vet Med Assoc 1989;194:1028.

Klimper KR, Arora N, Leppla SH. Anthrax toxin lethal factor contains a zinc metalloprotease consensus sequence which is required for lethal toxin activity. Molec Microbiol 1994;13:1093.

LaForce FM. Anthrax. Clin Infect Dis 1994;19:1009.

Lin CG, Kao YT, Liu WT, et al. Cytotoxic effects of anthrax lethal toxin on macrophage-like cell line J774A.1. Curr Microbiol 1996;33:224.

Logan NA. *Bacillus* species of medical and veterinary importance. J Med Microbiol 1988;25:157.

Little SE, Knudson GB. Comparative efficacy of *Bacillus anthracis* live spore vaccine and protective antigen vaccine against anthrax in the guinea pig. Infect Immun 1986;52:509.

Menard A, Altendorf K, Breves D, et al. The vacuolar ATPase proton pump is required for the cytotoxicity of *Bacillus anthracis* lethal toxin. FEBS Lett 1996;386:161.

Mock M, Ullmann A. Calmodulin-activated bacterial adenylate cyclases as virulence factors. Trends Microbiol 1993;1:187.

Ramisse V, Patra G, Garrigue H, et al. Identification and characterization of *Bacillus anthracis* by multiplex PCR analysis of sequences on plasmids pXO1 and pXO2 and chromosomal DNA. FEMS Microbiol Lett 1996;145:9.

Sirard JC, Mock M, Fouet A. The three *Bacillus anthracis* toxin genes are coordinately regulated by bicarbonate and temperature. J Bacteriol 1994;176:5188.

Uchida I, Hornung JM, Thorne CB, et al. Cloning and characterization of a gene whose product is a trans-activator of anthrax toxin synthesis. J Bacteriol 1993;175:5329.

Van Ness GB. Ecology of anthrax. Science 1971;122:1303.

Vietri NJ, Marrero R, Hoover TA, Welkos SL. Identification and characterization of a trans-activator involved in the regulation of encapsulation by *Bacillus anthracis*. Gene 1995;152:1.

Bacillus cereus

Agata N, Ohta M, Mori M. Production of an emetic toxin, cereulide, is associated with a specific class of *Bacillus cereus*. Curr Microbiol 1996;33:67.

Beecher DJ, Schoeni JL, Wong ACL. Enterotoxic activity of hemolysin BL from *Bacillus cereus*. Infect Immun 1995;63:4423.

Granum PE, Andersson A, Gayther C, et al. Evidence for a further enterotoxin complex produced by *Bacillus cereus*. FEMS Microbiol Lett 1996;141:145.

Granum PE, Lund T. *Bacillus cereus* and its food poisoning toxins. FEMS Microbiol Lett 1997;157:223.

Jones TO, Turnbull RCB. Bovine mastitis caused by *Bacillus cereus*. Vet Rec 1981;108:271.

Perrin D, Greenfield J, Ward GE. Acute *Bacillus cereus* mastitis in dairy cattle associated with use of contaminated antibiotics. Can Vet J 1976;17:244.

Schuh JA, Weinstock D. Bovine abortion caused by *Bacillus cereus*. J Am Vet Med Assoc 1985;187:1047.

Sears CL, Kaper JB. Enteric bacterial toxins: mechanisms of action and linkage to intestinal secretion. Microbiol Rev 1996;60:167.

46 Pathogenic Actinomycetes (Actinomyces and Nocardia)

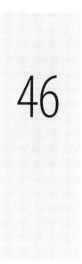

ERNST L. BIBERSTEIN   DWIGHT C. HIRSH

Actinomycetes are gram-positive bacteria that can grow in branching filaments. Apart from this pattern, the genera *Actinomyces* and *Nocardia* have little in common. However, their morphologic resemblance and similarities in pathogenic patterns justify their consideration under a common heading. Table 46.1 summarizes their differential characteristics.

ACTINOMYCES SPP.

DESCRIPTIVE FEATURES

Morphology and Staining

Actinomyces spp. are gram-positive diphtheroid or filamentous rods, about 0.5 μm in width. Branching filaments, often beaded due to uneven staining, are most readily demonstrable in pathologic specimens (Fig 46.1). In culture, diphtheroid forms predominate.

Structure and Composition

Actinomyces spp. have distinctive cell wall constituents (see Table 46.1). Surface fibrils in *A. viscosus* may be adhesins for host cells or other bacteria ("coaggregation"). Surface antigens are related to chemotactic and mitogenic activities.

Each named species of *Actinomyces* has group antigens and several serologic subtypes. Interspecific cross-reactivity occurs least with immunofluorescence.

Growth Characteristics

Animal *Actinomyces* spp. are capnophilic or facultative anaerobes. All require rich media, preferably containing serum or blood. No growth occurs on Sabouraud's agar or at room temperature. Development of macroscopic colonies may require several days' incubation at 37°C. Colonial morphology varies between and within species. *Actinomyces bovis* forms granular to smooth microcolonies within 24 hours. Typical macrocolonies, detectable after 48 hours, never attain a diameter much beyond 1 mm. *Actinomyces viscosus* produces flat, smooth to granular colonies up to 2 mm in diameter. Some unclassified animal-derived *Actinomyces* show patterns of the type species *A. israelii* of humans. Early growth (24 hours) is a microscopic meshwork of filaments (spider colonies). Later, colonies develop ridges and valleys ("molar tooth"). Hemolysis is rare. In thioglycolate broth, growth may be diffuse (*A. bovis*) or clumped ("bread crumbs," *A. israelii*).

Biochemical Activities

Actinomyces spp. are catalase negative, with some exceptions (e.g., *A. viscosus*).

Resistance

Actinomyces spp. are readily killed by heat and disinfectants and require frequent passage to survive in culture.

ECOLOGY

Reservoir

Actinomyces spp. are found on oral mucous membranes and tooth surfaces and secondarily in the gastrointestinal tract.

Transmission

Most actinomycotic infections are endogenous, that is, they are caused by introduction of a commensal strain into susceptible tissue of its host. Bites are another means of transmission (rare).

Pathogenesis

Pathology. Actinomycosis evokes pyogranulomatous reactions by unknown mechanisms. Bacterial colonies form in tissue, triggering suppurative responses in the immediate vicinity. Peripheral to this, granulation, mononuclear infiltration, and fibrosis furnish the granulomatous elements. Sinus tracts carry exudate to the outside; the exudate often contains "sulfur granules": colonial masses surrounded by a microscopic fringe of "clubs" consisting of mineral and possibly antigen-antibody complexes. They are also called *rosettes* (Fig 46.2). Alternatively, *Actinomyces* spp. may be found, usually in mixed culture, in abscesses, empyemas, or suppurative serositis.

Disease Patterns. In "lumpy jaw" of cattle, *A. bovis* and (exceptionally) *A. israelii* are introduced from an oral reservoir into the alveolar or paralveolar region of the jaw initiating a chronic rarefying osteomyelitis. This leads eventually to replacement of normal bone by porous bone, which is laid down irregularly and honeycombed with sinus tracts containing pus. There may be dislodgement of teeth, inability to chew, and mandibular fractures. The lesion expands but has little tendency for vascular dissemination. Similar infections occur in humans and marsupials.

Actinomyces spp. participate in soft tissue infections of many species. In horses they are found in supra-atlantal and supraspinous bursitis (poll evil and fistulous withers, respectively), usually alongside other bacteria (e.g., *Brucella abortus*). An unspeciated *Actinomyces* is sometimes isolated from cervical abscesses, mimicking *Streptococcus equi* infections.

Actinomyces spp. are common isolates from suppurative serositides of small carnivores. In dogs, actinomycosis may be associated with foreign bodies, particularly migrating grass awns, especially of the genus *Hordeum* ("foxtails"), which sometimes lodge near vertebrae, causing actinomycotic discospondylitis. Cutaneous actinomycosis in dogs is a rare nodulo-ulcerative lymphangitis. *Actinomyces viscosus*, *A. hordeovulneris*, or unnamed forms are usually implicated.

A pyogranulomatous mastitis of sows is attributed to *Actinomyces* spp. (*A. bovis*, "*A. suis*"). *Actinomyces naeslundii* is implicated in porcine abortions.

Epidemiology

Actinomycosis is noncommunicable, except via bites (which are rare). Contamination of bursae or body cavities may be hematogenous or result from perforations (of the alimentary tract, body wall). Actinomycosis associated with foxtails occurs in outdoor dogs in semiarid areas.

Actinomyces spp. occur in goats, sheep, wild ruminants, monkeys, rabbits, squirrels, hamsters, marsupials, and birds. Except for occasional isolations of *A. israelii* in dogs and cattle, there is little to suggest interspecific transmission of *Actinomyces* spp.

Table 46.1.   Contrasting Characteristics of *Actinomyces* and Common Pathogenic *Nocardia*

Characteristic	Actinomyces	Nocardia
Source	Endogenous	Exogenous
Atmospheric requirements	Anaerobic/microaerophilic	Aerobic
Catalase	− or +	+
Growth on Sabouraud's agar	−	+
Acid-fastness	−	+
Penicillin	Susceptible	Resistant[a]
Cell wall contains meso DAP[b]	−	+
Lysine	+	−
Mycolic acid	−	+
Lymph node involvement	Rare	Common
Granules in exudate ("sulfur granules")	Common	Rare

[a] "*Nocardia nova*" are susceptible to penicillin.
[b] Diaminopimelic acid.

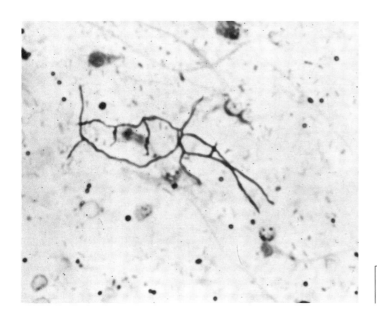

FIGURE 46.1.   Actinomyces *spp. in aspirate from retrobulbar abscess in a horse. Gram stain, 1000×.*

IMMUNOLOGIC FACTORS

Infected humans show cell-mediated and humoral immune responses.

Circulating antibody, produced during infection, confers no protection. Specific resistance, if any, is probably cell mediated. Actinomyces is killed by phagocytes. No artificial immunization is available.

LABORATORY DIAGNOSIS

Sample Collection

Aspirates from unopened lesions or tissues, preferably including granules, are optimal.

Direct Examination

Suspected exudates are examined for "sulfur granules": yellowish particles, varying in firmness, up to several millimeters in diameter. Granules are washed in saline and placed on a slide in a drop of saline. A cover slip is gently pressed down. The preparation is examined under subdued light (see Fig 46.2). Rosettes are suggestive of actinomycosis, especially if bacterial-sized filaments extend into the clubbed fringe.

Crushed granules, exudate, or tissue impressions are stained with Gram and acid-fast stain (Kinyoun's). Branching, gram-positive, beaded, non-acid-fast filaments suggest *Actinomyces* spp. (see Fig 46.1).

Isolation and Identification

Most strains obtained from animals do not require anaerobic incubation but benefit from increased carbon dioxide. Granules offer the best chance of isolation from the usually mixed flora. Colonies develop in 48 hours or more. Organisms of suggestive morphology and staining characteristics are tested for catalase activity. Isolates grown on blood agar sometimes give false-positive catalase results.

Precise identification includes cell wall analysis (see Table 46.1) and biochemical tests. Many animal isolates cannot be assigned to existing species.

TREATMENT AND CONTROL

In bovine actinomycosis, iodine compounds given orally (4 to 8 gm) daily or intravenously (75 mg/kg) weekly are used. Treatment must be interrupted when signs of toxicity appear (hypersalivation, anorexia, vomiting) but can be resumed some weeks later. Accessible soft tissue lesions can be drained or excised.

Penicillin and aminoglycoside combinations are often used on bovine actinomycosis. The contribution of aminoglycoside is uncertain. Isoniazid per os has been advocated. Bacteriologic cure of lumpy jaw will not restore normal bone structure, but the process can be arrested by systemic medication aided by drainage, lavage (iodine), and debridement of lesions.

In dogs and cats, surgery (drainage, lavage, excision, removal of foreign bodies) is required, supplemented by

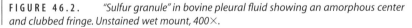

FIGURE 46.2.   *"Sulfur granule" in bovine pleural fluid showing an amorphous center and clubbed fringe. Unstained wet mount, 400×.*

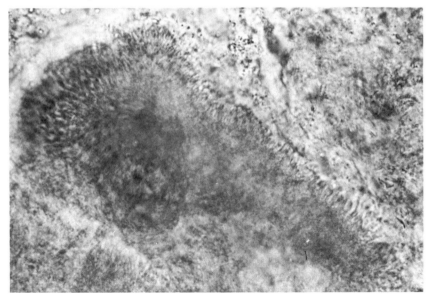

long-term antimicrobic therapy. A penicillin derivative (e.g., ampicillin) is the drug of choice. Alternatives are erythromycin, rifampin, cephaloridine, and minocycline. Aminoglycosides and fluoroquinolones are ineffective. Remnants of plant awns together with the propensity of *Actinomyces* spp. to form cell-wall-deficient variants (L-forms) make treatment of this condition difficult.

Where foxtails are prevalent, conscientious grooming is a critical preventive step.

NOCARDIA

Nocardiae are aerobic, saprophytic actinomycetes present in most environments. Generalized suppurative and pyo-granulomatous processes occur in immunosuppressed and massively exposed individuals. Of three main species, *N. asteroides*, *N. brasiliensis*, and *N. otitidiscaviarum* (synonym *N. caviae*), *N. asteroides* accounts for most cases. *Nocardia asteroides* is probably a heterogenous collection of nocardiae. *"Nocardia nova"* is a part of this collection and is the most frequent nocardiae isolated from affected dogs and cats. Probably all animals are susceptible to infection. Dogs are most often affected. In dairy cattle, nocardial mastitis is economically important. Nocardiosis occurs in humans, cats, horses, goats, sheep, swine, nonhuman primates, rabbits, nondomestic ruminants and carnivores, marine mammals, birds, and fish.

DESCRIPTIVE FEATURES

Morphology and Staining

Gram-stained *Nocardia* spp. can be indistinguishable from *Actinomyces* spp. (Fig 46.3). The three species named

exhibit varying degrees of acid-fastness. Nocardiae alternate between the coccobacillary (resting phase), and the actively growing filamentous forms.

Structure and Composition

The cell wall architecture and constituents are typical of the coryneform group (see Chapter 23). Mycolic acids and other nocardial lipids are possible virulence factors.

No exotoxins are known, but a superoxide dismutase acts as a virulence factor. Soluble antigens — largely protein — are type-specific.

Growth Characteristics

Pathogenic nocardiae are obligate aerobes growing on simple media (e.g., Sabouraud's) over a wide temperature range (10 to 50°C). Colonies, which appear after several days, are opaque and variously pigmented. The colony surface, waxy to powdery to velvety depending on the abundance of aerial growth, becomes wrinkled with age. Colonial diameters may reach several centimeters. In broth, a surface pellicle or sediment is produced, but little turbidity.

Biochemical activities include catalase production, acidification of various carbohydrates, and usually urea hydrolysis. Differential substrate utilization serves to identify pathogenic *Nocardia* spp.

Resistance

Nocardiae thrive in the environment. *Nocardia asteroides* withstands 60°C for several hours, and *N. otitidiscaviarum* 50°C. *Nocardia brasiliensis* is less tolerant. All are susceptible to chlorine disinfectants (100 ppm/5 min) and benzalkonium chloride (100 ppm/10 min).

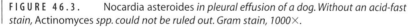

FIGURE 46.3.   Nocardia asteroides *in pleural effusion of a dog. Without an acid-fast stain,* Actinomyces *spp. could not be ruled out. Gram stain, 1000×.*

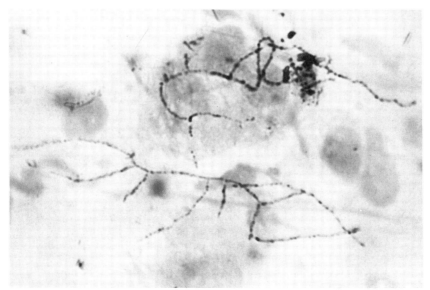

Variability

Colonial dissociation is seen in single strains of *N. asteroides*. Serotypes are based on soluble antigens.

ECOLOGY

Reservoir

Pathogenic nocardiae are saprophytes found in many climates in soils and water, either as indigenous flora or contaminants.

Transmission

Three main routes of infection are inhalation, trauma, and ingestion. Dust, soil, and plant material serve as vehicles. Bovine mastitis is introduced and disseminated by equipment and personnel.

Pathogenesis

Pathogenic Mechanisms. Pathogenic nocardiae survive within phagocytic vacuoles by preventing phagolysosome formation. This is attributed to a surface lipid. Other cell wall lipids may trigger granulomatous reactions. Variations between strains and growth phases in cell envelope constituents are paralleled by changes in virulence and infectivity.

Superoxide dismutase and lysosomal enzyme inhibition protect *N. asteroides* against phagocytic killing.

Pathology. Nocardiosis is a predominantly suppurative process with variable granulomatous features. Lymph nodes are consistently involved. Hematogenous dissemination may result in osteomyelitis and widespread abscess formation. Central nervous involvement is rare in animals. In dogs, the common form is thoracic empyema with granulomatous serositis. Exudates are sanguinopurulent and sometimes contain small (<1 mm diameter), soft granules consisting of bacteria, neutrophils, and debris ("sulfur granule-like"). They usually lack the microstructure of sulfur granules.

Disease Patterns. Infections can be regional or disseminated. Local wound infections may extend to regional lymph nodes or spread by contiguousness. Dogs and cats develop debilitating, febrile illness. Pneumonia and suppurative pleuritis with empyema is the common finding. Dissemination occurs to liver, kidneys, bones, joints, and, rarely, the central nervous system. Case fatality rate exceeds 50%.

Bovine nocardial mastitis is often introduced with udder infusions. Onset is sudden with fever, anorexia, and abnormal milk secretion. The affected gland is swollen, hot, and painful. Discharging fistulous tracts may develop. Lymphadenopathy is common, and there is occasional dissemination. The affected gland usually becomes nonfunctional. Fatalities (5% to 10%) may occur during the acute stage or upon rupture of the udder.

In horses, rare local or general infections are seen, the latter secondary to profound constitutional disturbances (equine Cushing's, combined immunodeficient foals).

In swine, sheep, cattle, and goats, pneumonia, abortion, and lymphadenitis are seen in addition to mastitis.

Cases observed in birds, whales, and dolphins were mostly respiratory with signs of dissemination.

Nocardial mycetoma ("actinomycotic mycetoma," see Chapter 41) has been reported in dogs and cats.

Bovine farcy is a chronic suppurative infection usually starting at the lower limbs. It involves the lymphatics of the extremities or head region and the associated lymph nodes. Ulcers and discharging sinuses form along the path of infection. Affected animals remain in general good health unless dissemination to internal organs occurs. The disease is restricted to the tropics and attributed to *N. asteroides* ("*N. farcinica*") or *Mycobacterium farcinogenes*.

Epidemiology

Pathogenic nocardiae occur worldwide, suggesting constant exposure. In humans, disease is associated largely with immunodeficiencies. This association is established in horses. In dogs and cats, disease occurs as sequel to immunosuppressive virus infection: canine distemper and feline leukemia, respectively. Canine nocardiosis is most common in pups.

Bovine nocardial mastitis is most often traceable to unsatisfactory hygienic practices. Typically infection is introduced during the "dry period," with intramammary mastitis therapy. Acute mastitis is triggered when onset of lactation flushes the organism from limited foci through the lactiferous duct system. Alternatively, nocardiosis appears spontaneously in one animal and spreads in the course of milking operations.

IMMUNOLOGIC ASPECTS

Antibody and cell-mediated immune responses, including hypersensitivity, commonly develop during nocardial infections. Yet severe nocardiosis in several species is associated with immunosuppression, particularly of cell-mediated responses.

Antibody apparently confers little protection. Specific resistance is largely cell mediated.

No practical immunization method is presently available.

LABORATORY DIAGNOSIS

Branching, gram-positive, acid-fast beaded filaments, along with shorter, coccobacillary forms, are found in smears made from nocardia-infected sampler, impressions, and sections. Granules occur in *N. brasilensis* and *N. otitidiscaviarum*, but rarely in *N. asteroides* infections.

Specimens for culture should not be chilled or frozen. Nocardial colonies on blood agar, incubated at 37°C, will be dull opaque, waxy to velvety, and hard to dislodge by loop or needle. Nocardial morphology is confirmed by stains. Acid-fastness may be lost on culture. Catalase tests are positive, and the agent fails to grow serially under anaerobic conditions.

Serologic (immunodiffusion, complement fixation, enzyme-linked immunosorbent assays) and cutaneous hypersensitivity tests employing extracellular antigen to detect *N. asteroides* infection in cattle and dogs are of uncertain sensitivity and are not generally available.

TREATMENT AND CONTROL

Antimicrobic therapy of nocardial mastitis may produce temporary clinical relief and cessation of shedding, but no permanent cures. Control involves removal of infected animals, thorough disinfection of premises and equipment, and scrupulous stabling and milking hygiene.

In other forms of nocardiosis, trimethoprim-sulfonamide therapy has produced impressive results, especially when combined with surgery.

Alternative drugs include minocycline and doxycycline. Nocardiae are fairly resistant to the fluoroquinolones. "*Nocardia nova*" responds to the penicillins and macrolides (erythromycin, clarithromycin), and the tetracyclines (doxycycline, minocycline).

Abscesses, empyemas, and serosal effusions are treated by drainage and lavage. Granulomatous proliferations require excision.

SELECTED REFERENCES

Actinomyces

Bestetti G. Morphology of the "sulphur granules" (Drusen) in some actinomycotic infections. A light and electron microscopic study. Vet Pathol 1978;15:506.

Brennan KE, Ihrke PI. Grass awn migration in dogs and cats: a retrospective study of 182 cases. J Am Vet Med Assoc 1983;182:1201.

Buchanan AM. Morphological variants developing in L-form cultures of two strains of *Actinomyces* spp. of canine origin. Vet Microbiol 1982;7:587.

Buchanan AM, Davis DC, Pedersen NC, Beaman BL. Recovery of microorganisms from synovial and pleural fluids of animals using hyperosmolar media. Vet Microbiol 1982;7:19.

Buchanan AM, Scott JL. *Actinomyces hordeovulneris*, a canine pathogen that produces L-phase variants spontaneously with coincident calcium deposition. Am J Vet Res 1984;45: 2552.

Buchanan AM, Scott JL, Gerencser MA, et al. *Actinomyces hordeovulneris* sp. nov. an agent of canine actinomycosis. Int J Syst Bacteriol 1984;34:439.

Cisar JO, Vatter AE, Mcintire EC. Identification of virulence-associated antigen on the surface fibrils of *Actinomyces viscosus*. Infect Immun 1978;19:312.

Davenport AA, Carter GR, Beneke ES. *Actinomyces viscosus* in relation to the other actinomycetes and actinomycosis. Vet Bull 1975;45:313.

Dunbar M, Vulgamott SC. Thoracic and vertebral osteomyelitis caused by actinomycosis in a dog. Vet Med Small Anim Clin 1981;76:1159.

Engel D, VanEpps D, Claggett J. In vivo and in vitro studies on possible pathogenic mechanisms of *Actinomyces viscosus*. Infect Immun 1976;14:548.

Hardie EM, Barsanti JA. Treatment of canine actinomycosis. J Am Vet Med Assoc 1982;180:537.

Kolenbrander PE, London J. Adhere today, here tomorrow: oral bacterial adherence. J Bacteriol 1993;175:3247.

Palmer NC, Kierstead M, Wilson RW. Abortion in swine associated with *Actinomyces* spp. Can Vet J 1979;20:199.

Wallach JD. Lumpy jaw in captive kangaroos. Int Zoo Yearbook 1972;11:13.

Nocardia

Anderson KL, Wileke JR. Potentiated sulfonamides in the treatment of pulmonary nocardiosis. J Vet Pharm Ther 1980; 3:217.

Beaman BL, Beaman L. *Nocardia* species: host parasite relationships. Clin Microbiol Rev 1994;7:213.

Biberstein EL, Jang SS, Hirsh DC. *Nocardia asteroides* infection in horses. A review. J Am Vet Med Assoc 1985;186:273.

Davenport DJ, Johnson GC. Cutaneous nocardiosis in a cat. J Am Vet Med Assoc 1986;188:728.

Deem RL, Beaman BL, Gershwin ME. Adoptive transfer of immunity to *Nocardia asteroides* in nude mice. Infect Immun 1983;38:914.

Dewsnup DH, Wright DN. In vitro susceptibility of *Nocardia asteroides* to 25 antimicrobial agents. Antimicrob Agents Chemother 1984;25:165.

Lerner PI. Nocardiosis. Clin Infect Dis 1996;22:891.

Marino DJ, Jaggy A. Nocardiosis. A literature review with selected case reports in two dogs. J Vet Intern Med 1993;7:4.

McNeil MM, Brown JM. The medically important aerobic actinomycetes: epidemiology and microbiology. Clin Microbiol Rev 1994;7:357.

Wallace RJ, Brown BA, Tsukamura M, et al. Clinical and laboratory features of *Nocardia nova*. J Clin Microbiol 1991;29:2407.

Yano I, Imaeda T, Tsukamura M. Characterization of *Nocardia nova*. Int J Syst Bacteriol 1990;40:170.

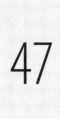

47 *Agents of Systemic Mycoses*

Ernst L. Biberstein

The agents of most systemic (or "deep") mycoses are saprophytes. Morphologically and ecologically diverse, they share some disease-related features.

1. Many are dimorphic, that is, their saprophytic and parasitic phases differ morphologically. *Coccidioides, Histoplasma, Blastomyces,* and *Paracoccidioides* grow as molds in their inanimate habitat. In tissue, *Coccidioides* produces sporangia, whereas the others grow as budding yeasts.
2. Infection is usually by inhalation.
3. Host factors are often the decisive disease determinants. Some mycoses (aspergillosis, zygomycosis) are seen primarily in immunocompromised animals.
4. Lesions tend to be pyogranulomatous. After primary pulmonary infection, the course of disease is determined by the effectiveness of cell-mediated immune responses. If these are inadequate, dissemination may occur to bone, skin, central nervous system, or abdominal viscera.
5. Systemic mycoses are noncontagious. Although the agent is often demonstrably shed, it fails to infect individuals in contact.

COCCIDIOIDES IMMITIS

Coccidioides immitis, the agent of coccidioidomycosis, occurs only in the western hemisphere in the Lower Sonoran Life Zone, apparently as a result of that area's peculiar soil properties and temperature and rainfall patterns. Of domestic animals, dogs are most frequently affected, although horses are occasionally affected as well. Infections also occur in cats, swine, sheep, cattle, human and nonhuman primates, and some 30 species of nondomestic mammals.

DESCRIPTIVE FEATURES

Morphology, Structure, and Composition

In the soil, *C. immitis* is a mold made up of slender septate hyphae that give rise, on thicker secondary branches, to chains of infectious arthroconidia (arthrospores, arthroaleuriospores, arthroaleurioconidia). These are

bulging, thick-walled cells, 2.5 to 4.0 μm × 3.0 to 6.0 μm, separated by empty cells (disjunctors), through which breaks occur when arthroconidia are dispersed (Fig 47.1).

In tissue, arthroconidia grow into spherical sporangia with birefringent walls, "spherules" (10 μm to 80 μm diameter), which by internal cleavage produce several hundred "endospores" (2 μm to 5 μm diameter) (Fig 47.2). The walls disintegrate, allowing dissemination of endospores, each of which may repeat the cycle or, on a nonliving substrate, give rise to mycelial growth. Though only arthroconidia are naturally infectious, endospores can experimentally initiate disease. Sexual spores are not known.

"Coccidioidin" in supernatants of mycelial *C. immitis* broth cultures is largely polysaccharide, but contains some amino acid nitrogen. It is used in cutaneous hypersensitivity and serologic tests. "Spherulin," a lysate of cultured spherules, is also used in skin tests. Both are leukotactic.

Growth Characteristics

Coccidioides immitis grows on simple media over a broad temperature range. On Sabouraud's or blood agar, growth is mycelial. Over several days, initially dull gray colonies develop with sparse aerial mycelium, which gradually becomes more abundant. Arthroconidia are produced in 5 to 7 days. Bovine blood agar is hemolyzed. Much colonial variability exists.

The sporangial phase is produced at 40°C in media containing casein hydrolysate, glucose, biotin, glutathione, and a salt mixture.

Arthroconidia resist drying and tolerate heat and salinity better than do competing soil organisms. In summer heat, *C. immitis* survives in soil layers nearer the surface than its competitors. When conditions favor growth again after rains, *C. immitis* repopulates the superficial soil layers first, ensuring its widespread dispersal.

ECOLOGY

Reservoir

Coccidioides immitis inhabits the soil in the Lower Sonoran Life Zone, including parts of the southwestern United States, Mexico, Central America, the northern and western rim states of South America, Argentina, and Paraguay. High prevalence is associated with an annual

FIGURE 47.1. Coccidioides immitis. *Teased preparation from a 5-day-old culture on Sabouraud's agar. Lactophenol cotton blue mount. Thick-walled barrel- or brick-shaped arthroconidia alternate with empty cells. On lower left, an isolated arthroconidium with fragments of adjacent cells (disjunctors, hyaline pegs) attached. 400×.*

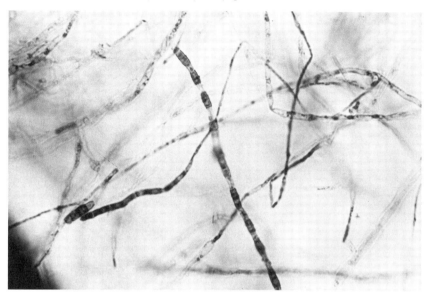

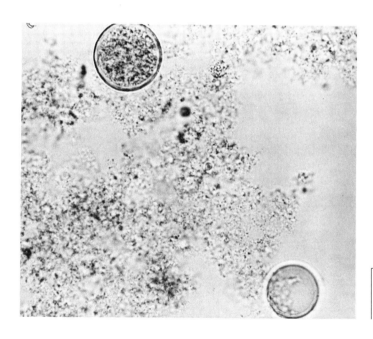

FIGURE 47.2. Coccidioides immitis. *Transtracheal aspirate from a dog. Unstained. Top left: mature spherule (sporangium) with endospores. Bottom right: immature spherule. 400×.*

rainfall of 5 to 20 inches and mean summer and winter temperatures of over 80°F and 45°F, respectively.

Transmission

Infection is mainly by inhalation of dust. Primary cutaneous infections are rare.

Pathogenesis

Mechanisms and Pathology. Relevant cell products include proteases, T suppressor cell activator, and leukotactic agents.

Leukocytes in vitro encourage arthroconidial metamorphosis to spherules.

The agent triggers an inflammatory response in the lung, is engulfed but not killed by phagocytes, and is conveyed to the hilar lymph node, where another inflammatory focus develops. Inflammation is stimulated in part by a potent serine protease (among several other proteases), which is liberated during the growth of the fungus in vivo (digests elastin, collagen, and immunoglobulins). Normally, cell-mediated immune responses arrest the process at this stage following stimulation of T_{H1} lymphocytes that activate macrophages. With inadequate cell-mediated immunity, dissemination can occur to bones, skin, abdominal viscera, heart, genital tract, and eye (and rarely in animals to brain and meninges). Gross lesions are white granulomas varying from miliary nodules to irregular masses. Peritoneal, pleural, and pericardial effusions occur. Microscopically, the predominant response is pyogranulomatous: to arthroconidia and endospores, the response is suppurative; and to spherules, the response is proliferative, with epithelioid cells the chief component, admixed with giant cells, lymphocytes, and neutrophils (Fig 47.3).

Disease Patterns.   Disseminated disease of dogs is the pattern seen most commonly by veterinarians. The complaints are lassitude, anorexia, and loss of condition. There may be respiratory signs (including cough), fever, lameness due to bone involvement, or discharging sinuses from deep lesions. In other species (horses, cats), there may be less osseous and more visceral involvement. In cattle, sheep, and swine, the disease is usually asymptomatic, limited to lungs and regional lymph nodes and undiagnosed until slaughter.

Epidemiology

In all species, overt disease is the exception. Highest prevalence of canine systemic coccidioidomycosis is observed in male dogs, 4 to 7 years of age, with peak occurrence of illnesses January to March and May to July. These peaks may represent seasonal stress and increased exposure, respectively. Geographic and climatic factors have been mentioned. An early report described young Boxer dogs and Doberman pinschers as particularly susceptible.

IMMUNOLOGIC ASPECTS

Cell-mediated hypersensitivity, as determined by skin tests, develops within one or more weeks of exposure and can persist indefinitely. Its presence is an indicator of resistance to progressive disease. Its absence is the rule in disseminated infections, and its return is a favorable sign. IgM antibody, demonstrable by tube precipitin or latex particle test, appears temporarily after infection and usually disappears again. IgG antibody titers (specific for the chitinase enzyme the fungus uses to break open a mature spherule releasing endospores), which are detectable by complement fixation and immunodiffusion tests, rise in disseminated disease and remain high (1 : >16) until the infection is brought under control. Natural killer cells inhibit growth in vivo.

No vaccines are presently available.

LABORATORY DIAGNOSIS

Direct Examination of Specimens

Animal fluids and tissues are examined for spherules by wet mount in saline containing 10% KOH. Spherules are 10 to 80 μm in diameter, have a thick wall (<2 μm), and contain endospores when mature (see Fig 47.2). Free endospores look indistinct in wet mounts but are recognizable in fixed smears stained by a fungal stain.

Stained tissue sections (hematoxylin and eosin [H&E], Gomori methanamine silver, Gridley) show both the agent and the characteristic lesion (see Fig 47.3).

FIGURE 47.3.   *Coccidioides immitis in lung tissue of a Bengal tiger. Hematoxylin-eosin stain. Note prominence of neutrophils in exudate. 400×. (Photograph courtesy of Dr. Roy Henrickson.)*

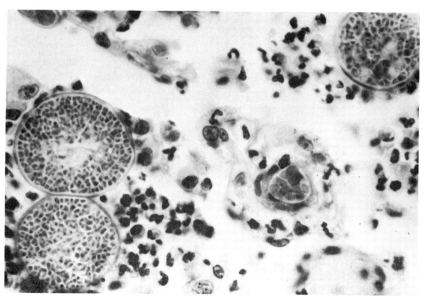

Culture

Blood agar and Sabouraud's agar with antibiotics are inoculated, tape-sealed, and incubated at 37°C and 25°C, respectively. All processing of cultures is done under a microbiological safety hood. Mycelial growth should be evident within a week and is examined for presence of arthroconidia in a lactophenol cotton blue wet mount. The isolate can be reconverted to the sporangial phase by animal inoculation or cultivation in a spherule medium.

A commercially available "exoantigen" test kit furnishes prepared antisera to *C. immitis, Histoplasma capsulatum,* and *Blastomyces dermatitidis* to be tested against extracts of suspect cultures in an immunodiffusion agar plate, where precipitation lines develop between extracts and their homologous antisera.

Immunodiagnosis

The coccidioidin skin test has been used in animal surveys.

The complement fixation (CF) and immunodiffusion tests detect disseminated disease. Because it is quantifiable, the CF test gauges progress and cure of infection more sensitively.

TREATMENT AND CONTROL

Amphotericin B has been the mainstay of anticoccidioidal therapy in humans. Limitations are its toxicity and the intravenous route of administration, requiring hospitalization or frequent visits. Liposomal preparations of amphotericin B show promise because of lower toxicity, which makes possible higher doses. Ketoconazole and itraconazole are used in small animals. Given orally over a period of months, they have effected apparently permanent cures. Toxic effects are relatively minor except during pregnancy, when fetal deaths may occur. The complement fixation titer is used to monitor the effect of treatment.

Vaccines are not available.

HISTOPLASMA CAPSULATUM VAR. CAPSULATUM

Histoplasmosis shares pathogenic and immunologic features with coccidioidomycosis. It differs in its geographic distribution. Affected species include humans, dogs, and cats. Infection in other hosts (cattle, horses, swine, wildlife) is rarely clinical.

DESCRIPTIVE FEATURES

Morphology, Structure, and Composition

The free-living *H. capsulatum* consists of septate hyphae bearing spherical to pyriform microconidia 2 to 4 μm in diameter, and "tuberculate" macroconidia, thick-walled spheroidal cells, 8 to 14 μm in diameter, studded with fingerlike projections (Fig 47.4). In animal hosts or appropriate culture, the mold becomes a yeast consisting of oval, singly budding cells that measure 2 to 3 μm × 3 to 4 μm. A sexual, ascomycetous state, *Ajellomyces capsulatus,* has been described.

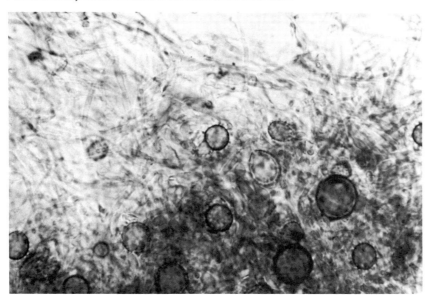

FIGURE 47.4.   Histoplasma capsulatum, *mycelial phase. Teased preparation from a 7-day culture on Sabouraud's agar at 25°C. Lactophenol cotton blue mount. "Tuberculate" macroconidia and hyphae. The "tubercles" appear as projections from the thick cell walls, most obviously on the conidium in the center of the field. 400×.*

Histoplasmins, which are used in immunodiagnosis, are obtained from mycelial culture filtrates. They contain polysaccharides, with variable admixtures of glycoproteins and cellular breakdown products. Mycelial and yeast phases differ in cellular constituents, some of which (e.g., cell wall glucan) have been related to virulence.

Growth Characteristics

Histoplasma capsulatum grows on common laboratory media over a broad temperature range. The optimum for mycelial growth is 25° to 30°C. The cottony aerial mycelium is white (A), brown (B), or intermediate (see below). Pigmentation parallels abundance of macroconidia. The yeast phase requires richer media (e.g., glucose cysteine blood agar) and temperatures of 34° to 37°C. Growth may take over a week before characteristic colonies are seen.

Histoplasma capsulatum survives at ambient temperatures for months and at refrigerator temperature for years. It withstands freezing and thawing and tolerates heating for more than an hour at 45°C.

Variability

Serologic variants appear to be related to geographic distribution. All share at least one antigen, which is common to several fungal species and may account for some cross-reactivity. B to A variation occurs during artificial cultivation and can be prevented by maintenance of cultures in the yeast phase.

ECOLOGY

Reservoir

Although most concentrated in the Mississippi and Ohio River watersheds, *H. capsulatum* occurs sporadically worldwide. It is found in the top soil layers, especially in the presence of bird and bat guano, which provide both enrichment and inoculum. Birds are mainly passive carriers, whereas bats undergo intestinal infections. *Histoblasma capsulatum* is favored by neutral to alkaline soil environments with annual rainfall between 35 and 50 inches and mean temperatures between 68°F and 90°F.

Transmission

Transmission is mostly by inhalation, possibly by ingestion, and, rarely, by wound infection.

Pathogenesis

Early events and lesions resemble those of tuberculosis. Thoracic lymph nodes become enlarged, and lungs may contain grayish-white nodules. The histologic response varies from suppurative to granulomatous inflammation. Caseation necrosis and calcification are common.

The yeast attaches to macrophages by way of the CD18 receptor. It is immediately phagocytosed, a respiratory burst occurs, and a phagolysosome results following fusion with lysosomes. The agent multiplies within the phagolysosome, ultimately killing the cell. Survival within the phagolysosome is thought to be related to secretion of proteins by the yeast, which raises the intraphagolysosome pH and thereby decreases the effectiveness of acid hydrolases. Within infected macrophages, colonies of thick-walled yeast cells measuring less than 4mm in one dimension are observed. Budding is inconspicuous.

In disseminated cases, lymph nodes and parenchymatous organs are enlarged and may contain gross nodular lesions. There may be ulcerations of skin and mucous membranes, abdominal and pleural effusions, and involvement of the central nervous system (including eyes), skin, and bone marrow. The inflammatory exudate consists of macrophage elements colonized by yeast cells (Fig 47.5).

Dogs may develop a primary pulmonary form with coughing, fever, regional lymphadenopathy, and radiographic abnormalities. The more common form in dogs is disseminated disease, marked by lethargy, anorexia, weight loss, diarrhea, dehydration, and anemia. Hepatomegaly, splenomegaly, mesenteric lymphadenitis, and ascites may cause abdominal distention.

Comparable patterns have rarely been observed in cats.

Disease patterns in humans parallel those described.

Epidemiology

Subclinical infections with histoplasmosis are common in dogs and cats — and humans — in endemic areas. Clinical disease is most prevalent in dogs aged 2 to 7 years, in early autumn (September to November) and later winter to early spring (February to April). No sex predilection is reported, but pointers, weimaraners, and Brittany spaniels were found to be at greatest risk. Disseminated histoplasmosis in humans and dogs is found in association with immunosuppression.

IMMUNOLOGIC ASPECTS

Recovery and resistance are considered to be governed by cell-mediated immune responses, while circulating antibodies have no apparent protective function. Recovery from histoplasmosis appears to confer immunity.

No vaccines are available.

LABORATORY DIAGNOSIS

Direct Examination

Smears of buffy coat, sediment of aspirates, and tissue impressions are stained with a Romanovsky-type or specific fungal stain and searched for intraphagocytic yeast cells (see Fig 47.5).

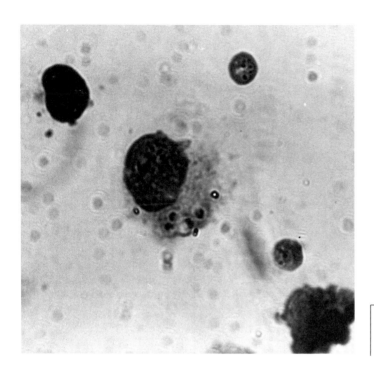

FIGURE 47.5. *Histoplasma capsulatum, yeast phase. Sediment of peritoneal exudate from a dog. Wright-Giemsa stain. Four yeast cells within a macrophage. 1000×.*

In sections stained with H & E, *H. capsulatum* appears as tiny dots surrounded by haloes. A duplicate fungal stain (e.g., periodic acid–Schiff [PAS], Gridley, or Gomori) can be helpful.

Immunofluorescence has been used to identify the yeast in tissue and exudates.

Culture

Specimens are planted on blood agar and Sabouraud's agar (with inhibitors) and incubated in jars or plastic bags at room temperature for up to 3 months. Colonial growth may look reddish-wrinkled before the appearance of cottony brownish to white mycelium.

Microconidia and macroconidia are demonstrated in lactophenol cotton blue wet mounts. Dimorphism must be proven by conversion to the yeast phase in culture or by IV injection of mice. Mice will die within a few weeks. Their macrophages will contain the yeast forms.

The exoantigen test can be used on suspect mycelial cultures of *H. capsulatum*.

Immunodiagnosis

Histoplasmin skin and CF tests using antigens of either mycelial or yeast origin have not been reliable diagnostic aids in animal infections. The position of the precipitin band in immunodiffusion tests differentiates early and recovered human cases (near serum well) from active and progressive ones (near antigen well). Limited use of these tests on animals has given erratic results.

A recently described radioimmunoassay for antigen detection has not been tested in animals.

TREATMENT AND CONTROL

Azoles (ketaconazole, itraconazole, fluconazole) and amphotericin B have been used successfully in the treatment of some cases of canine histoplasmosis. Monitoring of renal function is mandatory when giving amphotericin B.

Relapses are common. The prognosis for disseminated cases is grave.

BLASTOMYCES DERMATITIDIS

Blastomycosis is endemic in the eastern third of North America. Cases of the disease are reported from Africa, Asia, and Europe. Affected hosts are humans and dogs and, rarely, horses, cats, and wildlife species.

DESCRIPTIVE FEATURES

Morphology, Structure, and Composition

In the saprophytic phase of *B. dermatitidis*, its hyphae produce conidiophores with spherical or oval smooth-walled conidia, 2 μm to 10 μm in diameter. On blood agar at 37°C, the agent is a thick-walled yeast, 8 μm to 15 μm in diameter, that reproduces by single buds attached by a broad base (Fig 47.6). The fungus has a sexual form, *Ajellomyces dermatitidis*.

Cell wall extracts contain 3 to 10 parts of polysaccharide to 1 part of protein. Protein is highest in the mycelial

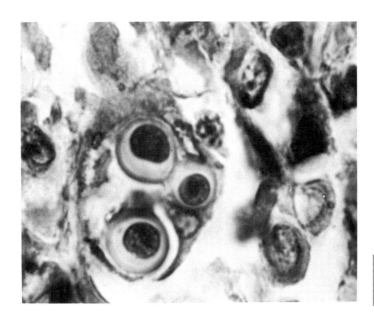

FIGURE 47.6.   Blastomyces dermatitidis, *yeast phase, in lung of dog. Hematoxylin-eosin stain. Note bud (lower right of upper yeast cell) attached by broad base to mother cell. 1000×.*

phase, while chitin is highest in the yeast phase. The lipid content of *B. dermatitidis* is higher than in other fungi. Lipid, protein, and chitin levels vary directly with virulence.

Virulent strains express a protein adhesin, WI-1.

Extracellular enzymes include proteases, phosphatases, esterases, and glycosidases. An alpha esterase and catalase evokes immune responses in natural infections. Culture filtrates are leukotactic for human neutrophils.

Growth Characteristics

Blastomyces dermatitidis grows on most media at room temperature and 37°C. Colonies develop from within 2 to over 7 days. Mold colonies, formed at ambient temperatures, are cottony white to tan depending on the abundance of conidia. Yeast colonies develop on blood agar at 37°C. They are opaque off-white to tan, with rough surface and a pasty consistency.

Neither phase survives in soil for significant periods. Survival and growth are observed on woody substrates.

The two recognized serotypes are related to geographic strain origin.

ECOLOGY

Reservoir

There is limited evidence of natural reservoirs. Moisture, low pH, animal wastes, and decaying vegetation appear to favor colonization. Humidity promotes release of conidia.

Transmission

Blastomycosis most commonly begins by respiratory exposure. Percutaneous infection probably occurs in dogs.

Pathogenesis

Conidia change to the yeast form in host tissue. The adhesin WI-1, expressed by conidia, is used to target respiratory epithelium. After traversing the epithelium, the change from conidia to yeast also results in a repression of WI-1 expression. In dogs, an inflammatory response involving macrophages and neutrophils and resulting in pyogranulomatous lesions occurs in the terminal bronchioles, followed by similar reactions in satellite lymph nodes. Blastomycosis is more often progressive than histoplasmosis and coccidioidomycosis. Dissemination involves superficial lymph nodes, skin, bones, bone marrow, eyes, viscera, mammary glands, and urogenital tract. The nodular lesions can be tubercle-like, with mononuclear cell types predominating, or there may be significant suppurative admixtures. Liquefaction and caseation occur, but calcification and encapsulation are exceptional.

Signs include skin lesions and respiratory distress with fever, depression, anorexia, and weight loss. Locomotor disturbances result from bone or joint infection or — rarely — central nervous system involvement. Ocular disease is common in disseminated blastomycosis. Most dogs with multiple organ system involvement die within months. Evidence for a benign form is uncertain. Blastomyces induce macrophages to produce elevated amounts of calcitriol resulting in hypercalcemia.

The disease in cats resembles that in dogs.

Epidemiology

Highest prevalence in dogs is from spring to fall. Male dogs less than 4 years of age are most often affected. A differential breed susceptibility has not been found. Though generally noncontagious, one human infection resulted from a dog bite. Risk factors for infection include proximity to waterways and excavation.

IMMUNOLOGIC ASPECTS

Impaired cell-mediated responsiveness may explain canine disseminated blastomycosis.

Humoral and cell-mediated responses occur as a result of infection. Cell-mediated immunity in mice is decisive in determining resistance. Artificial immunization is not available.

LABORATORY DIAGNOSIS

Blastomyces dermatitidis can be demonstrated in wet mounts of exudates and tissue smears as thick-walled yeast cells with single buds attached by a broad base. In section, intracellular yeasts may be found (see Fig 47.6).

Cultures on Sabouraud's agar (with inhibitors) are incubated at ambient temperature for up to 3 weeks. It is difficult to obtain the yeast form on primary isolation but it is relatively easy to convert the mold to the yeast phase by increasing the temperature to 37°C.

For "exoantigen" demonstration a commercial kit is available.

Blastomycin skin and complement fixation tests lack acceptable sensitivity and specificity. The agar gel double diffusion test appears to be specific (96%) and sensitive (91%).

TREATMENT AND CONTROL

Blastomycosis responds to amphotericin B and ketoconazole (or both together), and to itraconazole. Fluconazole is moderately effective.

CRYPTOCOCCUS NEOFORMANS

Cryptococcosis affects animals and humans worldwide. The most frequently affected domestic animal is the cat. In all species, there is the tendency for the central nervous system to become involved.

DESCRIPTIVE FEATURES

Morphology

Cryptococcus neoformans is a yeast. The spherical cells (3.5 µm to 7.0 µm diameter) produce usually single buds attached by slender stalks and surrounded by polysaccharide capsules (Fig 47.7).

Strains of *C. neoformans* have been experimentally converted to a mycelial, sexually reproducing phase, *Filobasidiella neoformans*, a basidiomycete.

Growth Characteristics

Cryptococcus neoformans grows on common laboratory media at ambient or body temperatures. Other *Cryptococcus* spp. cannot grow consistently at 37°C. Encapsulation is optimal on chocolate agar plates incubated under 5% carbon dioxide at 37°C. Colonial growth may be apparent within 2 days or require several weeks. Colonies are grayish white to white and mucoid and can reach diameters of several centimeters.

Biochemical Reactions

Cryptococcus spp. hydrolyze urea. Their carbohydrate assimilation patterns are utilized in identification

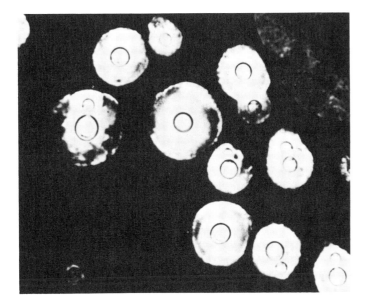

FIGURE 47.7. Cryptococcus neoformans *in nasal granuloma of a mouflon. India ink wet mount showing encapsulated budding spherical yeast cells. 400×. (Photograph courtesy of Dr. Roy Henrickson.)*

procedures. *Cryptococcus neoformans* (but few other *Cryptococcus* spp.) can utilize creatinine and produces melanin-pigmented colonies on media containing diphenolic and polyphenolic compounds. These substances are used in media for selective recovery of *C. neoformans*.

Resistance

Cycloheximide concentrations used in fungal isolation media inhibit *C. neoformans*. Replication ceases above 40°C. Highly alkaline environments kill the agent.

Variability

Four antigenic types, A and D, B and C, based on capsular polysaccharides, constitute the varieties *neoformans* and *gattii*, respectively, which differ biochemically, morphologically, and epidemiologically. Variety *neoformans* predominates in the temperate zone except for an area in Southern California, where variety *gattii* is prominent.

ECOLOGY

Reservoir

Cryptococcus neoformans lives in surface dust and dirt. In soil it is outcompeted by the resident microbiota. In dried pigeon droppings, which are rich in creatinine and inhibit other microorganisms, *C. neoformans* var. *neoformans* reaches high concentrations and survives for more than a year at much reduced capsular and cell size. *Cryptococcus neoformans* var. *gattii* lives in association with the flower buds of the red river gum tree (*Eucalyptus canaldulensis*). *Cryptococcus neoformans* var. *neoformans* has also been associated with decaying wood in hollows of a variety of different species of trees.

Transmission

The route of infection is usually respiratory, rarely percutaneous. Cryptococcosis is noncontagious.

Pathogenesis

In an environment where moisture and nutrients are plentiful, *C. neoformans* makes little if any capsular material. In arid conditions, the capsule collapses and protects the yeast from dehydration. In either case, the size (approximately 3 μm) is small enough to make it to the lung alveoli. At physiologic concentrations of bicarbonate, CO_2, and free iron, a capsule is produced. The cryptococcal capsule is a very efficient activator of the alternate complement pathway resulting in the deposition of C3b on the surface. Thus opsonized the yeast will adhere to the surface of phagocytic cells, but is poorly phagocytosed even in the presence of anticapsular antibody. Capsular polysaccharide increases participation of suppressor T lymphocytes and decreases antigen processing leading to a poor antibody response. Capsular poly-

saccharide also diminishes the chemoattractive effects of the anaphylotoxins C3a and C5a generated by activation of the alternate complement pathway. In the event phagocytosis occurs, the respiratory burst is diminished (capsule). Encapsulated cryptococci are poorly killed inside a nonactivated phagocytic cell. This may be due in part to the production of melanin by the yeast (from phenols by phenoloxidase) and the production of mannitol. Both of these substances are free radical scavengers and may reduce the hostile environment within the phagolysosome by inactivating hydroxyl radicals, superoxides, and singlet oxygen radicals. Thus, inflammatory responses are minimal and cryptococci grow into large space-occupying "myxomatous" masses, consisting of capsular slime, yeast cells, and few inflammatory cells. Eventually these "masses" acquire histiocytes, epithelioid cells, and some giant cells.

Development of pulmonary lesions is erratic. Infections often localize in the central nervous system (CNS) following dissemination from the lungs and are manifested by neurologic signs (perhaps due to lower complement concentrations in the CNS and to high concentrations of catechols, a substrate for phenoloxidase). Eye involvement, leading to chorioretinitis and blindness, is relatively common.

In cats and dogs, the animals most often clinically affected, ulcerative lesions of the mucous membranes in nose, mouth, pharynx, and sinuses or myxomatous nasal polyps are also common. They may arise from local infections. Most skin lesions are probably hematogenous.

In cattle, the important form of cryptococcosis is mastitis, often initiated during intramammary medication. There is gross swelling, hardening of the gland, and gradual changes in the secretions. Destruction of the lactiferous epithelium is extensive. Several glands may be irreversibly damaged. The disease rarely advances beyond regional lymph nodes.

Epidemiology

Cryptococcus can probably affect any mammal. Its occurrence is sporadic and worldwide. Birds, particularly pigeons, often carry the agent in their intestinal contents and contribute to its reservoir (see above). They are rarely affected clinically, and then mostly on mucous surfaces.

Human cryptococcosis is often associated with immunosuppression (organ transplants, Hodgkin's disease, pregnancy, AIDS) or intensive exposure. Attempts to relate animal infections to similar circumstances have been speculative.

Bovine cryptococcal mastitis usually starts as an inoculation infection.

IMMUNOLOGIC ASPECTS

Immunosuppression is a predisposing factor. The capsular polysaccharides produce immune paralysis, complement depletion, and antibody masking.

Humoral and cell-mediated phenomena (T$_{H1}$ subset resulting in macrophage activation) evidently contribute to defense against cryptococcal infection. Macrophages participate in disposal of the agent. There is some evidence that T-lymphocytes (CD4$^+$ and CD8$^+$) as well as natural killer cells are able to kill or inhibit *C. neoformans* directly.

Results of experimental immunization have been equivocal. No vaccines are available.

Cryptococcosis does not appear to be a disease in cats infected with feline immunodeficiency virus (FIV) as it is in human patients infected with human immunodeficiency virus (HIV). FIV-positive cats respond to appropriate antifungal therapy; human patients respond poorly if at all.

LABORATORY DIAGNOSIS

Direct Examination

A small amount of sediment from exudates, tracheobronchial washes, and cerebrospinal fluids is mixed with an equal amount of India ink on a slide and a cover slip is added. Microscopically, the encapsulated organisms appear as bright circular lacunae in a dark field, containing the yeast cells in their centers (see Fig 47.7). Fungal stains delineate the cell wall but not the capsule, which is stainable by mucicarmine.

In sections processed by the usual histologic methods, the capsules are unstained halos separating the yeast cells from tissue constituents or from each other.

Culture

Blood agar and Sabouraud's agar cultures (without cycloheximide) are incubated, respectively, at 37°C and room temperature. Suggestive colonies are examined by India ink wet mount. If found to consist of encapsulated yeasts, *C. neoformans* is confirmed by demonstration of urease activity, absence of lactose, melibiose and nitrate assimilation, and lethality for mice upon intracerebral or intraperitoneal injection.

Selective media incorporating antibacterial and antifungal drugs, creatinine and diphenyl, are used for environmental sampling.

Some normal dogs and cats harbor small numbers of *C. neoformans* in their nasal cavities. Therefore, care should be taken when interpreting culture results from samples obtained from this site. Examination of direct smears (the numbers of yeast in smears from clinically normal animals would be too low to see) and/or analysis of serum for capsular antigen are helpful adjuncts to culture. Capsular antigen is not detectable in serum of normal dogs, regardless of whether they harbor *C. neoformans* in their nasal passages.

Immunodiagnosis

Antigen demonstration in serum and cerebrospinal fluid is attempted in diagnosis and assessment of patient progress. Latex particle suspensions coated with anticapsular antibody are marketed as slide agglutination test kits.

Antibody is irregularly demonstrable because of the "sponging" action of circulating antigens. Its presence (demonstrated by indirect IFA or by latex particles coated with capsular polysaccharide) is a favorable sign of decreasing antigen levels.

TREATMENT AND CONTROL

The treatment of choice for dogs and cats is fluconazole. Alternative therapy is 5-fluorocytosine, but its efficacy should be tested periodically as strains may be resistant or become resistant.

Therapy should be continued until clinical signs are resolved and antigen disappears from serum and cerebrospinal fluid.

Contaminated surfaces (pigeon lofts, attics) can be disinfected with lime solution (1 lb hydrated lime/3 gal water) prior to physical cleanup. Dirt removed is placed in containers and covered with hydrated lime powder, which can also be used on exposed floors and beams. Masks are worn during the operation.

ASPERGILLUS SPP.

Aspergilli are ubiquitous saprophytic molds with opportunistic pathogenic patterns depending on impaired, overwhelmed, or bypassed host defenses. Of some 900 species, *A. fumigatus* is most frequent in animal and human infections.

DESCRIPTIVE FEATURES

Morphology and Composition

Aspergillus spp. are molds consisting of septate hyphae and characteristic asexual fruiting structures that are borne on condiophores, which are hyphal branches originating by a foot cell in the vegetative mycelium and ending in an expanded vesicle. This is covered by a layer or layers of flask-shaped phialides, from which chains of pigmented conidia, the asexual reproductive units, arise (Fig 47.8). They give the fungal colony its color.

In tissue, only mycelium is seen. In aerated cavities (e.g., nasal passages, air sacs, cavitary lesions), fruiting structures may be found.

Fruiting bodies are important diagnostic features of *Aspergillus* spp. by which species are identified.

Aspergillus fumigatus, the leading pathogenic species, produces "endotoxins," hemolysins, and proteolytic enzymes.

Mycotoxins are considered separately (Chapter 48).

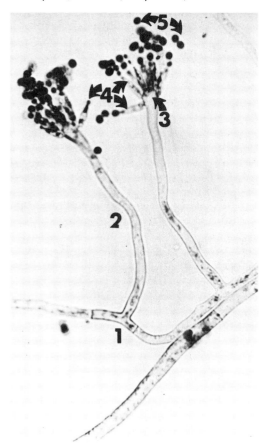

FIGURE 47.8.   Aspergillus clavatus. *Lactophenol cotton blue mount from slide culture on Sabouraud's agar. 1 = foot cell, 2 = conidiophore, 3 = vesicle, 4 = phialides, 5 = conidia. 400×.*

Growth Characteristics

Aspergilli grow on all common laboratory media over a wide range of temperatures (up to 50°C). Their biochemical activities have not been clearly related to virulence or utilized diagnostically.

Aspergilli thrive in the environment. Some are highly resistant to heat and drying. Most do not grow in cycloheximide-containing fungal media.

ECOLOGY

Reservoir

Aspergilli are present in soil, vegetation, feed, and secondarily in air and water and objects exposed to them. *Aspergillus fumigatus* becomes predominant over competing microbiota in fermented plant material (e.g., hay, silage, compost). Animal disease outbreaks are often traced to such sources.

Transmission

Aspergillosis is acquired from environmental sources, generally by inhalation or ingestion. Most *Aspergillus*

mastitis follows intramammary inoculation. Intrauterine infections in cattle result from dissemination of subclinical lung or intestinal infections. In poultry, egg transmission occurs.

Pathogenesis

Mechanism.   Toxic constituents can induce hemorrhagic lesions. Elastase activity may cause tissue damage. Allergenic factors, which are recognized in human aspergilloses, are insufficiently documented in animal disease.

Pathology.   In pulmonary infection, suppurative exudate accumulates in bronchioles and adjacent parenchyma. It surrounds colonies of mycelial growth, which may extend into blood vessels and produce infected thrombi and vasculitis, leading to dissemination. Infection may also spread directly into adjacent air spaces. Granulomas develop; they are grossly visible as grayish white nodules and consist of mononuclear cells and fibroblasts. In old lesions, colonies may be fringed by acidophilic clubs (asteroid bodies) resembling actinomycosis (see Fig 46.2).

Lesions in avian lungs are caseous nodules. On serous membranes, caseous foci are covered by macroscopic mold colonies, accompanied by thickening of the membranes (e.g., air sacs) (Fig 47.9). The cellular response is acute suppurative to chronic granulomatous.

Bovine abortion results from hematogenous seeding of placentomes, which is possibly a response to a growth factor in placental tissue. There is hyphal invasion of blood vessels producing vasculitis and a necrotizing, hemorrhagic placentitis. The fetus undergoes disseminated infection with signs of emaciation and dehydration. Lymph nodes, viscera, and brain may be involved. Ringworm-like plaques on the skin are often seen.

On mucosal surfaces (e.g., nasal passage, trachea) mold colonies form on top of necrotic tissue, which is surrounded by a hemorrhagic zone.

Disease Patterns.   Pulmonary and disseminated infections, frequently involving kidneys and central nervous system, occur in most species.

1. Avian aspergillosis, which affects many species of birds, sometimes in epidemics, reflects heavy exposure or severe stress on domestic flocks or pet bird operations, or the effects of oil spills on marine birds. The disease is usually a respiratory tract infection, sometimes with hematogenous dissemination. Signs are inappetence, listlessness, weight loss, dyspnea, sometimes diarrhea, and abnormal behavior and posture. The eyes are often affected. Mortality may approach 50%, especially in young birds. In mild cases, only gasping and hyperpnea may be seen. The course varies from a day to several weeks.
2. Bovine abortions usually occur late in pregnancy and resemble abortions due to other causes. Fetal skin plaques occur also in other mycotic abortions.

FIGURE 47.9. *Aspergillosis in a waterfowl (grebe). The exposed air sac in the center contains one large mold colony (arrow) and a smaller one on the upper left. The air sac on the lower right (★) has had a portion removed (★), revealing luxuriant mold growth within. (Photograph courtesy of Dr. Murray Fowler.)*

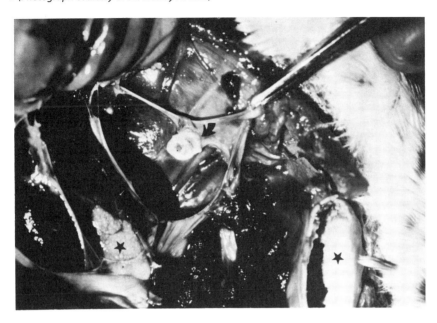

3. Aspergillosis of mucous membranes occurs in dogs in nasal passages or paranasal sinuses. It is manifested by sneezing and unilateral or bilateral persistent nasal discharge that is unresponsive to medical treatment. Vague upper respiratory signs may point to an aspergillosis of the equine guttural pouch.

4. Intestinal aspergillosis, presenting as diarrhea, occurs in calves, foals, and cats.

5. In horses, *Aspergillus* infection of the cornea is the leading cause of keratomycosis.

6. Mastitis due to *A. fumigatus* is reported at an increased rate, especially from Europe. It is usually chronic progressive, producing abscesses in the udder.

7. *Aspergillus terreus* and *A. deflectus* cause disseminated aspergillosis in dogs, particularly German shepherd dogs. Osteomyelitis is a common feature.

Epidemiology

Intensity of exposure is a significant feature in animal aspergillosis. Bovine abortion outbreaks are often related to moldy fodder. Aspergillosis in chicken flocks commonly coincides with the use of heavily contaminated litter.

Stress aspects are usually recognizable in outbreaks. Avian aspergillosis is seen under conditions of poor husbandry. In oiled seabirds, there is severely impaired thermal regulation. In pregnant cows, advanced gestation combined with low-quality feed and poor weather and housing add up to severe challenge.

Canine nasal aspergillosis occurs especially in young dogs of dolichocephalic breeds. Some T cell deficiency may exist.

In keratomycosis of horses, the frequent history of topical antibacterial and steroid treatment suggests immunosuppression and impaired colonization resistance.

IMMUNOLOGIC ASPECTS

Circulating antibody with no demonstrably protective role may be present in dogs with nasal aspergillosis (see under *Treatment, Control, and Prevention*, p. 268). Cell-mediated immunity may be related to resistance.

Immunization procedures are not available.

LABORATORY DIAGNOSIS

Direct Examination

Mycelium, fruiting heads, and conidia can often be demonstrated in samples either in wet mounts in 10% KOH or with calcofluor white. For fixed-stained smears, fungal stains (PAS) are best, Giemsa satisfactory, and Gram of limited use. Septate branching hyphae constitute strong evidence of aspergillosis. Other fungi (*Penicillium, Pseudallescheria, Paecilomyces*) present a similar picture but are much rarer. Conidia may occur in air passages or other exposed sites in the absence of infection.

In stained tissue sections, septate hyphae dividing dichotomously at acute angles are the only structures seen.

Isolation and Identification

Aspergillus is readily cultured. Because it is a ubiquitous contaminant, interpretation of positive cultures is often problematic. Presence of the agent must always be correlated with pathologic and clinical findings. Identification of agents rests upon morphologic features and growth characteristics of isolates.

Immunodiagnosis

Serologic tests are useful adjuncts to the diagnosis of aspergillosis. Because the tests that are available are species specific, it is necessary to know which *Aspergillus* to expect. For example, *A. fumigatus* is most commonly seen in nasal aspergillosis of dogs, whereas disseminated aspergillosis in that species is either *A. deflectus* or *A. terreus*. An immunodiffusion kit for antibody detection is commercially available for detection of antibodies to *A. fumigatus*.

TREATMENT, CONTROL, AND PREVENTION

Aspergillosis in birds is generally not treated.

The nasal form in dogs is treated topically with instillation of clortrimazole or enilconazole into the nasal passages and sinuses. Itraconazole has been successfully used to treat nasal aspergillosis when topical treatment was not possible.

Itraconazole has been beneficial in treating disseminated aspergillosis.

There is no established treatment for mammary aspergillosis.

For intestinal infections in pigs, foals, and calves, oral nystatin is recommended.

Keratomycosis is treated topically with antimycotic ointments and solutions.

Avoidance of massive exposure requires elimination of cattle feed, particularly hay and silage that has undergone noticeable deterioration. *Aspergillus fumigatus* only reaches high concentrations under conditions of "biologic heat" generation, after other microbiota are eliminated. With poultry litter, proper storage and frequent changes of litter can prevent such buildup.

OTHER SAPROPHYTIC FUNGAL PATHOGENS

Penicillium spp. also produce septate mycelium and conidia in chains, but their conidiophores, unlike those of aspergilli, are branched, creating a broomlike structure (Fig 47.10). The colonies grow at rates comparable to *Aspergillus* and develop a blue-green pigmentation. *Penicillium* spp. are occasional causes of a nasal mycosis in dogs.

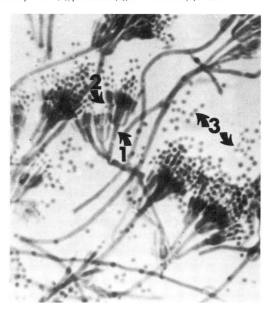

FIGURE 47.10.   Penicillium *sp. lactophenol cotton blue mount from slide culture on Sabouraud's agar. Note branched conidiophores (1), phialides (2), and conidia (3). 400×.*

Scedosporium apiospermum is prominent as a mycetoma agent (see Chapter 41). It is a fast-growing organism filling a tube or petri dish within a few days with dirty-white ("singed cotton") mycelium. Oval to club-shaped conidia are produced on septate hyphae. A sexual state, *Pseudallescheria boydii* evident by large (≤200 μm diameter) spherical "ascocarps," can usually be demonstrated.

Pseudallescheria boydii causes visceral mycetoma and pneumonia in dogs, ocular disease and abortion in horses, and mastitis and abortion in cattle.

Paecilomyces spp. resemble penicillium except that the terminal portions of the conidiophore taper to a point on which chains of short spindle-shaped conidia arise. Pigmentation varies. Disseminated canine and feline paecilomycosis with bone involvement and a respiratory epidemic in captive turtles have been reported.

Zygomycetes have broad (up to 10 μm) nonseptate mycelium. Asexual reproduction in the genera of greatest importance is by sporangiospores, produced in balloon-like sporangia over 20 micrometers in diameter.

1. In *Rhizopus* spp., sporangia are carried on sporangiophores that arise from hyphae at a cluster of rootlike rhizoids that bind colonies to their substrate. Hyphal stolons join adjacent rhizoids (Fig 47.11). In *Absidia* spp., sporangiophores arise from stolons between rhizoids. *Mucor* has no rhizoids. Its sporangiophores are branches of the mycelium. Sporangiophores of *Mortierella* originate at rhizoids and branch repeatedly before tapering to a point where the sporangium is formed. In the other genera, the sporangiophore expands into a *columella* at the base of the sporangium.

FIGURE 47.11. Rhizopus *sp. Lactophenol cotton blue mount from slide culture on Sabouraud's agar. (1) rhizoid, (2) sporangiophore, (3) sporangium (several are collapsed). 400×.*

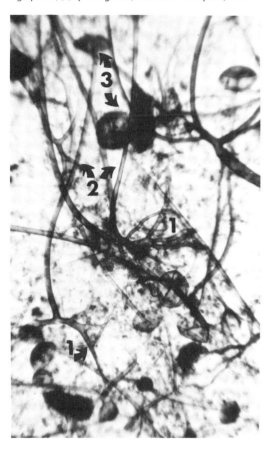

2. The zygomycetes named grow rapidly into fluffy colonies dotted with black (sporangia), filling a petri dish within a few days. They are inhibited by cycloheximide.

3. The agents named cause mycotic bovine abortions resembling, in most respects, those due to aspergillosis.

4. Gastrointestinal infections, marked by ulcerative lesions and mesenteric lymphadenitis, occur in ruminants, swine, and dogs, as do respiratory and hematogenous infections affecting various viscera and the central nervous system. They are secondary to stress, such as dietary changes and inadequacies, antibiotic suppression of the gastrointestinal flora, concurrent infections, recent parturition, or trauma.

5. A usually fatal pneumonia due to *Mortierella wolfii*, occurring in cattle shortly after abortions, is seen in New Zealand.

Canine gastrointestinal "phycomycosis" in warm climates, often due to *Pythium* spp., causes lesions in the stomach or gut wall similar to those of skin and subcutaneous pythiosis (see Chapter 41). No effective treatment exists. Copper sulfate added to drinking water may reduce exposure. Resection of the affected bowel segment is sometimes curative.

Rhinosporidium seeberi causes a granulomatous mucocutaneous infection affecting humans, horses, cattle, mules, dogs, goats, and some wild waterfowl. The agent produces sporangia up to several hundred micrometers in diameter, containing sporangiospores 7 μm in size (Fig 47.12). It has been propagated only in tissue culture. A saprophytic (aquatic) reservoir is assumed.

Rhinosporidiosis commonly produces single or multiple polyps in nasal (or other) epithelium. The condition is mostly seen in the tropics or subtropics. Treatment is by excision of polyps.

FIGURE 47.12. Rhinosporidium seeberi *in nasal polyp of dog. Hematoxylin-eosin stain. A maturing sporangium with spores; several immature sporangia. About 300×. (Section obtained through courtesy of Dr. W. Spengler.)*

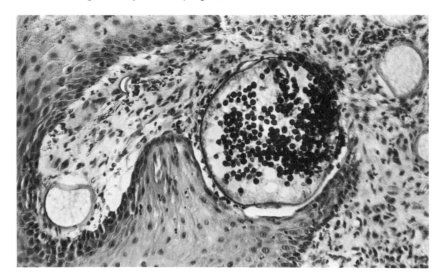

Mycotic nasal granulomas in cattle may be due to other agents, especially the fungi mentioned under phaeohyphomycosis. In horses, the zygomycetes *Conidiobolus* and *Basidiobolus* spp. may cause similar lesions.

PNEUMOCYSTIS CARINII

Pneumocystis carinii, an organism that has suffered through years of taxonomic uncertainty, is a fungus (based on DNA sequences of the 16S-like rRNA gene, and the genes encoding a number of proteins). This fungus has only been isolated from affected hosts (dogs, horses, pigs). *Pneumocystis carinii* consists of a number of morphologically similar varieties, each of which is host-specific (it does not appear to be a zoonosis). Spread is by way of aerosol. Affected hosts are almost always immunocompromised, though there are reports of animals (mainly foals) that have pneumocystis pneumonia without an obvious underlying condition.

The fungus has not been grown in a cell-free culture system. Diagnosis is made by examination of material that has been strained with a Romanovsky-type stain (e.g., Giemsa stain).

Treatment includes (in order of preference) trimethoprim-sulfonamides, dapsone, atovaquone, pentamidine, or clindamycin.

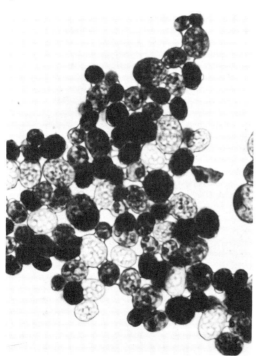

FIGURE 47.13.   *Prototheca sp. in bovine mastitis. Wright stain. The less intensely stained organisms show evidence of endosporulation. 1000×.*

PROTOTHECOSIS

Prototheca is an alga lacking chlorophyll. It multiplies by endosporulation, producing roughly spherical cells that are 8 μm to 25 μm in diameter (Fig 47.13). *Prototheca zopfii* and *P. wickerhamii* are occasionally pathogenic. They grow on fungal media (without cycloheximide) at 25°C and 37°C, respectively, into white to tannish dull colonies in less than a week and are differentiated serologically and by carbohydrate assimilation tests.

Prototheca spp. are widespread in nature. Exposure is by ingestion, percutaneously, or, in dairy cows, by intramammary injection.

Disease occurs in dogs, cats, cattle, deer, bats, snakes, fish, and humans. In dogs, it is usually disseminated and accompanied by hemorrhagic diarrhea. Central nervous system involvement and eye lesions are frequent. In cats and humans, cases to date have been cutaneous. Immunodeficiency is suspected. In cattle, chronic progressive mastitis develops. Tissue reactions are pyogranulomatous.

The agent is easily cultured and can be demonstrated in unstained wet mounts from specimens or in fixed smears stained with a Romanovsky-type or fungal stain.

Amphotericin B and ketoconazole are used on humans. The agents are susceptible to the aminoglycosides in vitro. Treatment of animals has not been effective, although liposomal formulations of amphotericin B show promise.

SELECTED REFERENCES

General

Bodey GP. Azole antifungal agents. Clin Infect Dis 1992;14:S161.

Deepe GS, Bullock WE. Immunological aspects of fungal pathogenesis. Eur J Clin Microbiol Infect Dis 1990;9:377.

Hogan LH, Klein BS, Levitz SM. Virulence factors of medically important fungi. Clin Microbiol Rev 1996;9:469.

Kozel TR. Activation of the complement system by pathogenic fungi. Clin Microbiol Rev 1996;9:34.

Wolf AM. Systemic mycoses. J Am Vet Med Assoc 1989;194:1192.

Coccidioides immitis

Armstrong PJ, DiBartola SR. Canine coccidioidomycosis: a literature review and report of eight cases. J Am Anim Hosp Assoc 1983;19:938.

Cox RA, Kennell W. Suppression of T lymphocyte response by *Coccidioides immitis* antigen. Infect Immun 1988;56:1424.

Elcomin AE, Egeberg MC. A fungicide effective against *Coccidioides immitis* in the soil. In: Ajello L, ed. Coccidioidomycosis. Tucson: University of Arizona, 1967:319–322.

Johnson SM, Pappagianis D. The coccidioidal complement fixation and immunodiffusion-complement fixation antigen is a chitinase. Infect Immun 1992;60:2588.

Magee DM, Cox RA. Interleukin-12 regulation of host defenses against *Coccidioides immitis*. Infect Immun 1996;64:3609.

Pappagianis D, Zimmer BL. Serology of coccidioidomycosis. Clin Microbiol Rev 1990;3:247.

Stevens DA. Coccidioidomycosis. N Engl J Med 1995;332:1077.

Thilstead JR, Shifrine M. Delayed cutaneous hypersensitivity in the dog: reaction to tuberculin, purified protein derivative, and coccidioidin. Am J Vet Res 1978;39:1702.

Wolf AM. Primary cutaneous coccidioidomycosis in a dog and a cat. J Am Vet Med Assoc 1979;174:504.

Wolf AM, Pappagianis D. Canine coccidioidomycosis treatment with a new antifungal agent: ketoconazole. Calif Vet 1981; 35:25.

Histoplasma capsulatum

Clinkenbeard KD, Cowell RL, Tyler RD. Disseminated histoplasmosis in cats: 12 cases (1981–1986). J Am Vet Med Assoc 1987;190:1445.

Deepe GS. The immune response to *Histoplasma capsulatum*: unearthing its secrets. J Lab Clin Med 1994;123:201.

Eissenberg LG, Goldman WE, Schlesinger PH. *Histoplasma capsulatus* modulates the acidification of phagolysosomes. J Exp Med 1993;177:1605.

Gomez FJ, Gomez AM, Deepe GS. An 80-kilodalton antigen from *Histoplasma capsulatum* that has homology to heat shock protein 70 induces cell-mediated immune responses and protection in mice. Infect Immun 1992;60:2565.

Jackson JA. Immunodiagnosis of systemic mycoses in animals: a review. J Am Vet Med Assoc 1986;188:702.

Kaufman L, Standard PG. Specific and rapid identification of medically important fungi by exoantigen detection. Annu Rev Microbiol 1987;41:209.

Lane TE, Otero GC, Wu-Hsieh BA, Howard DH. Expression of inducible nitric oxide synthase by stimulated macrophages correlates with their antihistoplasma activity. Infect Immun 1994;62:1478.

Maresca B, Kobayashi GS. Dimorphism in *Histoplasma capsulatum*: a model for the study of cell differentiation in pathogenic fungi. Microbiol Rev 1989;53:186.

Mitchell M, Stark DR. Disseminated canine histoplasmosis: a clinical survey of 24 cases in Texas. Can Vet J 1980;21:95.

Newman SL, Gootee L, Morris R, Bullock WE. Digestion of *Histoplasma capsulatum* yeasts by human macrophages. J Immunol 1992;149:574.

Stickle JE, Hribernik TN. Clinicopathological observations in disseminated histoplasmosis in dogs. J Am Anim Hosp Assoc 1978;14:105.

Wheat LJ, Kohler RB, Twari R. Diagnosis of disseminated histoplasmosis by detection of *Histoplasma capsulatum* antigen in serum and urine specimens. N Engl J Med 1986;314:83.

Blastomyces dermatitidis

Baumgardner DJ, Burdick JS. An outbreak of human and canine blastomycosis. Rev Infect Dis 1991;13:898.

Baumgardner DJ, Paretsky DP, Yopp AC. The epidemiology of blastomycosis in dogs: north central Wisconsin, USA. J Med Vet Mycol 1995;33:171.

Bloom JD, Hamor RE, Gerding PA. Ocular blastomycosis in dogs: 73 cases, 108 eyes (1985–1993). J Am Vet Med Assoc 1996; 209:1271.

Breider MA, Walker TL, Legendre AM, VanEe RT. Blastomycosis in cats: five cases (1979–1986). J Am Vet Med Assoc 1988; 193:570.

Buyukmihci N. Ocular lesions of blastomycosis in the dog. J Am Vet Med Assoc 1982;180:426.

Buyukmihci NC, Moore PF. Microscopic lesions of spontaneous ocular blastomycosis in dogs. J Comp Pathol 1987;97:321.

Dow SW, Legendre AM, Stiff M, Greene C. Hypercalcemia associated with blastomycosis in dogs. J Am Vet Med Assoc 1986;188:706.

Dunbar M, Pyle RL, Boring JG, McCoy CP. Treatment of canine blastomycosis with ketoconazole. J Am Vet Med Assoc 1983; 182:156.

Graham WR. Primary inoculation blastomycosis in a veterinarian. J Am Acad Dermatol 1982;7:785.

Jackson JA. Immunodiagnosis of systemic mycoses of animals: a review. J Am Vet Med Assoc 1986;188:702.

Klein BS, Hogan LH, Newman SL. Cell surface molecules of *Blastomyces dermatitidis*. ASM News 1997;63:140.

Legendre AM, Becker PU. Immunologic changes in acute canine blastomycosis. Am J Vet Res 1982;43:2050.

Legendre AM, Selcer BA, Edwards DF, Stevens R. Treatment of canine blastomycosis with amphotericin B and ketoconazole. J Am Vet Med Assoc 1984;184:1249.

Legendre AM, Walker M, Buyukmihci N, Stevens R. Canine blastomycosis: a review of 47 clinical cases. J Am Vet Med Assoc 1981;178:1163.

Nafe LA, Turk JR, Carter JD. Central nervous system involvement of blastomycosis in the dog. J Am Anim Hosp Assoc 1983; 19:933.

Neunzig RJ. Epidemiology, diagnosis and treatment of canine and feline blastomycosis. Vet Med Small Anim Clin 1983; 78:1081.

Pappas PG, Bradsher RW, Chapman SW, et al. Treatment of blastomycosis with fluconazole: a pilot study. Clin Infect Dis 1995;20:267.

St. Georgiev V. Treatment and experimental therapeutics of blastomycosis. Int J Antimicrob Agents 1995;6:1.

Turner S, Kaufman L, Jalbert M. Diagnostic assessment of an enzyme-linked immunosorbent assay for human and canine blastomycosis. J Clin Microbiol 1986;23:294.

Cryptococcus neoformans

Blackstock R, Hall NK, Hernandez NC. Characterization of a suppressor factor that regulates phagocytosis by macrophages in murine cryptococcosis. Infect Immun 1989;57:1773.

Buchanan KL, Murphy JW. Characterization of cellular infiltrates and cytokine production during the expression phase of the anticryptococcal delayed-type hypersensitivity response. Infect Immun 1993;61:2854.

Dong ZM, Murphy JW. Intravascular cryptococcal culture filtrate (CneF) and its major component, glucuronoxylomannan, are potent inhibitors of leukocyte accumulation. Infect Immun 1995;63:770.

Flatland B, Greene RT, Lappin MR. Clinical and serologic evaluation of cats with cryptococcosis. J Am Vet Assoc 1996; 209:1110.

Glaser CA, Angulo FJ, Rooney JA. Animal-associated opportunistic infections among persons infected with the human immunodeficiency virus. Clin Infect Dis 1994;18:14.

Hidore MR, Nabavi N, Sonleitner F, Murphy JW. Murine natural killer cells are fungicidal to *Cryptococcus neoformans*. Infect Immun 1991;59:1747.

Innes JRM, Seibold HR, Arentzen WR. The pathology of bovine mastitis caused by *Cryptococcus neoformans*. Am J Vet Res 1952;13:49.

Jackson JA. Immunodiagnosis of systemic mycosis in animals: a review. J Am Vet Med Assoc 1986;188:702.

Kwon-Chung KJ, Kozel TR, Edman JC, et al. Recent advances in biology and immunology of *Cryptococcus neoformans*. J Med Vet Mycol 1992;30:133.

Lazera MS, Pires FD, Camillo-Coura L, et al. Natural habitat of *Cryptococcus neoformans* var *neoformans* in decaying wood forming hollows in living trees. J Med Vet Mycol 1996;34:127.

Levitz SM. The ecology of *Cryptococcus neoformans* and the epidemiology of cryptococcosis. Rev Infect Dis 1991;13:1163.

Levitz SM, Dupont MP, Smai EH. Direct activity of human T lymphocytes and natural killer cells against *Cryptococcus neoformans*. Infect Immun 1994;62:194.

Malik R, Wigney DI, Muir DB, et al. Cryptococcosis in cats: clinical and mycological assessment of 29 cases and evaluation of treatment using orally administered fluconazole. J Med Vet Mycol 1992;30:133.

Malik R, Wigney DI, Muir DB, Love DN. Asymptomatic carriage of *Cryptococcus neoformans* in the nasal cavity of dogs and cats. J Med Vet Mycol 1997;35:27.

Miller MF, Mitchell TG, Storkus WJ, Dawson JR. Human natural killer cells do not inhibit growth of *Cryptococcus neoformans* in the absence of antibody. Infect Immun 1990;58:639.

Muth SM, Murphy JW. Direct anticryptococcal activity of lymphocytes from *Cryptococcal neoformans*-immunized mice. Infect Immun 1995;63:1637.

Naslund PK, Miller WC, Granger DL. *Cryptococcus neoformans* fails to induce nitric oxide synthase in primed murine macrophage-like cells. Infect Immun 1995;63:1298.

Rosskopf WJ, Woerpel RW. Cryptococcosis in a thick-billed parrot. Avian/Exotic Pract 1984;1:14.

Walker C, Malik R, Canfield PJ. Analysis of leucocytes and lymphocyte subsets in cats with naturally-occurring cryptococcosis but differing feline immunodeficiency virus status. Aust Vet J 1995;72:93.

Walter JE, Coffee EG. Control of *Cryptococcus neoformans* in pigeon coops by alkalinization. Am J Epidemiol 1968;87:173.

Wang Y, Aisen P, Casadevall A. *Cryptococcus neoformans* melanin and virulence: mechanism of action. Infect Immun 1995;63:3131.

Aspergillus spp.

Dyar RM, Fletcher QJ, Page RK. Aspergillosis in turkeys associated with use of contaminated litter. Avian Dis 1984;28:250.

Farnsworth RJ. Significance of fungal mastitis. J Am Vet Med Assoc 1977;170:1173.

Greet TRC. Outcome of treatment of 35 cases of guttural pouch mycosis. Equine Vet J 1987;19:483.

Jang SS, Dorr TE, Biberstein EL, Wong A. *Aspergillus deflectus* infection in 4 dogs. J Med Vet Mycol 1996;24:95.

Kelly SE, Shaw SE, Clark WT. Long-term survival of four dogs with disseminated *Aspergillus terreus* infection treated with itraconazole. Aust Vet J 1995;72:311.

Knudtson WU, Kirkbride CA. Fungi associated with bovine abortion in the northern plains states (USA). J Vet Diagn Invest 1992;4:181.

Kothary MH, Chase T, MacMillan JD. Correlation of elastase production by some strains of *Aspergillus fumigatus* with ability to cause pulmonary invasive aspergillosis in mice. Infect Immun 1984;43:320.

Mathews KG, Koblik PD, Richardson EF, et al. Computed tomographic assessment of noninvasive intranasal infusions in dogs with fungal rhinitis. Vet Surg 1996;25:309.

McCausland IP, Slee KJ, Hirst FS. Mycotic abortion in cattle. Aust Vet J 1987;64:129.

McCullough SM, McKiernan BC, Grodsky BS. Endoscopically placed tubes for administration of enilconazole for treatment of nasal aspergillosis in dogs. J Am Vet Med Assoc 1998;212:67.

Ossent R. Systemic aspergillosis and mucormycosis in 23 cats. Vet Rec 1987;120:330.

Richard RL, Thurston JR. Rapid hematogenous dissemination of *Aspergillus fumigatus* and *Aspergillus flavus* spores in turkey poults following aerosol exposure. Avian Dis 1983;27:1025.

Richardson EF, Mathews KG. Distribution of topical agents in the frontal sinuses and nasal cavity of dogs: comparison between current protocols for treatment of nasal aspergillosis and a new noninvasive technique. Vet Surg 1995;24:476.

Schallibaum M, Nicolet J, Konig H. *Aspergillus nidulans* and *Aspergillus fumigatus* as causal agents of bovine mastitis. Sabouraudia 1980;18:33.

Sheridan JJ. The relationship of systemic phycomycosis and aspergillosis in cattle showing clinical signs of disease to the occurrence of lesions in different organs. Vet Res Comm 1981;5:1.

Watt PR, Robbins GM, Galloway AM, O'Boyle DA. Disseminated opportunistic fungal disease in dogs: 10 cases (1982–1990). J Am Vet Med Assoc 1995;207:67.

White LO, Smith H. Placental localization of *Aspergillus fumigatus* in bovine mycotic abortion: enhancement of spore germination in vitro by fetal tissue extracts. J Med Microbiol 1974;7:27.

Other Saprophytic Fungal Pathogens

Ader PL. Phycomycosis in 15 dogs and 2 cats. J Am Vet Med Assoc 1979;174:1216.

Allison N, McDonald RK, Guist SR, Bentinck-Smith J. Eumycotic mycetoma caused by *Pseudoallescheria boydii* in a dog. J Am Vet Med Assoc 1989;194:797.

Allison N, Willard MD, Bentinck-Smith S, Davis K. Nasal rhinosporidiosis in 2 dogs. J Am Vet Med Assoc 1986;188:869.

Baszler T, Chandler FN, Bertog RW, et al. Disseminated pseudallescheriasis in a dog. Vet Pathol 1988;25:95.

Harvey CE, O'Brien JA, Felsburg PJ, et al. Nasal penicilliosis in six dogs. J Am Vet Med Assoc 1981;178:1084.

Littman MR, Goldschmidt MH. Systemic paecilomycosis in a dog. J Am Vet Med Assoc 1987;191:445.

MacDonald SM, Corbel MJ. *Mortierella wolfii* infection in cattle in Britain. Vet Rec 1981;109:419.

McKenzie RA, Connole MD. Mycotic nasal granuloma in cattle. Aust Vet J 1977;53:268.

Miller RI. Gastrointestinal phycomycosis in 63 dogs. J Am Vet Med Assoc 1985;186:473.

Patton CS. *Helminthosporium spiciferum* as the cause of dermal and nasal maduromycosis in a cow. Cornell Vet 1977;67:236.

Pepin GA. Bovine mycotic abortion. Vet Annual 1983;23:79.

Sheridan JJ. Bovine mycotic abortion, with particular reference to the occurrence of the disease in Ireland. Ir Vet J 1980;34:75.

Pneumocystis carinii

Bille-Hansen V, Jorsal SE, Henriksen SA, Settnes OP. *Pneumocystis carinii* pneumonia in Danish piglets. Vet Rec 1990;20:407.

Cailliez JC, Seguy N, Denis CM, et al. *Pneumocystis carinii*: an atypical fungal micro-organism. J Med Vet Mycol 1996;34:227.

Ewing PJ, Cowell RL, Tyler RD, et al. *Pneumocystis carinii* pneumonia in foals. J Am Vet Med Assoc 1994;204:929.

Farrow BR, Watson AD, Hartley WJ, Huxtable CR. Pneumocystis pneumonia in the dog. J Comp Pathol 1972;82:447.

Fishman JA. Treatment of infection due to *Pneumocystis carinii*. Antimicrob Agents Chemother 1998;42:1309.

Peters SE, Whitwell AEWKE, Hopkin JM. *Pneumocystis carinii* pneumonia in thoroughbred foals: identification of a genetically distinct organism by DNA amplification. J Clin Microbiol 1994;32:213.

Stringer JR. *Pneumocystis carinii*: what is it, exactly? Clin Microbiol Rev 1996;9:489.

Protothecosis

Arnold R, Ahearn DG. The systematics of the genus *Prototheca* with a description of a new species, *P. filamenta*. Mycologia 1972;64:265.

Dillberger JE, Homer B, Daubert D, Altman NH, et al. Protothecosis in two cats. J Am Vet Med Assoc 1988;192:1557.

McDonald JS, Richard JL, Cheville NE. Natural and experimental bovine intramammary infection with *Prototheca zopfii*. Am J Vet Res 1984;45:492.

Migaki G, Font RL, Sauer RM, et al. Canine protothecosis: review of the literature and report of an additional case. J Am Vet Med Assoc 1982;181:794.

Sudman SM. Protothecosis — a critical review. Am J Clin Pathol 1974;61:10.

48 *Mycotoxins*

Francis D. Galey

Mycotoxins are metabolites produced by fungi that may be found in grains and forages. A *mycotoxicosis* is a disease caused by those toxins, unlike a *mycosis*, which is a disease caused by fungal growth (not due to its toxins). Mycotoxins may be divided into two general classes. *Endomycotoxins* are constituents of a fungus such as those found in mushrooms and will not be discussed here. This discussion will concern the *exomycotoxins*, which are elaborated into the substrate. Exomycotoxins may be present even after a fungus has ceased to grow. Thus, the absence of a fungus does not rule out the presence of a potentially toxic metabolite in a substrate.

Mycotoxins are of worldwide veterinary and public health concern. Diseases caused by mycotoxins include acute and chronic poisoning, alteration of the immune system, loss of production, carcinogenicity, and teratogenicity.

Many genera and species of fungi are toxigenic. A given mycotoxin may be elaborated by more than one fungal species. For example, aflatoxin may be produced by different strains of *Aspergillus* or *Penicillium* spp. Some genera of fungi may produce more than one toxin. For example, various *Fusarium* spp. may produce trichothecenes, fumonisin, fusaric acid, moniliformin, and other toxins. A given fungus is not always toxic (many are ubiquitous) and fungi will only produce toxins under certain environmental conditions. Thus, finding the fungus alone is rarely significant and diagnosis requires chemical identification of the toxin.

Colonization and toxin elaboration may occur in the field or in storage. Basic requirements for colonization include a substrate with sufficient nutrients (why fruits and seeds are commonly infested), moisture content in feed above 14%, relative humidity over 70%, appropriate temperature (varies with species of fungus), and oxygen. Damage to fruits or plants favors colonization. The requirements for toxin elaboration may vary from those needed for colonization. For example, alternating warm and cool ambient temperatures tend to favor the formation of some trichothecene mycotoxins.

Mycotoxins are found in a variety of matrices, including grain or forages. Although many have been identified, many more, as yet unidentified toxins, may exist. For example, moldy hay has been implicated as a cause of many problems, including gastrointestinal disturbances and photosensitization, yet the toxins have not been identified. Some mycotoxins have related, toxic metabolites that are not routinely screened. A classic example is provided by deoxynivalenol (DON or "vomitoxin"). Pure DON will cause toxicosis in swine when present at over 10 ppm in feed, whereas as little as 0.5 ppm has been associated with toxicosis in the field, most likely because of the presence of other, related toxins at the same time.

Feed contaminated with mycotoxins may not be visibly moldy. Diagnosis of mycotoxicosis usually requires identification of the toxin in a suspected feed source. To date, few reliable tests exist for testing of mycotoxins in animal-related samples. The sampling technique is critical because toxin levels will vary greatly within a lot of feed. The methodology used to test various matrices for mycotoxins varies depending on the compound. Quick screens, like thin-layer chromatography and immunoassay, exist for common grain mycotoxins such as aflatoxins and DON. However, inaccurate positive results and matrix-related problems are common. Thus, further analytical chemistry is needed to verify findings. Techniques that are used include gas or high-performance liquid chromatography, coupled with a variety of detection methods including mass spectrometry. Samples for testing should be representative of a lot and frozen for storage.

Some important mycotoxins of livestock are discussed below.

AFLATOXINS

Many fungal species can produce aflatoxins, including *Aspergillus flavus* ("A" + "fla" + toxin), *A. parasiticus,* and various species of *Penicillium, Rhizopus, Mucor,* and *Streptomyces.* Colonization and toxin production occur in grains such as corn, cottonseed, and peanuts in all phases of production from growth through storage. Aflatoxins are produced in soybeans and other small grains mainly during storage. Aflatoxin production can occur when the climate is warm and conditions are moist. Crop damage will encourage toxin formation. Although many aflatoxins exist, the major toxins of concern include aflatoxins B_1, B_2, G_1, and G_2 (based on fluorescence color). The major marker metabolite in milk and meat is aflatoxin M_1. Aflatoxin is bioactivated in liver to the toxic 8,9 epoxide. The bioactivated toxin acts by binding such biological molecules as essential proteins, blockade of RNA polymerase and ribosomal translocase (inhibiting protein synthesis), and formation of DNA adducts.

Aflatoxin can cause peracute signs, chronic toxicity, or oncogenesis depending on the species and age of animal, and the amount and duration of aflatoxin exposure. All animals may be affected by aflatoxins. Species differences largely result from the balance between microsomal bioactivation vs. microsomal and cytosolic deactivation rates in the liver. Birds and trout are extremely sensitive to aflatoxins, with as little as 1 ppb (0.001 ppm) in the diet being carcinogenic in trout. Young swine and pregnant sows are also sensitive to aflatoxins, followed by calves (0.2 ppm in feed for 16 weeks caused mild liver damage), horses (0.4 to 0.6 ppm), fat pigs, mature cattle (0.66 ppm in feed caused mild liver damage after 20 weeks), and lastly, sheep. Levels over 1 ppm in feed may cause severe liver damage and acute death in livestock. As little as 0.15 ppm or less of aflatoxin in the feed may lead to actionable aflatoxin residues in meat and milk. Action levels for aflatoxin residues are 0.0005 ppm in meat and milk, and 0.02 ppm in feed.

Signs of peracute toxicosis include hemorrhage, bloody diarrhea, and rapid onset of death. Lesions in those cases include hemorrhage and prolonged prothrombin times. Subacute toxicosis results in liver damage with icterus, anorexia, ataxia, reproductive failure including abortion, impaired immune function, weakness, tremors, slowed rumen motility, coma, and death. Liver failure due to aflatoxicosis may result in anemia, ascites, pallor, elevated liver-associated enzymes (e.g., alkaline phosphatase, aspartate transaminase, total bilirubin), and decreased albumin and total protein levels. Lesions include a pale, yellow liver with centrilobular to portal liver fatty degeneration and necrosis and biliary hyperplasia. The pattern of liver damage is animal species-specific. Chronic toxicity is associated with decreased growth rates, decreased feed efficiency, rough hair coats, ill thrift, increased incidence of disease, and liver fibrosis with regenerative nodules. Diagnosis is supported by testing of feed and liver samples for aflatoxins.

Aflatoxin B$_1$ is also a very potent carcinogen. Aflatoxins are distributed to tissues (especially liver) and milk of food animals, leading to significant concerns about residue, as mentioned above. Alfatoxin is cleared from the liver by 1 week after withdrawal of contaminated feed. Dairy cows can "decontaminate" aflatoxin to below the 0.0005 ppm action level in milk if the maximum level of aflatoxin in feed is below 0.1 ppm (up to a 300:1 dilution).

Beyond providing aflatoxin-free feed and therapy for liver failure, treatment for aflatoxicosis centers on prevention. Feed has been ammoniated to prevent colonization and growth of fungi. In emergencies, farmers may dilute feeds to nontoxic levels or feed lower levels to less sensitive species, which may be risky given possible uneven levels of aflatoxin in a lot of feed. Feeding of low levels of aflatoxins may be possible when fed in combination with hydrated sodium calcium aluminosilicate binders to prevent aflatoxin absorption, toxicosis, and contamination in milk and meat.

TRICHOTHECENES

The trichothecene mycotoxins are found worldwide in various grains and forages. Chemically, the toxins are tetracyclic sesquiterpenoid toxins. At least six genera of fungi produce the toxins, the most important of which are various *Fusarium* spp., *Mycothecium* spp., *Stachybotrys atra*, and *Trichothecium roseum*. Growth of these fungi and toxin production is favored by undulating, warm–cool temperatures. Thus, a cool, wet, delayed harvest would favor higher toxin production. Trichothecenes may be present in combination with zearalenone.

Agriculturally, among the 100 or so known related toxins, the most important trichothecenes are deoxynivalenol (DON or "vomitoxin"), T-2 toxin, stachybotryotoxin (can be in forage), and diacetoxyscirpenol (DAS). Potent inhibitors of protein synthesis, trichothecenes block all three major translational processes including initiation, elongation, and termination of ribosomal translation. The damage to protein synthesis adversely affects the gastrointestinal, hematologic, immunologic, and nervous systems. Historically, disease due to related compounds has been called "alimentary toxic aleukia," referring to the impact on those systems.

All species of animals are sensitive to the trichothecenes. As with any poison, mycotoxicosis from this class of compounds depends on the specific toxin, its concentration, and the species exposed. For example, cattle and other ruminants are much more resistant to DON than are monogastric animals like pigs or dogs. Additionally, the toxicity of naturally contaminated grain is often much greater than that reported for experimental toxicity studies using pure compounds, probably because related trichothecenes are often present in the field along with the toxin being assayed. For example, as mentioned above, 10 ppm of pure DON is needed to cause feed refusal experimentally in swine, whereas 0.5 ppm in field-contaminated grain may lead to feed refusal.

General, dose-dependent signs of trichothecene toxicity include feed refusal, reduced weight gains, severe gastroenteritis with vomition and diarrhea, coagulopathy and shock, skin necrosis (from direct contact), decreased reproductive performance, and altered immune responses. Severe trichothecene toxicosis primarily reflects shock and/or hemorrhagic gastroenteritis. Affected animals in those cases may have anemia and leukopenia. Bilirubin may be increased secondary to feed refusal. DON, the most clinically important trichothecene, usually causes feed refusal, increased incidence of disease, and related production losses. Other trichothecenes are likely to cause the more severe, acute signs of hemorrhagic gastroenteritis, shock, and death. Lesions in those cases may be extensive, involving the gastrointestinal, lymphoid, cardiovascular, and other systems. Testing for trichothecenes in feed is diagnostically useful.

DON toxicosis is treated by providing mycotoxin-free feed. In addition to nonspecific therapy for signs, animals with acute trichothecene toxicosis may benefit from decontamination with activated charcoal, therapy with corticosteroids and fluids for acute shock, and antibiotic treatment to minimize secondary infections from skin and gastrointestinal (GI) lesions. The trichothecenes are rapidly metabolized and would not be expected to be a residue hazard after 12 to 24 hours postexposure.

FUMONISIN

Fumonisins are mycotoxins produced by *Fusarium* spp., especially *F. moniliforme* and occasionally *F. proliferatum*. These toxins are hepatotoxic, pneumotoxic, neurotoxic, and carcinogenic. Mycotoxins, with a similar structure, called *AAL-toxins*, are produced by *Alternaria* spp. (e.g., *A. alternata*) and other molds. Fumonisins are responsible for the neurological disease known as "moldy corn poisoning of horses" or "equine leukoencephalomalacia." Swine may suffer from pulmonary edema and chronic nodular pulmonary disease with cardiovascular damage. In addition to the more species-specific effects, fumonisins cause liver disease in almost all animals. *Fusarium moniliforme* is ubiquitous in the environment, so culturing the mold is not diagnostic.

Fumonisins (fumonisin B_1 is most common) act largely by interfering with sphingolipid biosynthesis. The toxins structurally inhibit enzymes important for acylation of ceramide (e.g., ceramide synthase). That inhibition causes accumulation of sphinganine, which has toxic cellular effects, and an increase in the sphinganine-sphingosine ratio. Found in high concentrations in liver and brain, complex sphingolipids are critical for cell growth, differentiation, and transformation. Additionally, fumonisins may also be directly toxic to endothelial surfaces such as those in the lung and brain.

Fumonisins are produced mainly on corn, especially screenings. Although other species can be affected, horses and swine are most sensitive to fumonisin's effects. Ruminants and poultry are resistant. Fumonisin B_1 at levels of 10 ppm or greater in corn may lead to toxicosis in horses. Levels of 40 ppm or more may cause disease in swine. Clinical signs in horses appear suddenly after 7 to 90 days of ingesting toxic corn or corn screenings and may include depression, confusion, ataxia, sweating, apparent blindness, head pressing, recumbency, convulsions, and death within 5 days of onset of signs. Rabbits have experimentally developed neurologic signs after being dosed with fumonisin.

Morbidity is generally low but mortality high for animals with neurotoxicosis from fumonisins. Signs of fumonisin toxicosis in swine include poor weight gain, depression, icterus, dyspnea, and death. Lesions include pulmonary edema and centrilobular hepatic necrosis. Hepatotoxicosis is common for most species of animals due to fumonisin exposure. Clinical pathology changes include transient increases in serum enzymes associated with liver damage. The pathognomonic lesion of fumonisin toxicosis in horses is leukoencephalomalacia, which is characterized by liquefactive necrosis of white matter of the brain leaving fluid-filled cavities (often grossly visible). Acutely affected horses may have cen-

trilobular hepatic necrosis, which may be present with or without the brain lesion. Swine have lesions of pulmonary edema. Fumonisin is a potent hepatocarcinogen in laboratory animals. Diagnosis of fumonisin toxicosis is aided by analysis of corn or corn-based feeds for the mycotoxin.

Prevention of fumonisin toxicosis is accomplished by avoiding corn, or at least eliminating corn screenings, in the diet of horses. Poor oral bioavailability, rapid elimination of fumonisin in bile, a relatively short elimination half-life, and a lack of transfer to milk and eggs have minimized the hazard of fumonisin-related food residues in most species. The toxins do, however, accumulate in swine liver and kidney, requiring several weeks of withdrawal from contaminated feed to ensure a lack of residue in those tissues.

STAGGERS MYCOTOXINS

Some forages contain alkaloidal mycotoxins that cause a neurological dysfunction in livestock that is commonly called *staggers*. Implicated forages include perennial ryegrass (*Lolium perenne*) infested with *Neophytodium* (formerly *Acremonium*) *lolia* in leaf sheaths, ergotized Dallis grass (*Paspalum dilatatum*, seed fungus is *Claviceps paspali*), Bermuda grass (*Cynodon dactylon*, mold unknown), moldy walnuts and dairy products (*Juglans* spp., walnut mold is *Penicillium* spp.), and although not a forage, *Aspergillus* spp. in grain. The alkaloids are indole-based paxallines and include lolitrems (perennial ryegrass), paspalitrems (Dallis grass), penitrems (moldy walnuts), and aflatrems (*Aspergillus*). The mechanism of action of those toxins is incompletely understood but may involve enhanced release of excitatory amino acid neurotransmitters perhaps via inhibition of calcium-dependent potassium channels.

The toxicity of tremorgenic forages depends on grazing habits and climate. Perennial ryegrass is hazardous late in the season when grass is grazed closely to the ground, since lolitrems are found in the lower leaf sheaths. Dallis grass is hazardous when ergotized seed heads are grazed. All species exposed to the staggers toxins may be affected. Dried perennial ryegrass and perennial ryegrass seeds may retain toxicity. Signs of staggers appear within 7 days of initial grazing of toxic grass and within hours for penitrems in moldy walnuts or dairy products. Animals appear normal at rest or may have a fine tremor in the ear and head. When stimulated, affected animals have a characteristic stiff, spastic gait, followed by spasms and tetanic seizures. Opisthotonus occurs in severe cases. Recovery from an episode may be rapid for perennial ryegrass, Dallis grass, and Bermuda grass staggers if uncomplicated. Losses occur, however, due to injuries, drowning, becoming trapped during seizure episodes, and other forms of misadventure. For most staggers toxins, seizure episodes dissipate within 2 weeks after removal from the toxic forages. Unlike the grass staggers, penitrem toxicosis is often fatal if patients do not receive adequate therapy.

Lesions of staggers are minimal, although degeneration of cerebellar Purkinje cells has been reported for longer-standing or severe cases of perennial ryegrass staggers. Diagnosis of staggers syndromes is helped by ruling out other tremorgenic syndromes, identification of the fungus (e.g., for perennial ryegrass), and identification of the toxin in the plant (e.g., lolitrem B in perennial ryegrass). If standards for the forage toxins are not available for analysis, bioassay using an extract of the forage in the laboratory can be diagnostic. Other causes of tremorgenic syndromes in livestock include the tryptamine alkaloids of *Phalaris* grass and tunicamycauracil compounds from annual grass staggers (*Clavibacter* sp. bacterial toxin).

Alternate forage should be provided for affected animals until new pasture growth is available. Some managers move animals away from the toxic pasture during the sensitive periods. Affected animals are placed in areas where misadventure can be minimized. Mowing the seed heads is suggested to minimize effects of ergotized Dallis grass. Therapy for penitrem toxicosis includes control of seizures and decontamination of the GI tract with adsorbents like activated charcoal.

Fescue Toxicosis

Fescue toxicosis is common throughout the United States. Tall fescue grass (*Festuca arundinacea*) infested by *Neophytodium* (formerly *Acremonium*) *coenophialum* and strains of perennial ryegrass (*Lolium perenne*) infested by *Neophytodium lolia* (also produces staggers toxins) produce ergot-like alkaloids such as ergovaline and pyrrolizidine alkaloids. The ergovaline and related alkaloids act by agonistic stimulation of dopaminergic neurotransmission at the D-2 receptor and thus inhibiting prolactin.

The impact of grazing endophyte-infected tall fescue depends on the ambient temperatures and the reproductive status of exposed livestock. Livestock suffer from "summer syndrome," characterized by increased rectal temperatures, lethargy, ill thrift, failure to gain weight, and intolerance to heat during warm periods. During cool conditions, cattle may develop typical ergot-type lesions of dry gangrene in the distal extremities. Perhaps the most devastating aspect of tall fescue toxicosis is reproductive failure characterized by agalactia, prolonged gestation, weak/stillbirths, and thickened placentas in horses and cattle.

Lesions of fescue toxicosis are nonspecific. Serum prolactin and progesterone concentrations are decreased in exposed animals. Postmortem, fat necrosis with foci of hard nodules in the omental region may be present in animals with "summer syndrome" and ergot-like gangrene is present in distal extremities for animals with "fescue foot." Diagnosis of tall fescue toxicosis is helped by demonstration of the endophyte or toxins in grass.

Pregnant animals should be removed from tall fescue pastures 30 to 60 days before parturition. Some farms have successfully used herbicides to kill the tall fescue,

planted an annual crop the next year, and then followed by planting of endophyte-free tall fescue, which is now available.

Zearalenone

Zearalenones are polyphenolic, estrogenic mycotoxins produced in corn and other grains by various *Fusarium* spp. (especially *F. roseum*) under similar warm–cool climatic cycles as for trichothecenes. For example, zearalenone is often produced along with DON. The primary biological effect of zearalenones is hyperestrogenism with infertility. Prepuberal animals, especially swine, are the most sensitive animals to zearalenone. Cattle, sheep, and poultry are relatively resistant. Zearalenol, a zearalenone metabolite, has been used as an estrogenic growth promoter in cattle.

Corn contaminated with zearalenone may cause toxicosis at levels as low as 1 ppm. Like the trichothecenes, this level is well below the toxicity of pure toxin, suggesting the presence of other estrogenic metabolites in field samples. Zearalenone can be metabolized to the more toxic zearalenol. Zearalenone causes chronic hyperestrogenism with vulvar swelling, prolapsed rectum, enlarged mammary glands, low fertility, and feminization in swine and cattle (at much higher levels). Although zearalenone may be distributed to milk and meat, medically significant residues would not be expected in products from animals exposed to grain with natural zearalenone contamination.

Slaframine

Slaframine is an indolizidine alkaloid mycotoxin produced by black batch mold (*Rhizoctonia leguminicola*) contamination in moldy red clover (*Trifolium repens*) grass and hay. Moldy red clover hay also can contain small amounts of swainsonine, the related indolizidine alkaloid that is the principal toxin in locoweeds. Like aflatoxins, slaframine is bioactivated in the liver of exposed animals to a toxic form. That active metabolite is thought to be a quaternary amine that mimics acetylcholine causing cholinergic effects. Clinically, slaframine causes excessive salivation, diarrhea, decreased milk production, weight loss, abortion, and bloat in affected cattle and horses. Signs may persist for several days after consumption of the moldy forage has ceased.

Ergot

Classical ergot results from parasitism of developing grass or grain flowers by *Claviceps purpurea*. *Ergot* refers to the formation of a dark, fungal sclerotium on the seed heads. Several wild grasses and grains such as rye, triticale, wheat, oat, and barley may be affected. Affected grains contain a series of alkaloids including ergotamine, ergonovine, and ergotaxine. The ergot alkaloids are similar to those found in fescue grass.

The ergot alkaloids have a variety of neurologic and cardiovascular effects. For example, lysergic acid neurotoxins are ergot alkaloids. Historically, ergotism caused epidemics of pain, cramps, and numbing of extremities as part of development of dry gangrene. The numbness in humans was referred to as "Saint Anthony's fire." Ergotism in livestock may result in ataxia, convulsions, lameness, dyspnea, diarrhea, dry gangrene of the extremities much like "fescue foot," abortion, neonatal mortality, reduced lactation, poor weight gains, lowered production, and lowered feed intake. Some ergot alkaloids have been used medicinally for the uterotropic effects.

OCHRATOXIN

Ochratoxin is an isocoumarin derivative of phenylalanine. The ochratoxins are produced by several species of *Aspergillus* and *Penicillium* and are favored by cool temperatures and high moisture. Although several mechanisms of action have been demonstrated for ochratoxin, it primarily acts as a competitive inhibitor of phenylalanyl transfer RNA synthetase, inhibiting protein synthesis. The toxin also interferes with carbohydrate metabolism, causes lipid peroxidation, and may be genotoxic in some models. This toxin has caused kidney disease in Europe, historically referred to as "Endemic Balkan Nephropathy."

Feeding of over 0.2 to 4.0 ppm in grain to livestock can cause nephropathy. Monogastric animals such as swine and horses are more sensitive than ruminants. Young ruminants, however, may be susceptible to levels of ochratoxin above 2 to 40 ppm in the grain. Liver damage, enteritis, reduced growth rates, and abortion have also been reported. Some possibility exists that ochratoxin may also act as a carcinogen in mice and in vitro.

Citrinin, another nephrotoxic mycotoxin, might be found along with ochratoxin in a contaminated grain sample. Ochratoxin has a long half-life in pigs relative to other species and is widely distributed to the tissues. Therefore, like aflatoxin, ochratoxin is considered to be a food safety hazard. Swine that have been exposed to ochratoxin should be fed clean feed for at least 4 weeks before slaughter to ensure freedom from residues. Residues in food products from cattle and poultry are possible but much less likely to be of concern.

DICUMAROL

White and yellow sweet clovers, *Melilotus alba* and *M. officinalis*, respectively, produce glucosides containing coumarin. *Penicillium* spp. in moldy hay or silage dimerize the aglycone to dicumarol, which inhibits vitamin K epoxide reductase. Failure of that enzyme leads to failure of vitamin K-sensitive clotting factors, which ultimately leads to hemorrhagic disease.

In one study, feeding of moldy sweet clover hay that contained 30 ppm of dicumarol to cattle for 130 days resulted in bleeding disorders. From the same study, 70 ppm resulted in toxicosis after as little as 17 days of daily exposure. Moldy sweet clover poisoning in cattle results in widespread, vitamin K-responsive hemorrhage. Clinical toxicosis is hazardous to pregnant bovine heifers during late-term pregnancy due to hemorrhagic abortions.

Dicumarol toxicosis is responsive to treatment with vitamin K. Proper preparation of hay and silage will minimize the opportunity for *Penicillium* to dimerize the coumarin to dicumarol. Many ranchers avoid feeding sweet clover forages to pregnant heifers, especially late in gestation.

SUBSTITUTED FURANS

Moldy sweet potatoes (*Ipomoea batatas*) and moldy green beans (*Phaseolus vulgaris*) can contain mycotoxins that are toxic to the lungs. The syndrome that is produced, severe interstitial edema, is very similar to the diseases caused by lush pastures that are high in tryptophan or toxic *Perilla frutescens* plants. *Fusarium solani* in sweet potatoes and *Fusarium semitectum* in green beans are the toxigenic molds. Apparently, a synergy exists between the plant and mold in producing these pneumotoxins, somewhat like the relationship described above for dicumarol. The toxins are substituted furans such as 4-ipomeanol and are apparently metabolized by the mixed function oxidases in pulmonary Type 1 pneumocytes and nonciliated bronchiolar epithelial cells (CLARA) to highly cytotoxic free radicals, leading to damage to local alveolar and, perhaps most importantly, endothelial cells.

Feeding of moldy sweet potatoes or moldy green beans is hazardous in many livestock species. Clinical effects of these pneumotoxins include sudden onset of rapid breathing, severe dyspnea with an expiratory grunt, frothing at the mouth, lowered head, and open-mouth breathing. Some animals may be found dead in the pasture without evidence of other clinical signs.

Affected cattle have wet, heavy lungs with variable amounts of emphysema. Histologically, the lungs have severe interstitial edema. No specific treatment for toxic interstitial pneumonia is available.

SPORIDESMIN

Spores of *Pithomyces chartarum*, a fungus that grows in the dead litter material from ryegrass pastures, produce the family of mycotoxins called *sporidesmins*. The most important form is sporidesmin A. This mold and toxin is mostly of importance in New Zealand, although reports have suggested that the disease may occur in the United States in Oregon. Warm, wet weather favors the formation of the toxins. Sporidesmin has a disulfide bridge that generates tissue oxidants.

Sporidesmin is mainly a secondary photosensitizing agent. Thus, primary liver damage results in secondary skin necrosis because phylloerythrin metabolites of chlorophyll pigments in grass are no longer properly eliminated from the liver and are therefore circulated throughout, including to the skin. The lesions involve unpigmented and unprotected skin areas. Sheep mostly suffer from ear and face lesions. The crusting facial lesions are referred to as "facial eczema." Dairy cattle are affected in the udder and unpigmented areas. Therapy with zinc salts may be of benefit in protecting animals from this disease.

some effects being very specific (e.g., leukoencephalomalacia in horses) or nonspecific (e.g., poor production with DON). Diagnosis is made difficult by not only variable concentration and variable effects but also by the need to use very specific chemistry tests to identify the toxins. Although desirable, many of the kits and quick tests have proven to be unreliable in the field for many matrices.

Finally, the possibility of many related and potentially toxic cocontaminants, the potential for the presence of as yet undiscovered toxins, and the possiblity of interactions and mixtures make management and study of mycotoxicosis a continuing challenge.

SUMMARY

A variety of mycotoxins have diverse effects on biological systems. Known mycotoxins of major importance are discussed above. Many others, known and unknown, have a variety of toxicities and effects in animals. For example, citrinin is a nephrotoxin produced by various *Penicillium* and *Aspergillus* spp. Although citrinin toxicosis has not been recognized in the field, it may contribute to nephrotoxicity of ochratoxin when present as a cocontaminant in feed. Patulin is a toxic contaminant of apple products. Livestock deaths associated with liver and kidney lesions have been attributed to that toxin. Cyclopiazonic acid is an indole acid produced by a variety of *Aspergillus* and *Penicillium* spp. Cyclopiazonic acid has neurologic and muscular effects, although no clinical cases have been blamed on this toxin. Kojic acid is a fungal metabolite that is produced often in conjunction with aflatoxin. It is not particularly toxic. However, kojic acid does fluoresce, a property that has led to the use of black lights to diagnose moldy feeds. Unfortunately, this practice has proven to be very unreliable and nonspecific. Additional toxins from *Fusaria* are moniliformin, which is associated with cardiotoxicity in poultry; fusarochromanone, which is associated with tibial dyschondroplasia in poultry; and fusaric acid, which is a potential neurotoxin that has relatively low overall toxicity.

Mycotoxins often occur as mixtures, perhaps with additive or synergistic effects. For example, aflatoxin and fumonisin both are toxic to liver and may occur together. Citrinin may act in concert with ochratoxin to produce nephrotoxicity. Cyclopiazonic acid has been linked with aflatoxicosis as a cause of "Turkey X disease" in England. As mentioned above, deoxynivalenol and zearalenone often occur together in mixtures.

Many mycotoxins also occur as families of related, possibly toxic compounds. For example, multiple forms of fumonisin (B_1, B_2, etc.), aflatoxins, and trichothecenes exist. Confusion is generated when feed has tested to have a nontoxic level of one member of the family (e.g., DON) yet obvious signs of toxicosis are present clinically (e.g., DON-related metabolites).

Mycotoxins present a special challenge to animal and crop industries. Their potential for sporadic occurrence in concentrated "hot spots" in batches of feed make diagnosis an art. The variety of clinical effects is great, with

SELECTED REFERENCES

Bucci TJ, Hansen DK, LaBorde JB. Leukoencephalomalacia and hemorrhage in the brain of rabbits gavaged with mycotoxin fumonisin B_1. Nat Toxins 1996;4:51.

Carr SB, Jacobson DR. Bovine physiological responses to toxic fescue and related conditions for application in a bioassay. J Dairy Sci 1969;52:1792.

Casper HH, Alsad AD, Monson SB. Dicoumarol levels in sweet clover toxic to cattle. Proceedings of the Annual Meeting of the American Association of Veterinary Laboratory Diagnosticians, pp 41–48, 1982.

Cheeke PR. Natural toxicants in feeds, forages, and poisonous plants. 2nd ed. Danville, CT: Interstate, 1997.

Colvin BM, Cooley AJ, Beaver RW. Fumonisin toxicosis in swine: clinical and pathologic findings. J Vet Diagn Invest 1993;5:232.

Galey FD, Tracy ML, Craigmill AL, et al. Staggers induced by consumption of perennial ryegrass in cattle and sheep from Northern California. J Am Vet Med Assoc 1991;199:466.

Gallagher RT, White EP, Mortimer PH. Ryegrass staggers: isolation of potent neurotoxins lolitrem A and lolitrem B for staggers-producing pastures. N Z Vet J 1981;29:189.

Hagler WM, Benlow RF. Salivary syndrome in horses: identification of slaframine in red clover hay. Appl Environ Microbiol 1981;42:1067.

Harvey RB, Kubena LF, Phillips TD, et al. Prevention of aflatoxicosis by addition of hydrated sodium aluminosilicates to the diets of growing barrows. Am J Vet Res 1989;50:416.

Kerr LA, Linnabary RD. Atypical bovine pulmonary emphysema — another cause. 31st Annual Meeting of the American Association of Veterinary Laboratory Diagnosticians. Little Rock, Arkansas, October 1988:74. Abstract.

Kuiper-Goodman T. Risk assessment of ochratoxin A: an update. Food Addit Contam 1996;13(suppl):53.

Li X, Castleman WL. Ultrastructural morphogenesis of 4 ipomeanol-induced bronchiolitis and interstitial pneumonia in calves. Vet Pathol 1990;27:141.

McCann JS, Caudle AB, Thompson FN, et al. Influence of endophyte-infected tall fescue on serum prolactin and progesterone in gravid mares. J Anim Sci 1992;70:217.

Marasas WFO, Kellerman TS, Gelderblom WCA, et al. Leukoencephalomalacia in a horse induced by fumonisin B_1 isolated from *Fusarium moniliforme*. Onderspoort J Vet Res 1988;55:197.

Osweiler GD, Carson TL, Buck WB, Van Gelder GA. Clinical and diagnostic veterinary toxicology. Dubuque, IA: Kendall/Hunt, 1985:409.

Osweiler GD, Trample DW. Aflatoxicosis in feedlot cattle. J Am Vet Med Assoc 1985;187:636.

Riley RT, Wang E, Shroeder JJ, et al. Evidence for disruption of sphingolipid metabolism as a contributing factor in the toxicity and carcinogenicity of fumonisins. Nat Toxins 1996; 4:3.

Rotter BA, Prelusky DB, Pestka JJ. Toxicology of deoxynivalenol (vomitoxin). J Toxicol Environ Health 1996;48:1.

Wang E, Norred WP, Bacon CW, et al. Inhibition of sphingolipid biosynthesis by fumonisins. J Biol Chem 1991;266:14486.

49   *The Yersiniae*

ERNST L. BIBERSTEIN   DWIGHT C. HIRSH

The genus *Yersinia* belongs to the family *Enterobacteriaceae*. There are 11 species, one of which, *Y. ruckeri*, affects only fish. *Yersinia pseudotuberculosis* attacks mainly birds and rodents but occasionally domestic animals and primates. Plague, caused by *Y. pestis*, is a rodent-based zoonosis. The zoonotic aspects of *Y. enterocolitica*, *Y. intermedia*, *Y. frederiksenii*, and *Y. kristensenii* are uncertain. *Yersinia aldovae*, *Y. rohdei*, *Y. mollaretii*, and *Y. bercovieri* are without known pathogenic potential.

DESCRIPTIVE FEATURES

Morphology and Staining

Cells are gram-negative coccobacilli. Bipolarity is common in tissue smears. Most species are flagellated at ambient temperatures.

Cellular Composition and Products of Medical Importance

Yersinia enterocolitica and *Y. pseudotuberculosis* possess the chromosomally encoded proteins Ail (*a*ttachment *i*nvasion *l*ocus), and Inv (*inv*asion). These proteins are responsible for adhesion to target cell integrin proteins (Inv, Ail), as well as resistance to complement activity (Ail). Adhesion triggers actin cytoskeletal changes resulting in "ruffles" that entrap attached yersiniae resulting in their internalization. A number of plasmid-encoded, virulence-associated proteins are made under conditions of low calcium ion concentrations at 37°C. Whether low calcium ion concentration is actually the in vivo signal is uncertain. It is more likely that low calcium ion concentration mimics another, as yet unknown, in vivo cue. These plasmids are pYV (*y*ersinal *v*irulence in *Y. enterocolitica*), pCAD (*ca*lcium *d*ependence in *Y. pseudotuberculosis*), and pCD1 (*c*alcium *d*ependence in *Y. pestis*). Important products encoded by genes residing on these plasmids include Yops (*y*ersinia *o*uter membrane *p*roteins, a misnomer — they are not outer membrane proteins); YadA (*y*ersinia *ad*herence protein); LcrV (*l*ow *c*alcium *r*esponse *v*irulence); and YpkA (*y*ersinia *p*rotein *k*inase). Yops are produced and secreted (Type III secretory pathway) by all the virulent yersiniae. They are responsible for depolymerization of actin and disruption of signal transduction resulting in the inhibition of phagocytosis and the oxidative burst. YadA is produced by *Y. enterocolitica* and *Y. pseudotuberculosis* and is responsible for adherence to target cell integrins and invasion as well as resistance to complement. LcrV (at one time known as *V antigen*) is produced by all of the pathogenic yersiniae and is responsible for interfering with phagocytosis. YpkA is produced by *Y. pseudotuberculosis* and interferes with the signal transduction events necessary for effective phagocytosis, as does YopJ, which induces apoptosis in phagocytic cells. Antigen W, once thought to be a virulence-associated protein in *Y. pestis*, has been shown to be a complex of LcrV and the heat shock protein GroEL. Transcription of the calcium responsive proteins is also temperature regulated. At 26°C, transcription of Yops, LcrV, and YpkA is repressed, while at 37°C transcription is derepressed.

Yersinia pestis produces a protein Pla (*pl*asminogen *a*ctivator or Pla protease) responsible for coagulase, fibrinolytic and C3 degradative activity. Transcription of the gene, *pla*, which resides on a plasmid pPCP1 (*p*esticin, *c*oagulase, *p*lasminogen activation), is higher at 37°C, but is not calcium dependent. Pesticin, a bacteriocin produced by *Y. pestis*, does not appear to function as a virulence determinant. What role Pla plays in the pathogenesis of *Y. pestis* disease is unclear.

Yersinia pestis contains a third plasmid pMT1 (*m*ouse *t*oxin), which contains a gene encoding a protein lethal for rodents and a gene responsible for the protein that makes up the capsular structure F1. The gene encoding F1 (*caf1*, for *c*apsular *a*ntigen *F1*) is transcribed at 37°C and not at 26°C and is not calcium dependent. F1 is related to virulence.

A fibrillar structure composed of a protein produced at low pH (pH 6 antigen) is produced by *Y. pestis*. Some have hypothesized that this structure serves as an adhesin (there is limited homology with the *Escherichia coli* adhesin PapG) for entry into phagocytic cells in order to deliver Yops. Transient survival within phagocytic cells may be due to GsrA, a protein induced following phagocytosis (see Chapter 17). pH 6 antigen is not calcium nor temperature dependent.

Virulent yersiniae produce a siderophore termed *yersiniabactin* (Ybt), which is needed to acquire iron from host iron-binding proteins.

Yersinia pestis colonies bind hemoglobin or Congo red dye. This phenotype is known as Hms (*hem*in *s*torage). The gene encoding the Hms phenotype, *hms*, is located in a larger segment of chromosome that is termed Pgm (for *pigm*ented phenotype — colonies of *Y. pestis* appear pigmented when grown on hemin-containing medium, they are not, but adsorb hemin from the medium). The Hms phenotype is related in some unknown fashion to blockage in the flea, without which transfer of the agent occurs poorly, if at all.

Growth Characteristics

Yersiniae grow on ordinary laboratory media, including MacConkey agar, although they grow slower than most members of the family *Enterobacteriaceae.* Colony diameters range from under 1 mm (*Y. pestis*) up to 1.5 mm for most other yersiniae. They are not hemolytic when grown on blood agar.

In biochemical activities and resistance, yersiniae resemble other members of the family *Enterobacteriaceae.*

Variability

Yersinia pestis is serologically uniform. Other yersiniae have serotypes based on somatic and flagellar antigens, some of which are shared with other yersiniae and with other members of the family *Enterobacteriaceae.*

YERSINIA PESTIS (PLAGUE BACILLUS)

ECOLOGY

Reservoir

Tolerant rodents in endemic areas (see below) constitute the plague reservoir. They rarely develop fatal disease and are called *maintenance* or *enzootic* hosts. In coastal California, the meadow mouse *Microtus californicus* is such a host.

Transmission

Transmission is by fleas. They may carry infection to more susceptible, epizootic or amplification hosts, such as ground squirrels or rats. When these die, still other hosts, such as humans, are attacked. Infected mammals may spread plague by the airborne route. Oral acquisition is by predation, cannibalism, and scavenging.

Pathogenesis

Ingested *Y. pestis* in fleas proliferate until they block the flea's proventriculus. "Blocked" fleas infect the feeding wound when attempting to feed. The bacteria, thus introduced, lack Yops, LcrV, F1, do not produce YpkA, and are killed when ingested by neutrophils. In mononuclear phagocytes, at mammalian temperatures, they synthesize these proteins, acquiring resistance to further phagocytosis and intracellular killing by polymorphonuclear neutrophil leukocytes (PMNs).

Multiplication, intracellularly and extracellularly, elicits hemorrhagic inflammatory lesions, followed by local lymph node involvement ("bubo"). The infection commonly becomes septicemic and, if untreated, terminates fatally. This form is called *bubonic plague.*

Some individuals develop plague pneumonia and shed *Y. pestis* in sputum. Others contract primary pneumonic plague from this source and transmit it by the same route. Under epidemic conditions this form is nearly always fatal.

Among domestic animals, the cat acquires natural clinical infection, often apparently by ingestion. Signs include regional (particularly mandibular) lymphadenitis, fever, depression, anorexia, sneezing, coughing, and occasionally central nervous system disturbances. Most cases end fatally. Lesions, mainly in the respiratory and alimentary tracts, include lymphadenitis, tonsillitis, cranial and cervical edema, and pneumonia.

Human plague has been traced to feline infections. Suspected inoculation routes are via cuts, bites, scratches, and airborne and flea-borne pathways, although the latter is unlikely since the cat flea (*Ctenocephalides felis*) does not become blocked.

Epidemiology

Plague spread by animals, usually via fleas, is called *zootic.* Plague, usually pneumonic, spreading among people is called *demic.* Depending on the environment, plague can be *sylvatic* (rural) or *urban.* Plague is concentrated in certain endemic areas in southern and southeastern Asia, southern and west central Africa, western North America, and north central South America. Endemicity largely parallels presence of enzootic and epizootic rodent hosts. Human plague epidemics have historically been precipitated by importation of infected rats on board ships coming from endemic regions.

In endemic areas, infections are clustered during the warm months. "Off-season" plague affects mostly persons handling infected rabbits, coyotes, bobcats, and occasionally house cats.

IMMUNOLOGIC ASPECTS

Specific resistance to plague probably requires antibody and cell-mediated responses. F1 antigen (capsule) evokes opsonin formation. Disposal of intracellular organisms depends on activated macrophages. Immunity following recovery is good, but temporary.

LABORATORY DIAGNOSIS

Diagnostic attempts should be supervised by qualified public health personnel (see below). Samples from affected sites (i.e., edematous tissues, lymph nodes, and nasopharynx), transtracheal aspirates, cerebrospinal fluid, and blood (for culture and serology) are collected.

Direct smears are examined following immunofluorescent, "bipolar" (Wayson's), and Gram staining. Culture is done on blood or infusion agar. Identification is confirmed by immunofluorescence or bacteriophage susceptibility. Mice or guinea pigs injected subcutaneously with *Y. pestis* die within 3 to 8 days.

Serologic tests (hemagglutination, hemagglutination-inhibition, enzyme-linked immunosorbent assay [ELISA]) are useful only retrospectively in diagnosis of clinical cases.

TREATMENT AND CONTROL

If plague is suspected in domestic cats, the following recommendations from the Centers for Disease Control apply:

1. Arrange immediately with local and state public health officials for laboratory diagnostic assistance and steps to prevent spread and contamination.
2. Place all suspect cats in strict isolation.
3. When handling such cats, wear gown, mask, and gloves.
4. Treat every suspect for fleas (5% carbaryl dust for residual effect).

Flea elimination should precede rodent control.

Aminoglycosides, chloramphenicol, fluoroquinolones, and tetracycline are effective antimicrobics.

No vaccines for animals are available. Protection of humans by bacterins is transient.

YERSINIA PSEUDOTUBERCULOSIS

Yersinia pseudotuberculosis is closely related to *Y. pestis*.

ECOLOGY

Reservoir

Yersinia pseudotuberculosis is a parasite of wild rodents, lagomorphs, and birds, but it infects other mammals and reptiles and persists in the environment. The cat is the most commonly infected domestic mammal. Minor epidemics occur among sheep, pigs, nonhuman primates, fowl, and pet birds.

Transmission

Exposure is primarily through ingestion.

Pathogenesis

After ingestion, *Y. pseudotuberculosis* follows the same steps of attachment and invasion as outlined for *Y. enterocolitica* (Chapter 17). The result is enteritis and septicemia.

Yersinia pseudotuberculosis causes intestinal infections with formation of necrotic foci in the intestinal wall, abdominal lymph nodes, and viscera, particularly liver and spleen. There may be vomiting, diarrhea, or constipation, and weight loss, pale to subicteric mucous membranes, and depression. Fever is inconsistent. Few cases are diagnosed clinically antemortem. Mastitis is seen in cattle and abortion in ruminants and monkeys. In immunocompetent humans, the disease is generally an enteritis and abdominal lymphadenitis that is self-limiting or responsive to treatment.

Epidemiology

Pseudotuberculosis occurs worldwide. Cases tend to cluster in the cold months. In cats, prevalence is biased toward adult, rural, outdoor cats.

IMMUNOLOGIC ASPECTS

Natural infection is said to leave surviving individuals immune. Avirulent live vaccine protects against homologous challenge. It is not available commercially.

LABORATORY DIAGNOSIS

Diagnosis involves isolation of the agent antemortem from feces or lymph node aspirates. Isolation, particularly from mixed sources, is enhanced by cold enrichment, that is, incubation of a 10% mixture of inoculum in a minimal medium for several weeks at 4°C.

TREATMENT AND CONTROL

Pseudotuberculosis responds to the same antimicrobics as plague.

YERSINIA RUCKERI

"Enteric redmouth" is a hemorrhagic inflammation of the perioral subcutis of freshwater fish, particularly rainbow trout. Infection is systemic and causes significant mortality in hatcheries of North America, Australia, and Europe. The agent is disseminated by asymptomatic carrier fish and possibly riparian mammals (muskrats). Outbreaks appear to be related to massive exposure.

Outbreaks are brought under control with antimicrobics (e.g., sulfonamides, tetracycline, trimethoprim-sulfonamide) and prevented with bacterins.

Other yersiniae (particularly *Y. enterocolitica*, Chapter 17) are frequently recovered from animals (especially swine) and animal products, but rarely from diseased animals.

SELECTED REFERENCES

Austin B, Austin DA. *Yersinia ruckeri*. In: Bacterial fish pathogens. New York: Wiley, 1987:207–217.

Bonacorsi SP, Scavizzi MR, Guiyoule A, et al. Assessment of a fluoroquinolone, three beta-lactams, two aminoglycosides, and a cycline in treatment of murine *Yersinia pestis* infection. Antimicrob Agents Chemother 1994;38:481.

Bullock GL, Anderson DR. Immunization against *Yersinia ruckeri*. Symposium on fish vaccination. Office Internationale des Epizooties, 12 Rue de Prony, 75017 Paris, France, 1984:151–166.

Carlson ME. *Yersinia pestis* infection in cats. Feline Pract 1996;24:22.

Fasano A. Cellular microbiology: how enteric pathogens socialize with their intestinal host. ASM News 1997;63:259.

Finlay BB, Cossart P. Exploitation of mammalian host cell functions by bacterial pathogens. Science 1997;276:718.

Finlay BB, Falkow S. Common themes in microbial pathogenicity revisited. Microbiol Molec Biol Rev 1997;61:136.

Lee CA. Pathogenicity islands and the evolution of bacterial pathogens. Infect Agents Dis 1996;5:1.

Monack DM, Mecsas J, Ghori N, Falkow S. Yersinia signals macrophages to undergo apoptosis and YopJ is necessary for this cell death. Proc Nat Acad Sci USA 1997;94:10385.

Orloski KA, Eidson M. *Yersinia pestis* infection in three dogs. J Am Vet Med Assoc 1995;207:316.

Perry RD, Fetherston JD. *Yersinia pestis* — etiologic agent of plague. Clin Microbiol Rev 1997;10:35.

Rosenberg DR, Lerche NW, Henrickson RV. *Yersinia pseudotuberculosis* in a group of *Macaca fasciculatus*. J Am Vet Med Assoc 1980;177:818.

Slee KJ, Brightling R, Seiler RJ. Enteritis in cattle due to *Yersinia pseudotuberculosis* infection. Aust Vet J 1988;65:271.

Smith MD, Vinh DX, Hoa NTT, et al. In vitro antimicrobial susceptibilities of strains of *Yersinia pestis*. Antimicrob Agents Chemother 1995;39:2153.

Zhang C. Bacterial signalling involving eukaryotic-type protein kinases. Molec Microbiol 1996;20:9.

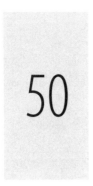

50 Francisella tularensis

ERNST L. BIBERSTEIN

Francisella tularensis, a noted pathogen of humans under limited epidemiologic conditions, occasionally infects domestic animals (sheep, horses, swine, carnivores). *Francisella philomiragia* and *F. tularensis* biogroup *novicida* (syn. *F. novicida*), are of uncertain animal pathogenicity.

DESCRIPTIVE FEATURES

Morphology and Staining

Francisella tularensis are gram-negative coccobacilli. They measure less than 1 μm in any dimension and can pass filter membranes of 600 nm porosity. In older cultures, more pleomorphism develops. Fresh isolates have a capsule high in lipid and amino acids. Giemsa stain is preferred. A cell wall antigen cross-reacts with *Brucella* spp.

Growth Characteristics

Francisella tularensis is a fastidious aerobe. The preferred medium is glucose-cysteine-blood-agar. Two to four days of incubation produce grayish, viscous, oxidase-negative colonies 1 to 4 mm in diameter. Tests for acidification of certain carbohydrates and citrulline ureidase activity permit subdivision of the *F. tularensis* into biotypes A and B, which differ in geographic distribution, host specificity, and virulence for humans.

Francisella tularensis survives cold temperatures for months in water, soil, and animal tissues.

ECOLOGY

Reservoir

The reservoirs of *F. tularensis* are infected lagomorphs (hares, rabbits; type A) and rodents (type B).

Transmission

The more virulent biotype A (*tularensis*) is predominant in North America and is transmitted largely by ticks and hemophagous insects. The milder biotype B (*palaearctica*) is predominant in Eurasia, and surface waters contaminated by rodents are sources of infection. Ingestion of infected prey spreads *F. tularensis* to animals. Sheep on the western range are infected by way of ticks. Transmission by animal bite has been documented. Humans are commonly infected by contact (percutaneous, conjunctival, inhalation, ingestion) with uncooked rabbit tissue.

Pathogenesis

From mucous membranes or arthropod bite, *F. tularensis* invades neighboring tissue, causing a local ulcerative inflammatory lesion. A facultatively intracellular parasite (growing within phagosomes of macrophages, inhibiting phagosome-lysosome fusion), it spreads to lymph nodes and possibly beyond, producing necrotic foci. In animals, probably only disseminated disease is noticed. Clinical signs resemble those of other acute systemic illnesses.

Epidemiology

Tularemia is a northern disease, its southern limits being Mexico and Mediterranean Africa. Seasonal peaks reflect vector activity and contact with the reservoir. Water-borne infections predominate in fall and winter.

IMMUNOLOGIC ASPECTS

Solid, largely cell-mediated immunity follows recovery in humans. Animals in endemic areas carry antibody. Its relation to immunity is unrelated. Live attenuated vaccines are used in humans at risk.

LABORATORY DIAGNOSIS

Demonstration of the organism in exudates is by polychrome stains, immunofluorescence, and culture. Isolation is facilitated by injection of suspect material into mice or guinea pigs.

Rising serum tube agglutination titers (1:≥80) are evidence of infection.

TREATMENT AND CONTROL

Streptomycin is the preferred drug for treating human tularemia. Tetracycline has been effective in animals. Fluoroquinolones appear to be effective, but whether they are as effective as aminoglycosides is unclear. Control measures are aimed at limiting tick exposure and access to contaminated feed and water.

SELECTED REFERENCES

Anthony LSD, Burke RD, Nano FE. Growth of *Francisella* spp. in rodent macrophages. Infect Immun 1991;59:3291.

Baldwin CJ, Panciera RJ, Morton RJ, et al. Acute tularemia in three domestic cats. J Am Vet Med Assoc 1991;199:1602.

Bevanger L, Maeland JA, Naess AI. Agglutinins and antibodies to *Francisella tularensis* outer membrane antigens in the early diagnosis of disease during an outbreak of tularemia. J Clin Microbiol 1988;26:433.

Earnvik A. Nature of protective immunity to *Francisella tularensis*. Rev Infect Dis 1989;11:440.

Fortier AH, Leiby DA, Narayanan RB, et al. Growth of *Francisella tularensis* LVS in macrophages: the acidic intracellular compartment provides essential iron required for growth. Infect Immun 1995;63:1478.

Hollis DG, Weaver RE, Steigerwalt AG, et al. *Francisella philomiragia* comb. nov. (formerly *Yersinia philomiragia*) and *Francisella tularensis* biogroup *novicida* (formerly *Francisella novicida*) associated with human disease. J Clin Microbiol 1989;27:1601.

Olsufjev NG, Meshcheryakova IS. Subspecific taxonomy of *Francisella tularensis*. McCoy and Chapin 1912. Int J Syst Bacteriol 1983;33:872.

Risi DF, Pombo DJ. Relapse of tularemia after aminoglycoside therapy: case report and discussion of therapeutic options. Clin Infect Dis 1995;20:174.

Sjostedt AJ, Conlan W, North RJ. Neutrophils are critical for host defense against primary infection with the facultative intracellular bacterium *Francisella tularensis* in mice and participate in defense against reinfection. Infect Immun 1994;62:2779.

Sjostedt A, Tarnvik A, Sandstrom G. *Francisella tularensis*: host-parasite interaction. FEMS Immunol Med Microbiol 1996;13:181.

51 Borrelia *spp.*

RANCE B. LEFEBVRE

Borreliae are spirochetes transmitted and maintained primarily by ticks. The infections they cause have blood-borne phases accompanied or followed by general and localizing manifestations.

Animal pathogens include *B. anserina*, the fowl spirochetosis agent; *B. theileri*, a mild pathogen mainly of cattle; and *B. burgdorferi* sensu lato, comprised of three genospecies, the cause of Lyme disease in dogs, horses, cattle, and humans. Tick-borne relapsing fever borreliae of humans occur asymptomatically in feral mammals, birds, and reptiles. Characterization of *B. coriaceae* as agent of epizootic bovine abortion is at present speculative.

DESCRIPTIVE FEATURES

Morphology and Staining

Borreliae measure 0.2 to 0.5 μm × 8 to 30 μm and are gram negative. For demonstration by light microscopy, polychrome strains (Giemsa, Wright's) are best. Dark field examination reveals spirals and motility.

Cellular Anatomy and Composition

Borreliae have a structure like other spirochetes, with an outer sheath encasing the axial fibrils consisting of 15 to 20 endoflagella (depending on species).

Borrelia spp. are unique among prokaryotes in that they have a linear double-stranded chromosome of approximately 900 kbp and a multiplicity of linear and circular plasmids that may in fact constitute components of the genome. Genes expressing major outer surface proteins may be found on any of the genetic elements.

Growth Characteristics

Of the *Borrelia* spp. pathogenic for animals, *B. anserina* is propagated in embryonated hen's eggs, and *B. burgdorferi* sensu lato is cultivated at 33°C on modified Kelly's medium (BSK), an enriched serum broth made selective by inclusion of kanamycin and 5-fluorouracil.

The organisms are slow-growing microaerophiles (doubling times: 12 to 18 hours). They ferment glucose and possibly other carbohydrates.

Survival of borreliae is about a week at room temperature in blood clots, several months at 4°C, and indefinite at less than 20°C.

Variability

A number of genes encoding outer surface proteins have been identified in several *Borrelia* species. The spirochetes control the expression of these genes at the transcriptional level. The antigenic variability available to the spirochetes is utilized for immune evasion in the relapsing fever borreliae. Lyme disease spirochetes are also equipped to express a wide range of outer surface proteins both at the intragenic and intergenic level. Though not utilized like the relapsing fever borreliae, an immune evasion function may still be involved in their maintenance and expression in these spirochetes.

ECOLOGY

Reservoir and Transmission

Pathogenic borreliae of animals are vectored by ticks. Ticks become infected at some stage in their life cycle by feeding on infected animals. Some vertical (transovarian, maternal) transmission occurs. Other arthropods may serve as short-term vectors. Infection occurs by wound contamination, usually during feeding by infected ticks. Passage via placenta, milk, and urine has been documented. During an outbreak in birds, infection may occur by coprophagia and cannibalism.

Pathogenesis

Endotoxin is incriminated in the pathogenesis of relapsing fever and probably other borrelioses. Hemolysin activity has been described in Lyme disease spirochetes.

ANIMAL BORRELIOSES

BORRELIA ANSERINA

Borrelia anserina causes fowl spirochetosis in chickens, turkeys, geese, ducks, pheasants, pigeons, canaries, and some species of wild birds. Onset of disease is marked by fever, depression, and anorexia. Affected birds are cyanotic and develop a greenish diarrhea. Later signs may include paralysis and anemia. Mortality ranges from 10% to almost 100%. Necropsy reveals splenomegaly and widespread hemorrhages. The enlarged liver may contain necrotic foci. Peripheral blood is often sterile.

Avian spirochetosis occurs on all continents and in all ages of birds. The young suffer high mortality rates and die at earlier, septicemic stages of infection. Following an outbreak, the agent generally disappears from the flock within 30 days.

The leading vector, *Argas persicus*, can remain infected for over a year and can pass the agent transovarially.

Temporary immunity, apparently antibody mediated, follows recovery. Antisera confer protection for several weeks. Inactivated vaccines made from infected blood or egg-propagated *B. anserina* are beneficial.

Spirochetes are demonstrable in blood by darkfield microscopy, stained smear, or immunofluorescence. Suspect material (i.e., blood, spleen, or liver suspension) may be inoculated into the yolk sac of 5-to-6-day embryonated eggs. Spirochetes will appear within 2 or 3 days. Antigen or antibody may be demonstrated in agar gel diffusion tests.

Borrelia anserina is susceptible to penicillin, tetracycline, chloramphenicol, streptomycin, kanamycin, and tylosin. Immune serum has protective potential and bacterins produce long-lasting immunity.

Control of ectoparasites is essential.

BORRELIA THEILERI

Borrelia theileri causes a mild febrile anemia, most often in African and Australian cattle, and occasionally in sheep and horses. The disease is associated with several species of ixodid ticks. The pathogenic mechanism(s) is not understood. Most information comes from field cases, which may be complicated by other tick-borne infections. Although not routinely treated, animals respond to tetracycline. Tick control is advisable.

LYME BORRELIOSIS

Lyme disease is caused by *B. burgdorferi* sensu lato, a pathogenic spirochete. Genetic analysis now defines three genospecies, *B. burgdorferi* sensu stricto, *B. garinii*, and *B. afzelii*. *Borrelia burgdorferi* sensu stricto is the predominant pathogen of North America.

Distribution and Transmission

Endemic areas include the Atlantic states; Minnesota and Wisconsin; parts of the American South and far West; most of continental Europe and Britain; Russia; Asia; Japan; and parts of New South Wales in Australia. May through October is the time of peak prevalence. Increasing spread of the disease is attributed to increased deer populations, increasing human movement into rural areas, and the dissemination of infected ticks by migratory birds. The agent is harbored by several ixodid ticks (primarily *Ixodes scapularis* and *I. pacificus* in North America). The tick has a 2-year life cycle comprised of a larval, nymph, and adult stage, requiring a blood meal at each molt. Deer mice and white-footed mice and other small rodents serve as reservoirs for the spirochete. *Borreli burgdorferi* has been isolated from the urine of dogs and cows as well as milk from infected cows, potentially serving as alternate routes for exposure and infection.

Human Lyme borreliosis, caused by *B. burgdorferi*, typically begins with a skin lesion (erythema migrans) often followed weeks or months later by neural, cardiac, and arthritic complications. Endotoxin, hemolysin, immune complexes, and immunosuppression may be involved in pathogenesis.

In animals, dogs are most often affected, with manifestations of polyarthritis, fever, and anorexia the most common ailment. Malaise, lymphadenopathy, carditis, and renal disease have also been noted in dogs.

Borreliosis in horses and cattle have also been reported. Abortions were observed cattle. In horses, polyarthritis, ocular and neural involvement, and foal mortality have been reported.

Diagnosis

Diagnosis involves demonstration of the agent in tissues and fluids (darkfield, immunofluorescence microscopy), antibody in serum or other fluids (indirect immunofluorescent test, enzyme-linked immunosorbent assay [ELISA]), or DNA amplification of tissue or fluid samples using genus specific DNA primers and the polymerase chain reaction (PCR).

Culture is laborious and often unrewarding. However, culturing ear punch biopsies from infected dogs and mice has proven to be reliable. Culture of synovial fluid from affected joints is also possible. BSKII is a good isolation medium. The spirochetes grow best at 33°C.

TREATMENT AND CONTROL

Tetracycline, doxycycline, enrofloxacin, erythromycin, and penicillin are generally effective, although not invariably so. Tick control is vital.

IMMUNOLOGIC FACTORS

A humoral immune response appears essential for protection against *B. burgdorferi* infection. Most animals appear to self-immunize with no apparent clinical manifestations subsequent to exposure to the spirochete.

Artificial Immunization

Antibodies produced in response to vaccination with *B. burgdorferi* have proven effective in preventing infection of laboratory animals. These observations have led to the development of a commercially available whole cell bacterin for use in canines. Protective immunity, however, appears to be of short duration and limited in range. Moreover, the potential for the induction of an autoimmune response has shifted the focus from a whole cell vaccine to a subunit vaccine approach. Two subunit vaccines have recently become commercially available.

SELECTED REFERENCES

Barbour A, Hayes SF. Biology of *Borrelia* species. Microbiol Rev 1986;50:381.

Burgess E, Gendron-Fitzpatrick A, Wright WQ. Arthritis and systemic disease caused by *Borrelia burgdorferi* in a cow. J Am Vet Med Assoc 1987;191:1468.

Cohen ND. Borreliosis (Lyme disease) in horses. Equine Vet Educ 1996;4:213.

Gross WB. Spirochetosis. In: Hofstad MS, et al, eds. Diseases of poultry. 8th ed. Ames, IA: Iowa State, 1984.

Johnson RC, Hyde FW, Schmid GP, Brenner DJ. *Borrelia burgdorferi* sp. nov.: etiologic agent of Lyme disease. Int J Syst Bacteriol 1984;34:496.

Johnson SE, Klein GC, Schmid GP, et al. Lyme disease: a selective medium for isolation of the suspected etiological agent, a spirochete. J Clin Microbiol 1984;19:81.

Levy SA. Lyme borreliosis in dogs. Canine Pract 1992;17:5.

Madigan JE, Teitler J. *Borrelia burgdorferi* borreliosis. J Am Vet Med Assoc 1988;192:892.

Magnarelli LA, Anderson JF, Schreier AB, Ficke CM. Clinical and serologic studies of canine borreliosis. J Am Vet Med Assoc 1987;191:1089.

Schmid GR. The global distribution of Lyme disease. Rev Inf Dis 1985;7:41.

Schwann TG. Ticks and *Borrelia*: model systems of investigating pathogen-arthropod interactions. Infect Agents Dis 1996;5:167.

Smibert RM. Spirochetosis. In: Hitchner SB, et al, eds. Isolation and identification of avian pathogens. College Station, TX: American Association for Avian Pathology, 1975:66–69.

Smith RD, Miranpuri GS, Adams JH, Ahrens EH. *Borrelia theileri*: isolation from ticks (*Boophilus microplus*) and tick-borne transmission between splenectimized calves. Am J Vet Res 1985;46:1396.

Von Stedingk LV, Olsson I, Hanson HS, et al. Polymerase chain reaction for detection of *Borrelia burgdorferi* DNA in skin lesions of early and late Lyme borreliosis. Eur J Clin Microbiol 1995;14:1.

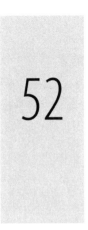

52 Streptobacillus moniliformis

Ernst L. Biberstein

The taxonomic position of *Streptobacillus moniliformis* (*Actinobacillus multiformis*, *Haverhillia moniliformis*, and *Streptothrix muris ratti*), an agent of rat-bite fever, is uncertain. In rodents, it causes respiratory infections, and in rodents, turkeys, and humans, systemic infections that commonly localize in joints.

DESCRIPTIVE FEATURES

Streptobacillus moniliformis is a nonmotile, gram-negative, pleomorphic rod that often grows in long, beaded filaments bearing knobby irregularities. Its cellular proteins vary with geographic and pathologic sources. It requires blood or serum-enriched media and incubation for 48 hours or more to produce visible gray, mucoid colonies. Dissociation into cell wall-deficient L-forms produces mycoplasma-like colonies that are recognizable among the conventional colonies. It is a facultative anaerobe, oxidase and catalase negative, and ferments glucose and some other carbohydrates. Its resistance is not remarkable.

ECOLOGY

The reservoir is the pharynx of rodents, particularly rats, and possibly small carnivores and swine. Infection is endogenous (rodents) by bite or other contact with contaminated material, including ingestion, as in milk-borne "Haverhill fever" among humans.

Lesions are inflammatory and often purulent or necrotic. Rats and mice develop bronchopneumonia and guinea pigs cervical lymphadenitis. In turkeys and mice, septicemic infections lead to polyarthritis or synovitis and often death.

In humans, prostrating fever, accompanied by a rash on the extremities, precedes localization in joints, lymph nodes, lungs, or heart valves. Mortality rates may approximate 10% in untreated cases.

IMMUNOLOGIC ASPECTS

Little is known about immunity. Antibodies are produced during infection.

LABORATORY DIAGNOSIS

Diagnosis requires demonstration of the agent. It can be visualized directly by immunofluorescent reagents and cultivated in thioglycollate broth and blood agar or other rich media in a moist chamber. Identification is by the morphologic and biochemical traits. The agent produces a unique array of cell wall fatty acids that can be determined chromatographically. Production of L-form colonies is favored by special media (e.g., Rogosa's).

TREATMENT AND CONTROL

The obvious preventive measure is avoidance of direct and indirect contact with likely carriers. Effective antimicrobics include penicillin and tetracycline.

SELECTED REFERENCES

Costas M, Owen RJ. Numerical analysis of electrophoretic protein patterns of *Streptobacillus moniliformis* strains from human, murine, and avian infections. J Med Microbiol 1987; 23:303.

Edwards R, Finch RG. Characterization and antibiotic susceptibilities of *Streptobacillus moniliformis*. J Med Microbiol 1986; 21:39.

Jenkins SG. Rat bite fever. Clin Microbiol Newslett 1988;10:57.

Pins MR, Holden JM, Yang JM, et al. Isolation of presumptive *Streptobacillus moniliformis* from abscesses associated with the female genital tract. Clin Infect Dis 1996;22:471.

Rowbotham TJ. Rapid identification of *Streptobacillus moniliformis*. Lancet 1983;2:567. Letter.

Wullenweber M. *Streptobacillus moniliformis* — a zoonotic pathogen. Taxonomic considerations, host species, diagnosis, therapy, geographical distribution. Lab Anim 1995;29:1.

Yamamoto R, Clark GT. *Streptobacillus moniliformis* infections in turkeys. Vet Rec 1966;79:95.

53

Rickettsial Agents of Animal Disease; the Rickettsieae

ERNST L. BIBERSTEIN   DWIGHT C. HIRSH

Rickettsiales are minute obligate intracellular gram-negative bacteria. Their cell walls and energy-generating capability distinguish the genera *Rickettsia* and *Coxiella* from mycoplasmas and chlamydiae, respectively. Other members of the *Rickettsiales* grow on lifeless media, and still others lack cell walls. All multiply by binary fission and are associated with invertebrate vectors.

Three families are of veterinary interest. The family *Rickettsiaceae* includes parasites of the vascular endothelium (tribe *Rickettsieae*) and phagocytic cells (tribe *Ehrlichiaeae*). *Bartonellaceae* are epicellular parasites and *Anaplasmataceae* are parasites of erythrocytes.

DESCRIPTIVE FEATURES

Cell Morphology and Staining

Cells measure up to 0.5 μm by 1.0 μm. Although structurally gram negative, preferred stains are Gimenez's, Macchiavello's, or Giemsa stains. The former two stain rickettsiae red, the latter purple. Electron microscopically and chemically, rickettsiae resemble other gram-negative bacteria. Endotoxic activity is present. Cells are non-motile. The life cycle of *Coxiella burnetii* includes an endospore-like phase.

Members of the tribe *Rickettsieae*, except *C. burnetii*, cross-react with somatic antigens of certain *Proteus* (OX) strains, a phenomenon (Weil-Felix reaction) utilized in the diagnosis of rickettsial infections. This approach generally lacks species specificity. Rickettsial antigens used in complement fixation, immunofluorescence, enzyme-linked immunosorbent assay (ELISA), and indirect hemagglutination tests can be group-specific or species-specific: extracts tend to give group reactions, while cell suspensions approximate species specificity.

Growth Characteristics

Rickettsiae are propagated in yolk sacs of chick embryos, cell cultures, and laboratory animals, notably guinea pigs or mice. The optimal temperature is 33°C to 35°C, at which the generation time is about 9 hours. In cell culture, good growth may require incubation for several weeks, depending on the rickettsial species involved.

Glutamate is the key nutrient for rickettsiae, which utilize it with the aid of transaminases, dehydrogenases, and enzymes of the citric acid cycle. There is little glycolytic activity. Rickettsial adenosine diphosphate (ADP) is readily exchanged for host adenosine triphosphate (ATP) across cell membranes. This "leakiness" of rickettsiae causes loss of critical metabolites, infectivity, and viability when agents are removed to extracellular sites, but is probably an adaptation to intracellular existence rather than its cause, which is unknown. *Coxiella burnetii* survives extracellularly for months, classical pasteurization at 63°C for 30 minutes, and occasionally even "flash" pasteurization (71.6°C for 10 to 20 seconds).

Variability

Antigenic variability of *Orientia* (*Rickettsia*) has frustrated development of a scrub typhus vaccine. *Coxiella burnetii* dissociates in culture from phase I to a less virulent phase II due to the loss of lipopolysaccharide antigens.

ECOLOGY

Reservoir and Transmission

Rickettsiales are basically parasites of arthropods. Some can be passed transovarially in ticks and mites. The pathogenic and ecologic relationships of the most important members of the tribe *Rickettsieae* are shown in Table 53.1.

Pathogenesis

Mechanism and Pathology. Toxicity, neutralizable by antiserum, is characteristic of viable rickettsiae. They enter endothelial cells through endocytosis actively initiated by metabolizing rickettsial cells. They escape from the phagolysosome and multiply in the cytoplasm, and, in the case of spotted fever rickettsiae, in the nucleus. Replication results in endothelial cell necrosis and vasculitis, which leads to vascular disturbances, hemorrhages, edema, perfusion inadequacies, thrombosis, and necrosis. *Coxiella burnetii* multiplies within the phagolysosome, thanks to an enzyme system adapted to the low pH prevailing there (<5.0).

Table 53.1.   Some Diseases Due to *Rickettsieae*: Agents, Reservoirs, Vectors, Hosts

Disease	Causative Agent	Vertebrate Reservoir	Vectors	Transovarian Passage	Clinically Affected Hosts
Epidemic typhus					
Classical	*Rickettsia prowazekii*	Humans (recovered)	Lice	−	Humans, lice
Sylvatic	*R. prowazekii*	Eastern flying squirrels	Fleas	−	Humans, lice
Endemic (murine) typhus	*R. typhi*	Rats, opossums, cats	Fleas	−	Humans
Endemic (murine) typhus-like	*R. felis* (ELB agent)	Opossums, cats	Fleas	−	Humans
Scrub typhus	*Orientia tsutsugamushi*	Mice, rats	Mites	+	Humans
Rocky Mountain spotted fever	*R. rickettsii*	Various feral mammals	Ticks	+	Humans (dogs, sheep)[a]
Q fever	*Coxiella burnetii*	Many mammals (birds?, fish?)	Arthropods,[b] ticks, mites, insects	?	Humans (ruminants)

[a] Occasionally affected.
[b] Airborne transmission commonly occurs in absence of vectors.

Disease Patterns and Epidemiology.   Only two species are significantly associated with animal disease.

Rickettsia rickettsii.   The agent of Rocky Mountain spotted fever (RMSF), *Rickettsia rickettsii* infects dogs in endemic areas. It is carried naturally by some 20 species of ixodid ticks and is capable of producing febrile, rarely fatal disease in dogs. Early signs are high fever (>40°C), anorexia, vomiting, diarrhea, infected or hemorrhagic mucous membranes, and tenderness over lymph nodes, joints, and muscles. Purpuric and central nervous disturbances may occur later. These, and heart and kidney involvement, may account for fatalities.

Serologic surveys suggest that most canine RMSF infections go unnoticed. Other tick-borne diseases (ehrlichiosis, babesiosis, borreliosis) should be considered along with RMSF in tick-infested dogs.

RMSF is limited to the New World. Most cases occur in the eastern United States, reflecting population densities and distribution of the principal vectors, *Dermacentor andersoni* (West) and *D. variabilis* (East). Seasonal prevalence parallels adult tick activity: *D. andersoni* is active in spring and early summer, while *D. variabilis* is active from midspring to late summer.

Coxiella burnetii.   The agent of Q fever, *C. burnetii* survives in the environment, unlike other Rickettsieae, and can be disseminated by the airborne route. Survival may be related to the "small-cell-variant," endospore-like growth phase. Natural hosts include some 125 mammalian species and many species of arthropods: ticks, mites, fleas, lice, and flies, some of which support a sylvatic cycle of *C. burnetii*.

Domestic ruminants are infected through inhalation, ingestion, or arthropod bite. After hematogenous dissemination, infection persists particularly in the lactating mammary gland and the pregnant uterus. At parturition, which is usually normal and produces viable young, rickettsiae are abundantly shed. Sporadic — rarely epidemic — abortions due to *C. burnetii* are associated with placentitis. Sometimes the birth of weak lambs is blamed on Q fever infection. While neonatal infection is common, its clinical impact is uncertain.

The ruminant infections are of greatest concern because of their public health implications. Respiratory exposure from the contaminated environment constitutes a greater hazard to humans than ingestion of infected dairy products. The human disease is usually an influenza-like respiratory illness, from which complete recovery is the rule; but mortality is high in cases of pneumonia, hepatic infection, or endocarditis.

Q fever occurs worldwide. Most human cases suggest origin from domestic ruminant sources. Outbreaks have been related to wind currents carrying infection from infected dairies. Many cases are occupationally linked to handling of sheep, cattle, and goats. Parturient cats and dogs have been implicated as rare sources of human infection.

IMMUNOLOGIC ASPECTS

Immune complexes have been suspected in the pathogenesis of late vascular manifestations of RMSF. Humoral and cell-mediated responses occur. The latter especially are significant for removal of the agents by activated macrophages. No vaccines for animal rickettsioses are available. There is considerable interest in the development of a phase I Q fever vaccine, which has proven effective experimentally in ruminants and humans.

LABORATORY DIAGNOSIS

Direct demonstration of rickettsiae in cells is best done by direct immunofluorescence. In ruminant placentas, this establishes the presence of Q fever rickettsiae but not the cause of abortion. The use of Gimenez or other stains will not differentiate between *C. burnetii* and *Chlamydia psittaci*.

Isolation involves use of guinea pigs and mice, embryonated eggs, or cell culture. In surviving animals, a blood sample may contain antibody 2 to 3 weeks later. In eggs, tissue culture, and experimental animal tissues, direct immunofluorescent staining will identify an isolate.

Serology (complement fixation, microagglutination) is useful when paired samples can be obtained, and in recent infections a significant increase in antibody level is observed in the sample collected 10 to 14 days after the first. The Weil-Felix reaction is a helpful screening test for RMSF (not Q fever). Conclusions should be confirmed by specific rickettsial tests.

TREATMENT AND CONTROL

Rickettsia rickettsii is susceptible to chloramphenicol, tetracyclines, and fluoroquinolones. Long-term tetracycline feeding has been used in attempts to control mammary excretion of *C. burnetii,* which has met with mixed results.

Prevention of RMSF in dogs requires tick control. Transmission depends on prolonged feeding and may be reduced by prompt tick removal.

Vaccination of female ruminants may reduce the Q fever reservoir.

SELECTED REFERENCES

Ascher MS, Berman MA, Ruppanner R. Initial clinical and immunological evaluation of a new phase I Q fever vaccine and skin test in humans. J Infect Dis 1983;148:214.

Azad AF, Radulovic S, Higgins JA, et al. Flea-borne rickettsioses: ecologic considerations. Emer Infect Dis 1997;3:319.

Behymer D, Riemann H. *Coxiella burnetii* infection. J Am Vet Med Assoc 1989;194:764.

Birtles RJ, Harrison TG, Saunders NA, Molyneux DH. Proposals to unify the genera *Grahamella* and *Bartonella* with descriptions of *Bartonella talpae* comb. nov., *Bartonella peromysci* comb. nov., and three new species, *Bartonella grahamii* sp. nov., *Bartonella taylorii* sp. nov., and *Bartonella doshiae* sp. nov. Int J Syst Bacteriol 1995;45:1.

Brenner DJ, O'Connor SP, Winkler HH, Steigerwalt AG. Proposals to unify the genera *Bartonella* and *Rochalimaea*, with descriptions of *Bartonella quintana* comb. nov., *Bartonella vinsonii* comb. nov., *Bartonella henselae* comb. nov., and *Bartonella elizabethae* comb. nov., and to remove the family *Bartonellaceae* from the order *Rickettsiales*. Int J Syst Bacteriol 1993;43:777.

Breitschwerdt EB. Clinical, hematologic and humoral responses in female dogs inoculated with *Rickettsia rickettsii* and *Rickettsia montana.* Am J Vet Res 1988;49:70.

Brooks DL. Q fever vaccination of sheep. Challenge of immunity in ewes. Am J Vet Res 1986;47:1235.

Buhariwalla F, Cann B, Marrie TJ. A dog-related outbreak of Q fever. Clin Infect Dis 1996;23:753.

Greene CE. Rocky Mountain spotted fever. J Am Vet Med Assoc 1987;191:666.

Hackstadt T. The biology of rickettsiae. Infect Agents Dis 1996;5:127.

Heinzen RA, Scidmore MA, Rockey DD, Hackstadt T. Differential interaction with endocytic and exocytic pathways distinguish parasitophorous vacuoles of *Coxiella burnetii* and *Chlamydia trachomatis.* Infect Immun 1996;64:796.

Marrie TJ. Exposure to parturient cats: a risk factor for acquisition of Q fever in maritime Canada. J Infect Dis 1988;158:101.

Raoult D, Marrie T. Q fever. Clin Infect Dis 1995;20:489.

Weisburg WG, Dobson ME, Samuel JE, et al. Phylogenetic diversity of the Rickettsiae. J Bacteriol 1989;171:4202.

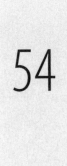

54 Ehrlichieae: Ehrlichia, Cowdria, *and* Neorickettsia

Ernst L. Biberstein   Dwight C. Hirsh

Descriptive Features

Ehrlichieae are rickettsial parasites of white blood cells. They multiply within membrane-lined intracytoplasmic vesicles. Colonies (morulae), less than 4 µm in diameter, which consist of "elementary bodies" smaller than 1 µm in diameter, are demonstrable by stained blood smears (Fig 54.1) or immunofluorescence. A cell wall is present.

Twelve species of *Ehrlichia* are described: *E. bovis, E. canis, E. chaffeensis, E. equi, E. ewingii, E. muris, E. ondiri, E. ovina, E. phagocytophila, E. platys, E. risticii,* and *E. sennetsu*. The agent of human granulocytic erhlichiosis (HGE) is almost identical to *E. equi. Ehrlichia canis, E. chaffeensis, E. muris, E. risticii, E. sennetsu,* and *Cowdria ruminantium* have been propagated in cell culture. Those known to be tick-borne (*E. canis, E. phagocytophila,* and *C. ruminantium*) are passed transstadially but not transovarially. Little is known concerning their metabolic activities.

The genus *Ehrlichia* has been called "phylogenetically incoherent" and can be grouped (in anticipation of a change in species?) by genetic relatedness based upon the sequence of 16S rRNA: *E. canis* group (*E. canis, E. chaffeensis, E. muris, E. ewingii*); *E. phagocytophila* group (*E. phagocytophila, E. equi,* HGE agent, *E. platys, Anaplasma*); and *E. sennetsu* group (*E. sennetsu, E. risticii, Neorickettsia helminthoeca*).

Blood may remain infectious for 10 days at room temperature, 14 days at refrigerator temperature, and 1.5 years at −80°C.

Ehrlichia Canis

Ecology

The brown dog tick, *Rhipicephalus sanguineus,* is reservoir and vector of *E. canis*. Although dogs (and presumably other canid hosts) may remain bacteremic for years, their blood is infectious for ticks generally for 2 weeks or less during the acute disease.

Immune-mediated and endotoxin-like phenomena are suspected pathogenic mechanisms.

Acute onset of canine ehrlichiosis (tropical canine pancytopenia) follows an incubation period of 1 to 3 weeks, during which the agent proliferates by binary fission within mononuclear cells. The acute stage, lasting several weeks, is characterized by vasculitis and thrombocytopenia. Intravascular coagulation may occur, and leukopenia and anemia are common. In the chronic form, which may follow a long quiescent period, reduction of all blood cell types may contribute to hemorrhages, edema, serosal effusions, anemia, secondary infections, and the enlargement of spleen, liver, and lymph nodes seen at this stage. Hyperglobulinemia and widespread plasma cell infiltration suggest immunologic mechanisms.

Uncomplicated *E. canis* infection is often mild and marked by moderate fever, depression, inappetence, weight loss, pale mucous membranes, dyspnea, and lymphadenopathy. In severe chronic ehrlichiosis, these signs will be greatly aggravated and coupled with bleeding tendencies, including epistaxis. Complications include central nervous system (CNS) disturbances, glomerulonephritis, interstitial pneumonia, secondary infections, and unrelated tick-borne diseases (e.g., babesiosis).

Canine neutrophilic ehrlichiosis (*E. ewingii*) is usually milder and has been observed in association with polyarthritis. It may be due to *E. equi* as well.

The long and variable course makes it difficult to relate ehrlichiosis to a particular season. Puppies and German shepherd dogs are most severely affected. The infection is concentrated in tropical and subtropical latitudes, but occurs on all continents except Australia. Human cases are reported in the United States.

Immunologic Aspects

Cellular and humoral autoimmune responses to infected mononuclear cells and platelets are suspected to contribute to blood cell destruction and bone marrow depression.

Resistance to superinfection, antibody and cell-mediated, seems to depend upon persistent infection.

Laboratory Diagnosis

Giemsa-stained smears of buffy coat are examined for intramonocytic morulae. These are scarce and found mainly during the acute stage.

FIGURE 54.1. Ehrlichia equi *(arrows) in smear of buffy coat from horse. Wright stain, 1000×.*

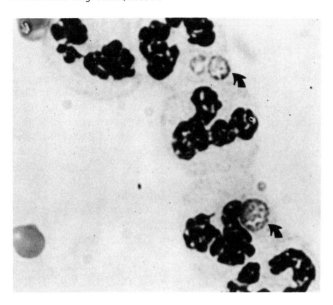

A simple culture technique involves incubation of supernatant of a heparinized suspect blood sample on cover slips in Leighton tubes.

Serodiagnosis by indirect immunofluorescence is carried out in specialized laboratories.

TREATMENT AND CONTROL

Tetracycline is effective in early cases but less so in advanced cases. Imidocarb dipropionate has also been recommended. Disease produced by *E. canis* does not respond to fluoroquinolones.

For prevention, tick control is optimal. Treatment with low-level tetracycline for up to 2 years has been suggested as a means of producing uninfected dog populations incapable of infecting new tick generations.

EHRLICHIA PLATYS

Ehrlichia platys parasitizes canine thrombocytes causing an essentially nonclinical cyclic thrombocytopenia.

EHRLICHIA EQUI

ECOLOGY

The natural host of *E. equi* is the horse. Donkeys, sheep, goats, dogs, cats, and monkeys can be experimentally infected. Ticks are suspected vectors and *Ixodes pacificus* (western black-legged tick) is the most likely.

The affected cells are granulocytes. The basic lesion is a vasculitis associated with thromboses and thrombocytopenia. Edema and hemorrhages are typically found in the distal limbs. Vascular changes are also pronounced in testes and ovaries.

Clinically, the infection is often inapparent in young foals and most severe in old horses, where fever, inappetence, hemorrhages, edema, anemia, icterus, and locomotor problems are seen. Fatalities are due to rare secondary complications, such as respiratory infections or falls.

The disease has been found mainly in California in winter and early spring. Dogs in certain areas of California (Marin County) are clinically affected following infection with *E. equi*.

IMMUNOLOGIC ASPECTS

Recovered horses are refractory to reinfection. Antibody is produced in the course of infection. No vaccines exist.

LABORATORY DIAGNOSIS

Morulae in neutrophils can be demonstrated in stained blood and buffy coat films most readily 48 hours after onset (see Fig 54.1). An indirect immunofluorescent antibody test has been developed.

TREATMENT

Tetracycline is effective. The first dose can be given intravenously followed by daily doses intravenously or orally for 1 week.

EHRLICHIA PHAGOCYTOPHILA

ECOLOGY

Ehrlichia phagocytophila occurs in granulocytes and monocytes of ruminants in different parts of Europe. The vector tick is *Ixodes ricinus*.

The pathogenesis of "tick-borne fever" (TBF) resembles that of other ehrlichioses. Thrombocytopenia occurs early. Leukopenia successively affects lymphocytes and neutrophils. Lesions include splenomegaly and hemorrhages along the intestinal tract. Histologically, a striking lack of lymphoid elements is observed.

There is febrile response accompanied by depression, accelerated breathing, and a drop in milk yield. Ewes and cows may abort. The disease is mildest in young animals. A heightened susceptibility to secondary infections may be due to parasitization of neutrophils, leukopenia, and a lymphopenia affecting B lymphocytes selectively. Tick pyemia is commonly linked with TBF.

IMMUNOLOGIC ASPECTS

Little is known about immunity. Recurring illnesses may occur in successive years. Resistance has been correlated with complement-fixing antibody.

LABORATORY DIAGNOSIS

Morulae are demonstrable by stained blood smears or immunofluorescence. A complement fixation test has been described.

TREATMENT AND CONTROL

Tetracycline is effective. Reduction of exposure to ticks is desirable.

EHRLICHIA RISTICII

Potomac horse fever, an acute equine diarrheal syndrome first noted in horses in Montgomery County, Maryland, is a monocytic ehrlichiosis caused by *E. risticii* and resembles other ehrlichioses in producing fever, listlessness, anorexia, and variable leukopenia. Distinctive features are intestinal involvement and, as a late complication, laminitis. Uterine infection has been observed. The fatality rate of clinical diarrheal cases is 20% to 30%. Ulcerative gastroenteritis is the most notable lesion at necropsy.

The agent appears to be noncontagious from June to October and transmissible by injection and feeding of infectious material. Its distribution includes most of North America. No reservoir host or vector is known. Dogs and cats can be experimentally infected.

Immunologic factors are not fully understood. Antibody cross-reactive with *E. sennetsu*, but not with *E. equi*, has been demonstrated in affected horses. Antibody reactive with *E. risticii* occurs in sheep, goats, dogs, and cats of endemic regions. Recovered horses are immune.

Microbiologic diagnosis involves demonstration of the agent in monocytes. Serologic diagnosis is by an indirect fluorescent antibody test or by enzyme-linked immunosorbent assay (ELISA).

Tetracycline, if given early, has been credited with reducing mortality to under 10%. An effective bacterin is commercially available.

OTHER EHRLICHIA

Ehrlichia bovis and *E. ovina* parasitize bovine or ovine mononuclear cells, while *E. ondiri* also invades granulocytes. The latter causes bovine petechial fever (Ondiri disease) in the highlands of East Africa, a disease

marked by fever, lowered milk yield, mucosal hemorrhages, and variable early mortality. Arthropod vectors are assumed.

COWDRIA RUMINANTIUM

"African heartwater disease" affects mostly ruminants. The agent, *Cowdria ruminantium*, resembles *Ehrlichia* but multiplies in cells lining the sinusoids of lymph nodes, disseminates to the bloodstream, and colonizes endothelial cells. There is little cellular inflammatory response to their presence, but widespread edema, effusions, and epithelial and endothelial hemorrhage. Pericardial effusion, which gave the disease its name, is inconsistent. Spleen, lymph nodes, and usually liver are grossly enlarged, and rickettsiae occur in endothelial cells, most noticeably of cerebrocortical capillaries.

Clinical signs vary. In the peracute form, a fever of several hours' duration precedes collapse and death under convulsions. In the acute form, fever precedes nervous disturbances by several hours. Death within 2 to 10 days is the rule in sheep and likely in cattle. A subclinical form is also recognized.

The disease is passed only by parenteral introduction of blood. Tick hosts are *Amblyomma* spp. Strains, though serologically uniform, vary in virulence and host populations differ in susceptibility. Newborn animals are resistant.

The agent disappears within 2 months after recovery, but immunity — probably cell mediated — persists for up to 5 years. Young calves and lambs (<4 weeks) or goats (<6 weeks) are vaccinated with virulent rickettsiae. Older animals are immunized by infection followed by antimicrobial therapy.

Specific diagnosis is by demonstration of the agent in tissues (smear of cerebral cortex, stained with Giemsa stain). Infected cerebral extracts will flocculate with specific antibody providing the basis of a diagnostic test on currently infected animals.

Tetracycline treatment is effective. Tick control and vaccination are useful preventive steps.

NEORICKETTSIA HELMINTHOECA

Salmon ("poisoning") disease affects lymphoreticular tissues of canids and is characterized by fever, swollen lymph nodes, and often a hemorrhagic enteritis. Its agent, *Neorickettsia helminthoeca*, is associated with the fluke *Nanophyetus salmincola* and its endemicity is limited by the range of the snail intermediate hosts of *N. salmincola*.

DESCRIPTIVE FEATURES

Neorickettsia helminthoeca multiplies in the cytoplasm of macrophages, forming frequently multiple morulae. Individual neorickettsiae may be dispersed through the cytoplasm. They are coccobacilli measuring usually less than 0.5mm in any dimension and are demonstrable by Giemsa stain. The agent is unrelated serologically to *E. canis* and does not induce immunity to the closely related, epidemiologically identical Elokomin fluke fever agent.

It has been propagated in cell cultures.

ECOLOGY

Reservoir and Transmission

The reservoir of *N. helminthoeca* is the fluke *N. salmincola*, whose life cycle includes passage through a fish. Dogs are infected by eating fluke-infected fish.

Pathogenesis

From the ingested fish kidney, metacercarial flukes emerge in the dog's intestine, develop into adults, attach, and release into the tissues *N. helminthoeca*, which colonizes lymphoid aggregates throughout the body. Enlargement of lymphoid organs results from proliferation of reticuloendothelial components. A nonsuppurative meningoencephalitis is common.

Within 5 days to several weeks of exposure, dogs develop high fever, anorexia, depression, and weight loss. Vomiting and persistent, eventually hemorrhagic, diarrhea are typical. Death in up to 90% of untreated cases occurs in less than 2 weeks.

Epidemiology

Salmon disease is endemic in coastal areas of northernmost California, Oregon, and south central Washington: the range of the snail *Oxytrema silicula*. Infections in nonendemic areas are due to planting of infected fish. Dogs are the definitive hosts of the fluke, harboring the adults in their intestine. Eggs are shed, embryonate, and hatch miracidia that invade the snail. Cercaria emerge from the snail and invade a fish, becoming sessile metacercaria encysted in the kidney. Upon being ingested by the definitive host, they become adults within 6 days. Uninfected flukes produce little disturbance in dogs. Infected flukes produce disease only in canids.

Elokomin fluke fever, a mild form of salmon disease, attacks canids, ferrets, raccoons, and bears.

IMMUNOLOGIC ASPECTS

Dogs recovered from salmon disease are immune. They remain susceptible to Elokomin fluke fever.

LABORATORY DIAGNOSIS

Presence of eggs of *N. salmincola* in the feces of a dog showing pertinent clinical signs constitutes strong evidence of salmon disease. Demonstration of rickettsiae in lymph node aspirates is definitive (Fig 54.2).

TREATMENT AND CONTROL

Penicillin, tetracycline, chloramphenicol, and various sulfonamides given parenterally are usually effective. Supportive treatment is essential.

The best preventive measure is the exclusion of infected salmon from the canine diet. Flukes and agent are killed by cooking and by freezing at −20°C for 24 hours.

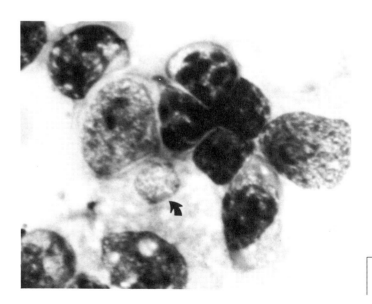

FIGURE 54.2.   *Neorickettsia helminthoeca colony (morula; arrow) in canine lymph node impression. 1000×.*

SELECTED REFERENCES

Anderson BE, Dawson JE, Jones DC, Wilson KH. *Ehrlichia chaffeensis*, a new species associated with human ehrlichiosis. J Clin Microbiol 1991;29:2838.

Anderson BE, Greene CE, Jones DC, Dawson JE. *Ehrlichia ewingii* sp. nov., the etiologic agent of canine granulocytic ehrlichiosis. Int J Syst Bacteriol 1992;42:299.

Barlough JE, Madigan JE, DeRock E, et al. Protection against *Ehrlichia equi* is conferred by prior infection with human granulocytotropic *Ehrlichia* (HGE agent). J Clin Microbiol 1995;33:3333.

Breider MA, Henton JE. Equine monocytic ehrlichiosis (Potomac horse fever). Vet Clin North Am Eqine Pract 1987;9:20.

Codner EC, Farris-Smith LL. Characterization of the subclinical phase of ehrlichiosis in dogs. J Am Vet Med Assoc 1986;189:47.

Dumler JS, Asanovich KM, Bakken JS, et al. Serologic cross-reactions among *Ehrlichia equi, Ehrlichia phagocytophila*, and human granulocytic *Ehrlichia*. J Clin Microbiol 1995;33:1098.

Gorham JR, Foreyt WJ. Salmon poisoning disease. In: Greene CE, ed. Clinical microbiology and infectious diseases of the dog and cat. Philadelphia: WB Saunders, 1984:538–544.

Greene CE, Burgdorfer W, Cavagnolo R, et al. Rocky Mountain spotted fever in dogs and its differentiation from canine ehrlichiosis. J Am Vet Med Assoc 1985;186:465.

Hackstadt T. The biology of rickettsiae. Infect Agents Dis 1996;5:127.

Hildebrandt RK, Huxsoll DL, Walker JS, et al. Pathology of canine ehrlichiosis (tropical canine pancytopenia). Am J Vet Res 1973;34:1309.

Kuehn NF, Baunt SD. Clinical and hematologic findings in canine ehrlichiosis. J Am Vet Med Assoc 1985;186:355.

Madewell BT, Gribble DH. Infection in two dogs with an agent resembling *Ehrlichia equi*. J Am Vet Med Assoc 1982;180:572.

Madigan JE, Gribble DH. Equine ehrlichiosis in northern California: 49 cases (1969–1981). J Am Vet Med Assoc 1987;109:445.

Madigan JE. Equine ehrlichiosis. Vet Clin North Am Equine Pract 1993;9:423.

Madigan JE, Barlough JE, Dumler JS, et al. Equine granulocytic ehrlichiosis in Connecticut caused by an agent resembling the human granulocytotropic ehrlichia. J Clin Microbiol 1996;34:434.

Madigan JE, Richter PJ, Kimsey RB, et al. Transmission and passage in horses of the agent of human granulocytic ehrlichiosis. J Infect Dis 1995;172:1141.

Madigan JE, Rikihisa Y, Palmer JE, et al. Evidence for a high rate of false-positive results with the indirect fluorescent antibody test for *Ehrlichia risticii* antibody in horses. J Am Vet Med Assoc 1995;207:1448.

Maeda K, Markowitz N, Hawley RC, et al. Human infection with *Ehrlichia canis*, a leukocytic rickettsia. N Engl J Med 1987;316:853.

Magnarelli LA, Dumler JS. Ehrlichioses: emerging infectious diseases in tick-infested areas. Clin Microbiol Newslett 1996;18:81.

Mahan SM. Review of the molecular biology of *Cowdria ruminantium*. Vet Parasitol 1995;57:51.

Mebus CA, Logan LL. Heartwater disease of domestic and wild ruminants. J Am Vet Med Assoc 1988;192:950.

Pretzman CI. Enzyme-linked immunosorbent assay for Potomac horse fever disease. J Clin Microbiol 1987;25:31.

Pretzman C, Ralph D, Stothard DR, et al. 16S rRNA gene sequence of *Neorickettsia helminthoeca* and its phylogenetic alignment with members of the genus *Ehrlichia*. Int J Syst Bacteriol 1995;45:207.

Price JE, Sayer RD. Canine ehrlichiosis. Curr Vet Ther 1983;8:1197.

Richter PJ, Kimsey RB, Madigan JE, et al. *Ixodes pacificus* (Acari: Ixodidae) as a vector of *Ehrlichia equi* (Rickettsiales: Ehrlichieae). J Med Entomol 1996;33:1.

Rikihisa Y. The tribe *Ehrlichieae* and ehrlichial diseases. Clin Microbiol Rev 1991;4:286.

van Vliet AH, Jongejan F, van der Zeijst BA. Phylogenetic position of *Cowdria ruminantium* (Rickettsiales) determined by analysis of amplified 16S ribosomal DNA sequences. Int J Syst Bacteriol 1992;42:494.

55 Bartonellaceae

Bruno B. Chomel

Bartonellaceae are thin, gram-negative, slightly curved rods. Until recently, the genus *Bartonella* consisted of only one species, *B. bacilliformis*. It has recently been proposed to combine all the species of the three genera *Bartonella*, *Rochalimaea*, and *Grahamella* into the family *Bartonellaceae* and the genus *Bartonella*; the family *Bartonellaceae* has also been removed from the order *Rickettsiales*. They are members of the alpha-2 subgroup of the alpha-proteobacteria. Most of these bacteria are erythrocyte-adherent bacilli.

The present family consists of eleven species, of which four are human pathogens. *Bartonella bacilliformis* is the etiologic agent of Oroya fever, an acute bacteremic infection characterized by sepsis and hemolysis, and of verruga peruana, mainly a cutaneous nodular vascular eruption representing chronic infection. *Bartonella quintana*, the agent of trench fever, has also been found to be one of the agents of bacillary angiomatosis (BA), a vascular proliferative lesion observed mainly in immunocompromised individuals. Bacillary angiomatosis can also be caused by *B. henselae*, a newly discovered bacterium. *Bartonella henselae* causes cat scratch disease (CSD) in immunocompetent individuals. The fourth human pathogen is also a newly discovered bacterium, *B. elizabethae*. This bacterium was isolated in an immunocompetent individual suffering from endocarditis. The seven other *Bartonella* — *B. grahami, B. vinsoni, B. doshiae, B. taylorii, B. peromysci, B. talpae,* and *B. clarridgeiae* — have only been isolated from the blood of various animal species. New *Bartonella* species have recently been isolated from various wild rodents, rabbits, felids, canids, and cervids. Except for *B. vinsoni* var. *berkhoffii*, found in a case of canine endocarditis, these species are not known to induce any specific disease in the infected animal.

DESCRIPTIVE FEATURES

Morphology and Staining

Bartonellaceae are fastidious, aerobic, thin, gram-negative coccobacillary or slightly curved rods ($0.6\,\mu m \times 1.0\,\mu m$) that take from 5 to 15 days and up to 45 days on original culture to form visible colonies on most rich blood-containing media, as they are highly hemin dependent. In infected tissues, Warthin-Starry silver impregnation stain reveals small bacilli, which tend to appear as clumps of tightly compacted organisms. Similarly, small organisms can be identified in red blood cells by May-Grünwald Giemsa coloration.

Cellular Composition

Bartonella bacilliformis and *B. clarridgeiae* are the only members of the genus that are motile by means of unipolar flagella. *Bartonella quintana* and *B. henselae* have a twitching motility associated to fimbriae or pili. Because of the slow growth of these bacteria, standard biochemical methods for identification may not be applicable. The *Bartonella* are oxidase and catalase negative. Measurement of preformed enzymes and standard testing have revealed differences between species. Most species are biochemically inert except for the production of peptidases. The MicroScan Rapid Anaerobe Panel (Baxter Diagnostics, Deerfield, IL) has been reported to provide species identification. Whole cell fatty acid (CFA) analysis for the genus has proven useful for identification because bartonellae have a unique and characteristic whole cell fatty acid composition. The *Bartonella* have gas-liquid chromatography profiles consisting mainly of $C_{18:0'}$, $C_{18:1'}$, and $C_{16:0}$ acid. Molecular genetic methods such as restriction fragment length polymorphism (RFLP) of genes encoding citrate synthase, 16S rRNA or 16S–23S rRNA spacer region, and more recently analysis based on polymerase chain reaction (PCR) of random, repetitive extragenic palindromic sequences have been used to distinguish strains and species of *Bartonella*. RFLP or sequence analysis of 16S rRNA genes after PCR amplification both directly from specimens or pure cultures have been largely used for detecting and characterizing *Bartonella*.

Growth Characteristics

Traditionally, *Bartonella* are cultivated in semisolid nutrient agar containing fresh rabbit blood (or sheep or horse blood) at 35°C (except for *B. bacilliformia*, which grows best at 28°C in 5% CO_2). On primary isolation, some *Bartonella*, such as *B. henselae, B. clarridgeiae, B. vinsoni,* or *B. elizabethae* have colonies with a white, rough, dry, raised appearance and pit the medium. They are hard to break up or transfer. Other *Bartonella* such as *B. quintana* have colonies that are usually smaller, gray, translucent, and somewhat gummy or slightly mucoid.

ECOLOGY

Reservoir and Transmission

Most *Bartonella* species are vector-borne organisms. *Bartonella bacilliformis* is transmitted by a sandfly (*Lutzomia* spp.) limited to the Andean mountain region of Peru, Ecuador, and Colombia. *Bartonella quintana*, the agent of trench fever, was found to be transmitted by the human body louse, *Pediculus humanus;* however, no specific reservoir nor vector has been identified in cases of bacillary angiomatosis caused by this species. Most cases of BA caused by *B. henselae* and almost all cases of CSD have now been associated to cat scratch exposure. The domestic cat is a healthy carrier of *B. henselae* and *B. clarridgieae* and constitutes the main reservoir of these organisms. *Bartonella henselae* infection is transmitted from cat to cat mainly by the cat flea, *Ctenocephalides felis*, but its role seems limited in human infection. *Bartonella vinsonii* was isolated from Canadian meadow voles (*Microtus pennsylvanicus*) and was successfully transmitted to a hamster by ear mites, *Trombicula microti*. A recent report seems to involve the dog tick, *Rhipicephalus sanguineous*, in the transmission of *B. vinsonii* var. *berkhoffii* to dogs. *Bartonella grahamii* was transmitted by the rodent flea, *Xenopsylla cheopis*, to bank voles. No specific reservoir or vector has yet been identified in the transmission of *B. elizabethae*.

Bartonella doshiae, B. grahamii, and *B. taylorii* were isolated from meadow voles (*Microtus agrestis*), bank voles (*Clethrionomys glareolus*), and field mice (*Apodemus*), respectively. *Bartonella* (formerly *Grahamella*) *talpae* was isolated from a mole (*Talpa europaea*) and *B.* (formerly *Grahamella*) *peromysci* was isolated from meadow voles.

Pathogenesis

Mechanisms.   *Bartonella quintana* and *B. henselae* are clinically associated with proliferative neovascular lesions. The pathogenesis of bacillary angiomatosis lesions involves injury and proliferation of the vascular endothelium both with *B. henselae* and *B. quintana*. These organisms induce endothelial cell proliferation and migration in vitro, and a protein fraction was identified as the angiogenic factor. *Bartonella* infection (in vitro) stimulated endothelial cell proliferation and induced obvious morphological changes due to modifications of the cytoskeleton.

Bartonella henselae seems to share with *B. bacilliformis* a common mechanism for mediating pathogenesis. A bacteriophage-like particle similar to the bacteriophage observed in *B. bacilliformis* has been found in culture supernatant from *B. henselae*. This particle has at least three associated proteins and contains 14 kbp linear DNA segments that are heterogeneous in sequence. It has been speculated that an ancestor of *B. henselae* and *B. bacilliformis* acquired the ability to mediate angioproliferation as a means of enhancing its dissemination or its acquisition of nutrients within the host. It is possible that a common transducting phage may be the mechanism of

genetic exchange by which the two organisms acquired this pathogenic trait.

Disease Patterns and Epidemiology

Humans.   In CSD, 1 to 3 weeks elapse between the scratch or bite of a cat and the appearance of clinical signs. In 50% of the cases, a small skin lesion, often resembling an insect bite, appears at the inoculation site, usually the hand or forearm, and evolves from a papule to a vesicle and partially healed ulcers. These lesions resolve within a few days to a few weeks. Lymphadenitis develops approximately 3 weeks after exposure and is generally unilateral. It commonly appears in the epitrochlear, axillary, or cervical lymph nodes. Swelling of the lymph node is usually painful and persists for several weeks to several months. In 25% of the cases, suppuration occurs. The large majority of the cases show signs of systemic infection: fever, chills, malaise, anorexia, headaches. In general, the disease is benign and heals spontaneously without sequelae. Atypical manifestations of CSD occur in 5% to 10% of the cases. The most common of these is Parinaud's oculoglandular syndrome (periauricular lymphadenopathy and palpebral conjunctivitis), but also meningitis, encephalitis, osteolytic lesions, and thrombocytopenic purpura may occur. Encephalopathy is one of the most serious complications of CSD which usually occurs 2 to 6 weeks after the onset of lymphadenopathy. However, it usually resolves with complete recovery and few or no sequelae. New clinical presentations associated with *B. henselae* infection have been reported in immunocompetent persons, including neuroretinitis or bacteremia as a cause of chronic fatigue syndrome, and a case of aggressive *B. henselae* endocarditis in a cat owner.

There were an estimated 22,000 human cases of CSD in the United States in 1992, some 2000 of whom were hospitalized. The estimated annual health cost of CSD was more than $12 million. From 55% to 80% of CSD patients are under the age of 20 years. There is a seasonal pattern, with most cases seen in autumn and winter.

For BA in immunocompromised persons, the symptoms are very different from CSD. Bacillary angiomatosis, also called *epithelioid angiomatosis*, is a vascular proliferative disease of the skin characterized by multiple, blood-filled, cystic tumors. It is usually characterized by violaceous or colorless papular and nodular skin lesions that clinically may suggest Kaposi's sarcoma, but histologically resemble epithelioid hemangiomas. When visceral parenchymal organs are involved, the condition is referred to as *bacillary peliosis hepatis*, *splenic peliosis*, or *systemic BA*. Fever, weight loss, malaise, and enlargement of affected organs may develop in people with disseminated BA. Endocarditis has also been reported.

Cats.   No clinical signs of CSD have been reported in cats under natural conditions, but infection is very common, especially in young kittens. In California, a 40% prevalence of bacteremic cats was found in the San Francisco–Sacramento area. Bacteremia usually lasts a few weeks to a few months. The organisms have been reported to be intraerythrocytic and pili may be a pathogenic determinant for *Bartonella* species. Cats can yield more than 1 million colony-forming units (CFU) per milliliter of blood. Direct transmission from cat to cat as well as vertical transmission from bacteremic female cats to kittens was unsuccessful in various experiments. Transmission from cat to cat was successfully achieved by depositing infected fleas collected from bacteremic cats onto noninfected kittens. Presence of *B. henselae* DNA was found in infected fleas. Seroprevalence studies clearly demonstrate that prevalence is the highest in cat populations living in warm and humid areas where flea infestation is usually higher.

Dogs. *Bartonella vinsonii* var. *berkhoffii* has been isolated from the heart valve of a dog with endocarditis. Serologic studies indicate that *Bartonella* infection in dogs is rare (less than 5%).

IMMUNOLOGIC ASPECTS

Infection by *Bartonella* organisms stimulates both a cellular and humoral response. *Bartonella henselae* and *B. quintana* induce proliferation and migration of endothelial cells. These effects are due to a trypsin-sensitive factor that appears to be associated with the bacterial cell wall or membrane or heavy intracellular molecules.

In infected individuals, specific antibodies can be detected a few days to a few weeks after infection. Most of the clinical cases of CSD or BA are associated with elevated titers against *B. henselae* or *B. quintana*, the latter often inducing higher antibody titers. Immunity is usually long lasting in cases of CSD.

In cats, *B. henselae* antibodies detected by immunofluorescent test (IFA) or enzyme-linked immunosorbent assay (ELISA) appear 2 to 3 weeks after experimental inoculation and usually persist for several months. Most of the infected cats are bacteremic for several weeks despite high antibody titers. Chronic bacteremia, despite a humoral immune response, is commonly observed among cats. There is no direct correlation between antibody titer and the magnitude of bacteremia; however, cats with IFA serologic titers of 512 or more are more likely to be bacteremic than cats with lower titers.

LABORATORY DIAGNOSIS

For years, the diagnosis of CSD was based on clinical criteria, history of exposure to a cat, failure to isolate other bacteria, and/or histologic examination of biopsies of lymph nodes. A skin test using antigen prepared from pasteurized exudate from lymph nodes of patients with CSD was also used in diagnosing CSD, but this test was not standardized and elicited concerns about the safety of such a product. In the past few years, serologic tests such as IFA or ELISA and techniques to isolate the organism from human and cat specimens have been developed. Because *B. henselae* is an intraerythrocytic bacterium,

cell lysis using a lysis centrifugation technique greatly facilitates bacterial isolation from the blood. For blood culture from cats, 1.5 mL of blood is drawn into lysis-centrifugation tubes (Isostat Microbial System, Wampole Laboratories). More recently, cat blood collection in EDTA tubes kept frozen at $-70°C$ for a few days or weeks has been a preferred alternative because of easier handling and lower cost. The tubes are centrifuged and the pellet spread onto heat infusion agar plates containing 5% fresh rabbit blood, which are maintained at 35°C in a high humidity chamber with 5% CO_2 for 3 or 4 weeks. Colonies will develop usually in a few days from cat blood, although some strains may require a few weeks.

Other means of isolation of *Bartonella* have been with use of Bactec blood-culture system or BacT/Alert blood culture system. Identification of isolates as *Bartonella* can be performed by using enzyme-based identification systems, but is usually confirmed by DNA amplification using PCR-RFLP analysis. Several restriction endonucleases, such as TaqI and HhaI for citrate synthase gene, are used to digest the single product amplified by specific primers. PCR has also been used to identify *B. henselae* in tissue or CSD skin test antigens, in absence of culture.

Evidence of infection can be detected in humans or animals by looking for antibodies by IFA or ELISA. An IFA titer of at least 1:64 is considered positive. *Bartonella henselae* antibodies can be detected despite concurrent bacteremia in cats and sometimes in humans.

TREATMENT

In humans, antimicrobial treatment is generally indicated for patients with bacillary angiomatosis, bacillary peliosis, or relapsing bacteremia. Treatment with erythromycin, rifampicin, or doxycycline for at least 2 to 3 months in immunocompromised people is recommended, but relapses can occur. In such cases, patients should receive life-long treatment with these antibiotics. For CSD, antimicrobial treatment is not generally indicated, as most typical cases do not respond to antimicrobial administration. Intravenous administration of gentamicin and doxycycline and oral administration of erythromycin have been used successfully in the treatment of disseminated CSD and therapy of patients with neuroretinitis.

In cats, antibiotic treatment (doxycycline, 25 mg to 50 mg twice daily; lincomycin, 100 mg twice a day for 3 weeks) of cats may suppress bacteremia. Various antibiotics (doxycycline, erythromycin, enrofloxacin) have been shown to reduce the level of bacteremia in experimentally infected cats but do not eliminate infection and the level of bacteremia may surpass the initial level a few weeks after the cessation of treatment.

PREVENTION

A large reservoir for *B. henselae* and possibly for *B. clarridgeiae* exists among the 57 million pet cats residing in one-third of homes in the United States, and negative publicity about the perceived hazards of cat ownership is likely, especially for immunocompromised people. Seronegative cats are likely not to be bacteremic, but young kittens, especially impounded kittens and flea-infested kittens, are more likely to be bacteremic. Therefore, people who want to acquire a pet cat, especially if they are immunocompromised, should seek a cat raised in a cattery, if possible, an adult cat coming from a flea-controlled environment. Serologic testing could be performed and only seronegative cats adopted. Unfortunately, there is no correlation between seropositivity and bacteremia. Bacteremia can also be transient with relapses.

Declawing the cats has also been suggested but has a limited value, as infection can be transmitted from cat to cat by fleas. Flea control, therefore, appears to be one of the major control measures to prevent cat infection and its spread from cat to cat. The most effective means of preventing *B. henselae* infection are common sense, hygiene, flea control, and, possibly, modification of behavior of the cat owners themselves. Wash hands after handling pets and clean any cuts, bites, or scratches promptly with soap and water.

SELECTED REFERENCES

Abbott RC, Chomel BB, Kasten RW, et al. Experimental and natural infection with *Bartonella henselae* in domestic cats. Comp Immun Microbiol Infect Dis 1997;20:41.

Anderson B, Goldsmith C, Johnson A, et al. Bacteriophage-like particle of *Rochalimaea henselae*. Molec Microbiol 1994;13:67.

Anderson B, Kelly C, Threlkel R, Edwards K. Detection of *Rochalimaea henselae* in cat scratch disease skin test antigens. J Infect Dis 1993;168:1034.

Anderson B, Sims K, Regnery R, et al. Detection of *Rochalimaea henselae* DNA in specimens from cat scratch patients by PCR. J Clin Microbiol 1994;32:942.

Barka NE, Hadfield T, Patnaik M, et al. EIA for detection of *Rochalimaea henselae*-reactive IgG, IgM, and IgA antibodies in patients with suspected cat-scratch disease. J Infect Dis 1993;67:1503. Letter.

Batterman HJ, Peek JA, Loutit JS, et al. *Bartonella henselae* and *Bartonella quintana* adherence to and entry into cultured human epithelial cells. Infect Immun 1995;63:4553.

Breitschwerdt E, Kordick DL. Bartonellosis. J Am Vet Med Assoc 1995;206:1928.

Breitschwerdt EB, Kordick DL, Malarkey DE, et al. Endocarditis in a dog due to infection with a novel *Bartonella* subspecies. J Clin Microbiol 1995;3:154.

Brenner DJ, O'Connor SP, Winkler HH, Steigerwalt AG. Proposals to unify the genera *Bartonella* and *Rochalimaea*, with descriptions of *Bartonella quintana* comb. nov., *Bartonella vinsoni* comb. nov., *Bartonella henselae* comb. nov., and *Bartonella elizabethae* comb. nov., and to remove the family *Bartonellaceae* from the order *Rickettsiales*. Int J Syst Bacteriol 1993;43:777.

Carithers HA. Cat scratch disease. An overview based on a study of 1200 patients. Am J Dis Child 1985;139:1124.

Childs JE, Olson JG, Wolf A, et al. Prevalence of antibodies to *Rochalimaea* species (cat scratch disease agent) in cats. Vet Rec 1995;136:519.

Childs JE, Rooney JA, Cooper JL, et al. Epidemiologic observations on infection with *Rochalimaea* species among cats living in Baltimore, Md. J Am Vet Med Assoc 1994;204:1775.

Chomel BB, Abbott RC, Kasten RW, et al. *Bartonella henselae* prevalence in domestic cats in California: risk factors and association between bacteremia and antibody titers. J Clin Microbiol 1995;33:2445.

Chomel BB, Kasten RW, Floyd-Hawkins KA, et al. Experimental transmission of *Bartonella henselae* by the cat flea. J Clin Microbiol 1996;34:1952.

Clarridge JE III, Raich TJ, Pirwani D, et al. Strategy to detect and identify *Bartonella* species in routine clinical laboratory yields *Bartonella henselae* from human immunodeficiency virus-positive patient and unique *Bartonella* strain from his cat. J Clin Microbiol 1995;33:2107.

Conley T, Slater L, Hamilton K. *Rochalimaea* species stimulate human endothelial cell proliferation and migration in vitro. J Lab Clin Med 1994;24:521.

Debré R, Lamy M, Jammet ML, et al. La maladie des griffes de chat. Bull Mem Soc Méd Hosp Paris 1950;66:76.

Demers DM, Bass JW, Vincent JM, et al. Cat-scratch disease in Hawaii: etiology and seroepidemiology. J Pediatr 1995;127:23.

Dolan MJ, Wong MT, Regnery RL, et al. Syndrome of *Rochalimaea henselae* adenitis suggesting cat scratch disease. Ann Intern Med 1993;118:331.

English CK, Wear DJ, Margileth AM, et al. Cat scratch disease. Isolation and culture of the bacterial agent. JAMA 1988;259:1347.

Foley JE, Chomel B, Kikuchi Y, et al. Seroprevalence of *Bartonella henselae* in cattery cats: association with cattery hygiene and flea infestation. Vet Quart 1998;20:1.

Groves MG, Harrington KS. *Rochalimaea henselae* infections: newly recognized zoonoses transmitted by domestic cats. J Am Vet Med Assoc 1944;204:267.

Hensel DM, Slater LN. The genus *Bartonella*. Clin Microbiol Newslett 1995;17:9.

Holmes AH, Greenough TC, Balady GJ, et al. *Bartonella henselae* endocarditis in an immunocompetent adult. Clin Infect Dis 1995;21:1004.

Jackson LA, Perkins BA, Wenger JD. Cat scratch disease in the United States: an analysis of three national data bases. Am J Public Health 1993;83:1707.

Jameson P, Green C, Regnery R, et al. Prevalence of *Bartonella henselae* antibodies in pet cats throughout regions of North America. J Infect Dis 1995;172:1145.

Koehler JE, Glaser CA, Tappero JT. *Rochalimaea henselae* infection: a new zoonosis with the domestic cat as reservoir. JAMA 1994;271:531.

Koehler JE, Leboit PE, Egbert BM, Berger TG. Cutaneous vascular lesions and disseminated cat scratch disease in patients with acquired immuno-deficiency syndrome (AIDS) and AIDS-related complex. Ann Intern Med 1988;109:449.

Koehler JE, Quinn FD, Berger TG, et al. Isolation of *Rochalimaea* species from cutaneous and osseous lesions of bacillary angiomatosis. N Engl J Med 1992;327:1625.

Kordick DL, Breitschwerdt EB. Intraerythrocytic presence of *Bartonella henselae*. J Clin Microbiol 1995;33:1655.

Kordick DL, Wilson KH, Sexton DJ, et al. Prolonged *Bartonella* bacteremia in cats associated with cat-scratch disease patients. J Clin Microbiol 1995;33:3245.

Lawson PA, Collins MD. Description of *Bartonella clarridgeiae* sp. nov. isolated from the cat of a patient with *B. henselae* septicemia. Med Microbiol Lett 1996;5:64.

Leboit PE, Berger TG, Egbert BM, et al. Epithelioid haemangioma-like vascular proliferation in AIDS: manifestation of cat scratch disease bacillus infection? Lancet 1988;1:960.

Margilet AM. Antibiotic therapy for cat scratch disease: clinical study of therapeutic outcome in 268 patients and a review of the literature. Pediatr Infect Dis J 1992;11:474.

Maurin M, Raoult D. Antimicrobial susceptibility of *Rochalimaea quintana, R. vinsoni*, and the newly recognized *Rochalimaea henselae*. J Antimicrob Chemother 1993;32:587.

Noah DL, Bresee JS, Gorensek MJ, et al. Cluster of five children with acute encephalopathy associated with cat-scratch disease in South Florida. Pediatr Infect Dis J 1995;14:866.

Palamry J, Teysseire N, Dussert C, Raoult D. Image cytometry and topographical analysis of proliferation of endothelial cells in vitro during *Bartonella (Rochalimaea)* infection. Anal Cell Pathol 1996;11:13.

Regnery RL, Anderson BE, Clarridge JE III, et al. Characterization of a novel *Rochalimaea* species, *R. henselae*, sp. nov., isolated from blood of a febrile, HIV-positive patient. J Clin Microbiol 1992;30:265.

Regnery RL, Childs JE, Koehler JE. Infections associated with *Bartonella* species in persons infected with human immunodeficiency virus. Clin Infect Dis 1995;21(S1):S94.

Regnery RL, Martin M, Olson JG. Naturally occurring *Rochalimaea henselae* infection in domestic cat. Lancet 1992;340:557. Letter.

Regnery RL, Olson JG, Perkins BA, Bibb W. Serological response to *Rochalimaea henselae* antigen in suspected cat scratch disease. Lancet 1992;339:1443.

Relman DA, Lepp PW, Sadler KN, Schmidt TM. Phylogenic relationships among the agent of bacillary angiomatosis, *Bartonella bacilliformis* and other alpha-proteobacteria. Molec Microbiol 1992;6:1801.

Relman DA, Loutit JS, Schmidt TM, et al. The agent of bacillary angiomatosis: an approach to the identification of uncultured pathogens. N Engl J Med 1990;323:1573.

Schwartzman WA, Patnaik M, Angulo FJ, et al. *Bartonella (Rochalimaea)* antibodies, dementia, and cat ownership among men infected with human deficiency virus. Clin Infect Dis 1995;21:954.

Slater LN, Welch DF, Hensel D, Coody DW. A newly recognized fastidious gram-negative pathogen as a cause of fever and bacteremia. N Engl J Med 1990;323:1587.

Slater LN, Welch DF, Min KW. *Rochalimaea henselae* causes bacillary angiomatosis and peliosis hepatitis. Arch Intern Med 1992;152:602.

Stoler MH, Bonfiglio TA, Steigbigel RT, Pereira M. An atypical subcutaneous infection associated with acquired immune deficiency syndrome. Am J Clin Pathol 1983;80:714.

Tappero JW, Mohle-Boetani J, Koehler JE, et al. The epidemiology of bacillary angiomatosis and bacillary peliosis. JAMA 1993;269:770.

Wear DJ, Margileth AM, Hadfield TL, et al. Cat scratch disease: a bacterial infection. Science 1983;221:1403.

Welch DF, Pickett DA, Slater LN, et al. *Rochalimaea henselae* sp. nov., a cause of septicemia, bacillary angiomatosis, and parenchymal bacillary peliosis. J Clin Microbiol 1992;30:275.

Wong MT, Dolan MJ, Lattuada CP, et al. Neuroretinitis, aseptic meningitis, and lymphadenitis associated with *Bartonella (Rochalimaea) henselae* infection in immunocompetent patients and patients infected with human immunodeficiency virus type I. Clin Infect Dis 1995;21:352.

Zangwill KM, Hamilton DH, Perkins BA, et al. Cat scratch disease in Connecticut: epidemiology, risk factors, and evaluation of a new diagnostic test. N Engl J Med 1993;329:8.

56 Anaplasmataceae

ERNST L. BIBERSTEIN

Anaplasmataceae includes the genera *Anaplasma, Haemobartonella, Eperythrozoon,* and *Aegyptianella,* which differ in morphology, host specificity, and location on erythrocytes. *Anaplasmataceae* parasitize erythrocytes in several classes of vertebrates and may cause anemias.

Of four *Anaplasma* species, only *A. marginale* is a significant pathogen. *Anaplasma ovis* rarely causes anaplasmosis of sheep and is infective for goats and deer. *Anaplasma caudatum,* which has a tail-like appendage, has been seen in bovine infections alongside *A. marginale.* Its significance is uncertain. *Anaplasma centrale,* also found in cattle, is of interest as an immunizing agent against *A. marginale.*

ANAPLASMA MARGINALE

DESCRIPTIVE FEATURES

In Giemsa-stained blood smears, *A. marginale* appears as purple spots (≤1 mm) near the periphery of erythrocytes (Fig 56.1). These marginal or inclusion bodies are membrane-lined vacuoles containing up to 10 initial bodies (≤400 nm each) enclosed in a two-layered membrane. Initial bodies contain DNA and RNA but lack cell walls.

The organism has been serially propagated in a tick cell culture. It is aerobic, catalase positive, and utilizes exogenous amino acids. It can be preserved by deep-freezing (−70°C). There is antigenic strain variability involving mainly the major surface proteins (Msp) and cross-reactivity with other *Anaplasmataceae.*

ECOLOGY

Infected ruminants are the reservoir of *A. marginale.* Although many species can be infected, few regularly develop disease. Some, such as deer, may be naturally infected and serve as a source of bovine anaplasmosis. The infection occurs on all continents.

Transmission is by parenteral introduction of infected blood, in nature probably most often by ticks and bloodsucking flying insects, but also by contaminated instruments and transplacental and conjunctival exposure.

Initial bodies enter erythrocytes by endocytosis after adhering to the cell surface by way of Msp-1 and multiply by binary fission within the endosome. New initial bodies are released from the erythrocyte surface, possibly to contiguous cells, without discernible cell damage. Anemia dominates the clinical picture. The mechanism may be an immune response to parasitized erythrocytes, resulting in indiscriminate erythrocyte removal by the macrophage system and causing anemia, icterus, bile stasis, splenomegaly, and hepatomegaly. There is little intravascular hemolysis and no hemoglobinuria.

Illnesses, following incubation periods of up to 5 weeks, range from subclinical to peracutely fatal. Signs include anemia, fever, anorexia, depression, weakness, constipation, and abortion. Severity often varies directly with age and duration from hours to weeks. In mature cattle (>3 years), fatality rates may reach 50%.

Disease is generally seen in cattle 1 year of age or older. Recovered animals, which remain infected, constitute the main reservoir. Other possible sources are infected wild ruminants. Long-term carriage occurs in ticks.

IMMUNOLOGIC FACTORS

Humoral and cell-mediated responses develop. Antibody response is directed also to host antigens, and probably plays a role in pathogenesis. Immunity following recovery may not be permanent.

Resistance of calves outlasts maternal antibody and can be terminated by splenectomy. Specific resistance is probably cell-mediated.

Artificial immunization prevents disease, although not infection. "Premunition" involves exposure of calves, which typically results in subclinical infection and resistance to subsequent exposure. It may produce immediate or delayed clinical disease. Vector control to prevent spread to susceptible stock is required.

Infection with *A. centrale,* resulting in an usually mild disease, induces resistance to *A. marginale.* Inactivated *A. marginale* in adjuvant produces immunity of several months' duration subject to reinforcement through natural exposure. The erythrocyte constituents of this vaccine account for occasional immunohemolytic problems in neonatal calves nursing immunized animals.

LABORATORY DIAGNOSIS

Anaplasma marginale is demonstrable by routine blood stains, acridine orange, or immunofluorescence. The

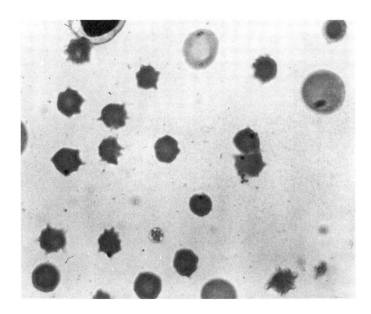

FIGURE 56.1. Anaplasma marginale *in bovine erythrocytes. Wright stain, 1000×.*

latter is most specific and sensitive. Acridine orange produces nonspecific staining of nucleic acids, whereas routine blood stains may not detect infection beyond the first few weeks. Methods utilizing molecular biological techniques (such as the polymerase chain reaction [PCR]) have been developed and are more sensitive than methods utilizing observation of stained smears. A nucleic acid probe has been developed.

Serologic methods include complement fixation, capillary agglutination, radioimmunoassay, enzyme-linked immunosorbent assay (ELISA), and a card agglutination test for field use. All are useful in detecting subclinical cases.

Anaplasma marginale expresses at least five major surface proteins (Msp), all of which display antigenic variation due in large part to the polymorphic nature of the encoding *msp* genes. The antigenic variations may explain the chronic nature of anaplasmosis. Antibodies to Msp do not influence the development of the microorganism while in the tick.

The definitive method of diagnosis requires injection of suspect blood into splenectomized calves.

Treatment and Control

Tetracycline is effective against *A. marginale*. Clinical cases are treated by injection; the carrier state is treated by feed medication for up to 2 months. Vaccination and vector control are helpful.

Aegyptianella

A tick-borne anemia of poultry, found in Mediterranean countries, South Africa, and Southeast Asia, is due to *Aegyptianella pullorum*, an anaplasma-like organism found in erythrocytes, leukocytes, mononuclear phagocytes,

and plasma. Similar organisms occur in wild birds and reptiles. Initial and inclusion bodies resemble those of *A. marginale*. *Aegyptianella pullorum* is susceptible to tetracyclines and thiosemicarbazone.

Eperythrozoon and Haemobartonella

Eperythrozoon and *Haemobartonella* consist of pleomorphic basophilic bodies — rings, cocci, and rods — ranging from 200 nm to 3 μm (Fig 56.2). In *Eperythrozoon*, rings and cocci predominate, whereas rods are common with *Haemobartonella*. Cytochemical tests show high levels of DNA and RNA. The organisms are attached to the surface of erythrocytes without visible membrane damage. A two-layered membrane, but no cell wall, encloses the organisms.

They have not been propagated in vitro.

Most species are host-specific. Latent infections are the rule, but hemolytic disease occurs in young or stressed animals, for example, in pigs due to *Eperythrozoon suis*. The spleen appears to be important in maintaining latency and protecting against exogenous infection. Arthropod vectors are suspected.

Feline Infectious Anemia

Haemobartonella felis is transmitted via blood (possibly among fighting tomcats) and by bloodsucking arthropods. Maternal transmission occurs.

Autoimmune phenomena appear during infection (hemagglutination, positive Coombs' test). Intravascular hemolysis is negligible. Red cell loss occurs by erythrophagocytosis via the mononuclear phagocyte system. Splenectomy does not dramatically influence the course.

The disease is a normocytic, hemolytic, febrile anemia beginning days to weeks after exposure. There is weakness,

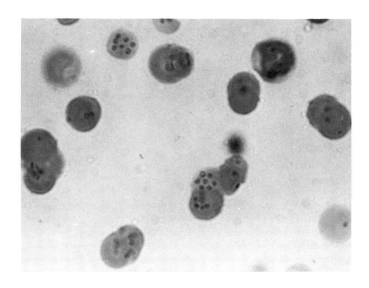

FIGURE 56.2. Haemobartonella felis *on feline erythrocytes. Note coccal and ring forms. Wright stain, 1000×.*

pallor, jaundice, and splenomegaly. Cases may be acute or chronic, and when untreated are about 33% fatal.

Young adult males are preferably affected. Seasonal peaks possibly reflect mating activity. A frequent presence of other infections, such as feline leukemia or feline immunodeficiency virus, has been noted.

Antibody is produced. Its protective role is undetermined. Infection persists and may be manifested by periodic illness.

Demonstrability of the agent is inconsistent. Giemsa-stained smears should be checked daily for 1 week. An indirect fluorescent antibody test has been described. Molecular biologic tests (PCR; DNA probe) have been developed.

Tetracycline is the drug of choice. Corticosteroid therapy for suppression of immunopathologic reactions may be considered. Supportive treatment is often required.

SELECTED REFERENCES

Alleman AR, Palmer GH, McGuire TC, et al. *Anaplasma marginale* major surface protein 3 is encoded by a polymorphic, multigene family. Infect Immun 1997;65:156.

Barbet AF. Recent developments in the molecular biology of anaplasmosis. Vet Parasitol 1995;57:43.

Bobade RA, Nash AS, Rogerson R. Feline haemobartonellosis: clinical haematological and pathological studies in natural infections and the relationship to infection with feline leukemia virus. Vet Rec 1982;122:32.

Eckblad WR, McGonigle RA. Acquired cellular responsiveness in cattle cleared of *Anaplasma marginale* 28 months earlier. Vet Immunol Immunopathol 1983;4:659.

Eriks IS, Palmer GH, McGuire TC, et al. Detection and quantitation of *Anaplasma marginale* in carrier cattle using a nucleic acid probe. J Clin Microbiol 1989;27:279.

Gale KR, Dimmock CM, Gartside M, Leatch G. *Anaplasma marginale:* detection of carrier cattle by PCR-ELISA. Int J Parasitol 1996;26:1103.

Ge NL, Kocan KM, Murphy GL, Blouin EF. Detection of *Anaplasma marginale* DNA in bovine erythrocytes by slot-blot

and in situ hybridization with a PCR-mediated digoxigenin-labeled DNA probe. J Vet Diagn Invest 1995;7:465.

Grindem CT, Corbett WT, Tomkins MT. Risk factors for *Haemobartonella felis* infection in cats. J Am Vet Med Assoc 1990; 196:96.

Hayes HM, Priester WA. Feline infectious anemia. Risk by age, sex and breed; prior disease; seasonal occurrence; mortality. J Small Anim Pract 1973;14:797.

Hoskins JD. Canine haemobartonellosis, canine hepatozoonosis, and feline cytauxzoonosis. Vet Clin North Am Small Anim Pract 1991;21:129.

Kocan KM. Targeting ticks for control of selected hemoparasitic diseases of cattle. Vet Parasitol 1995;57:121.

Kocan KM, Blouin EF, Palmer GH, et al. Strategies to interrupt the development of *Anaplasma marginale* in its tick vector. The effect of bovine-derived antibodies. Ann NY Acad Sci 1996;791:157.

Kocan KM, Stiller D, Goff WL, et al. Development of *Anaplasma marginale* in male *Dermacentor andersoni* transferred from parasitemic to susceptible cattle. Am J Vet Res 1992;53: 499.

Kreier JR, Ristic M. The biology of hemotrophic bacteria. Annu Rev Microbiol 1981;35:325.

Kuttler KL, Johnson LW, Simpson JE. Chemotherapy to eliminate *Anaplasma marginale* under field and laboratory conditions. Proc US Anim Health Assoc 1980;84:73.

Lincoln SD, Zaugg JL, Maas J. Bovine anaplasmosis: susceptibility of seronegative cows from an infected herd to experimental infection with *Anaplasma marginale.* J Am Vet Med Assoc 1987;190:171.

Maede Y, Hata R. Studies on feline haemobartonellosis: the mechanism of anemia produced by infection with *Haemobartonella felis.* Jpn J Vet Sci 1975;37:49.

Magonigle RA, Newby TJ. Elimination of naturally acquired chronic *Anaplasma marginale* infections with longacting oxytetracycline injectable. Am J Vet Res 1982;43:2170.

McGarey DJ, Barbet AF, Palmer GH, et al. Putative adhesins of *Anaplasma marginale:* major surface polypeptides 1a and 1b. Infect Immun 1994;62:4594.

Munderloh UG, Blouin EF, Kocan KM, et al. Establishment of the tick (Acari: Ixodidae)-borne cattle pathogen *Anaplasma marginale* (Rickettsiales: Anaplasmataceae) in tick cell culture. J Med Entomol 1996;33:656.

Palmer GH, Oberle SM, Barbet AF, et al. Immunization of cattle with a 36-kilodalton surface protein induces protection against homologous and heterologous *Anaplasma marginale* challenge. Infect Immun 1988;56:1526.

Palmer GH, McElwain TF. Molecular basis for vaccine development against anaplasmosis and babesiosis. Vet Parasitol 1995; 57:233.

Pedersen NC, Yamamoto JK, Ishida T, Hansen H. Feline immunodeficiency virus infection. Vet Immunol Immunopathol 1989;21:111.

Visser ES, McGuire TC, Palmer GH, et al. The *Anaplasma marginale* msp5 gene encodes a 19-kilodalton protein conserved in all recognized *Anaplasma* species. Infect Immun 1992; 60:5139.

Wyatt CR, Davis WC, Knowles DP, et al. Effect on intraerythrocytic *Anaplasma marginale* of soluble factors from infected calf blood mononuclear cells. Infect Immun 1996;64:4846.

PART III

Viruses

57

General Properties of Viruses

Janet S. Butel   Joseph L. Melnick

Yuan Chung Zee

DEFINITIONS

Viruses are the smallest infectious agents (20 nm to 300 nm in diameter); they contain one kind of nucleic acid (RNA or DNA) as their genome. The nucleic acid is encased in a protein shell, which may be surrounded by a lipid-containing membrane. The entire infectious unit is termed a *virion*. Viruses replicate only in living cells. The viral nucleic acid contains information necessary for programming the infected host cell to synthesize a number of virus-specific macromolecules required for production of viral progeny. During the replicative cycle, numerous copies of viral nucleic acid and coat proteins are produced. The coat proteins assemble together to form the *capsid*, which encases and stabilizes the viral nucleic acid against the extracellular environment and facilitates the attachment and penetration of the virus upon contact with new susceptible cells.

The following criteria are consistent among viruses:

1. The genome of a virus is composed of one type of nucleic acid, RNA or DNA.
2. A virus reproduces only from its nucleic acid.
3. A virus does not possess genetic information for the synthesis of enzymes responsible for energy metabolism.
4. A virus utilizes host ribosomal and transfer RNA for synthesis of viral proteins.

The host range for a given virus may be extremely limited, but viruses are known to infect unicellular organisms such as mycoplasmas, bacteria, and algae, as well as all higher plants and animals.

Some useful definitions in viral structure are as follows:

Capsid: The protein shell, or coat, that encloses the nucleic acid genome. Empty capsids may be byproducts of the replicative cycle of viruses with icosahedral symmetry.

Nucleocapsid: The capsid together with the enclosed nucleic acid.

Structural units: The basic protein building blocks of the coat. They are usually a collection of more than one nonidentical polypeptides.

Capsomeres: Morphologic units seen in the electron microscope on the surface of icosahedral viral particles. Capsomeres represent clusters of poly-

peptides, but the morphologic units do not necessarily correspond to the chemically defined structural units.

Envelope: A lipid-containing membrane that surrounds some viral particles. It is acquired during viral maturation by a budding process through a cellular membrane. Virus-encoded glycoproteins are exposed on the surface of the envelope.

Virion: The complete viral particle, which in some instances (adenoviruses, parvoviruses, picornaviruses) may be identical with the nucleocapsid. In more complex virions (herpesviruses, orthomyxoviruses), this includes the nucleocapsid plus a surrounding envelope. This structure, the virion, serves to transfer the viral nucleic acid from one cell to another.

Defective virus: A viral particle that is functionally deficient in some aspect of replication. Defective virus may interfere with the replication of normal virus.

Viral structures are illustrated in Figure 57.1.

CLASSIFICATION OF VIRUSES

Basis of Classification

The following properties, listed in order of preference or importance, have been used as a basis for the classification of viruses. The amount of information available in each category is not uniform for all viruses. Concerning some agents, knowledge is available for only a few of the properties listed.

1. Nucleic acid type: RNA or DNA; single-stranded or double-stranded; strategy of replication.
2. Size and morphology, including type of symmetry, number of capsomeres, and presence or absence of envelopes.
3. Presence of specific enzymes, particularly RNA and DNA polymerases concerned with genome replication, and neuraminidase necessary for release of certain viral particles (influenza) from the cells in which they were formed.
4. Susceptibility to physical and chemical agents, especially ether.
5. Immunologic properties.
6. Natural methods of transmission.

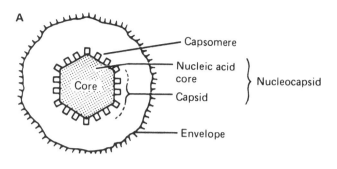

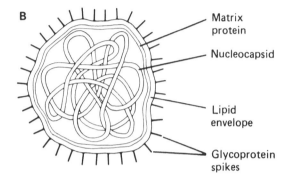

FIGURE 57.1. *Schematic diagram illustrating the components of the complete viral particle (the virion). A: Enveloped virus with icosahedral symmetry. B: Virus with helical symmetry.*

7. Host, tissue, and cell tropisms.
8. Pathology; inclusion body formation.
9. Symptomatology.

Classification by Biologic, Chemical, and Physical Properties

Viruses can be clearly separated into major groupings, called *families*, on the basis of the type of nucleic acid genome and the size, shape, substructure, and mode of replication of the virus particle. Table 57.1 shows one scheme used for classification. Within each family, subdivisions, called *genera*, are usually based on physiochemical or serologic differences. Properties of the major families of animal viruses are also summarized in Table 57.1.

Viroids are small infectious agents causing diseases of plants. They are nucleic acid molecules (MW 70,000 to 120,000) without a protein coat. Plant viroids are single-stranded, covalently closed, circular RNA molecules consisting of about 360 nucleotides and comprising a highly base-paired rodlike structure with unique properties. Each is arranged into 26 double-stranded regions separated by 25 regions of unpaired bases embodied in single-stranded internal loops; there is a loop at each end of the rodlike molecule. These features provide the viroid RNA molecule with structural, thermodynamic, and kinetic properties very similar to those of a double-stranded DNA molecule of the same molecular weight and guanine-plus-cytosine (G + C) content. Viroids replicate by an entirely novel mechanism in which infecting viroid RNA molecules are copied by the host enzyme normally responsible for synthesis of nuclear precursors to messenger RNA. Viroid RNA has not been shown to encode any protein products; the devastating plant diseases induced by viroids occur by an unknown mechanism. To date, viroids have been detected only in plants.

Prions are proteinaceous infectious particles that cause several degenerative nervous disorders of animals (e.g., scrapie, mink encephalopathy, bovine spongiform encephalopathy) and maybe of humans (e.g., Creutzfeldt-Jakob disease, kuru). The infective agents so far do not fit the definition of a virus. These diseases of the central nervous system are characterized by 1) a very long incubation period, 2) production of characteristic histopathology in the central nervous system (CNS), and 3) absence of association with any morphologically identifiable viral particles.

Most studies on prions have been carried out with the scrapie agent, which causes a transmissible, degenerative neurological disease of sheep and goats. There are few definitive data documenting any scrapie-specific nucleic acid in highly infectious preparations. The scrapie agent is resistant to heat, to a variety of chemical and physical agents (e.g., psoralens, ultraviolet light, and ionizing radiation), and to procedures that inactivate nucleic acids. A sialoglycoprotein (27–30 kilodalton [KdA]) has been shown to be the major component of infectious preparations of scrapie. A cellular gene that encodes scrapie 27–30 KdA sialoglycoprotein has been identified, indicating that the prion protein is a constituent of normal cells. A 33–35 KdA protein designated as PrP^{sc}, scrapie isoform of the prion protein, has been recovered from animal brains infected with scrapie. This protein (PrP^{sc}) has the same amino acid sequence as a protein (PrP^{c}) found in the membrane of normal neurons of uninfected animals. The only difference between these two proteins is their conformation. The genes for the infectious prion proteins of most subacute spongiform encephalopathies have been sequenced. It appears that changes of host range may be

Table 57.1. Families of Animal Viruses That Contain Members Able to Infect Animals

Nucleic Acid Core	Capsid Symmetry	Virion: Enveloped or Naked	Ether Sensitivity	Number of Capsomeres	Virus Particle Size (nm)[a]	Size of Nucleic Acid in Virion (kb/kbp)	Physical Type of Nucleic Acid[b]	Virus Family
DNA	Icosahedral	Naked	Resistant	32	18–26	5.6	ss	Parvoviridae
				72	45–55	5–8	ds circular	Papovaviridae
				252	80–110	36–38	ds	Adenoviridae
		Enveloped	Sensitive	162	150–200	124–235	ds	Herpesviridae
					120–300		ds	Iridoviridae
	Complex	Complex coats	Resistant[c]		230 × 400	130–375	ds	Poxviridae
RNA	Icosahedral	Naked	Resistant	32	28–30	7.2–8.4	ss	Picornaviridae
					28–30	7.2–7.9	ss	Astroviridae
				32	27–38	7.4–7.7	ss	Caliciviridae
				32	55–60	6.0	ds segmented	Birnaviridae
				132[d]	60–80	16–27	ds segmented	Reoviridae
		Enveloped	Sensitive	42	50–70	9.7–11.8	ss	Togaviridae
	Unknown	Enveloped	Sensitive		45–60	9.5–12.5	ss	Flaviviridae
	or complex				50–300	10–14	ss segmented	Arenaviridae
					80–220	20–30	ss	Coronaviridae
					80–100	7–11[e]	ss diploid	Retroviridae
	Helical	Enveloped	Sensitive		80–120	11–21	ss segmented	Bunyaviridae
					80–120	10–13.6	ss segmented	Orthomyxoviridae
					150–300	16–20	ss	Paramyxoviridae
					75 × 180	13–16	ss	Rhabdoviridae

[a] Diameter, or diameter × length.

[b] ss = single-stranded; ds = double-stranded.

[c] The genus *Orthopoxvirus*, which includes the better-studied poxviruses (e.g., vaccinia), is ether-resistant; some of the poxviruses belonging to other genera are ether-sensitive.

[d] Reoviruses possess a double protein capsid shell in which the exact number and spatial arrangement of capsomeres are difficult to determine. Rotaviruses appear to have 132 capsomeres.

[e] Size of monomer.

due to posttranslational configurational changes in the prion proteins of the new host. Further studies are needed to establish the precise nature and the mechanism of replication of the scrapie agent.

PRINCIPLES OF VIRAL STRUCTURE

Types of Symmetry of Viral Particles

Electron microscopy, cryoelectron microscopy, and x-ray diffraction techniques have made it possible to resolve fine differences in the basic morphology of viruses. The study of viral symmetry with the electron microscope requires the use of heavy metal stains (e.g., potassium phosphotungstate) to emphasize surface structure. The heavy metal permeates the viral particle as a cloud and brings out the surface structure of viruses by virtue of "negative staining."

Viral architecture can be grouped into three types based on the arrangement of morphologic subunits: 1) those with cubic symmetry (e.g., adenoviruses), 2) those with helical symmetry (e.g., orthomyxoviruses), and 3) those with complex structures (e.g., poxviruses). Genetic economy requires that a viral structure be made from many identical molecules of one or a few proteins.

Cubic Symmetry

All cubic symmetry observed with animal viruses to date is of the icosahedral pattern, the most efficient arrangement for subunits in a closed shell. Knowledge of the rules guiding icosahedral symmetry makes it possible to determine the number of capsomeres in a particle, an important characteristic in viral classification. The icosahedron has 20 faces (each an equilateral triangle), 12 vertices, and fivefold, threefold, and twofold axes of rotational symmetry. Capsomeres can be arranged to comply with icosahedral symmetry in a limited number of ways, expressed by the formula $N = 10(n - 1)^2 + 2$, where N is the total number of capsomeres and n the number of capsomeres on one side of each equilateral triangle.

Icosahedral structures can be built from one simple, asymmetric building unit, arranged as 12 pentamer

FIGURE 57.2. *(a) Representation of the capsomere arrangement of an adenovirus particle, as viewed through the twofold axis of symmetry. (b) Arrangement of capsomere group of nine, obtained by treatment of an adenovirus with sodium lauryl sulfate. (c) Orientation of the capsomere group of nine on the adenovirus particle. If the model were marked to show the maximum number of small triangles formed on one face of the icosahedron by drawing a line between each adjacent morphologic subunit, it would yield the triangulation number of the adenovirus particle, which is 25.*

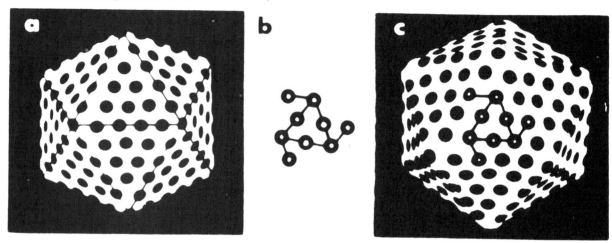

(vertex) units and X number of hexamer units. The polypeptides that comprise the pentamers and hexamers of the capsid may be the same or different, depending on the particular virus. The smallest and most basic capsid is that of the phage ϕX-174, which simply consists of 12 pentamer units.

An example of icosahedral symmetry is seen in Figure 57.2. The adenovirus (n = 6) model illustrated shows the six capsomeres along one edge (Fig 57.2a). Degradation of this virus with sodium lauryl sulfate releases the capsomeres in groups of nine (Fig 57.2b, c) and possibly groups of six. The groups of nine lie on the faces and include one capsomere from each of the three edges of the face, and the groups of six would be from the vertices. The groups of nine form the faces of the 20 triangular facets, which account for 180 subunits, and the groups of six that form the 12 vertices account for 72 capsomeres; thus the total is 252 capsomeres in the particle.

The viral nucleic acid is condensed within the isometric particles: virus-encoded "core" proteins or, in the case of papovaviruses, cellular histones are involved in condensing the nucleic acid into a form suitable for packaging. The rules governing incorporation of nucleic acid into isometric particles are unknown; presumably a "packaging sequence" is involved in assembly, although primary, secondary, and tertiary structures of the nucleic acid generally are not crucial. There are size constraints on the nucleic acid molecules that can be packaged into a given icosahedral capsid. Icosahedral capsids are formed independent of nucleic acid. Most preparations of isometric viruses will contain some

"empty" particles devoid of viral nucleic acid. Both DNA and RNA virus groups exhibit examples of cubic symmetry.

Helical Symmetry

In cases of helical symmetry, protein subunits are bound in a periodic way to the viral nucleic acid, winding it into a helix. The filamentous viral nucleic acid-protein complex (nucleocapsid) is then coiled inside a lipid-containing envelope. Thus, unlike icosahedral structures, there is a regular, periodic interaction between capsid protein and nucleic acid in viruses with helical symmetry. It is not possible for "empty" helical particles to form.

An example of helical symmetry is shown in Figures 57.3 and 57.4. Vesicular stomatitis virus, a member of the rhabdoviruses, is well characterized with respect to the interaction between the viral RNA and capsid protein. However, it is a rigid bullet-shaped rod. All known examples of animal viruses with helical symmetry contain RNA genomes, and with the exception of rhabdoviruses, have flexible nucleocapsids that are wound into a ball inside envelopes (see Figs 57.1B and 57.5).

Complex Structures

Some viral particles do not exhibit simple cubic or helical symmetry but are more complicated in structure. For example, poxviruses are brickshaped with ridges on the external surface and a core with lateral bodies inside (see Fig 57.5).

FIGURE 57.3. *Photograph of model showing proposed arrangement of internal components of vesicular stomatitis virus. On the left, the internal component is shown in the helical form. On the right, the helix is shown unwound in the form of an undulatory ribbon that tightens into an irregular helix at the free end. The subunits forming the latter are probably arranged with the long axis parallel to the axis of the helix. The subunits are shown here as rods attached at their midpoint to a wire representing the RNA molecule. (Reproduced with permission from Nakai T, Howatson AF. The fine structure of vesicular stomatitis virus. Virology 1968;35:268.)*

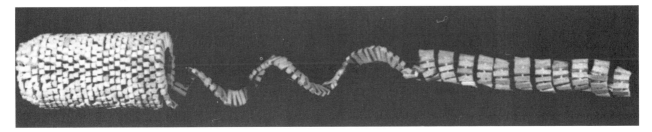

CHEMICAL COMPOSITION OF VIRUSES

Viral Protein

The structural proteins of viruses have several important functions. Their major purpose is to facilitate transfer of the viral nucleic acid from one host cell to another. They serve to protect the viral genome against inactivation by nucleases, participate in the attachment of the viral particle to a susceptible cell, and provide the structural symmetry of the viral particle.

The proteins determine the antigenic characteristics of the virus. The host's protective immune response is directed against antigenic determinants of proteins or glycoproteins exposed on the surface of the viral particle. Some surface proteins may also exhibit specific activities; for example, influenza virus hemagglutinin agglutinates red blood cells.

Some viruses carry enzymes (which are proteins) inside the virions. The enzymes are present in very small amounts and are probably not important in the structure of the viral particles; however, they are essential for initiation of the viral replicative cycle when the virion enters a host cell.

Examples include an RNA polymerase carried by viruses with negative-sense RNA genomes (e.g., orthomyxoviruses, rhabdoviruses) that is needed to copy the first mRNAs, and reverse transcriptase, an enzyme in retroviruses that makes a DNA copy of the viral RNA, an essential step in replication and transformation. At the extreme in this respect are the poxviruses, the cores of which contain a transcriptional system; at least 15 different enzymes are packaged in poxvirus particles.

Viral Nucleic Acid

Viruses contain a single kind of nucleic acid, either DNA or RNA, that encodes the genetic information necessary for replication of the virus. The genome may be single-stranded or double-stranded, circular or linear, and seg-

FIGURE 57.4. *Vesicular stomatitis virus treated with phosphotungstic acid. 321,000×. (Reproduced with permission from Hackett AJ. A possible morphological basis for the autointerference phenomenon in VSV. Virology 1964;24:51.)*

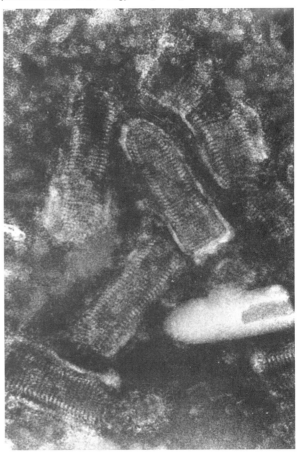

mented or nonsegmented. The type of nucleic acid, the strandedness, and the molecular weight are major characteristics used for classifying viruses into families (see Table 57.1).

The molecular weight of the viral DNA genome ranges from 1.5×10^6 (parvoviruses) to 200×10^6 (poxviruses). The molecular weight of the viral RNA genome ranges from 2×10^6 (picornaviruses) to 15×10^6 (reoviruses).

Most viral genomes are quite fragile once they are removed from their protective protein capsid, but some nucleic acid molecules have been examined in the electron microscope without disruption, and their lengths have been measured. If linear densities of approximately 2×10^6 per μm for double-stranded nucleic acid and 1×10^6 per μm for single-stranded forms are used, molecular weights of viral genomes can be calculated from direct measurements (see Table 57.1).

All major DNA virus groups in Table 57.1 have genomes that are single molecules of DNA and have a linear or circular configuration.

Viral RNAs exist in several forms. The RNA may be a single linear molecule (e.g., picornaviruses). For other viruses (e.g., orthomyxoviruses), the genome consists of several segments of RNA that may be loosely associated within the virion. The isolated RNA of picornaviruses and togaviruses, so-called positive-sense viruses, is infectious, and the entire molecule functions as an mRNA within the infected cell. The isolated RNA of the negative-sense RNA viruses, such as rhabdoviruses and orthomyxoviruses, is not infectious. For these virus families, the virions carry

FIGURE 57.5.   *Shapes and relative sizes of animal viruses of families that infect vertebrates. In some diagrams, certain internal structures of the particles are represented. (Reproduced with permission from Murphy FA, Fauquet CM, Bishop DHL. Virus taxonomy: Classification and nomenclature of viruses. Sixth report of the International Committee on Taxonomy of Viruses. New York: Springer-Verlag, 1994.*

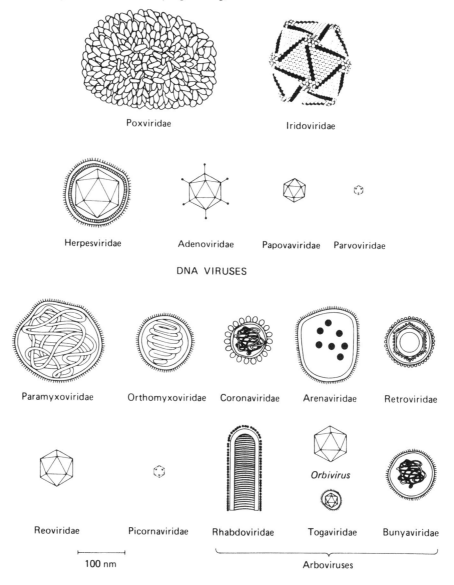

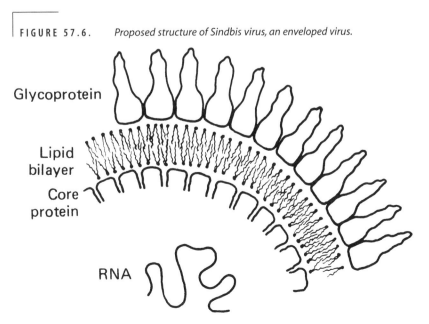

an RNA polymerase that in the cell transcribes the genome RNA molecules into several complementary RNA molecules, each of which may serve as an mRNA.

The sequence and composition of nucleotides of each viral nucleic acid are distinctive. One of the properties useful for characterizing a viral nucleic acid is its G + C content. DNA viral genomes can be analyzed and compared using restriction endonucleases, which are enzymes that cleave DNA at specific nucleotide sequences. Each genome will yield a characteristic pattern of DNA fragments after cleavage with a particular enzyme. Using molecularly cloned DNA copies of RNA, restriction maps also can be derived for RNA virus genomes. Molecular hybridization techniques (DNA to DNA, DNA to RNA, or RNA to RNA) permit the study of transcription of the viral genome within the infected cell as well as comparison of the relatedness of different viruses.

The number of genes in a virus can be approximated if one makes certain assumptions about 1) triplet codes, 2) the molecular weight of the genome, and 3) the average size of a protein. It must also be assumed in such calculations that there are no overlapping genes in the viral genome; this assumption has been proved incorrect for some viruses (papovaviruses, orthomyxoviruses). The number of proteins encoded by a virus can be estimated from the open reading frames deduced from the nucleic acid sequence. Many viral genomes have been sequenced. Although such estimates are not precise, the values serve to illustrate the varying complexities and relative coding capacities of different viral groups.

Viral Lipids

A number of different viruses contain lipid envelopes as part of their structure (e.g., Sindbis virus), as shown in Figure 57.6. The lipid is acquired when the viral nucleocapsid buds through a cellular membrane in the course of maturation. Budding occurs only at sites where virus-specific proteins have been inserted into the host cell membrane.

The specific phospholipid composition of a virion envelope is determined by the specific type of cell membrane involved in the budding process. For example, herpesviruses bud through the nuclear membrane of the host cell, and the phospholipid composition of the purified virus reflects the lipids of the nuclear membrane. The acquisition of a lipid-containing membrane is an integral step in virion morphogenesis in some viral groups.

Lipid-containing viruses are sensitive to treatment with ether and other organic solvents (see Table 57.1), indicating that disruption or loss of lipid results in loss of infectivity. Nonlipid-containing viruses are generally resistant to ether.

Viral Carbohydrates

Viral envelopes contain glycoproteins. In contrast to the lipids in viral membranes, which are derived from the host cell, the envelope glycoproteins are virus-coded. However, the sugars added to viral glycoproteins often reflect the host cell in which the virus is grown.

It is the surface glycoproteins of an enveloped virus that attach the viral particle to a target cell by interacting with a cellular receptor. The glycoproteins are also important viral antigens. As a result of their position at the outer surface of the virion, they are frequently involved in the interaction of the viral particle with neutralizing antibody. The three-dimensional structures of the externally exposed regions of both of the influenza viral membrane glycoproteins (hemagglutinin, neuraminidase) have been determined by x-ray crystallography. Such studies provide insights into the antigenic structure and functional activities of viral glycoproteins.

FIGURE 57.6.   *Proposed structure of Sindbis virus, an enveloped virus.*

CULTIVATION AND QUANTIFICATION OF VIRUSES

Cultivation of Viruses

At present, many viruses can be grown in cell cultures or in fertile eggs under strictly controlled conditions. Growth of virus in animals is still used for the primary isolation of certain viruses and for the study of the pathogenesis of viruses and of viral oncogenesis.

Chick Embryos.   Viral growth in an embryonated chick egg may result in the death of the embryo (e.g., encephalitis virus), the production of pocks or plaques on the chorioallantoic membrane (e.g., herpesvirus, smallpox virus, vaccinia virus), the development of hemagglutinins in the embryonic fluids or tissues (e.g., influenza virus), or the development of infective virus (e.g., Newcastle disease virus).

Tissue Cultures.   The availability of cells grown in vitro has facilitated the identification and cultivation of newly isolated and previously known viruses. There are three basic types of cell culture. Primary cultures are made by dispersing cells (usually with trypsin) from host tissues. In general, they are unable to grow for more than a few passages as secondary cultures. Diploid cell lines are secondary cultures that have undergone a change that allows their limited culture (up to 50 passages) but that retain their normal chromosome pattern. Continuous cell lines are cultures capable of more prolonged (perhaps indefinite) culture that have been derived from diploid cell lines or from malignant tissues. They invariably have altered and irregular numbers of chromosomes.

The type of cell culture used for viral cultivation depends on the sensitivity of the cells to that particular virus. In the clinical laboratory, multiplication of the virus can be followed by determining the following:

1. The cytopathic effect, or necrosis of cells in the tissue culture (e.g., foot-and-mouth virus, canine distemper virus, infectious bovine rhinotracheitis virus, canine parvovirus, canine infectious hepatitis virus).
2. The inhibition of cellular metabolism, or failure of virus-infected cells to produce acid (e.g., enteroviruses).
3. The appearance of a hemagglutinin (e.g., Newcastle disease virus, influenza virus) or complement-fixing antigen (e.g., foot-and-mouth virus, pseudorabies virus, canine distemper virus).
4. The adsorption of erythrocytes to infected cells, called *hemadsorption* (e.g., parainfluenzavirus, influenzavirus), due to the presence of viral-coded hemagglutinin in cellular membranes. This reaction becomes positive before cytopathic changes are visible, and in some cases it is the only means of detecting the presence of the virus.
5. Interference by a noncytopathogenic virus (e.g., bovine viral diarrhea virus) with replication and cytopathic effect of a second, indicator virus (e.g., Newcastle disease virus).
6. Morphologic transformation by an oncogenic virus (e.g., SV40, Rous sarcoma virus), usually accompanied by the loss of contact inhibition resulting in the piling up of cells into discrete foci.

Animals.   In the final analysis, no thorough knowledge of an animal virus has been realized except in instances where a susceptible laboratory animal exists for study of the virus; this is a self-evident truth, since all information about a virus derived from studies in tissue cultures or embryonated eggs must ultimately be translated into the course of events occurring within a susceptible animal host.

The ideal animal host for a study of a virus is, of course, the natural host of the virus; this is not always possible or practical, however, and quite often it is necessary to use whatever animal is susceptible to infection. Among the laboratory animals commonly employed for this purpose are mice, rats, rabbits, guinea pigs, hamsters, chickens, and monkeys. The choice of an animal is dictated by the nature of the virus under investigation, since not all animals are equally susceptible to all viruses; moreover, not all viruses have been successfully cultivated in experimental animals.

One of the most useful smaller laboratory animals is the mouse, which may be infected with a variety of viruses by various routes. The particular route to be used is determined by the ability of tissues to support viral multiplication — for example, influenza viruses are usually introduced intranasally; togaviruses are generally introduced intracerebrally. Note that the tissues of the CNS are sheltered tissues not normally exposed to infection. Consequently, many viruses, when introduced into such tissues, find a favorable environment for multiplication. The intracerebral inoculation of mice is thus a very useful procedure in virology. The usefulness of the mouse has been further extended through utilization of suckling mice, which apparently are susceptible to infection with a number of viruses that are normally incapable of infecting the adult animal.

Quantification of Viruses

Physical Methods.   Viral particles can be counted directly in the electron microscope by comparison with a standard suspension of latex particles of similar small size. A relatively concentrated preparation of virus is necessary for this procedure, however, and infectious virus particles cannot be distinguished from noninfectious ones.

Hemagglutination.   The red blood cells of humans and some animals can be agglutinated by different viruses. Both infective and noninfective particles give this reaction; thus, hemagglutination measures the total quantity of virus present.

Biologic Methods.   Quantal assays depend on the measurement of animal death, animal infection, or cytopathic effects in tissue culture upon end point dilution of the virus being tested. The titer is expressed as the 50% infectious dose (ID_{50}), which is the reciprocal of the dilution of virus that produces the effect in 50% of the cells or animals inoculated.

The most widely used assay for infectious virus is the plaque assay. Monolayers of host cells are inoculated with suitable dilutions of virus and after adsorption are overlaid with medium containing agar or carboxymethylcellulose to prevent virus spreading throughout the culture. After several days, the cells initially infected have produced virus that spreads only to surrounding cells, producing a small area of infection, or plaque. Under theoretical conditions, a single plaque can arise from a single infective viral particle, termed a *plaque-forming unit* (*PFU*). The cytopathic effect of infected cells within the plaque can be distinguished from uninfected cells of the monolayer, with or without suitable staining, and plaques can usually be counted macroscopically (Fig 57.7). The ratio of the number of viral particles to the number of plaques is always greater than 1. In most cases the ratio is about 1000 : 1. Major contributing factors are 1) the aggregation of viral particles, 2) the presence of anionic polysaccharides in the agar overlay that may be inhibitory to viral replication, and 3) the presence of defective noninfective particles in viral stocks.

Certain viruses, such as herpesvirus or poxvirus, form pocks when inoculated onto the chorioallantoic membrane of an embryonated egg. Such viruses can be quantitated by relating the number of pocks counted to the viral dilution.

PURIFICATION OF VIRUSES

Purification of Viral Particles

Once a system has been worked out for the cultivation and assay of a particular virus, it is often desirable to pursue investigations into the biochemical and biophysical properties of the viral particle. However, these investigations generally require substantial amounts of relatively homogeneous virus. In most cases, therefore, it is necessary to have not only a means of growing the virus to relatively high titer (and a means of determining this titer) but also one or more methods of obtaining an increasingly homogeneous and possibly more concentrated viral preparation.

Purification techniques can be loosely grouped into three categories: 1) methods based on physical properties, 2) methods based on biological properties, and 3) methods utilizing a combination of both. Physical methods commonly used include centrifugation, chromatography, electrophoresis, ultrafiltration, and phase distribution. Each of these techniques separates components of a suspension according to one or more physical properties and may or may not distinguish infectious from noninfectious particles depending on the method and the virus in question.

The biological method most frequently used in purification is agglutination of red blood cells. Agglutination of red blood cells of various species is a property shared by a number of viruses from a wide range of taxonomic classes and obviously could not be used to separate one of these hemagglutinating viruses from another.

The single most useful technique in viral purification is centrifugation. This is actually a group of techniques, the most commonly used of which are 1) differential centrifugation, 2) rate-zonal centrifugation, and 3) isopycnic centrifugation.

Differential centrifugation is the name given to alternating low-speed and high-speed sedimentation runs used to clarify viral suspensions of whole cells, nuclei, mitochondria, and other very large debris. These may be carried out using a number of general purpose machines, rotors, and tubes. When biological activity of the preparation is to be preserved, the runs are best carried out at

FIGURE 57.7. *Plaques produced in bovine kidney cell monolayers by vesicular stomatitis virus.*

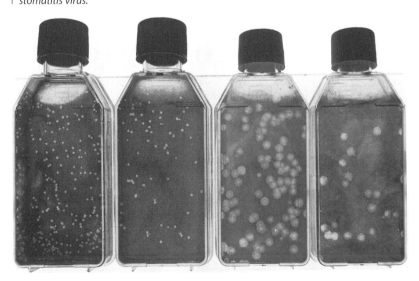

low temperature (4°C) as quickly as possible (20 to 30 minutes).

Rate-zonal centrifugation is also based on differential sedimentation rates and is so named because macromolecules having identical sedimentation rates move together in a zone down the centrifuge tube. This technique is most commonly used to separate two populations of viral particles with similar buoyant densities. These sedimentations may be performed in homogeneous liquids or in density gradients (as long as p solvent < p particle) and usually require a high-speed preparative ultracentrifuge, rotor, and tubes.

Isopycnic or *equilibrium density gradient centrifugation,* the third commonly used method, separates particles according to their buoyant density. Gradients are made from a variety of materials by a variety of methods but must always include within the range a point where p solvent = p particle. During the centrifugation, when the particles reach this point they will form a band. When all particles in the tube have reached the point at which p solvent = p particle, the tube is said to be at equilibrium (e.g., except for diffusion, no further changes take place). When the centrifugation is completed, the tubes are carefully removed and harvested, usually in droplet fractions, from either the top or the bottom of the tube.

REACTION TO PHYSICAL AND CHEMICAL PROPERTIES

Heat and Cold

There is great variability in the heat stability of different viruses. Icosahedral viruses tend to be stable, losing little infectivity after several hours at 37°C. Enveloped viruses are much more heat-labile, rapidly dropping in titer at 37°C. Viral infectivity is generally destroyed by heating at 50 to 60°C for 30 minutes, although there are some notable exceptions (e.g., hepatitis B virus, papovaviruses, scrapie agent).

Viruses can be preserved by storage at subfreezing temperatures, and some may withstand lyophilization and can thus be preserved in the dry state at 4°C or even at room temperature. Viruses that withstand lyophilization are more heat-resistant when heated in the dry state. Enveloped viruses tend to lose infectivity after prolonged storage even at −90°C and are particularly sensitive to repeated freezing and thawing.

Stabilization of Viruses by Salts

Many viruses can be stabilized by salts in concentrations of 1 mol/L, that is, the viruses are not inactivated even by heating at 50°C for 1 hour. The mechanism by which the salts stabilize viral preparations is not known. Viruses are preferentially stabilized by certain salts. $MgCl_2$, 1 mol/L, stabilizes picornaviruses and reoviruses; $MgSO_4$, 1 mol/L, stabilizes orthomyxoviruses and paramyxoviruses; and Na_2SO_4, 1 mol/L, stabilizes herpesviruses.

The stability of viruses is important in the preparation of vaccines. The ordinary nonstabilized poliovaccine must be stored at freezing temperatures to preserve its potency. With the addition of salts for stabilization of the virus, however, potency can be maintained for weeks at ambient temperatures, even in the high temperatures of the tropics.

pH

Viruses are usually stable between pH values of 5.0 and 9.0. Some viruses (e.g., enteroviruses) are resistant to acidic conditions. All viruses are destroyed by alkaline conditions. In hemagglutination reactions, variations of less than 1 pH unit may influence the result.

Radiation

Ultraviolet, x-ray, and high-energy particles inactivate viruses. The dose varies for different viruses. Infectivity is the most radiosensitive property, because replication requires expression of the entire genetic contents. Irradiated particles that are unable to replicate may still be able to express some specific functions in host cells.

Photodynamic Inactivation

Viruses are penetrable to a varying degree by vital dyes such as toluidine blue, neutral red, and proflavine. These dyes bind to the viral nucleic acid, and the virus then becomes susceptible to inactivation by visible light. Impenetrable viruses like poliovirus, when grown in the dark in the presence of vital dyes, incorporate the dye into their nucleic acid and are then susceptible to photodynamic inactivation. The coat antigen is unaffected by the process.

Neutral red is commonly used to stain plaque assays so that plaques are more readily seen. The assay plates must be protected from bright light once the neutral red has been added; otherwise, there is the risk that progeny virus will be inactivated and plaque development will cease.

Ether Susceptibility

Ether susceptibility can distinguish viruses that possess an envelope from those that do not. The viruses that are inactivated by ether include herpesvirus, orthomyxovirus, paramyxovirus, rhabdovirus, coronavirus, retrovirus, arenavirus, togavirus, flavivirus, and bunyavirus. The viruses that are resistant to ether include parvovirus, papovavirus, adenovirus, picornavirus, and reovirus. Poxviruses vary in sensitivity to ether.

Detergents

Nonionic detergents, for example, Nonidet P40 and Triton X-100, solubilize lipid constituents of viral membranes. The viral proteins in the envelope are released (undenatured). Anionic detergents, for example, sodium dodecyl sulfate, also solubilize viral envelopes; in addition, they disrupt capsids into separated polypeptides.

Formaldehyde

Formaldehyde destroys viral infectivity by reacting with nucleic acid. Viruses with single-stranded genomes are inactivated much more readily than those with double-stranded genomes. Formaldehyde has minimal adverse effects on the antigenicity of proteins and therefore has been used frequently in the production of inactivated viral vaccines.

Antibiotics and Other Antibacterial Agents

Antibacterial antibiotics and sulfonamides have no effect on viruses. Some antiviral drugs are available, however.

Quaternary ammonium compounds, in general, are not effective against viruses. Organic iodine compounds are also ineffective. Larger concentrations of chlorine are required to destroy viruses than to kill bacteria, especially in the presence of extraneous proteins. For example, the chlorine treatment of stools adequate to inactivate typhoid bacilli is inadequate to destroy poliomyelitis virus present in feces. Alcohols, such as isopropanol and ethanol, are relatively ineffective against certain viruses, especially picornaviruses. Clorox (bleach) remains the most effective viricidal agent for most known animal viruses.

REPLICATION OF VIRUSES

Viruses multiply only in living cells. The host cell must provide the energy and synthetic machinery and the low-molecular-weight precursors for the synthesis of viral proteins and nucleic acids. The viral nucleic acid carries the genetic specificity to code for all the virus-specific macromolecules in a highly organized fashion.

The unique feature of viral multiplication is that, soon after interaction with a host cell, the infecting virion is disrupted and its measurable infectivity lost. This phase of the growth cycle is called the *eclipse period*; its duration varies depending on both the particular virus and the host cell, and it ends with the formation of the first infectious progeny viral particles. The eclipse period is actually one of intense synthetic activity as the cell is redirected toward fulfilling the needs of the viral "pirate." In some cases, as soon as the viral nucleic acid enters the host cell, the cellular metabolism is redirected exclusively toward the synthesis of new viral particles. In other cases, the metabolic processes of the host cell are not altered significantly, although the cell synthesizes viral proteins and nucleic acids.

General Steps in Viral Replication Cycles

Viruses have evolved a variety of different strategies for accomplishing multiplication in parasitized host cells. Although the details vary from group to group, the general outline of the replication cycles is similar.

Attachment, Penetration, and Uncoating.   The first step in viral infection is interaction of a virion with a specific receptor site on the surface of a cell. Receptor molecules differ for different viruses; they are proteins in some cases (e.g., picornaviruses) and oligosaccharides in others (e.g., orthomyxoviruses and paramyxoviruses). The presence or absence of receptors plays an important determining role in cell tropism and viral pathogenesis; for example, poliovirus is able to attach only to cells in the CNS and intestinal tract of primates. Receptor binding is believed to reflect fortuitous configurational homologies between a virion surface structure and a cell surface component. For example, human immunodeficiency virus binds to the CD4 receptors on cells of the immune system, and it has been suggested that rabies virus interacts with acetylcholine receptors and that Epstein-Barr virus recognizes the receptor for the third component of complement on B cells. Each susceptible cell contains at least 100,000 receptor sites for a given virus.

After binding, the viral particle is taken up inside the cell. This step is referred to as *penetration, viropexis,* or *engulfment.* In some systems, this is accomplished by receptor-mediated endocytosis, with uptake of the ingested viral particles within endosomes. In other systems, the details of penetration are less clear. Uncoating occurs concomitant with or shortly after penetration. Uncoating is the physical separation of the viral nucleic acid (or in some cases internal nucleocapsids) from the outer structural components of the virion. The infectivity of the parental virus is lost at this point. Viruses are the only infectious agents for which dissolution of the infecting agent is an obligatory step in the replicative pathway.

Synthesis of Virus Components.   The synthetic phase of the viral replicative cycle ensues after uncoating of the viral genome. The essential theme in viral replication is that specific mRNAs must be transcribed from the viral nucleic acid for successful expression and duplication of genetic information. Once this is accomplished, viruses use cell components to translate the mRNA. Various classes of viruses use different pathways to synthesize the mRNAs depending upon the structure of the viral nucleic acid. Some viruses (e.g., rhabdovirus, orthomyxovirus, and paramyxovirus) carry RNA polymerases to synthesize mRNAs. RNA viruses of this type are called *negative-strand* (*negative-sense*) *viruses*, since their single-strand RNA genome is complementary to mRNA, which is conventionally designated *positive-strand* (*positive-sense*). Table 57.2 summarizes the various pathways of transcription (but not necessarily those of replication) of the nucleic acids of different classes of viruses.

In the course of viral replication, all the virus-specified macromolecules are synthesized in a highly organized sequence. In some viral infections, notably those involving double-stranded, DNA-containing viruses, early viral proteins are synthesized soon after infection and late proteins are made only late in infection, after viral DNA synthesis. Early genes may or may not be shut off when late products are made. In contrast, most if not all of the genetic information of RNA-containing viruses is expressed at the same time. In addition to these temporal controls, quantitative controls also exist, since not all

Table 57.2.   Pathways of Nucleic Acid Transcription for Various Viral Classes

Type of Viral Nucleic Acid	Intermediates	Type of mRNA	Example	Comments
±ds DNA	None	+mRNA	Most DNA viruses (e.g., herpesvirus, T4 bacteriophage)	
+ss DNA	±ds DNA	+mRNA	φ × bacteriophage	
±ds RNA	None	+mRNA	Reovirus	Virion contains RNA polymerase that transcribes each segment to mRNA.
+ss RNA	±ds RNA	+mRNA	Picornaviruses, togaviruses, flaviviruses	Viral nucleic acid is infectious and serves as mRNA. For togaviruses, smaller + mRNA is also formed for certain proteins.
−ss RNA	None	+mRNA	Rhabdoviruses, paramyxoviruses, orthomyxoviruses	Viral nucleic acid is not infectious; virion contains RNA polymerase that forms + mRNAs smaller than the genome. For orthomyxoviruses, + mRNAs are transcribed from each segment.
+ss RNA	−DNA, ± DNA	+mRNA	Retroviruses	Virion contains reverse transcriptase; viral RNA is not infectious, but complementary DNA from transformed cell is.

ds = double-stranded; ss = single-stranded; − indicates negative strand; + indicates positive strand; ± indicates a helix containing a positive and a negative

Table 57.3.   Comparison of Replication Strategies of Several Important RNA Viral Families

Characteristic	Grouping Based on Genomic RNA[a]					
	Positive-Strand Viruses			Negative-Strand Viruses		Double-Stranded Viruses
	Picornaviridae	Togaviridae	Retroviridae	Orthomyxoviridae	Paramyxo- and Rhabdoviridae	Reoviriade
Structure of genomic RNA	ss	ss	ss	ss	ss	ds
Sense of genomic RNA	Positive	Positive	Positive	Negative	Negative	
Segmented genome	0	0	0[b]	+	0	+
Genomic RNA infectious	+	+	0	0	0	0
Genomic RNA acts as messenger	+	+	+	0	0	0
Virion-associated polymerase	0	0	+[c]	+	+	+
Subgenomic messages	0	+	+	+	+	+
Polyprotein precursors	+	+	+	0	0	0

[a]   Abbreviations used: ss = single-stranded; ds = double-stranded; positive = same sense as mRNA; negative = complementary to mRNA; + = indicated property applies to that viral family; 0 = indicated property does not apply to that viral family.
[b]   Retroviruses contain a diploid genome (two copies of nonsegmented genomic RNA).
[c]   Retroviruses contain a reverse transcriptase (RNA-dependent DNA polymerase).

viral proteins are made in the same amounts. Virus-specific proteins may regulate the extent of transcription of genome or the translation of viral mRNA.

Small animal viruses and bacteriophages are good models for studies of gene expression. Their small size has enabled the total nucleotide sequence of many viruses to be elucidated. This has led to the discovery of overlapping genes in which some sequences in DNA are utilized in the synthesis of two different polypeptides, either by the use of two different reading frames or by two mRNA molecules using the same reading frames but different starting points. A viral system (adenovirus) first revealed the mRNA processing phenomenon called *splicing,* whereby the mRNA sequences that code for a given protein are generated from separated sequences in the template, with noncoding intervening sequences spliced out of the transcript.

The widest variation in strategies of gene expression is found among the RNA-containing viruses (Table 57.3). Some virions carry polymerases (orthomyxoviruses, reoviruses); some systems utilize subgenomic messages, sometimes generated by splicing (orthomyxoviruses, retroviruses); and some viruses synthesize large polyprotein precursors that are processed and cleaved to generate the final gene products (picornaviruses, retroviruses).

Table 57.4.   Summary of Replication Cycles of Major Viral Families

Virus Family	Type of Nucleic Acid Genome	Presence of Virion Envelope	Intracellular Location[a]				Duration of Multiplication Cycle (Hours)[b]
			Synthesis of Viral Proteins	Replication of Genome	Formation of Nucleocapsid	Virion Maturation	
Parvoviridae	DNA	0	C	N	N	N	
Papovaviridae	DNA	0	C	N	N	N	48
Adenoviridae	DNA	0	C	N	N	N	25
Hepadnaviridae	DNA	+	C	N	C	M-E	
Herpesviridae	DNA	+	C	N	N	M	15–72
Poxviridae	DNA	0	C	C	C	C	20
Picornaviridae	RNA	0	C	C	C	C	6–8
Reoviridae	RNA	0	C	C	C	C	15
Togaviridae	RNA	+	C	C	C	M-P	10–24
Flaviviridae	RNA	+	C	C	C	M-E	
Retroviridae	RNA	+	C	N	C	M-P	
Bunyaviridae	RNA	+	C	C	C	M-G	24
Orthomyxoviridae	RNA	+	C	N	N	M-P	15–30
Paramyxoviridae	RNA	+	C	C	C	M-P	10–48
Rhabdoviridae	RNA	+	C	C	C	M-P	6–10

[a] Abbreviations used: C = cytoplasm; N = nucleus; M = membranes; M-G = Golgi membranes; M-P = plasma membrane; M-E = endoplasmic reticulum membranes.
[b] The values shown for duration of the multiplication cycle are approximate; ranges indicate that various members within a given family replicate with different kinetics. Different host cell types also influence the kinetics of viral replication.

The extent to which virus-specific enzymes are involved in these processes varies from group to group. The larger viruses (herpesviruses, poxviruses) are more independent of cellular functions than are the smaller viruses. This is one reason the larger viruses are more susceptible to antiviral chemotherapy, because more virus-specific processes are available as targets for drug action.

The intracellular sites where the different events in viral replication take place vary from group to group (Table 57.4). A few generalizations are possible. Viral protein is synthesized in the cytoplasm on polyribosomes composed of virus-specific mRNA and host cell ribosomes. Viral DNA is usually replicated in the nucleus. Viral genomic RNA is generally duplicated in the cell cytoplasm, although there are exceptions.

Morphogenesis and Release.   Newly synthesized viral genomes and capsid polypeptides assemble together to form progeny viruses. Icosahedral capsids can condense in the absence of nucleic acid, whereas nucleocapsids of viruses with helical symmetry cannot form without viral RNA. There are no special mechanisms for the release of nonenveloped viruses; the infected cells eventually lyse and release the viral particles.

Enveloped viruses mature by a budding process (Fig 57.8). Virus-specific envelope glycoproteins are inserted into cellular membranes; viral nucleocapsids then bud through the membrane at these modified sites and in so doing acquire an envelope. Budding frequently occurs at

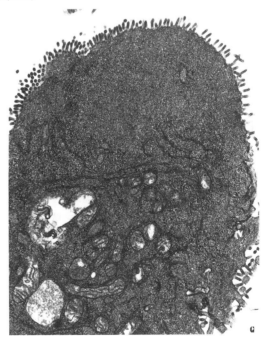

FIGURE 57.8.   *Vesicular stomatitis virus budding from plasma membrane of an infected L cell. 31,000×. (Reproduced with permission from Zee YC, Hackett AJ, Talena L. Vesicular stomatitis virus maturation sites in six different host cells. J Gen Virol 1970;7:95.)*

the plasma membrane but may involve other membranes in the cell. Enveloped viruses are not infectious until they have acquired their envelopes. Therefore, infectious progeny virions typically do not accumulate within the infected cell.

Viral maturation is sometimes an inefficient process. Excess amounts of viral components may accumulate and be involved in the formation of inclusion bodies in the cell. As a result of the profound deleterious effects of viral replication, cellular cytopathic effects eventually develop and the cell dies. There are instances, however, in which the cell is not damaged by the virus and long-term, persistent infections evolve.

Summary of Viral Replication

The molecular events discussed above are summarized in Figure 57.9. Viruses with genomes containing double-stranded nucleic acid proceed along most of the steps shown in the figure. Viruses with single-stranded nucleic acid genomes utilize only some of the steps. With RNA-containing viruses, the replicative cycle is not divided cleanly into early and late phases as it is with most DNA-containing viruses. Also, as noted above, not all viruses are enveloped in membranes.

VIRAL INTERFERENCE

Infection of either cell cultures or whole animals with two viruses often leads to inhibition of multiplication of one of the viruses, an effect called *interference*. Interference in animals is distinct from specific immunity. Furthermore, interference does not occur with all viral combinations; two viruses may infect and multiply within the same cell as efficiently as in single infections.

Several mechanisms have been elucidated as causes of interference:

1. One virus may inhibit the ability of the second to absorb to the cell, either by blocking its receptors (retroviruses, enteroviruses) or by destroying its receptors (orthomyxoviruses).
2. One virus may compete with the second for components of the replication apparatus (e.g., polymerase, translation initiation factor).
3. The first virus may cause the infected cell to produce an inhibitor (e.g., interferon) that prevents replication of the second virus.

When this phenomenon occurs between unrelated viruses, it is called *heterologous interference*. When it occurs

FIGURE 57.9. *Becker's diagram of molecular events in the replication of viruses. (Reproduced with permission from Jawetz E, Melnick JL, Adelberg EA. Review of medical microbiology. 17th ed. Norwalk, CT: Appleton and Lange, 1987.)*

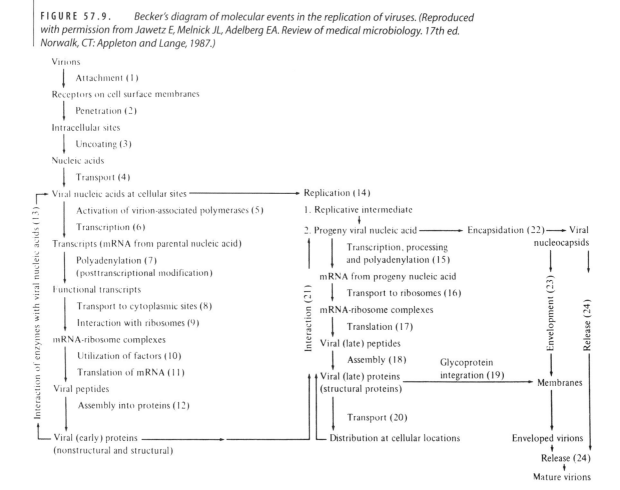

between related viruses, it is called *homologous interference*. Most viruses have the capacity to interfere with their own replication (*autointerference*). In this case, defective non-infectious particles are produced at the expense of complete virus when high multiplicities of infection are used. Autointerference may have a role in the establishment of persistent virus infections.

EFFECTS OF VIRAL REPLICATION ON CELLS

The effects of viral replication on affected cells are highly variable. The outcome of the cell-virus interaction varies from no detectable effect to profound morphologic and biochemical alterations that can lead to cell destruction. The various types of cell-virus interactions are summarized in Table 57.5. Some viruses are able to replicate in host cells without producing detectable effects. These steady-state infections or persistent infections are most frequently observed in cells infected with enveloped RNA viruses (e.g., bovine viral diarrhea virus, paramyxovirus SV5).

A large number of viruses can produce cell damage, which ultimately leads to the destruction of infected cells. Morphologic alterations of the infected cells, such as pyknosis and rounding of cells, precede cell lysis. These changes are collectively referred to as *cytopathic effect* (*CPE*). The mechanisms for CPE formation in infected cells are still unclear. Several factors, however, may play an important role in causing cell death: 1) depression or complete shutdown of cellular macromolecular synthesis either by viral structural proteins (e.g., adenovirus, reovirus) or by inhibitory proteins for cellular activity coded by the viral genome (e.g., poliovirus, herpesvirus), or 2) activation and release of lysosomal enzymes into cytoplasm of infected cells (e.g., adenoviruses).

In the course of many viral multiplications within cells, viral-specific structures called *inclusion bodies* may be produced. They become far larger than the individual viral particle and often have an affinity for acid dyes (e.g., eosin). They may be situated in the nucleus (herpesvirus), in the cytoplasm (poxvirus), or in both (measles virus). In many viral infections, the inclusion bodies are the site of development of the virions (the virus factories). In some infections (molluscum contagiosum), the inclusion body consists of masses of viral particles in the process of replication. In others (as in the intranuclear inclusion body of herpesvirus), the virus appears to have multiplied within the nucleus early in the infection, and the inclusion body appears to be a remnant of viral multiplication. Variations in the appearance of inclusion material depend largely upon the tissue fixative used.

The presence of inclusion bodies may be of considerable diagnostic aid. The intracytoplasmic inclusion in nerve cells, the Negri body, is pathognomonic for rabies.

Several viruses (e.g., respiratory syncytial virus, herpesvirus, visna virus, avian infectious bronchitis virus) cause fusion of infected cells leading to syncytia formation. The mechanism of virus-induced cell fusion is not fully understood. Cell transformation is induced by a number of RNA and DNA viruses (e.g., retroviruses, adenovirus, herpesvirus, polyomavirus). Transformed cells are characterized by loss of contact inhibition, altered morphology, indefinite growth, reduced serum requirement, chromosome aberrations, and antigenic alterations on cell surfaces.

VIRAL GENETICS

Genetic analysis is a powerful approach toward understanding the structure and function of the viral genome, its gene products, and their roles in infection and disease.

Variation in viral properties is of great importance in veterinary medicine. Viruses that have stable antigens on their surfaces (parvovirus, canine distemper virus) can be controlled by vaccination. Other viruses that exist as many antigenic types (rhinoviruses) or change constantly (equine influenza viruses) are difficult to control by vaccination; viral genetics may help develop more effective vaccines. Some types of viral infections recur repetitively (parainfluenza viruses, togaviruses) or persist (retroviruses, herpesviruses) in the presence of antibody and may be better controlled by antiviral drugs. Genetic analysis will help identify virus-specific processes that may be targets for the development of antiviral drugs.

The following terms are basic to a discussion of genetics: *Genotype* refers to the genetic constitution of an organism. *Phenotype* refers to the observable properties of an organism, which are produced by the genotype in cooperation with the environment. A *mutation* is a heritable change in the genotype. The *genome* is the sum of the genes of an organism.

MAPPING OF VIRAL GENOMES

Recent advances in animal viral genetics using restriction enzymes and other biochemical techniques have facilitated identification of viral gene products and the mapping of these on the viral genome. Biochemical and physical mapping can usually be done much more rapidly than genetic mapping using classic genetic techniques.

The technique of reassortment mapping has been used with influenza A viruses, which have a genome of eight

Table 57.5.   Types of Viral Effects on Cells

Virus	Cell	Type of Effect on Cells	Production of Virus
Bovine viral diarrhea virus	Bovine	None	+
Foot-and-mouth virus	Bovine	Cytopathic	+
Equine adenovirus	Equine	Inclusion bodies	+
Bovine respiratory syncytial virus	Bovine	Syncytia formation	+
Polyoma virus	Hamster	Transformation	−
Polyoma virus	Mouse	Cytopathic	+

FIGURE 57.10. *Illustration of principles of restriction endonuclease cleavage site analysis. The linear DNA (double-stranded) genomes of three hypothetical viruses to be compared are indicated as I, II, III. Suppose a specific nucleotide sequence, e.g., GAATTC, the cleavage site for nuclease EcoR1, occurs at four sites in each genome as indicated by small arrows. Genomes I and II are identical except for a substantial DNA insertion mutation in genome II. Genome III has none of the sequences in question located in positions analogous to genomes I or II. Cleavage of these DNAs at the sites marked by arrows results in five fragments (A to E) in each case. If these DNA fragments are separated according to size in adjacent tracks in a gel electrophoresis experiment, the result will be as diagrammed: fragments B, C, D, and E of samples I and II will comigrate and fragment A from each virus will differ. The fragments from genome III will comigrate with none of those from genomes I and II. It should be noted that knowledge of the cleavage site maps at the top is not essential to be able to deduce the fact that genomes I and II are related to each other but not to genome III. (Reproduced with permission from Summers WC, Yale J. Molecular epidemiology of DNA viruses: application of restriction endonuclease cleavage site analysis. Biol Med 1980;53:55.)*

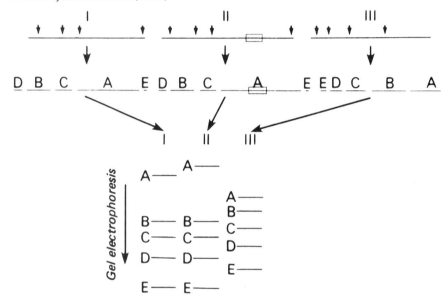

segments of RNA, each coding for one viral protein. Under suitable conditions, the RNA genome segments and the polypeptides of different influenza A viruses migrate at different rates in polyacrylamide gels, so that strains can be distinguished. By analyzing the recombinants (reassortants) formed between different influenza viruses, the RNA segment coding for each protein has been determined. Similar experiments with temperature-sensitive mutants have shown the biologic function of various polypeptides. Reassortants are being analyzed to determine which viral proteins are responsible for virulence in humans and animals.

The use of restriction endonucleases to identify specific strains or isolates of DNA viruses is illustrated in Figure 57.10. Viral DNA is isolated and incubated with a specific endonuclease until DNA sequences susceptible to the nuclease are cleaved. The fragments are then resolved on the basis of size by gel electrophoresis. The large fragments are most retarded by the sieving effect of the gel, so that an inverse relationship between size and migration is observed. The position of the DNA fragments can be determined by radioautography on x-ray film if the viral DNA is labeled. Such physical mapping techniques have been extremely useful in distinguishing viral types

in systems in which the viruses cannot be cultured (e.g., papillomaviruses).

Detailed physical maps can be prepared for DNA viruses by using a variety of restriction endonucleases. The position in the genome of given DNA sequences can be determined quite precisely.

Physical maps can be correlated with genetic maps if the latter are available. This allows viral gene products to be mapped to individual regions of the genome defined by the restriction enzyme fragments. Transcription of mRNAs throughout the replication cycle can be assigned to specific DNA fragments. Using mutagens, it is also possible to alter isolated fragments of viral DNA in order to introduce mutations into defined regions of the genome. Viral genome fragments generated by polymerase chain reaction (PCR) can be used in place of restriction enzyme fragments in mapping and mutagenesis studies.

SELECTED REFERENCES

Anderson WE, Diacumakos EG. Genetic engineering in mammalian cells. Sci Am 1981;245:106.

Boettiger D. Animal virus pseudotypes. Prog Med Virol 1979; 25:37.

Diener TO. Viroids. In: Maramorosch K, Murphy EA, Shatkin AJ, eds. Advances in virus research. Vol. 28. New York: Academic, 1983:241–283.

Fields BN, Knipe DM, Howley PM, et al. eds. Virology. 3rd ed. New York: Raven, 1996.

Harrison SC. Virus structure: high resolution perspectives. In: Maramorosch K, Murphy EA, Shatkin AJ, eds. Advances in virus research. Vol. 28. New York: Academic, 1983: 175–240.

Murphy FA, Fauquet CM, Bishop DHL, et al. Virus taxonomy. The classification and nomenclature of viruses. Sixth report of the international committee on taxonomy of viruses. New York: Springer-Verlag, 1994.

Prusiner SB. Biology and genetics of prion diseases. Annu Rev Microbiol 1994;48:655.

Prusiner SB, Scott M, Foster D. Transgenetic studies implicate interactions between homologous PrP isoforms in scrapie prion replication. Cell 1990;63:673.

Rossmann MG, Johnson JE. Icosahedral RNA virus structure. Annu Rev Biochem 1989;58:533.

58 Pathogenesis of Viral Diseases

YUAN CHUNG ZEE

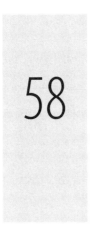

VIRUS–HOST RELATIONSHIPS

The outcomes of virus–host relationships vary depending on several factors, including the virus–cell interaction, species of the host, routes of viral exposure, modes of viral dissemination, and host resistance. Most viral-infected animal hosts that veterinarians see show clinical symptoms. It is important to recall that infection with a microorganism, in this case an animal virus, does not always result in clinical disease. The majority of virus–animal relationships end in asymptomatic or subclinical infection, and in some instances the virus is not even capable of establishing a relationship with the resistant animal host. The potential consequences of virus–animal relationships are shown in Table 58.1.

There are several major routes of viral entry into a host: the respiratory, alimentary, and urogenital routes and direct transmission (such as by an insect or animal bite). Successful establishment of viral infection depends on the presence of susceptible cell receptors and the physicochemical nature of the viral agent. Viruses infecting animals via the alimentary tract usually are resistant to low pH and enzymes in the digestive tract.

MODES OF DISSEMINATION OF VIRUSES WITHIN THE HOSTS

Viruses cause two basic patterns of infection: localized and generalized (Fig 58.1). In localized infections, viral multiplication and cellular damage remain localized near the site of entry (e.g., the skin or the mucous membranes of the respiratory, gastrointestinal, or genital tract), where the virus may spread from the first infected cells to neighboring cells by diffusion and cell contact. Rhinovirus infection of the nasal epithelial cells is a good example of a localized infection in which the virus does not spread to other parts of the respiratory tract. Other respiratory viruses, such as parainfluenza, influenza, and respiratory syncytial virus, replicate in cells at the portal of entry and also extend the infection to the cells of the trachea, bronchioles, and alveoli to produce bronchopneumonia of the infected species.

Generalized infections develop through several sequential steps: 1) the virus undergoes primary replication at the site of entry and in regional lymph nodes, 2) progeny virus spreads through blood (primary viremia) and lymphatics to additional parenchymal organs, where 3) further viral replication takes place, 4) virus is disseminated to the other target organs via a secondary viremia, and 5) it multiplies further in these target organs where it causes cellular damage, lesions, and clinical disease.

The asymptomatic period before the appearance of clinical disease is the incubation period. Overt disease begins only after virus becomes widely disseminated in the body and has attained maximum titers. It is at this stage of the infection that the veterinarian usually is first alerted. Canine distemper is a good example of a generalized infection. The canine distemper virus initiates the infection at the site of entry, but then disseminates through the blood or the lymphatic system to produce generalized infection with involvement of a variety of target organs (Fig 58.2). The sequence of events during the incubation period and development of signs of disease in experimental canine distemper infections indicate that the different clinical symptoms observed in the disease depend on which of the various organ systems are infected by the virus. Furthermore, not all viremic phases are characterized by free viruses in the blood. For some viruses, including the canine distemper virus, peripheral leukocytes and macrophages can serve as host cells. Infected peripheral white cells can serve as carriers to disseminate virus to target organs. Some viruses, such as hog cholera virus or parvovirus, can associate with red blood cells of the infected host. Viral particles in the blood are removed by phagocytic cells lining the reticuloendothelial system, and rate of removal is related to the size of the viral particles. Replication of virus in the parenchymal organs of vascular endothelial cells is necessary to maintain viremia for any period of time. The dissemination of virus to the central nervous system (CNS) can occur by viremia or, in the case of rabies, by transmission along peripheral nerves.

Viral infections that occur without producing overt disease are very common and have great epidemiologic importance in that they are a source for dissemination of virus and they confer immunity. Several factors are involved in producing inapparent infections: 1) the nature of the virus (e.g., virulent or attenuated strains), 2) degree of host immunity, 3) appearance of viral interference, and 4) failure of the virus to reach the target organ (e.g., due to the blood-brain barrier).

HOST RESPONSES TO VIRAL INFECTIONS

Resistance of intact organisms to viral infection depends to some extent on factors that act indiscriminately on all or many viruses and are therefore called *nonspecific*. These include hormonal factors, temperature, inhibitors other than antibody, and phagocytes. Phagocytosis is an important defense mechanism in bacterial infections. However, many viral agents are capable of attacking leukocytes and infecting macrophages, and thus these infected cells can serve as a vehicle to spread virus through the host.

HUMORAL AND CELLULAR IMMUNITY

In common with many biologically active substances, viruses are antigenic and stimulate production of classic circulating antibodies, which can be demonstrated by the

Table 58.1. Potential Consequences of Virus–Animal Relationships

1. Animal is resistant to viral infection → no relationship established
2. Asymptomatic of subclinical infection → recovery or persistent infection
3. Acute viral infection → death, recovery, or persistent infection
4. Chronic viral infection → recurrent clinical disease, or persistent infection
5. Tumor formation

usual serologic procedures. Thus, viruses may be studied in the same manner as bacteria by means of complement-fixation reactions, agglutination, precipitation, and gel diffusion techniques. The basic principles governing these tests are identical with those used in bacteriology and require no additional comment.

However, some serological reactions, such as viral neutralization, are unique for viruses and play an important role in terminating primary viral infection, limiting viremia, and preventing disease and reinfection. When preparations of virus are mixed with appropriate antisera and the mixtures are inoculated in susceptible hosts, infection will not occur if the antisera contain virus-neutralizing antibody. Three classes of immunoglobulins, IgG, IgM, and IgA, can serve as neutralizing antibodies. The interaction of virus and antibody, particularly antibodies specific to the viral antigens responsible for attachment to specific cell receptors, results in a virus-antibody complex formation. This formation blocks attachment of virus to cell receptors, and to a lesser extent prevents the penetration of virus into the susceptible cell. It is possible to recover infectious virus from such apparently inert virus-antibody mixtures by simple dilution or centrifugation, suggesting that the virus and antibody may be linked together in a loose combination in the initial stages of reaction.

The interaction between virus and antibody does not physically alter viral structure; however, the complement system and antiviral antibody can induce lysis of enveloped viruses as well as destroy the virus-infected cells.

Cellular immunity in viral infections, discussed in Chapter 2, is another important factor in host resistance to some viral infections. The destruction of virus-infected cells by immune lymphocytes can limit the dissemination of virus, particularly in instances where virus is trans-

FIGURE 58.1. *Modes of viral dissemination within the host.*

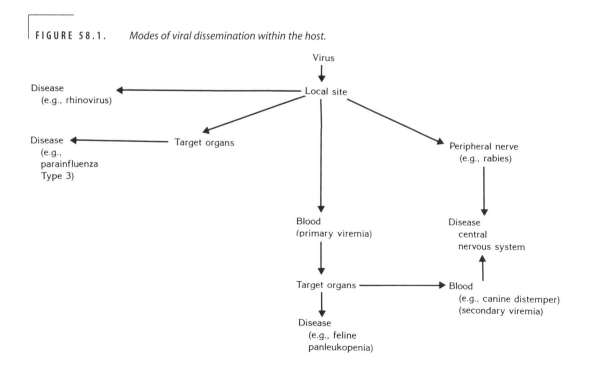

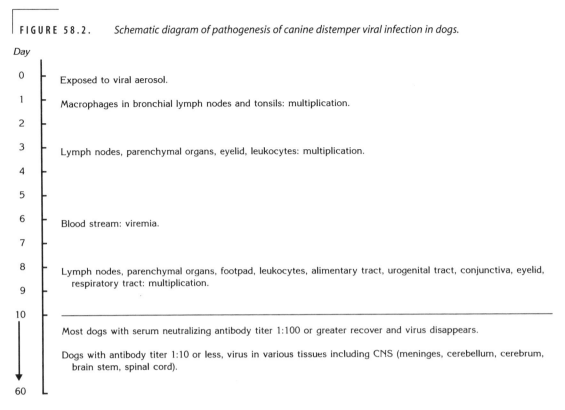

FIGURE 58.2.   *Schematic diagram of pathogenesis of canine distemper viral infection in dogs.*

Day	
0	Exposed to viral aerosol.
1	Macrophages in bronchial lymph nodes and tonsils: multiplication.
2	
3	Lymph nodes, parenchymal organs, eyelid, leukocytes: multiplication.
4	
5	
6	Blood stream: viremia.
7	
8	Lymph nodes, parenchymal organs, footpad, leukocytes, alimentary tract, urogenital tract, conjunctiva, eyelid, respiratory tract: multiplication.
9	
10	Most dogs with serum neutralizing antibody titer 1:100 or greater recover and virus disappears.
	Dogs with antibody titer 1:10 or less, virus in various tissues including CNS (meninges, cerebellum, cerebrum, brain stem, spinal cord).
60	

Figure 55.2. *Schematic diagram of pathogenesis of canine distemper viral infection in dogs.*

mitted from infected to noninfected cells through cell fusion. Recent evidence also indicates that macrophages play a role in host resistance to viral infections. Macrophages are a major part of an inflammatory response, and they can be activated either by interaction with viruses or by the soluble products produced by virus reacting with lymphocytes. Activated macrophages have been shown to participate in a wide range of host responses to viral infections, including phagocytosis of virus-antibody complexes, production of interferon, cytotoxicity for virus-infected cells, and immunoregulatory functions.

INTERFERON

Interferon is comprised of a group of cell proteins belonging to the superfamily of cytokines. They play an important role in modulating the immune system of the host animal, in the differentiation of certain cells, in conferring antiviral resistance on sensitive cells, and in exerting anticancer effects. The ability to induce interferon synthesis is a rather general property among different viruses. Synthetic polyribonucleotides have been found to be active interferon inducers. Numerous types of animal cells, upon interaction with an inducer, possess the ability to synthesize interferon. Any laboratory study of interferon requires the use of some method for its quantitative assay and so far the only way to assay interferon is by demonstrating its biologic activity — the induction of antiviral resistance in susceptible cells. The apparent interferon titer varies significantly, depending upon the type of cell culture and test virus used.

Most interferons fall into three categories: alpha, beta, and gamma (Table 58.2). All three types may be produced during the course of a viral infection. The mode of action of interferon in inhibiting viral replication has been widely investigated and two likely mechanisms have been proposed (Fig 58.3). One mechanism, it is suggested, involves the production in interferon-treated cells of a protein kinase (P1/eIF2alpha kinase), which in the presence of double-stranded RNA, blocks initiation of protein synthesis by phosphorylating the protein synthesis initiating factor eIF-2. The proposal for the other mechanism suggests that the interferon-treated cell produces an enzyme, 2′–5′ synthetase, which, in the presence of adenosine triphosphate (ATP) and dsRNA, synthesizes a group of oligoadenylates collectively known as 2′–5′A. 2′–5′A in turn activates a specific 2′3′A dependent endonuclease, which degrades viral RNA and cellular RNA preventing protein synthesis.

Besides its action on viral replication, interferon has other effects on cells. These include effects on cell multiplication and regulation of such cellular functions as phagocytosis, production of antibodies and lymphokines by lymphocytes, expression of cell surface antigens, and cytotoxicity of cellular immunity. Available evidence indicates that interferon plays an important role in host resistance to viral infection.

Table 58.2. Types of Interferon

Type of Interferon	Cell Source	Type of Inducer	Glycosylation	Action	Number of Subtypes
Alpha	Leukocytes	Viruses, synthetic dsRNA	No	Inhibits protein synthesis	More than 20
Beta	Fibroblasts, epithelial cells	Viruses, synthetic dsRNA	Yes	Inhibits protein synthesis	1
Gamma	Lymphocytes	Antigens, mitogens	Yes	Activates cytotoxic T cells, macrophages, NK cells	1

FIGURE 58.3. *Mechanisms of interferon action on protein synthesis.*

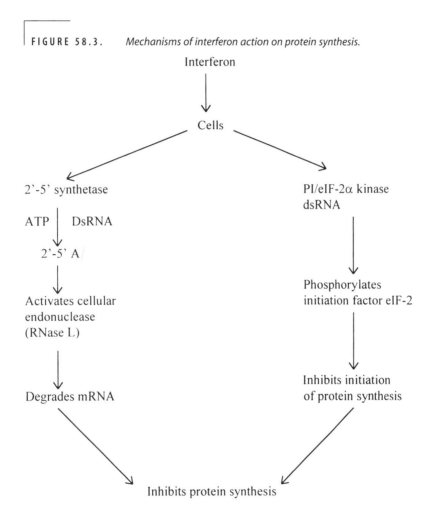

VIRAL IMMUNOSUPPRESSION

Several viruses of veterinary importance can infect lymphocytes, including canine distemper virus, feline panleukopenia virus, feline leukemia virus, bovine viral diarrhea virus, hog cholera virus, Newcastle disease virus, and infectious bursal disease virus of chickens. The destruction of lymphoid tissues by the viruses suppresses or compromises the immune response, subjecting the host to other opportunistic bacterial or viral infections. Recent studies have shown that the envelope protein P15E of retroviruses could cause profound immunosuppression and may be important in promoting tumor formation.

Many species of domestic animals (equine, bovine, ovine, porcine, canine, feline) suffer from immune deficiency diseases. Several mechanisms, including inherited deficiencies in the production of lymphocyte, neutrophil, and complement system and failure to acquire passive immunity, are responsible for this condition. Immunodeficient animals often suffer serious infections with ubiquitous viruses. A good example is the fatal respiratory tract infection of Arabian foals with combined immunodeficiency disorder (lack of production of functional T and B lymphocytes) by equine adenovirus.

Between 1974 and 1978, 12 reported cases of canine rabies were associated with the use of a modified live virus rabies vaccine in California. This finding led to the cancellation of approval for the use of this rabies vaccine in dogs by the California Department of Health. In view of the development of paralytic polio in immunodeficient humans vaccinated with modified live poliomyelitis viral vaccine, the dogs in this case could have been immunodeficient.

PERSISTENT VIRAL INFECTION

In inapparent persistent or latent infections, overt disease usually is not produced and virus is not eliminated from the host. This host–parasite equilibrium is achieved in different ways by different viruses and hosts: 1) by immunologic tolerance permitting a virus to replicate and persist without producing disease (e.g., lymphocyte chroniomeningitis viral infection of mice), 2) by association between a pathogenic virus and host organism that gives rise to signs of infection only when induced by some trigger mechanism (infectious bovine rhinotracheitis in cattle), and 3) by replication of viral nucleic acid without viral maturation (Shope papillomavirus in domestic rabbits).

SELECTED REFERENCES

Appel MJG. Pathogenesis of canine distemper. Am J Vet Res 1969; 30:1167.

Braciale TJ, ed. Viruses and the immune system. Semin Virol 1993;4:81.

Dimmock NJ. Neutralization of animal viruses. Curr Top Microbiol Immunol 1993;183:1.

Fields BN, Greene MI. Genetic and molecular mechanisms of viral pathogenesis: implications for prevention and treatment. Nature 1982;300:19.

Johnson HM, Bazer FW, Szente BE, Jarpe MA. How interferons fight disease. Sci Am 1994;270:68.

Marx JL. Persistent infections: the role of viruses. Science 1977; 196:151.

McChesney MB, Oldstone MBA. Viruses perturb lymphocyte functions: selected principles characterizing virus-induced immunosuppression. Annu Res Immunol 1987;5:279.

Mims CA. The pathogenetic basis of viral tropism. Am J Pathol 1989;135:447.

Oldstone MBA. Molecular anatomy of viral persistence. J Virol 1991;65:6381.

Perryman LE. Mechanisms of immune deficiency diseases of animals. J Am Vet Med Assoc 1982;181:1097.

Samuel CE. Antiviral actions of interferon: interferon-regulated cellular proteins and their surprisingly selective antiviral activities. Virology 1991;183:1.

59 *Parvoviridae*

YUAN CHUNG ZEE

Parvoviruses are nonenveloped, small (21 ± 4 nm in diameter), and contain a linear single-stranded DNA genome (MW 2.0 × 10^6 daltons). Some members of this group are the causative agents of specific diseases (Table 59.1). Three important animal diseases — feline panleukopenia, canine parvoviral disease, and Aleutian disease in mink — are caused by serologically and genetically related parvoviruses.

FELINE PANLEUKOPENIA

DISEASE

Feline panleukopenia is a highly contagious, acute viral infection of cats characterized by high fever (104°F to 105°F), anorexia, depression, and vomiting. The incubation period of the disease is usually 4 days. Cats of all ages are susceptible to infection. They can be infected by the oral or respiratory routes. Leukopenia and thrombocytopenia are common. Other frequent clinical signs are dehydration, diarrhea, and rapid loss of condition leading to death within a few days. Mortality is highest among kittens. Intrauterine infection with feline panleukopenia virus may lead to neonatal death or congenital abnormalities of the central nervous system (CNS) manifested by cerebellar ataxia seen in kittens 2 to 3 weeks after birth.

ETIOLOGIC AGENT

Physical, Chemical, and Antigenic Properties

Feline panleukopenia virus is a typical parvovirus with physical and chemical properties similar to those of the canine parvovirus and the mink enteritis virus. Feline panleukopenia virus is more resistant to heat, being inactivated at 80°C for two hours; canine parvovirus requires 1 hour.

Antigenically, it is not feasible to distinguish between feline panleukopenia virus and mink enteritis virus. DNA analysis with restriction endonucleases reveals no difference between feline panleukopenia virus and raccoon parvovirus, but it can differentiate between feline panleukopenia virus, canine parvovirus, and mink enteritis virus.

Resistance to Physical and Chemical Agents

Feline panleukopenia virus is very resistant to environmental factors and some commercial disinfectants. A 0.175% sodium hypochlorite solution (Clorox 1:30) is the most effective and practical virucidal disinfectant.

Infectivity for Other Species and Culture Systems

Feline panleukopenia virus infects predominantly domestic cats, although other members of the family *Felidae* can also be infected with this virus. In 1947 in Canada, a virus indistinguishable from feline panleukopenia virus was found to be responsible for outbreaks of severe enteritis in ranch mink. The same virus can produce disease in raccoons and in coatimundi. A previously nonexisting host-range mutant of feline panleukopenia virus, the canine parvovirus Type 2, has evolved in recent years to produce the canine parvoviral disease in dogs.

Feline panleukopenia virus grows in primary or continuous feline kidney cell cultures but not in canine cell cultures. It can be assayed by the plaque method in feline kidney cells under agarose overlay.

HOST–VIRUS RELATIONSHIP

Distribution, Reservoir, and Transmission

The disease in cats caused by feline panleukopenia virus is worldwide in incidence. Infected cats serve as the primary reservoir. Both infected cats suffering from acute disease and those having clinically inapparent infection excrete virus in their urine, feces, and body secretions. The infection spreads rapidly by contact with contaminated utensils, cages, and bedding.

Pathogenesis and Pathology

In kittens experimentally infected intranasally or orally with feline panleukopenia virus, cell-free viremia is present for 1 to 7 days after infection. Severe and prolonged leukopenia is seen in all infected animals. At 48 hours after inoculation, high titers of virus are detected in thymus, spleen, mesenteric lymph nodes, cerebellum, and cerebrospinal fluid. Virus is found in urine 2 to 22 days after inoculation and in feces at 22 days after inoculation. Virus disappears from most tissues in 2 weeks;

Table 59.1. Diseases Caused by Parvoviruses

Vernacular Name	Disease	Natural Host
Feline panleukopenia virus	Enteritis, ataxia	Cats
Mink enteritis virus	Enteritis	Mink
Canine parvovirus type 2	Enteritis, myocarditis	Dogs
Porcine parvovirus	Neonatal death, infertility	Swine
Bovine parvovirus	None	Cattle
Minute virus of canines (Type 1)	None	Dogs
Minute virus of mice	None	Mice
Aleutian mink disease	Aleutian disease	Mink
Kilham rat virus	None	Rats
Hemorrhagic encephalopathy	Hemorrhagic encephalopathy	Rats
Goose parvovirus	Hepatitis	Goose

however, in some instances, small amounts of virus may persist in some tissues, such as the kidney, for 1 year.

Macroscopic lesions prominently involve the intestine and the thymus. There are swelling and dilatation of the small intestine, and the thymus is reduced in size in young animals. Microscopic lesions most frequently observed in the intestinal tract are necrosis of the epithelium of the intestinal crypts and erosion of the epithelial villi. There is a marked depletion of lymphocytes in the follicles and paracortical tissue of lymph nodes, thymus, and spleen. Regenerative lymphoid hypoplasia may be present in the later phase of the disease. In cats with cerebellar ataxia from intrauterine infection, a loss of the granule cell layer, perivascular cuffing, and neuronal degeneration are found in the cerebellum.

Host Responses to Infection

Neutralizing antibodies first appear in cats 6 to 7 days after infection, reaching a maximum level by 10 to 12 days. Hemagglutination-inhibiting antibodies rise from the fourth day after infection, reaching a peak on the seventh day. These antibodies can persist in cats for several years. Maternal antibody with neutralizing titer of 30 or greater against feline panleukopenia virus protects kittens against viral infection, but it also interferes with active immunization by modified live or inactivated feline panleukopenia viral vaccines.

LABORATORY DIAGNOSIS

Clinical signs, the presence of leukopenia, and histopathological examination can be used for the presumptive diagnosis of feline panleukopenia. The diagnosis can be confirmed by one of the following laboratory methods: 1) isolation of feline panleukopenia virus from the feces or urine on feline kidney cells, 2) detection of viral antigen in infected tissues by immunofluorescence with a specific feline panleukopenia conjugate, 3) demon-

stration of a rising titer of neutralizing or hemagglutination-inhibiting antibody using paired serum samples.

TREATMENT AND CONTROL

There is no effective treatment for feline panleukopenia. Transfusion of concentrated leukocyte suspension to a leukopenic cat is helpful in some cases. Antiserum treatment is only effective in cats not showing signs of disease at the time of its administration.

Both inactivated and modified live feline panleukopenia viral vaccines are commercially available for veterinary use. These products elicit an immunity that is effective in preventing the disease.

CANINE PARVOVIRAL DISEASE

DISEASE

Parvoviral disease in dogs is an acute viral infection characterized by the sudden onset of diarrhea, vomiting, anorexia, and fever. Depression, lymphopenia, and dehydration are common among affected dogs. Mortality is higher in puppies than adults. Puppies sometimes develop myocarditis without clinical symptoms of enteritis.

The disease is found worldwide. It was first recognized in North America in 1978, and shortly afterward it was reported in Europe, Australia, and Asia. Canine parviral disease is probably caused by a "new" pathogen, the canine parvovirus Type 2, which is a variant of feline panleukopenia virus. Parvoviruses isolated from feline, raccoon, and fox probably have been circulating in countries around the world since before the twentieth century and variants of these parvoviruses emerged as ancestors to the canine parvovirus Type 2 in the early 1970s. Canine parvovirus Type 2 has continued to change in its new host, the dog. New variant forms of the virus have been recently identified by monoclonal antibody typing or by sequencing the DNA of the capsid protein genes. These new variants have been designated as canine parvovirus Type-2a and Type-2b. The minute virus of canines that does not produce disease in dogs has been designated as canine parvovirus Type 1.

ETIOLOGIC AGENT

Physical, Chemical, and Antigenic Properties

Canine parvovirus Type 2 is a nonenveloped spherical particle that has a diameter of 21 ± 3 nm (Fig 59.1). The virus has a sedimentation coefficient of 110 S and has a buoyant density of 1.38 to 1.44 g/cm^3 in CsCl. It resists heat inactivation at 60°C for 60 minutes and is stable at pH 3.0. The viral nucleic acid is a single-stranded DNA with 5000 nucleotides. The viral capsid is composed of

FIGURE 59.1. *Canine parvovirus in fecal materials. 200,000×. (Courtesy of LA Ibrahim and LC May.)*

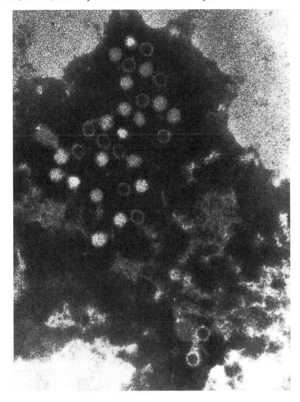

four polypeptides, which agglutinate red blood cells of pig and rhesus monkey. It is possible to distinguish between the canine parvovirus Type 2, the feline panleukopenia virus, and the mink enteritis virus by restriction endonuclease cleavage site analysis of the viral genome and by sequencing of the viral DNA.

Resistance to Physical and Chemical Agents

Parvovirus is very resistant to environmental factors, such as extremes of temperature, pH, and some disinfectants. The virus can persist for long periods in premises where infected dogs are kept and can be transmitted to other areas by fomites. It can be inactivated by common bleach such as Clorox (1:30).

Infectivity for Other Species and Culture Systems

Canine parvovirus Type 2 infects dogs of all breeds and other members of the family *Canidae*, such as maned wolf, crab-eating fox, coyote, and bush dog. Domestic cats without antibodies are susceptible to experimental infection but remain asymptomatic.

Canine parvovirus Type 2 can be propagated in primary cell cultures of canine or feline fetal lung and kidney. Continuous cell lines, such as canine cell line A72 and feline cell lines NLFK and CRFK, can be used to propagate the virus. Bovine cells and cells of mink, raccoon,

and African green monkey support the replication of canine parvovirus Type 2.

HOST–VIRUS RELATIONSHIP

Distribution, Reservoir, and Transmission

Parvoviral infection in dogs is prevalent in many areas of the world. Dogs and other *Canidae* are susceptible. Since canine parvovirus Type 2 appears to be a variant of feline panleukopenia virus, cats may be a potential reservoir.

There have been reports of humans suffering signs of enteritis after being associated with dogs infected with canine parvovirus Type 2. However, serologic surveys of such persons (who show signs of diarrhea and vomiting) and viral isolation attempts from feces and vomitus failed to yield any evidence for transmission of canine parvovirus to humans from dogs. Dogs infected with *Campylobacter jejuni* can have symptoms similar to those of parvoviral infection, and *Campylobacter jejuni* is transmitted from dogs to humans.

Dogs infected with parvovirus excrete infectious virus in their feces for up to 10 days after the onset of disease, and the disease can be transmitted from one animal to another by water or food contaminated with feces. Canine parvovirus Type 2 is very resistant to environmental factors and can persist under adverse conditions for a long period. Prompt disinfection (with Clorox) of premises where infected animals are being kept and vaccination of puppies with canine parvoviral vaccines prior to being introduced into such premises are important steps in preventing this disease.

Pathogenesis and Pathology

In experimental canine parvovirus Type 2 disease, cell-free viremia is detected on days 2 to 5 after oral inoculation of puppies. Viremia usually precedes intestinal epithelial infection and fecal virus excretion. The initial sites of viral replication are the thymus, tonsils, retropharyngeal and mesenteric lymph nodes, and spleen. Widespread viral infection of intestinal mucosa occurs on the sixth day after inoculation. Fecal excretion of virus first becomes detectable on the third day after infection and reaches a peak on days 4 to 7. Most infected dogs stop excreting virus by the twelfth day.

Macroscopic lesions of canine parvoviral infection occur usually in the jejunum and ileum when animals are examined during severe enteric disease. There is a thickening of the intestinal wall along with congestion and subserosal hemorrhage. Enlargement and edema of the mesenteric lymph nodes are common. In acute parvoviral myocarditis, the principal lesion is in the myocardium, which is mottled by white streaks. Pulmonary edema with perivascular edema is often present.

Microscopic lesions associated with canine parvoviral infection are confined to organs with a high number of rapidly proliferating cells, such as the small intestine, lymph nodes, and bone marrow. The most frequent findings in the small intestine are necrosis of crypt epithelium and atrophy of epithelial villi. Regeneration of intestinal epithelium occurs in dogs surviving the acute phase of enteric dysfunction. Lymphocytolysis in the thymic cortex and germinal centers of lymph nodes is common and results in cellular depletion. In the myocardial form of parvoviral infection, the ventricular myocardium shows myofiber loss, multifocal myofiber necrosis, and infiltration by mononuclear cells.

Host Response to Infection

Dogs infected with parvovirus develop high, long-lasting antibody titers, which can be detected by hemagglutination-inhibition or viral neutralization tests. The immune responses to parvoviral infection include both a humoral component of the lymphoid system and a secretory component of the intestinal mucosa. High levels of both sero-IgM and copro-IgM and moderate levels of sero-IgG and copro-IgA are detected as early as 3 days after infection, reaching maximum at 7 days. Serum antibody to canine parvovirus Type 2 can persist for 24 months. Local intestinal immunity is probably more important than humoral immunity in developing resistance to canine parvoviral enteritis.

LABORATORY DIAGNOSIS

Clinical symptoms, history, contrast radiography, and histopathological examinations are useful in a presumptive diagnosis of canine parvoviral disease. Laboratory procedures used to confirm the diagnosis include the following:

1. Isolation of canine parvovirus Type 2 from the feces of infected animals on susceptible cell cultures.
2. Detection of parvoviral antigen in the histological mucosal section, or fecal smear by the immunofluorescent antibody technique.
3. Demonstration of parvovirus in feces or infected tissue by electron microscopy or immunoelectron microscopy.
4. Identification of parvovirus in feces by hemagglutination test using swine red blood cells and the specific hemagglutination-inhibition by anticanine parvovirus antiserum.
5. Detection of parvovirus in feces by enzyme-linked immunosorbent assay (ELISA) using monoclonal antibodies to the canine parvovirus Type 2 hemagglutinating protein.
6. Demonstration of anticanine parvovirus antibody in serum by such serologic tests as hemagglutination inhibition, virus neutralization, or ELISA.
7. Identification of parvoviral nucleic acid in infected tissues by DNA hybridization.

The highest correlation is between the ELISA and the hemagglutination tests, and ELISA is the most sensitive and specific diagnostic test for canine parvoviral infec-

tion. Commercial ELISA test kits for detecting canine parvovirus in feces or canine parvovirus antibody in serum are now available for use by practitioners in the clinic.

TREATMENT AND CONTROL

Almost all severe cases of canine parvoviral disease show a marked decompensated metabolic acidosis. Treatment relies on replacing lost body fluids and correcting disturbed electrolyte balance and acidosis. Fluid therapy using a commercial 8.4% solution of sodium bicarbonate or lactated Ringer's solution is recommended. Intramuscular injection of a commercial dog hyperimmune serum (0.2 mg/kg body weight) is helpful in reducing the severity of the disease. The use of broad-spectrum antibiotics to prevent secondary bacterial infection is also indicated in most cases.

Vaccination of susceptible canine populations remains the best prophylaxis for canine parvoviral infection. Antibody levels correlate directly with the degree of protection. Currently, both inactivated and modified live parvoviral vaccines are commercially available. Inactivated parvoviral vaccine is generally prepared by treating virus with formalin, propiolactone, and binary ethylenimine (BEI) in serum-free media. Inactivated parvoviral vaccine induces active immunity but requires a booster dose in 2 to 3 weeks. The inactivated vaccine should have a high viral concentration and contain an effective adjuvant. Modified live parvoviral vaccine elicits the greatest antibody response, and a single dose of the vaccine can overcome maternal antibody to produce active immunity in puppies. Only a single dose of the live vaccine is needed to induce protection, and the efficacy of the vaccine is not diminished when it is mixed with other viral or bacterial vaccines. Inactivated or modified live feline panleukopenia vaccines also confer immunity to canine parvoviral infection, although they induce a lesser serum neutralizing antibody response than canine parvoviral vaccines. With the availability of commercial canine parvoviral vaccines, there is very little need to give feline panleukopenia vaccines for canine parvoviral infection.

PORCINE PARVOVIRAL INFECTION

DISEASE

The infection of swine by porcine parvovirus is widespread; the virus produces reproductive failure in swine and cutaneous lesions in piglets. Transplacental infection of fetuses leads to fetal death or mummification. Porcine parvovirus infection is a major cause of porcine fetal death. A rise in the number of sows returning to estrus after impregnation, followed by an increase in the number of stillborn and mummified piglets, frequently indicates parvoviral infection in a commercial swine herd.

ETIOLOGIC AGENT

Physical, Chemical, and Antigenic Properties

Porcine parvovirus is nonenveloped and has a diameter of 21 ± 1 nm. Purified virus has a buoyant density of 1.38 to 1.39 g/cm³ in CsCl. Porcine parvovirus has a single-stranded DNA genome, and its replicative form DNA is an infectious 5000-base pair molecule. The virus contains three major polypeptides.

There is only one serotype and porcine parvovirus is antigenically different from other parvoviruses. Restriction site mapping indicates homology among the genomes of porcine parvovirus, canine parvovirus, and feline panleukopenia virus. Porcine parvovirus agglutinates red blood cells of humans, monkeys, guinea pigs, chickens, rats, and mice.

Resistance to Physical and Chemical Agents

Porcine parvovirus is very resistant to heat, enzymes, and most commercial disinfectants. The virus is inactivated by heat at 73°C for 30 minutes or at 70°C for 1 hour, or by exposure to 0.5% sodium hypochlorite for 5 minutes, to 0.06% potassium dichloroisocyanurate for 5 minutes, or to 3% formaldehyde for 1 hour.

Infectivity for Other Species and Culture Systems

Porcine parvovirus apparently infects only swine. The virus can be propagated on primary or secondary cultures of fetal porcine kidney cells and swine testicle cells.

HOST–VIRUS RELATIONSHIP

Distribution, Reservoir, and Transmission

Serologic surveys of swine farms around the world indicate that porcine parvoviral infection is present in many herds. Infected swine serve as the reservoir of infection. Antibody to porcine parvovirus is widespread among warthog populations in Africa, which could act as a reservoir in that region. Infected swine develop a viremia and shed virus in oral secretions and feces. Since the porcine parvovirus can persist in the environment for long periods of time, contaminated premises can serve as the major reservoir and transmit the infection to susceptible animals. There is experimental evidence that rats can become infected with porcine parvovirus after systemic or oral exposure. However, rats do not shed enough virus to infect susceptible swine, and thus are an unlikely reservoir of porcine parvovirus.

PATHOGENESIS AND PATHOLOGY

Swine infected with porcine parvovirus produce antibodies without developing clinical disease or pathologic lesions. Fetal death occurs when gilts are infected transplacentally at 56 days of gestation. Litters of gilts exposed to porcine parvovirus at 70 days of gestation are also infected transplacentally, but the virus does not cause fetal death.

Macroscopic lesions are not seen in infected swine. Fetal resorption and mummification are the most frequent sequelae to fetal death. Microscopic lesions of infected fetuses consist primarily of extensive necrosis and mononuclear cell infiltration in many organs — the liver, heart, kidney, and cerebrum.

Host Responses to Infection

In piglets experimentally infected by porcine parvovirus via intranasal and oral inoculations, viremia is present between 2 and 6 days after infection, although no clinical disease is evident. Detectable hemagglutination inhibition antibody to porcine parvovirus in serum is demonstrated at 5 or 6 days. Infected sows have such antibodies in their blood and colostrum. The hemagglutination-inhibition titer of colostrum is five times higher than that of serum, piglets acquire HI antibodies via colostrum at 2 days after birth, and antibodies persist for 16 to 24 weeks. All piglets become seronegative by 26 weeks of age and susceptible to porcine parvoviral infection 1 week after they become seronegative.

LABORATORY DIAGNOSIS

An enzyme-linked immunosorbent assay (ELISA) for detection of parvovirus antigen in fetal tissues is a more specific and sensitive test than the fluorescent antibody and hemagglutination tests. A polymerase chain reaction (PCR) amplification method has also been developed for the detection of porcine parvovirus.

TREATMENT AND CONTROL

There is no treatment for reproductive failure produced by porcine parvovirus.

Vaccination remains the best method to ensure that gilts develop active immunity prior to being bred. Both vaccine inactivated by binary ethylenimine or formalin and modified live vaccine of porcine parvovirus can induce high hemagglutination-inhibition and neutralization antibodies in gilts. The vaccines have no adverse effects and are effective for preventing fetal loss in swine. A long-term vaccination program is a cost-effective method for controlling reproductive failure in pig herds infected with porcine parvovirus infection.

ALEUTIAN DISEASE IN MINK

DISEASE

Aleutian disease (AD) in mink is a chronic progressive disease characterized by anorexia, polydipsia, severe anemia, and hemorrhages. The disease has a long incubation period. Other pronounced characteristics of the disease in adult minks are plasmacytosis, uveitis, vascular damage, hypergammaglobulinemia, and glomerulonephritis, the last of which is caused by deposition of circulating immune complexes. In newborn mink kits, Aleutian disease virus (ADV) causes a fatal, acute interstitial pneumonitis. A genetic predisposition for the disease exists in Aleutian mink. It appears that mink homozygous for the recessive Aleutian gene has a genetic defect of preventing clearance of immune complexes from its circulation.

ETIOLOGIC AGENT

Physical, Chemical, and Antigenic Properties

Aleutian mink virus is 25 ± 1 nm in diameter and has a density of 1.42 to 1.44 g/cm^3 in CsCl. It contains a single-stranded DNA with a molecular weight of 1.4×10^6. Two major viral polypeptides have been identified. The Aleutian disease virus is antigenically unrelated to mink enteritis virus.

Resistance to Physical and Chemical Agents

Aleutian mink virus is inactivated by sodium hypochlorite, iodophor, glutaraldehyde, formalin, and a commercial disinfectant, O-Syl.

Infectivity for Other Species and Cell Systems

Aleutian disease virus infects mink of all types, although disease is more prevalent in the Aleutian mink. Ferrets can be infected with ADV, but they fail to develop clinical signs of the disease. The virus can be propagated in fetal mink kidney cell cultures or in feline cell lines.

HOST–VIRUS RELATIONSHIP

Distribution, Reservoir, and Transmission

Aleutian disease of mink is present in many mink ranches in the world. The virus is found in the blood, saliva, feces, and urine. Mink with overt clinical signs or with inapparent infection are the reservoirs of infection. The disease is transmitted by fecal–oral or respiratory routes.

Pathogenesis and Pathology

In mink experimentally infected with AD virus, viral antigen is first detected in cells of the intestine and kidney 3 to 6 days after infection. On day 6 or later, viral antigen is found in cells of spleen, liver, kidney, lymph nodes, and bone marrow. There is a significant increase in gamma globulin and anti-DNA antibody in sera of infected mink. The serum gamma globulin does not neutralize AD virus and formation of immune complexes has been detected in circulation as early as 2 weeks after infec-

tion. The glomerular deposition of immune complexes is the major cause of glomerulonephritis. Severity of glomerulonephritis is correlated with hypergammaglobulinemia, serum IgG, viral antibody titers, amount of immune complexes in serum, and amount of IgG deposited in glomeruli.

Enlarged kidneys and liver are seen in mink with AD. Microscopic lesions include plasmacytosis of the kidneys, liver, lymph nodes, and spleen, and fibrinoid degeneration of arteries. Dilation of the cerebrospinal canal is a prominent finding of newborn mink kids that have acquired AD in utero.

Host Responses to Infection

Hypergammaglobulinemia is the most prominent feature of mink infected with AD virus. In experimentally and naturally infected mink, most of the increased immunoglobulin and AD viral antibody is IgG. The first demonstrable AD viral antibody is IgM, and most infected mink have viral-specific IgM antibody for at least 85 days after infection. Aleutian disease viral infection also increases serum IgA levels. An excessive but ineffective humoral IgG response does not facilitate viral elimination.

LABORATORY DIAGNOSIS

A solid-phase radioimmune assay is the most sensitive test for detecting Aleutian disease viral antigen in tissues. With inhibition of antigen binding, the same radioimmune assay can be used to detect viral antibodies. Direct immunofluorescence and immunoperoxidase techniques can also be used to demonstrate AD viral antigen in tissues.

The counterimmunoelectrophoresis (CIE) test for detecting AD viral antibody is the best one available at present. With an efficacy of more than 90%, this test is commonly employed for finding positive reactors in mink ranches in North America and Europe.

TREATMENT AND CONTROL

No effective vaccines have been developed for the Aleutian disease of mink. Isolation and elimination of affected animals in mink ranches on the basis of serum CIE tests can be effective in controlling the disease.

SELECTED REFERENCES

Bloom ME, Kanno H, Mori S, Wolfinbarger JB. Aleutian mink disease: puzzles and paradigms. Infect Agents Dis 1994; 3:279.

Edwards EG, Fulker RH, Acree WM, Bandy DM. Use of a modified-live canine parvovirus vaccine in puppies with natural antibody. Vet Med Small Anim Clin 1982;77:1073.

Ishibashi K, Maede Y, Ohsugi T, et al. Serotherapy for dogs infected with canine parvovirus. Jpn J Vet Sci 1983;45:59.

Macartney L, McCandlish IA, Thompson H, Cornwell HJ. Canine parvovirus enteritis 1: clinical, hematological and pathological features of experimental infection. Vet Rec 1984; 115:201.

Mengeling WL. Porcine parvovirus infection. In: Lemans AD, et al., eds. Diseases of swine. 5th ed. Ames, IA: Iowa State University, 1981:352–366.

Nara PL. Systemic and local intestinal antibody response in dogs given both infective and inactivated canine parvovirus. Am J Vet Res 1983;44:1989.

Parrish CR. How canine parvovirus suddenly shifted host range. ASM News 1997;63:307.

Pollock RVH. The parvoviruses. Part 1. Feline panleukopenia virus and mink enteritis virus. Compend Cont Ed Pract Vet 1984;6:227.

Ridpath JF, Paul PS, Mengeling WL. Comparison of porcine parvovirus to other parvoviruses by restriction site mapping and hybridization analysis of Southern blots. J Gen Virol 1987; 68:895.

Senda M, Parrish CR, Harasawa R. Detection by PCR of wild-type canine parvovirus which contaminates dog vaccines. J Clin Microbiol 1995;33:110.

Siegel G. Canine parvovirus: origin and significance of a "new" pathogen. In: Berns KI, ed. The parvoviruses. New York: Plenum, 1984:363–383.

Teramoto YS, Mildbrand MM, Carlson J, et al. Comparison of enzyme-linked immunosorbent assay, DNA hybridization, hemagglutination, and electron microscopy for detection of canine parvovirus infections. J Clin Microbiol 1984; 20:373.

Wrathall AE, Cartwright SF, Wells DE, Jones PC. Maternally-derived antibodies to porcine parvovirus and their effect on active antibody production after vaccination with an inactivated oil-emulsion vaccine. Vet Rec 1987;120: 475.

60 *Iridoviridae*

JEFFREY L. STOTT

The Iridoviridae currently comprise five genera including those that infect insects (iridovirus and chloriridovirus) and three that infect frogs and/or fish (ranavirus, lymphocystivirus, and goldfish virus-like). From a veterinary perspective, the ranavirus and lymphocystivirus genera are the most important; ranaviruses are capable of causing high mortality in native and farmed fish populations and lymphocystivirus causes unsightly wart-like lesions in fish.

Iridoviruses have an icosahedral symmetry with an outer capsid composed primarily of a single protein subunit and a diameter ranging from 120 to 300 nm; capsid-associated fibrils have been described from some members of the family. An intermediate lipid membrane lies internal to the capsid and surrounds the viral core. A large number (in excess of 20) of virus-associated proteins have been described. The double-stranded DNA genome is circularly permuted and terminally redundant with many of the internal cytosine residues being highly methylated. Viral density ranges from 1.26 to 1.6 g/cm³. Definitive diagnosis is best made by viral isolation and/or characterization of the genome by molecular biology techniques.

Two strains of lymphocystis disease virus (LCDV) have been described with LCDV-1 being associated with flounder and LCDV-2 being associated with dabs. The disease was named from what has been described pathologically as lymphocystis cells. Clusters of these viral-infected hypertrophied cells (fibroblasts and osteoblasts) resemble neoplastic-like growths on the skin, peritoneum, and mesenteries. The lesions typically resolve with minimal mortality. In contrast, the ranavirus genus has been associated with high mortality in both farmed and free-ranging fish. These pathogenic iridoviruses causing fatal systemic disease are closely related to frog virus 3 (FV3), the latter serving as the prototype ranavirus. Members of this genus have been reported to cause epizootic hematopoietic necrosis and systemic hemorrhagic disease in fish.

AFRICAN SWINE FEVER VIRUS

African swine fever virus (ASFV) is an enveloped DNA virus with structural similarity to the iridoviruses. However, the genome of ASFV is not circularly permuted or terminally redundant, nor is it methylated.

DISEASE

African swine fever (ASF) is a highly contagious disease of domestic swine. Clinical signs in infected pigs range from peracute to chronic and inapparent. The peracute and acute diseases caused by ASF approach 100% mortality, and death may occur prior to development of clinical signs. Acute ASF closely resembles hog cholera. The disease is characterized by high fever and leukopenia, often followed by the appearance of red areas on the skin, weakness, accelerated respiration and pulse, vomiting, bloody diarrhea, and nasal and conjunctival discharges. Death usually occurs within 7 days following the onset of fever. Subacute ASF is characterized by death or recovery in 3 to 4 weeks. Affected pigs typically experience a high fever; abortion is common and may be the only sign of illness. Pigs with chronic ASF exhibit varying signs of illness, which often include stunting and emaciation, swollen joints and lameness, skin ulcerations, and pneumonia.

ETIOLOGIC AGENT

Physical, Chemical, and Antigenic Properties

African swine fever virus is an enveloped DNA virus with reported diameters ranging from 175 to 215 nm and a buoyant density of 1.7 g/cm³ in cesium chlolicle. The virus is structurally complex. It consists of concentric structures with an icosahedral symmetry; an inner nucleoid is enclosed within an envelope, which is in turn sequentially surrounded by the capsid and outer envelope. Figure 60.1 depicts electron micrographs of individual African swine viral particles. Five major structural proteins have been described, the remainder being considered minor components. While only one serotype of ASFV has been recognized, differences between isolates have been described, including variation in antigens, virulence, hemadsorption, and restriction endonuclease cleavage pattern; differences have also been identified by cross-protection and hemadsorption inhibition studies.

Resistance to Physical and Chemical Agents

African swine fever virus is extremely stable in tissues and excretions. The virus can withstand extreme pH ranges

FIGURE 60.1. *African swine fever virus in thin section of infected tissue culture cells. 58,000×. (Courtesy of IC Pang.)*

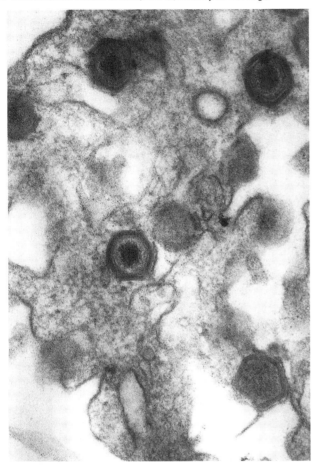

(pH 4 to 13), temperatures up to 56°C for 30 minutes, and freezing and thawing. Putrified blood maintains infectivity for 15 weeks at room temperature. The ASFV is inactivated by heating to 60°C for 20 minutes and by lipid solvents.

Infectivity for Other Species and Culture Systems

African swine fever virus is only known to occur naturally in pigs and argasid ticks of the genus *Ornithodoros*. Pigs appear to be the only mammalian species susceptible to ASF viral infection. Domestic pigs, warthogs, bush pigs, giant forest hogs, and European wild boars have all been described as susceptible to infection, with domestic and European wild boars commonly expressing clinical disease.

African swine fever virus can be propagated in vitro on cultures of swine bone marrow cells, monocytes, and alveolar macrophages. The virus can also be adapted to various established cell lines (pig kidney, VERO, and BHK).

HOST–VIRUS RELATIONSHIP

Distribution, Reservoir, and Transmission

African swine fever was first described in European domestic pigs in Kenya in the early 1900s. The first reported outbreak of ASF outside the African continent occurred in Portugal in 1957. Since that time, the disease has also been observed in Spain, France, Italy, Malta, Sardinia, Cuba, Brazil, the Dominican Republic, and Haiti. African swine fever has been described in most of the African countries south of the Sahara Desert and is also common in Portugal and Spain. The virus has apparently been eradicated in other European countries and from the Western Hemisphere as well.

Two reservoirs of ASFV are persistent or inapparent infections in the wild pig population and the argasid tick vector. The virus readily persists in the tick population as vertical transmission of the virus has been demonstrated.

Transmission of ASFV in nature is by tick bite, ingestion of infected tissues, or direct contact. Upon infection of domestic pigs, the virus is transmitted by direct contact. It is easily transmitted over long distances due to its stability in infected tissues and excrement and subsequent infection upon contact with susceptible animals.

Pathogenesis and Pathology

Following oral or nasal exposure of domestic pigs to ASF viruses, the upper respiratory tract is the primary site of viral replication with subsequent dissemination to adjacent lymph nodes. The viral infection becomes generalized by systemic spread via leukocytes, erythrocytes, or both in the lymph ducts and blood; this occurs within 3 days postinfection and corresponds closely with the onset of pyrexia. High titers of virus are found in tissues having large components of reticuloendothelial cells. Virus-associated lymphocyte apoptosis plays a role in lymphoid cell depletion in lymphoid organs. In newborn pigs, viral antigen was detected in endothelium and tunica media of blood vessels. This observation supports the contention that viral replication in these cells is directly responsible for the vascular necrosis and hemorrhages that occur.

The type and degree of macroscopic lesions observed in pigs with ASFV infection can be highly variable and have been described in the literature as depending on the type of infection — peracute, acute, subacute, or chronic. Pigs with peracute ASF often die before any signs of disease are obvious. In acute cases of ASF, lesions in the spleen and internal organs are commonly observed. Hemorrhages, often petechial in appearance, occur in internal organs, including the renal cortex, myocardium, subendocardial, and epicardial surfaces of the heart, mucosa of the urinary bladder, gastric and intestinal serosa, and lymph nodes. In addition to such lesions, fluids often accumulate in the pericardial, pleural, and peritoneal cavities. In subacute ASF, lesions are often less pronounced. The lymphatic system is often involved, however, with hemorrhages being common in the lymph nodes and kidneys. Additional lesions may include enlarged spleen due to hyperplasia, lobular consolidation in the cardiac and anterior lobes of the lung, interstitial pneumonia, mucosal hemorrhages in the large intestine, and bloody contents in the large intestine. Lesions observed in chronic ASF are also highly variable and may resemble the subacute disease. Lesions may include fibrinous pericarditis and pleuritis, firm foci in lobes of the lung that may result in caseous necrosis and calcification of the entire lobe.

Microscopic lesions are most pronounced in the lymphatic system. Degeneration of the lymphoid tissues is typical with lymphocytes undergoing apoptosis; the inducer of this programmed cell death is uncertain. Hyperplasia is often observed within the reticuloendothelial system (spleen, nodes, etc.) in chronic and subacute ASF. Kupffer cells often undergo necrosis.

Host Responses to Infection

Until a recent report, pigs infected with ASFV were considered not to produce classic neutralizing antibodies. However, neutralizing antibodies (monoclonal and convalescent) have been identified and bind a 72 kDa viral protein. Nonneutralizing antibodies develop in infected pigs, as determined by various assays including immunodiffusion, radioimmunoassay (RIA), enzyme-linked immunosorbent assay (ELISA), immunoelectrophoresis, and complement fixation (CF). Antibodies can be detected as early as 3 days postinfection by RIA. Antibodies specific for ASFV proteins have been demonstrated by radioimmune precipitation (RIP). Passive antibody transfer experiments have demonstrated varying degrees of protection to challenge by the homologous virus. Studies demonstrating in vitro complement-dependent antibody cytotoxicity (CDAC) and antibody-dependent cell-mediated cytotoxicity (ADCC) suggest that such a phenomenon may be responsible for protection induced by passive transfer of antibodies. It has been suggested that complement-mediated lysis reduced viremia and ADCC-conferred protection. Blocking antibodies have been identified that inhibit complete viral neutralization and may play a role in the establishment of persistent infection.

LABORATORY DIAGNOSIS

Laboratory tests are required to make a differential diagnosis between hog cholera and ASF. Tissues submitted include spleen, liver, lymph nodes, whole blood, and sera. The differential diagnosis is carried out by hemadsorption (HAd) inhibition to porcine leukocyte or bone marrow cultures. The alternative procedure, inoculation of hog cholera immune and susceptible pigs, is expensive. However, certain stains of ASF virus do not exhibit hemadsorption. Techniques based on polymerase chain reaction (PCR) can also be used to identify the presence of AHSV genomic material.

Serologic diagnosis can be conducted by ELISA, indirect fluorescent antibody (IFA) staining, immunoperoxidase plaque staining, HAd inhibition, immunoelectroosmophoresis, and complement fixation. Conducting multiple diagnostic tests is suggested since a single test may not be adequate to confirm infection under all conditions.

TREATMENT AND CONTROL

Effective treatment and prophylactic measures are currently unavailable for ASF. Eradication of the disease is only possible by slaughter and disposal of all exposed pigs. In certain areas, even these measures are not totally effective since the virus can persist in the tick and wild pig population. Premises that undergo eradication procedures must not only slaughter all pigs but also must be treated with insecticides and disinfectant containing ophenylphenol with surfactants and must remain free of livestock for at least a month. Prior to restocking, susceptible sentinel animals should be placed on the premises to confirm eradication of the virus. There is no effective vaccine at the present time.

SELECTED REFERENCES

Hess WR. African swine fever: a reassessment. Adv Vet Sci Comp Med 1981;25:39.

Mao J, Hedrick RP, Chinchar VG. Molecular characterization, sequence analysis and taxonomic position of newly isolated fish iridoviruses. Virology 1997;299:212.

Mebus CA. African swine fever. Adv Virus Res 1988;35:251.

Ramiro-Ibanez F, Ortega A, Brun A, et al. Apoptosis: a mechanism of cell killing and lymphoid organ impairment during acute African swine fever virus infection. J Gen Virol 1996;77:2209.

Tidona CA, Darai G. The complete DNA sequence of lymphocystis disease virus. Virology 1997;230:207.

Wardley RC, Wilkinson PJ. An immunological approach to vaccines against African swine fever virus. Vaccine 1985;3:54.

Williams T. The iridoviruses. Adv Virus Res 1996;46:345.

Zsak L, Onisk DV, Afonso CL, Rock DL. Virulent African swine fever virus isolates are neutralized by swine immune serum and by monoclonal antibodies recognizing a 72-kDa viral protein. Virology 1993;196:596.

61 Papovaviridae

Yuan Chung Zee

The family Papovaviridae has two genera: Papillomavirus and Polyomavirus. Polyomaviruses have not been associated with diseases of domestic animals with the exception of an avian polyomavirus that causes an acute generalized infection in fledgling budgerigars. The papillomaviruses are widespread among mammals. They have been found in cattle, sheep, goats, deer, elk, horses, rabbits, dogs, monkeys, pigs, opossums, mice, and elephants. Infectious papillomatoses (warts) are contagious in the animal in which they naturally occur. Many of these lesions may be regarded as either hyperplasia or benign neoplasms, since they do not metastasize and kill the host. However, papillomas may undergo malignant transformation in some animal species.

ETIOLOGIC AGENTS

Papillomaviruses are naked icosahedral capsids 50 nm to 55 nm in diameter (Fig 61.1). The virion has a density in CsCl of $1.34 \, g/cm^3$. The viral genome is a double-stranded, covalently closed, circular DNA molecule. Viral protein represents 88% of the mass of the particle, and as many as 10 polypeptides have been resolved in purified viral preparations. No serologic cross-reactivity among the major capsid proteins has been detected in papillomaviruses of different species. The propagation of papillomaviruses has not been very successful in cell culture. With the advent of recombinant DNA and polymerase chain reaction (PCR) technology, it is now feasible to clone and sequence papillomavirus DNA; thus far, no DNA sequence homology has been detected between selected members of this group.

PAPILLOMA TYPES

Papillomaviruses can generally be subdivided by tissue tropism and histopathologic effect. One group induces neoplasm of cutaneous stratified epithelium. Representatives of this group are equine, chaffinch, bovine Types 3 and 5, and the cottontail rabbit papillomaviruses. Canine oral and bovine papillomavirus Type 4 constitutes a second group that primarily induces hyperplasia of either nonstratified squamous epithelium or metaplastic squamous epithelium. A third group, consisting of bovine Types 1 and 2 and sheep and European elk papillomavirus, induces not only cutaneous papilloma but also an underlying fibroma of connective tissue (fibropapilloma). The deer fibromavirus represents the fourth group. It produces fibromas with a minimally hyperplastic cutaneous epithelium. In all histologic types, intact virus can be demonstrated only in the outer layers of keratinizing cells of the epithelium.

BOVINE PAPILLOMAVIRUS

Warts caused by bovine papillomavirus frequently occur in calves less than 2 years old. They appear most frequently on the head, especially in the region about the eyes. They may also appear on the sides of the neck and less commonly on other parts of the body. They develop from small, nodular growths slowly at first, and then grow rapidly into dry, horny, whitish, cauliflowerlike masses, which eventually fall off as a result of dry necrosis of their bases. Occasionally infectious papillomas occur in dairy herds, the tumors appearing only on the teats. These result in difficulty in milking and are spread in the milking process. Occasional fibroblastic tumors in the urinary bladder and the genital mucosa of cattle have been reported.

Bovine papillomavirus comprises at least five distinct viral types each producing a specific type of lesion. The viral types lack immunologic cross-reactivity and can be distinguished by the characteristic restriction endonuclease cleavage of their genomes.

Bovine papillomavirus Types 1 and 2 have a wide tissue range in cattle. Experimental inoculation of calves produces tumors of the urinary bladder and genital mucosa. However, Types 1 and 2 have been isolated from fibropapillomas on the head, neck, and flank of naturally infected cattle.

Bovine papillomavirus Types 1 and 2 have also been implicated in causing sarcoids, which are naturally occurring skin tumors of horses. The detection of bovine papillomavirus DNA sequences in equine sarcoids suggests this possibility.

Bovine papillomavirus Type 3 was isolated from cutaneous papillomas lacking a fibrous component. The virus is transmissible to the skin of cattle but not to other sites.

Infection with bovine papillomavirus Type 4 results in alimentary tract papillomatosis of cattle. Experimentally, the soft palate of calves is uniformly susceptible, but the skin is refractory.

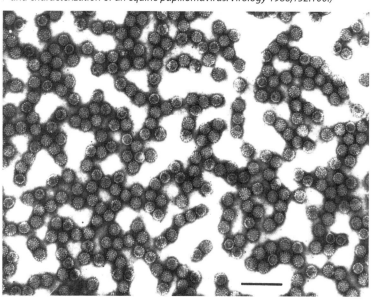

FIGURE 61.1. *Negatively stained preparations of equine papillomaviruses. 75,000×. (Reproduced with permission from Sundberg JP, O'Banion MK. Cloning and characterization of an equine papillomavirus. Virology 1986;152:100.)*

Three histologic types of lesions have been observed on the teats of cattle: 1) papilloma, 2) "rice grain" lesions consisting of white elongated protuberances, and 3) fibropapilloma. Bovine papillomavirus Type 5 has been associated with the "rice grain"-type lesions whereas the other lesions are probably caused by Types 1 or 2.

A new bovine papillomavirus, designated Type 6 (BPV-6), has been recently isolated from epithelial papillomas of the bovine udder. It is clearly distinguishable from all other bovine papillomaviruses based on DNA sequence homology and antigenic properties.

Bovine papillomaviruses (Types 1 and 2) are the only papillomaviruses shown to have a reproducible effect in tissue culture. Cytopathic changes develop in cultures of bovine conjunctival cells after infection with bovine papilloma extracts. These changes include altered cell morphology, piling-up, and increased acidity of the medium. Extracts of bovine papilloma have also been shown to induce morphologic transformation of primary embryonic bovine skin cells, mouse embryo cell cultures, and hamster embryo cells.

Bovine papillomavirus can be cultivated on the chorioallantoic membrane of developing chick embryos. Virus is concentrated in marked epithelial thickenings.

Host immune responses to papillomavirus infections are not well understood. In general, the infection is acquired by the young and warts persist for variable periods, after which they regress. The host is left immune to reinfection with the same virus. Calves produce IgM-precipitating antibodies within the first week after infection with bovine papillomavirus. These antibodies persist for 8 to 16 weeks. Precipitating antibodies of the IgG class appear at about 6 weeks and persist for at least 26 weeks after infection. The precipitin response does not correlate with either growth or regression of fibropapillomas. It has been reported that calves inoculated with BPV-transformed fetal bovine skin cells were resistant to challenge by BPV, whereas infected untransformed cells were unable to confer resistance. It is suggested that cell-mediated immunity plays a role in the rejection of viral warts and that the virus of virus-induced tumor factors may suppress cellular immunity in certain susceptible animals.

Treatment of bovine papillomatosis with finely ground wart tissue suspended in a 0.4% formalin solution has been used for many years to combat wart outbreaks. It is difficult to evaluate the procedure since the disease is self-limiting and its duration varies in individual animals. Studies indicate that a significant proportion of animals fail to reject their warts despite vaccination with autologous tumor preparations. Vaccination attempts with virus grown in embryonated eggs have met with variable success. There is recent evidence that cattle vaccinated with L2, the minor structural protein of bovine papillomavirus Type 4, did not develop alimentary papillomas when challenged with that virus type.

Bovine papillomavirus has been used in biotechnology to construct a shuttle vector system that can replicate in both bacteria and mammalian cells. Such vectors are useful in the study of the expression of cloned genes and of the molecular basis of cell mutations.

EQUINE PAPILLOMAVIRUS

Skin warts of horses are not as common as those affecting cattle. They develop most often on the nose and around the lips, appearing as small, elevated, horny masses, varying from a few to several hundred.

The virus is spread by direct contact of infectious material through wounds and cutaneous abrasions. The virus can be experimentally transmitted to horses by intradermal inoculation of a suspension of wart tissue, but not to calves, lambs, dogs, rabbits, or guinea pigs.

Equine papillomas are usually self-limiting and disappear spontaneously in 4 to 8 weeks. Natural infection provides solid immunity.

CANINE ORAL PAPILLOMAVIRUS

Canine papillomavirus induces warts in the mouths of dogs. The warts generally develop on the lips and spread to the buccal mucosa, tongue, palate, and pharynx. The warts are usually benign and disappear spontaneously after several months. Dogs recovered from the infection develop immunity to reinfection.

The infection is highly contagious, often spreading through all the dogs in a kennel. Warts have been experimentally transmitted by rubbing pieces of wart tissue on

scarified mucous membranes of susceptible dogs. Under such conditions the incubation period was from 4 to 6 weeks.

SELECTED REFERENCES

Campo MS. Infection by bovine papillomavirus and prospects for vaccination. Trends Microbiol 1995;3:92.

Chandrachud LM, Grindlay GJ, McGarvie GM, et al. Vaccination of cattle with the N-terminis of L2 is necessary and sufficient for preventing infection by bovine papillomavirus-4. Virology 1995;211:204.

Howley PH, Broker TR. Papillomaviruses: molecular and clinical aspects. UCLA symposia on molecular and cellular biology (new series). Vol. 32. New York: Alan R. Liss, 1986.

Jarrett WFH. The natural history of bovine papillomavirus infections. Adv Virol Oncol 1985;5:83.

Lancaster WD, Olson C. Animal papillomaviruses. Microbiol Rev 1982;46:19.

Pfister H. Papillomaviruses: general description, taxonomy, and classification. In: Salzman NP, Howle PM, eds. The *papovaviridae*. New York: Plenum, 1987:1–38.

Pfister H, Mesazaros J. Partial characterization of a canine oral papillomavirus. Virology 1980;104:243.

62   *Adenoviridae*

YUAN CHUNG ZEE

The family Adenoviridae is divided into two genera, Mastadenovirus and Aviadenovirus. Members of these two genera do not share the same group antigen. Adenoviruses are double-stranded DNA nonenveloped icosahedrons that are 70nm to 90nm in diameter and composed of 252 capsomers (Fig 62.1). They have been isolated from many species of animals; their host range is generally narrow. Table 62.1 lists the diseases of domestic animals caused by adenoviruses.

INFECTIOUS CANINE HEPATITIS

DISEASE

The first clinical symptom is high fever (104°F), which usually subsides after 24 hours. In some animals this may be the sole sign of illness. Other common signs include increased thirst, anorexia, tonsillitis, and congestion and hemorrhages of mucous membranes. Abdominal tenderness due to the swollen liver is frequently observed over the xiphoid region. Many affected dogs assume a "tucked-up" stance and are reluctant to move. During the acute phase of illness, dogs may develop conjunctivitis and photophobia. Subcutaneous edema of the head, neck, and trunk occurs rarely.

During early convalescence, usually 1 to 3 weeks after acute signs disappear, a transient corneal opacity may develop as a result of iridocyclitis and corneal edema.

In some dogs, petechial and ecchymotic hemorrhages occur in the skin, primarily over the abdomen. If hemorrhage is profuse, the prognosis is poor.

Most dogs with uncomplicated infections recover rapidly after about 4 to 7 days of illness. Appetite returns quickly but regain of lost weight is usually slow. Peracutely ill dogs die within a few hours after the onset of clinical signs.

ETIOLOGIC AGENT

Physical, Chemical, and Antigenic Properties

Infectious canine hepatitis (ICH) is caused by canine adenovirus Type 1 (CAV-1), which is antigenically related but distinct from canine adenovirus 2.

Canine adenovirus 1 is morphologically similar to other adenoviruses. Erythrocytes from various species, especially avian and the human O-type, agglutinate when mixed with viral suspensions. No cross-neutralization has been shown between CAV-1 and adenoviruses from other species.

Resistance to Physical and Chemical Agents

CAV-1 survives exposure to ether, acid, alcohols, and chloroform. It is stable for at least 30 minutes at a wide range of pH (3 to 9) when maintained at room temperature. Infectious virus can be demonstrated after 3 to 11 days at room temperature on soiled material. Viral infectivity is inactivated after 10 minutes at 50°C to 60°C. Steam cleaning and treatment with iodine, phenol, sodium hydroxide, or lysol are effective means of disinfection.

Infectivity for Other Species and Culture Systems

Canine adenovirus 1 causes clinical disease in dogs and other Canids. Raccoons, ferrets, and cats develop transient corneal edema after injection of virus into the anterior chamber of the eye, but they have limited susceptibility. Serologic evidence indicates that humans can be infected. Clinical signs do not develop. Canine adenovirus 1 propagates well in canine kidney cells.

Some CAV-1 and CAV-2 strains have been shown to be oncogenic when inoculated into hamsters but have not been associated with neoplastic disease in dogs.

HOST–VIRUS RELATIONSHIP

Distribution, Reservoir, and Transmission

Infectious canine hepatitis has a worldwide distribution with the fox as a reservoir host. In foxes, the disease is manifested primarily as encephalitis.

The disease is spread through the urine. After recovery from acute illness, a dog may retain virus in the kidneys and eliminate it in the urine for possibly more than one year.

Pathogenesis and Pathology

Following oronasal exposure, the virus localizes in the tonsils and spreads to regional lymph nodes and lym-

FIGURE 62.1. *Negatively stained preparations of avian adenovirus. 204,000×. (Courtesy of R. Nordhausen.)*

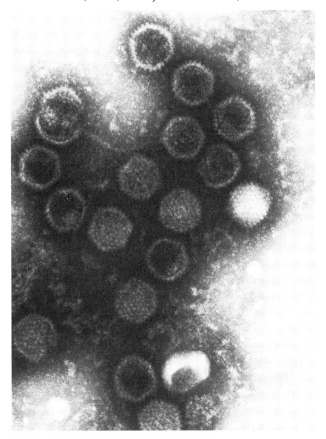

Table 62.1. Diseases of Domestic Animals Caused by Adenoviruses

Virus	Type of Disease
Mastadenovirus	
Bovine adenoviruses Types 1–10	Conjunctivitis, pneumonia, diarrhea, polyarthritis
Canine adenovirus Type 1 (CAV-1; infectious canine hepatitis)	Hemorrhagic and hepatic
Canine adenovirus Type 2	Respiratory
Equine adenovirus Types 1–2	Pneumonia
Ovine adenoviruses Types 1–6	Respiratory and enteric
Porcine adenoviruses Types 1–4	Diarrhea or meningoencephalitis, or both
Aviadenovirus	
Chicken adenoviruses Types 1–12	Respiratory disease, enteric disease, egg-drop syndrome, aplastic anemia, atrophy of the bursa of Fabricius
Turkey adenoviruses Types 1–4	Respiratory disease, enteritis, marble spleen disease

phatics before reaching the blood through the thoracic duct. Viremia, usually lasting 4 to 8 days, results in rapid dissemination of virus to all body tissues and secretions including saliva, urine, and feces. Hepatic parenchymal cells and vascular endothelial cells of many tissues are prime targets for viral replication and injury.

Lesions of the liver, kidney, and eye are associated with cytotoxic effects of the virus. Usually by the seventh day after infection, a sufficient antibody response clears the virus from the blood and liver, thereby restricting the extent of hepatic damage.

Dogs that die during the acute phase generally have edema and hemorrhage of superficial lymph nodes and cervical subcutaneous tissue. The abdominal cavity often contains fluid, which may vary in color from clear to bright red. Hemorrhages are present on all serosal surfaces. A fibrinous exudate may cover the liver, which can be swollen and congested. The sinusoids and major vessels in the lobules are dilated. Large nuclear inclusion bodies, Cowdry Type A, are present in many hepatic cells and may also occur in vascular endothelium and reticuloendothelial cells throughout the body.

The gallbladder may thicken and the spleen enlarge. The kidneys are often congested and contain intranuclear

inclusion bodies, especially in the glomeruli. In the brain, macroscopic and microscopic hemorrhages occur around the capillaries and are prominent in the thalamus, midbrain, and medulla.

Host Response to Infections

Recovery from ICH, regardless of the severity of illness, results in long-lasting immunity — as long as $5^1/_2$ years after experimental infection. Complement-fixing antibodies do not persist long after initial infection but neutralizing antibodies do. The neutralizing antibody titer is the most specific measure of a dog's resistance to ICH infection.

LABORATORY DIAGNOSIS

Clinically, ICH resembles canine distemper (CD), leptospirosis, and the effects of certain poisons, especially warfarin. In differential diagnosis, ICH is indicated if leukopenia and fever are present. Pain on palpation of the region of the liver suggests ICH. Unlike CD, ICH is rarely associated with neural disturbances. In liver function tests, significantly elevated values occur only in severely ill dogs. Retrospective diagnosis is indicated. The development of transient corneal opacity follows 1 to 3 weeks after recovery from a febrile illness.

Diagnosis can be confirmed by serologic testing (complement fixation, hemagglutination inhibition, enzyme-linked immunosorbent assay [ELISA], or viral isolation followed by immunofluorescent antibody testing).

TREATMENT AND CONTROL

Therapy for dogs developing ICH involves supportive and symptomatic treatment. Whole blood transfusions are required when hemorrhage has occurred. The recommended amount is 8 mL/lb of body weight by slow intravenous infusion, repeated every 48 hours as indicated. More than one transfusion is usually required.

Dextrose in physiologic saline solution should be given intravenously to restore fluid balance. Broad-spectrum antibiotics are advised to control bacterial complications.

Vaccines available for immunization include attenuated virus propagated in swine kidney or in embryonated duck eggs. The development of immunity is greater in older puppies because of the gradual loss of maternal antibody. Hence, if the dog is less than 12 weeks old, a second dose of vaccine should be given at 15 weeks of age. The exact age at which a puppy loses maternal antibodies depends upon the amount received from the dam. The rate of antibody decline in dogs is 50% every $8^1/_2$ days.

Vaccination success is directly related to the level of neutralizing antibody, which may persist for up to $3^1/_2$ years after vaccination with modified live virus.

Modified live vaccine virus may be disseminated in urine from vaccinated to susceptible dogs in kennels where dogs are in contact with each other. Apparently such virus does not revert to its former virulence. Modified live virus vaccines occasionally cause transient allergic corneal and iridal reactions 1 to 3 weeks after injection.

Tissue culture–propagated vaccines inactivated with formalin confer immunity for only relatively short periods, producing low antibody titers that decline rapidly even after a second injection.

The recommended schedule with any ICH vaccine involves at least two vaccinations, 3 to 4 weeks apart, at 8 to 10 and 12 to 14 weeks of age. Annual vaccination is recommended. The ICH vaccine is commonly given in combination with canine distemper vaccine and *Leptospira canicola* bacterin.

CANINE ADENOVIRUS TYPE 2

Canine adenovirus type 2 (CAV-2) has been isolated from dogs with acute cough and is one of several pathogens implicated in infectious tracheobronchitis (kennel cough). Experimental infection produces mild pharyngitis, tonsillitis, and tracheobronchitis. Virus is reported to persist in the respiratory tract for up to 28 days. Unlike CAV-1, CAV-2 does not produce generalized disease, is not excreted in the urine, and does not produce renal and ocular lesions.

The restriction endonuclease patterns obtained for the DNA of CAV-1 and CAV-2 are different.

CAV-2 is antigenically related to CAV-1 and CAV-2 vaccines have been developed as an alternative for ICH vaccine since they do not produce postvaccinal ocular and renal lesions.

BOVINE ADENOVIRUSES

The bovine adenoviruses (BAV) are currently classified into ten serotypes, which cause a variety of clinical signs including conjunctivitis, pneumonia, pneumoenteritis, diarrhea, and polyarthritis. Some types have been isolated from apparently normal cattle. Serologic surveys indicated widespread distribution of BAV throughout the world. Bovine adenovirus Types 3, 4, and 5 are associated with disease in the United States. There is no evidence that disease in humans is caused by bovine adenovirus.

Bovine adenovirus Type 3 is considered one of the important respiratory tract pathogens of cattle, particularly newborn calves. Clinical signs include pyrexia, respiratory distress, and nasal and conjunctival discharge. Gross pathologic lesions, primarily confined to the lungs, consist of consolidated areas with a distinct lobular distribution, collapse, and emphysema. Microscopically, there are proliferative bronchiolitis, necrosis with bronchiolar occlusion, and alveolar collapse. Typical intranuclear inclusions are found in a variety of tissues.

Calves inoculated with bovine adenoviruses develop neutralizing antibodies in 10 to 14 days, precipitating antibodies in 3 weeks; hemagglutinating antibodies reach maximum level at 7 days. Immunity after vaccination or natural infection is long-lasting.

Diagnosis requires viral isolation or serology. Virus is more often isolated from rectal than from nasal or conjunctival swabs. Most types do not produce characteristic cytopathogenic effects until after several blind passages.

The demonstration of a rising antibody titer (fourfold) with paired sera using serum neutralization, agar gel precipitation, fluorescent antibody, complement fixation, and hemagglutination inhibition have been employed for serologic diagnosis.

Although no vaccines are licensed for use in the United States, in Europe there is limited use of vaccines against BAV 1, 3, and 4.

EQUINE ADENOVIRUS

Adenovirus infection may cause disease of the upper respiratory tract, particularly in Arabian foals under 3 months of age, with combined immunodeficiency (CID). The morbidity in these foals is 10% to 15% and mortality approaches 100%. Immunocompetent foals normally develop subclinical or mild forms of disease. The course of disease is 10 to 56 days. Clinical signs include coughing, pneumonia, dyspnea, conjunctivitis, and fever. There is a persistent lymphopenia and neutropenia. Postmortem lesions include pulmonary atelectasis and pneumonia. Microscopic lesions include swelling, hyperplasia, intranuclear inclusions, and necrosis of epithelial cells of the entire respiratory tract and of transitional epithelium of the renal pelvis, ureter, urinary bladder, and urethra. Foals that recover develop significant antibody levels that provide prolonged immunity. The frequency of infection varies with the breed of horse. Serologic studies indicate that the prevalence of infection is 60% to 75% in different breeds and about 91% for Arabian horses.

There are two serotypes, as determined by serum neutralization. For laboratory diagnosis, virus may be isolated from infective tissue and nasal and ocular swab material in equine fetal kidney or equine fetal dermis cell cultures. The virus can be identified by electron microscopy or by immunofluorescent (IF) tests of infected cell cultures. Direct examination of tissue sections or exfoliated epithelial cells in respiratory and lacrimal secretions by IF can be used to detect the virus. Viral neutralization and hemagglutination-inhibition test are used to detect the presence and rise of antibody titers.

There is no commercially available vaccine.

OVINE ADENOVIRUSES

Adenoviruses have been isolated from the feces of apparently normal sheep and from lambs with respiratory disease. Six serotypes have been identified. All share common complement-fixing (CF) antigen. Rat erythrocytes are agglutinated by all serotypes but bovine erythrocytes are agglutinated only by serotype 4.

The pathogenic role of most of the ovine adenoviruses is uncertain. Some of the six serotypes produce a mild or inapparent infection associated with the respiratory and enteric tracts. A natural outbreak of pneumoenteritis with heavy mortality has been reported in suckling and fattening lambs.

AVIAN ADENOVIRUSES

Adenoviruses infect poultry and other avian species throughout the world. Some of the 12 avian serotypes have been associated with respiratory and enteric disease, inclusion body hepatitis, egg-drop syndrome, atrophy of the bursa of Fabricius, and the hemorrhagic-aplastic anemia syndrome. Other serotypes have come from apparently normal chickens.

Avian adenoviruses have been subdivided into three groups. The first group includes adenoviruses isolated from chickens, turkeys, geese, and other species sharing a common group antigen. The second group shares a different group antigen from the first group and includes viruses from marble spleen disease and turkey hemorrhagic enteritis. The third group includes viruses associated with egg-drop syndrome in chickens and ducks.

Avian adenoviruses resist inactivation by ether, chloroform, sodium deoxycholate, and trypsin. Some strains of avian adenoviruses are not inactivated by 2% phenol alcohol or 50% ethyl alcohol, but are inactivated by absolute alcohol. Strains of adenoviruses differ slightly in heat resistance at 56°C. Survival ranges from $^1/_2$ to 22 hours.

SELECTED REFERENCES

Bass EP, Gill MA, Beckenhauser WH. Evaluation of a canine adenovirus type 2 strain as a replacement for infectious canine hepatitis vaccine. J Am Vet Med Assoc 1980;177:234.

Ishibashi M, Yasue H. Adenoviruses of animals. In: Ginsberg HS, ed. The adenoviruses. New York: Plenum, 1984:497–562.

Kopotopoulos G, Cornwell HJC. Canine adenoviruses: a review. Vet Bull 1981;51:135.

Lehmkuhl HD, Catlip RC. Experimental infection of lambs with ovine adenovirus isolate RTS-151: clinical, microbiological, and serologic responses. Am J Vet Res 1984;45:260.

McFerran JB. Adenovirus infections. In: Calnek BW, ed. Diseases of poultry. 9th ed. Ames, IA: Iowa State University, 1991: 329–336.

McGuire TC, Perryman LE. Combined immunodeficiency of Arabian foals. In: Gershwin ME, Merchant B, eds. Immunologic defects in laboratory animals. New York: Plenum, 1981: 185–203.

63 Herpesviridae

ALEX A. ARDANS

The family Herpesviridae consists of viruses that have been isolated from a wide range of animal species, humans, catfish, and invertebrates such as oysters. Herpesviruses have been found in virtually every species that has been investigated. Within this group of viruses, there is wide variation in biological properties including pathogenicity, a propensity to form latent infections, and oncogenic potential. Herpesviruses are morphologically similar, with a double-stranded DNA core and an icosahedral capsid consisting of 162 capsomeres, surrounded by a granular zone composed of globular proteins (tegument) and encompassed by a lipid envelope (Fig 63.1). Herpesvirus nucleocapsids from different species have a similar polypeptide composition, with a major polypeptide, thought to be the major hexon protein, having a molecular weight (MW) of 140,000 to 160,000.

The family *Herpesviridae* consists of three major subfamilies, alpha-, beta-, and gammaherpesvirinae, which were initially distinguished by host range, duration of reproductive cycle, cytopathology, and latent infection characteristics. The alphaherpesvirinae have a variable host range, are generally highly cytopathic in cell culture, have a relatively short replicative cycle (<24 hours), and frequently cause latent viral infections in sensory ganglia. Betaherpesvirinae have a variable host range and a long replicative cycle; infected cells often become enlarged (cytomeglia). Latency can be established in numerous tissues. Gammaherpesvirinae, with some exceptions, tend to be specific for B or T lymphocytes, replicate in lymphoblastoid cells, and may cause lytic infections in certain types of epithelial and fibroblastic cells. Infection is frequently arrested at a prelytic stage with persistent and minimum expression of viral genome in the cell. Latency frequently is established in lymphoid tissue. Host range is narrow with experimental hosts usually limited to the order of the natural host.

The assignment of herpes viruses into the three major subfamilies, based on biologic criteria, may change as taxonomy should, in the future, be based on more objective molecular biology criteria. Based on biologic criteria, gallid herpesvirus 2 (Marek's disease) initially was classed as a gammaherpesvirus. Subsequently its gene arrangement data suggested it should be included with the alphaherpesvirinae. Others such as human herpesvirus 6, initially classified as gammaherpesvirus, are now more properly classified as a betaherpesvirus. Similarly, bovine herpesvirus 4, initially included with the betaherpesvirinae, has been demonstrated to share properties with the gammaherpesvirinae.

EQUINE HERPESVIRUS

DISEASE

There are five antigenically distinct equine herpesviruses: EHV-1 through EHV-5. EHV-1, EHV-3, and EHV-4 are typical alphaherpesviruses and EHV-2 and EHV-5, previously classified as betaherpesviruses, are now considered to be gammaherpesviruses. Three herpes viruses designated asinine herpes viruses have been isolated from donkeys AHV-1 and AHV-3 (alphaherpesvirus) and AHV-2 (gammaherpesvirus). EHV-1 has been associated with abortions, upper respiratory disease, and neurologic disease. EHV-2 has been isolated from cases of chronic pharyngitis, mild respiratory disease in young horses, severe respiratory disease in foals 3 to 4 months old, and from clinically normal horses. Venereal disease (coital exanthema) is a well-recognized clinical manifestation of EHV-3. EHV-4 shares a close antigenic relationship with EHV-1 and has been associated with respiratory disease and sporadic abortions. EHV-5 has been isolated from horses with upper respiratory diseases.

ETIOLOGIC AGENT

Physical, Chemical, and Antigen Properties

The equine herpesviruses have a typical herpes morphology and cannot be distinguished from each other. Most typically they range in size from 150 nm to 170 nm. The internal core contains a linear double-stranded DNA molecule.

Resistance to Physical and Chemical Agents

The equine herpesviruses are inactivated by ether, acid (pH 3), and exposure to heat of 56°C for 30 minutes.

Infectivity for Other Species and Culture Systems

Equine herpesviruses usually only infect horses. Ocular disease due to EHV-1 characterized by vitritis, retinitis, and optic neuritis leading to blindness has been described in new-world camelids (alpacas, llamas). Limited serologic surveys have not demonstrated widespread infection in these species. EHV-1 can be propagated in equine fetal kidney, rabbit kidney, and L (mouse fibroblast) cells,

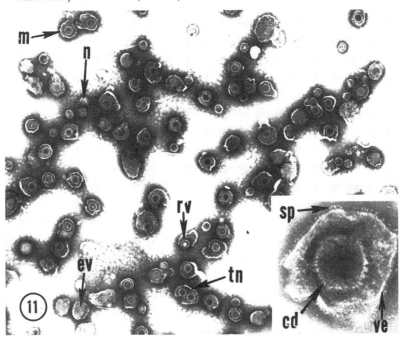

FIGURE 63.1. *Negatively stained preparation of infectious bovine rhinotracheitis virus. n = nucleocapsid, ev = envelope, rv = enveloped virus, tn = twin nucleocapsids. 17,000×. Inset: Minute projections on the envelope of a matured virus. sp = virus spikes, cd = virus core, ve = virus envelope. 100,000×. (Reproduced with permission from Talens LT, Zee YC. Purification and buoyant density of infectious bovine rhinotracheitis virus. Proc Exp Biol Med 1976;151:132.)*

resulting in formation of cytopathic effect and intranuclear inclusion bodies.

EQUINE HERPESVIRUS-1

DISEASE

Equine herpesvirus-1 (EHV-1) causes abortion in mares, respiratory tract disease in young horses, and occasional neurologic disease.

While abortion in mares may occur as early as 4 months of gestation, it most frequently occurs between the seventh and eleventh months of gestation and usually without any premonitory signs. Foals infected in utero may be born alive but are usually weak and die within 2 to 3 days. Myeloencephalitis with signs of ataxia and posterior paresis has been associated with certain strains of EHV-1.

HOST–VIRUS RELATIONSHIP

Distribution, Reservoir, and Transmission

EHV-1 is prevalent in horses worldwide. The virus appears to be maintained in the horse, but it is possible that dogs, foxes, and carrion birds may carry infection with frag-

ments of aborted fetuses from one farm to another. Respiratory disease is transmitted by droplet infection. In addition, transmission may also occur by direct contact with virus-laden aborted fetuses or placentas. The annual occurrence of respiratory disease in young horses suggests the existence of carriers and latent infections.

Pathogenesis and Pathology

The pathogenesis of EHV-1 abortions remains an enigma. Viremia in the presence of neutralizing antibodies has been detected in experimentally induced abortions and virus cultured from the buffy coat, but not from the cell-free plasma or from washed red-cell suspensions. The cell-associated virus may escape neutralization by antibody, but the mechanism by which the virus reaches the fetus is unknown.

Macroscopically, the most prominent lesions of the fetus are jaundice, mucous membrane petechiation, subcutaneous and pleural edema, splenic enlargement with prominent lymphoid follicles, and focal hepatic necrosis. Histologically there is bronchiolitis, pneumonitis, severe necrosis of the splenic white pulp, and focal hepatic necrosis, all accompanied by intranuclear inclusion bodies. The early fetus (<3 months) shows little or no response to the viral infection. However, the fetus in its last 4 months of gestation shows a marked ability to react in a specific manner to the presence of the virus. Lesions in the fetus less than 7 months of age differ from those in older fetuses, suggesting that the lesions represent a fetal response to the virus.

HOST RESPONSES TO INFECTION

Experimentally, within 24 hours after exposure to EHV-1, foals and mares demonstrate a leukopenia of 24 to 48 hours' duration. Virus persists in circulating leukocytes for as long as 9 days following infection. Abortion in mares may occur as long as 90 to 120 days following infection. Both complement-fixing and virus-neutralizing antibodies appear in the sera of infected horses. In general, complement-fixing antibodies are demonstrable for 6 months after infection, with virus-neutralizing antibodies persisting longer. IgG antibodies against the viral envelope neutralize virus, while those against the nucleocapsid do not. Experimentally pregnant mares with antibody to EHV-1 may abort when challenged with EHV-1. The lesions from which virus cannot be isolated suggest an antigen-antibody complex pathogenesis.

LABORATORY DIAGNOSIS

In case of abortions, diagnosis is based on characteristic lesions with intranuclear inclusions present in the fetal liver, spleen, lung, and thymus. The same tissues provide a good source of virus, which can be demonstrated by immunofluorescence on frozen section and by isolation. The virus is usually relatively easy to isolate. The mare's sera may, but does not invariably, demonstrate a rise in titer. Diagnosis of EHV-1-induced myeloencephalitis is difficult ante mortem because serology may be confusing and EHV-1 is rarely isolated. Histopathologically there is a vasculitis present also suggesting an antigen-antibody complex mechanism. On several occasions, myeloencephalitis has occurred in California horses exposed to mules returning from a mule event. With a specific enzyme-linked immunosorbent assay (ELISA) now available, it is possible to distinguish EHV-1 from EHV-4 serologically and a polymerase chain reaction (PCR) has been described for the diagnosis of EHV-1 abortion.

TREATMENT AND CONTROL

Limiting traffic in and out of brood-mare bands and weanling fields and minimizing stress to pregnant mares have been suggested to help prevent abortion disease. Vaccines, although widely used, have not been completely effective in eliminating abortion loss. A hamster-adapted live viral vaccine that was fully capable of causing disease in young animals and pregnant mares is no longer used. A modified live viral vaccine of cell culture origin, although capable of evoking antibody responses, has not proven effective. An inactivated cell culture vaccine, given at the fifth, seventh, and ninth months of gestation, was shown to be effective in field trials, but abortions have been seen in mares vaccinated with this product. More recently, combined EHV-1/EHV-4 inactivated vaccines are being used.

EQUINE HERPESVIRUS-2

DISEASE

Equine herpesvirus-2 (EHV-2) is prevalent in horses worldwide and has been isolated from both clinically healthy and ill horses. It has been isolated from cases of superficial and chronic lymphoid follicular hyperplasia (CLFG), mild respiratory disease in young animals, and foal pneumonia and from foals with keratoconjunctivitis. There is considerable skepticism, by some researchers, concerning its role in disease. Its role in pneumonia of young foals needs to be considered.

HOST–VIRUS RELATIONSHIP

Distribution, Reservoir, and Transmission

EHV-2, a heterogeneous group of viruses, has been isolated from horses worldwide. Both "healthy" and clinically ill horses act as a reservoir for the virus. In ponies experimentally inoculated with EHV-2, the virus was recovered up to 118 days postinoculation. EHV-2 has been associated with signs of upper respiratory tract disease, and the virus persisted for 418 days. Of a group of 30 foals with respiratory disease, virus has been isolated from 66%, but virus was isolated from only 5% of a group of 20 normal foals. It seems that the primary mode of transmission is via the respiratory tract.

Pathogenesis and Pathology

Little is known about the pathogenesis of EHV-2. Ninety-seven percent of horses less than 1 year old have antibodies to EHV-2, and the virus could be isolated from the leukocytes of 88.7% of normal horses. Similarly, virus could be isolated from 68 of 69 foals sampled once between 1 and 8 months of age. It is suggested that infection is initiated in tonsils, with replication in other sites based on an observed viremia and its cell-associated nature.

LABORATORY DIAGNOSIS

There are no specific diagnostic features associated with EHV-2 infection. The virus can be isolated from nasal and pharyngeal swabs and from blood buffy coats.

TREATMENT AND CONTROL

Control methods have not been established, and a vaccine is not available for EHV-2.

EQUINE HERPESVIRUS-3 (EQUINE COITAL EXANTHEMA)

DISEASE

Equine coital exanthema (ECE), is an acute, sexually transmitted disease characterized by the formation of papules, vesicles, pustules, and ulcers on the penis and prepuce of stallions and on the external genitalia and perineal skin of mares. The lesions usually heal after approximately 14 days, leaving depigmented patches on the vulva and erosions and ulcers on the prepuce and penis of the male. Lesions have occurred, infrequently, around the lips, external nares, nasal mucosa, and conjunctiva.

A unique characteristic of equine herpesvirus-3 (EHV-3) is its inability to grow in cell cultures other than those of equine origin.

Distribution, Reservoir, and Transmission

EHV-3 was first isolated in 1968 concurrently in the United States, Canada, and Australia. The only known reservoir for the virus is the horse and the usual mode of transmission is venereal, but EHV-3 can be spread without coitus. The vulva and vagina need not be damaged for infection to occur. It is plausible that veterinarians may spread the disease via fomites, or insects may act as mechanical carriers. It is suggested that in some infected stallions and mares, EHV-3 becomes latent in the non-breeding season and is reactivated during the breeding season.

Pathogenesis and Pathology

Little is known about the disease pathogenesis, but virus and an antibody increase can usually be demonstrated during development of the lesions. Perivascular and periglandular lymphocytic accumulations suggest that an immune-mediated reaction may play a role in pathogenesis.

Microscopic examination of vulvar tissue demonstrates shallow erosions along with occasional typical intranuclear inclusions scattered in germinal epithelium or in nuclear remnants in necrotic areas.

Host Responses to Infection

Antibodies usually appear during the acute stage of the disease.

LABORATORY DIAGNOSIS

Clinical signs, serologic tests, histopathologic examination, and viral isolation can be used in diagnosing ECE.

TREATMENT AND CONTROL

There is no EHV-3 vaccine available. Treatments include use of topical ointments to reduce pain and sexual rest for at least 3 weeks.

EQUINE HERPESVIRUS-4 (EQUINE RHINOPNEUMONITIS)

Clinical manifestations of equine herpesvirus-4 (EHV-4) are seen principally in foals and younger horses, with a seasonal peak of disease in fall and winter. Symptoms often include malaise and elevated temperature up to 105°F, which may persist for 2 to 5 days; watery nasal discharge, which becomes mucopurulent in the later stages; congested conjunctiva; and, infrequently, enlarged submandibular nodes.

The agent appears to have worldwide distribution; however, it is very infrequently isolated. Both inactivated and modified live vaccines are used but results are not uniformly favorable.

EQUINE HERPESVIRUS-5

In a study of multiple equine herpesvirus-5 (EHV-5) isolates, several were found to differ significantly genomically and in their protein composition. EHV-5 has been proposed for this group of viruses that were isolated from equine respiratory tracts. The role or significance of EHV-5 has not been described.

RUMINANT HERPES VIRUSES

Herpes viruses, representing alpha- and gammaherpesviruses, are responsible for a wide range of conditions in ruminants, including neurologic, genital, fetal, and respiratory diseases. Infections may range from inapparent to fatal in nature. Currently four different herpes viruses groups are classified as bovine herpes viruses. Based on restriction endonuclease patterns associated with disease, bovine herpesvirus-1 (BHV-1) isolates (alphaherpesviruses) were classified into three groups: BHV-1.1 (IBR virus) causes respiratory disease, BHV-1.2 (IPV virus) causes genital disease, and the third, originally classified as BHV-1.3, but reclassified as BHV-5, causes neurologic disease. Some confusion exists among the three groups as some researchers have reported neurologic disease with BHV-1.1 and respiratory disease with BHV-5. Restriction endonuclease pattern variation is known to occur with a single in vivo passage and may account for some of the reported discrepancies. BHV-2 (alphaherpesvirus) causes mammillitis. The role of BHV-4 (gammaherpesvirus) in clinical diseases is not clearly defined. BHV-5 (alphaherpesvirus) is associated with neurologic disease. There are two groups of herpesvirus classified as sheep herpes: OHV-1, which is associated with pulmonary adenomatosis, and OHV-2, which is classified as a gammaherpesvirus and is associated with malignant catarrhal fever. Two viruses (both gammaherpesviruses) previously designated BHV-3 have been designated Alcelaphine herpesvirus: AlHV-1 (African MCF, associated with wildebeest) and AlHV-2 (atypical MCF, associated with the hartebeest). An alphaherpesvirus, CpHV-1, has been associated with several clinical manifestations in goats. Two viruses, CerHV-1 and CerHV-2, have been isolated from deer.

BOVINE HERPESVIRUSES

BOVINE HERPESVIRUS-1

DISEASE

Bovine herpesvirus-1 (BHV-1) infection in cattle may present as ocular, genital, respiratory, and, infrequently, neurologic disease. Respiratory disease typically presents as rhinotracheitis (infectious bovine rhinotracheitis, IBR, BHV-1.1), which may lead to severe and often fatal bronchopneumonia. Conjunctivitis is common. Occasionally the cornea is involved and a panophthalmitis may occur. BHV-1 can infect genitalia, resulting in abortion, balanoposthitis, and vulvovaginitis (infectious pustular vulvovaginitis, IPV, BHV-1.2). Meningoencephalitis in young calves occurs infrequently with BHV-1. Neurologic isolates are most commonly designated BHV-5. BHV-1 has been isolated from vesicular lesions on the udder and teats of a cow.

ETIOLOGIC AGENT

Infectivity for Other Species and Culture Systems

Although cattle appear to be the major species affected by BHV-1, the virus has been incriminated in swine vaginitis and balanitis, and has been isolated from stillborn and newborn pigs. Approximately 11% of swine tested in Iowa and Texas had antibodies to IBR. The virus has been isolated from red deer with eye disease, and could be activated in Malaysian buffalo by steroid administration. It does not appear that BHV-1 virus is a significant pathogen of goats. Only 3% of 1146 serum samples of captive ruminants in U.S. zoos had antibodies to IBR virus.

BHV-1 virus can be grown in a wide variety of cells, including bovine, canine, feline, equine, ovine, rabbit, monkey, and human cells, where it produces a characteristic cytopathic effect.

HOST–VIRUS RELATIONSHIP

Distribution, Reservoir, and Transmission

The disease occurs worldwide. During the late 1950s, an apparently identical virus to IBR virus was isolated from infectious pustular vulvovaginitis (IPV). Although initially designated based on serologic characterization as IBR-IPV (BHV-1.2), the virus differs from the respiratory disease virus (BHV-1.1) in structural proteins and restriction endonuclease patterns.

It has been suggested that wildlife may play a role in disease transmission, but in light of demonstrated viral recrudescence, cattle must be considered the primary reservoir. Virus is transmitted by respiratory, genital, and conjunctival secretions of infected cattle.

Pathogenesis and Pathology

The virus replicates in the upper respiratory tract and spreads via the lacrimal ducts. Virus can be recovered from nasal secretions for almost 2 weeks following infection. Although viremia is difficult to demonstrate, experimental infections have yielded virus from various organs. Such spread is felt to result from leukocyte-associated virus.

Genital infections are most likely venereally transmitted. Lesions consisting of pustules and later fibronecrotic plaques are usually limited to the vulva and posterior vagina in the female. Similar lesions are seen on the prepuce of affected males. Respiratory disease has been produced with genital isolates, and genital lesions have been produced with respiratory isolates. Viral shedding was observed in cows 14 days after experimental genital infection and in males up to 19 days following infection. Virus was shed following prednisolone treatment in these cattle 2 and 7 months, respectively, following initial infection. These observations suggest that the virus may be maintained by periodic shedding when animals are subjected to stress. Although the frequency is low, occasional bulls are encountered that shed BHV-1 intermittently in semen. Insemination of cattle with such semen may result in endometritis, reduced conception, and shortened estrus periods. Experimentally, semen isolates can induce severe rhinotracheitis and vulvovaginitis in cattle. Natural outbreaks of simultaneous respiratory and genital disease are rare.

Abortion is often seen in pregnant cattle with IBR or occasionally following vaccination with modified live virus vaccine. The incubation period between infection of the dam and fetal death varies from 15 to 60 days. Since fetal death occurs several days before abortion, the fetus is often severely autolyzed. Fetal edema, especially of the fetal membranes, occurs along with extensive hemorrhagic edema in the perirenal tissue. Extensive hemorrhagic necrosis of the renal cortex is seen along with a focal necrosis in the liver and usually in the lymph nodes. Some necrosis may be observed in placentomes, which are usually good sources of virus for isolation attempts. Necrotic lesions occur in ovaries of cattle experimentally infected by nongenital routes.

Conjunctivitis is common in BHV-1 infection. Typically it presents with profuse lacrimation and occasionally extends into the cornea, resulting in a keratitis. In some cattle, a multifocal lymphoid hyperplasia may be seen in the palpebral conjunctiva.

Meningoencephalitis has been recorded in natural and experimental disease. Histopathologic lesions include those of a nonsuppurative meningoencephalitis, neuronal necrosis, focal malacia, and often intranuclear inclusion in astrocytes and neurones associated with lesions.

Latent infections have been demonstrated in the trigeminal ganglia of clinically normal cattle. Recrudescent shedding of virus has been observed naturally and in response to corticosteroid administration.

Host Response to Infection

The immune response to BHV-1 involves many factors in addition to the stimulation of neutralizing antibodies, most of which are directed toward surface glycoproteins. IgG and IgM antibodies appear 7 days following exposure. The IgG response during this primary phase is restricted primarily to the IgG-1 subclass. Secondary responses seen mainly in the IgG class are due to increase in IgG-2 antibody. Secondary intranasal exposure did not produce an increase in IgM antibody, whereas an increase in IgM levels was seen following abortion. The neutralization of extracellular virus prevents extracellular spread of virus stressing the importance of antibody at mucosal surfaces. Antibody can also play a role in the complement-mediated lysis of infected cells and in antibody dependent-cell cytotoxicity. The induction of cytokines can activate effector cells that destroy infected cells directly or through antibody interaction. These actions occur in concert with each other making it difficult to ascribe a level of importance to each. In vaccine considerations, it is important that consideration be given to a product's ability to both induce antibody and cell-mediated immunity.

LABORATORY DIAGNOSIS

The fibrinonecrotic plaques commonly present in the external nares and on the nasal septum are good sources of material for viral isolation. The conjunctival form can be tentatively diagnosed by the observation of multifocal white lesions in the palpebral conjunctiva. In their absence, viral isolation is needed. The virus can be readily isolated from the conjunctival swabs. Abortion may be difficult to diagnose as the fetus is often presented in an autolysed condition. If placenta is available and relatively fresh, isolation attempts can be made from the placentomes. While immunofluorescent staining techniques have been used on fetal tissue with varying degrees of success, immunoperoxidase staining that has been positive in IFA negative tissues has improved abortion diagnosis associated with BHV-1. Diagnosis based on serology may be difficult because animals often have high titers at

the time of abortion, regardless of cause, making it difficult to demonstrate rising titers. Detection of BHV-1 in semen is difficult by conventional methods. A PCR-based technique has been used to detect BHV-1 in semen.

TREATMENT AND CONTROL

A modified vaccine used intramuscularly was associated with reduction in disease but could cause abortion in pregnant cattle. An intranasal vaccine was shown to be safe for use in cattle. An intranasal IBR vaccine containing a temperature-sensitive mutant virus that will replicate only at the lower temperature found only in the upper airways of cattle is promoted as safe and effective for use in pregnant animals. Corticosteroid treatment of animals vaccinated with modified live vaccines has resulted in recrudesence of virus. Despite these uncertainties, modified live BHV-1 vaccines are widely used because of the potentially heavy economic loss resulting from infection.

Inactivated vaccines have not been consistently efficacious; however, newer products need to be evaluated. Subunit vaccines have been suggested as an alternative to modified live vaccine. Initial work demonstrated a detergent prepared subunit vaccine to prevent infection in exposed calves. Similarly, work with gene deletion mutants holds promise for successful vaccines that could contribute to eradication efforts.

Eradication

Countries with small cattle populations have used serology for eradication; however, common practices in larger countries prevent this approach to eradication. Appropriate serology used with genetically engineered vaccines may hold promise.

BOVINE HERPESVIRUS-2 (BOVINE MAMMILLITIS)

Bovine herpesvirus-2 (BHV-2) has been isolated from cattle with generalized skin disease (pseudolumpy skin disease [LSD] [Allerton, MN, RU strains]), mammillitis, and stomatitis.

BHV-2 will replicate in a wide range of cells, but bovine kidney cell culture is most widely used. Cattle appear to be primarily infected, with mild experimental disease produced in sheep, goats, and pigs.

BHV-2 has been isolated from cattle skin and mucosal infection in the United States, Africa, Europe, and Australia. Originally virus was isolated from South African cattle with generalized skin disease, subsequently termed *pseudolumpy skin disease*. Mammillitis due to BHV-2 was described in Africa and England, and subsequently in the United States. Stomatitis in bovine and buffalo calves has been described in association with calves nursing cows with mammillitis. Suggested modes of infection include transmission at milking, by insects, or activation of latent virus.

Intravenous exposure produces generalized skin lesions, which are characterized by a severe intercellular germinal cell edema in the epidermis along with syncytia with intranuclear inclusions. An epidermal mononuclear cell and neutrophil infiltrate is present along with mononuclear and lymphocytic dermal perivascular infiltration.

The diagnosis of pseudolumpy skin disease and mammillitis can be based on clinical signs and viral isolation in cell culture. Serology on paired samples will demonstrate an increase in antibody.

BOVINE HERPESVIRUS-4

Bovine herpesvirus-4 (BHV-4) consists of a group of viruses (Movar 33/63, 66-P-347, Rheims, DN-599) isolated from different clinical syndromes and normal cattle. Their importance as pathogens is unclear. Only strain DN-599 has been reported to produce conjunctivitis and respiratory disease. Viruses related to this group have been repeatedly isolated from cases of metritis in California cattle and are suspected of causing vaginitis in heifers. The American and European strains appear to be closely related. Latency has been suggested for this group as there appears to be reactivation in response to other inflammatory processes.

BOVINE HERPESVIRUS-5

Bovine nonsuppurative meningoencephalitis has been associated with bovine herpesvirus-5 (BHV-5) (previously designated BHV-1.3) infection. Isolates have been obtained in Argentina, Australia, Hungary, Japan, and the United States from cattle with sporadic cases of encephalitis. BHV-5 strongly cross-reacts with BHV-1 and currently the two cannot be distinguished serologically but can be differentiated by their restriction endonuclease patterns. It appears that BHV-5 has been circulating in cattle for at least 20 years, with only sporadic disease occurrences. Mortality is usually reported to be 100%. Lesions vary as to severity but usually consist of perivascular infiltrates throughout the brain, with neuronal necrosis, disruption of the neuropil, and gliosis. Experimental infections produce similar signs and lesions as those naturally occurring and BHV-5 can be reisolated from the brain.

ALCEPHALINE HERPESVIRUS-1 AND -2 (MALIGNANT CATARRHAL FEVER)

Malignant catarrhal fever (MCF), an often fatal infection of many species of bovidae and cervidae, exists as two epidemiologic entities: wildebeest-associated and sheep-associated MCF. Alcephaline herpesvirus-1 (AlHV-1) is responsible for wildebeest-derived (or African) MCF, which occurs when cattle and wildebeest graze together. An etiologic agent for sheep-associated (or European and

American) MCF has not been isolated; however, evidence based on competitive-inhibition ELISA and a PCR assay strongly suggested the presence of ovine herpesvirus-2 (OHV-2) in sheep-associated MCF. AlHV-2, which is associated with the hartebeest, has not been incriminated in naturally occurring disease of domestic cattle. A Minnesota virus isolated from clinical MCF cattle appears to be closely related to AlHV-1.

AlHV-1, a typical herpesvirus, has a distinct restriction endonuclease pattern. Infectivity is lost by freeze-thawing and sonication of infected cells. The virion is reported to range from 98 nm to 240 nm. Virus has been propagated in bovine thyroid and testicle cell culture.

The clinical disease is limited to cattle, buffalo, and several species of wild exotic ungulates (Pere David deer, banteng, gaurs). Disease is associated with mixing wildebeest and cattle during periods when the wildebeest are calving. Newborn wildebeest calves shed virus in nasal and ocular secretions up to 3 months of age. Viral shedding has been observed in adult wildebeest given corticosteroid. There is no evidence for congenital infection of sheep with OHV-2; rather, lambs appear to become infected during the first year of life. While sheep-associated MCF in cattle has been associated with lambing, it appears that the newborn lamb does not play the same role as the newborn wildebeest. It also appears that all domestic U.S. sheep carry OHV-2.

Diagnosis is made based on histopathology and a recently developed PCR test. Affected animals present with mucopurulent nasal and ocular discharge and corneal opacity. Oral lesions may be present, consisting of multiple erosions preceded by a diffuse hyperemia and profuse salivation. Central nervous disturbances are frequent and diarrhea is common.

Lesions are those of a lymphoproliferative disorder characterized by perivascular mononuclear infiltration, necrotizing vasculitis, and tissue lymphoid infiltration. Deposition of immunoglobulin, complement, and conglutinin has been seen in the glomeruli of affected cattle, suggesting an immune-mediated disease. Viral antigen was rarely detected, however, and virus-specific antibodies were not seen.

OVINE HERPESVIRUS

OVINE HERPESVIRUS-1

Ovine herpesvirus-1 (OVH-1) has been isolated from lung tissue of sheep with pulmonary adenomatosis ("jaagsiekte"). Although the virus causes experimental pneumonia in lambs, no solid evidence exists that it is responsible for pulmonary adenomatosis.

OVINE HERPESVIRUS-2

There are strong suggestions that sheep-associated malignant catarrhal of cattle is caused by ovine herpesvirus-2 (OHV-2). The virus has never been isolated;

however, OHV-2 DNA has been detected by PCR in cattle with MCF. It shares a close genomic relationship with AlHV-1.

Caprine Herpesvirus-1

A herpesvirus (previously designated BHV-6) was isolated from young goats (1 week) dying in California with enteric signs and necrosis and ulceration in the rumen, cecum, and colon. Signs of conjunctivitis and rhinitis were observed in Swiss goat kids. Although infection in adults usually is apparent, genital diseases may occur as vulvitis or valanoposthitis. An isolate from a California sheep fetus was determined by DNA analysis to be caprine herpesvirus (CpHV-1).

The California isolate replicates in canine, rabbit, feline, equine, bovine, and lamb cells. Virus is inactivated at 56°C within 5 minutes. The virus can be maintained at −70°C but rapidly loses its titer at −20°C. It is inactivated by ether, chloroform, and sodium deoxycholate. Buoyant density in CsCl was observed to be 1.282 g/cm³. A serologic relationship exists between BHV-1 and CpHV-1. Restriction endonuclease analysis demonstrates differences between BHV-1 and CpHV-1.

Virus could be isolated from vaginal secretions of does exposed intranasally, intramuscularly, and intravenously. Pregnant does abort, but no virus was isolated from the fetuses. Infections were severe in kids, with signs of conjunctivitis, rhinitis, and diarrhea. Fibronecrotic lesions on the nasal septum were remarkably similar to those of cattle with IBR.

Gross lesions are limited to the gastrointestinal tract with necrosis and ulceration in rumen, cecum, and colon. Intranuclear inclusions are present in epithelial cells near the necrotic areas.

The disease can be diagnosed by viral isolation from nasal secretions and fecal material. It appears to be rare, and no vaccine is available.

Pseudorabies (Aujeszky's Disease)

Disease

Pseudorabies in swine is most severe in younger animals. It commonly affects the nervous system and the mortality rate varies from 5% to 100%. Infection of sows during mid- to late pregnancy can result in abortion, fetal death, mummification, or stillbirths. In adult pigs, severe nervous disorders are rare, and pseudorabies usually presents as a rather vague illness of transient pyrexia, dullness, inappetence, incoordination, and ataxia. Respiratory disease can also be seen in pigs of various ages but is most common in grower and finishing pigs. Inapparent or mild disease may be missed or misdiagnosed in older swine. Natural disease occurs in other species, including cattle, sheep, dogs, cats, and raccoons, in which the clinical signs are usually neurologic and manifested by an intense pruritis.

Etiologic Agent

Physical, Chemical, and Antigenic Properties

The pseudorabies virus (PRV), an alphaherpesvirus, is about 180 nm in diameter and has an estimated buoyant density of 1.731 g/cm³ in CsCl. Its linear, double-stranded DNA molecule has a molecular weight of approximately 90×106. At least 20 polypeptides can be identified by polyacrylamide gel electrophoresis. Only one serotype has been identified; however, strain variability has been observed based on restriction endonuclease patterns of viruses from different geographic areas. Attenuated strains have been demonstrated to have a deletion in their genome, suggesting that specific regions are associated with virulence. Minor antigenic variations are seen upon serial passage of isolates.

Sensitivity to Physical and Chemical Agents

The PRV is fairly sensitive to high temperatures and is stable in cell culture fluid between a pH of 6 to 8 at cooler temperatures. Virus has been observed to survive in unchlorinated water for 7 days and for 2 days in an anaerobic lagoon. Chemicals that cleave chlorine appear to be the most effective disinfectants.

Infectivity for Other Species and Culture Systems

The disease occurs naturally in cattle, sheep, dogs, cats, and rats. In all but adult swine the disease is almost always fatal; hence, other animals are essentially "dead-end" hosts. Although one report exists of human infection, it is generally felt that PRV is not readily transmitted to humans.

The virus replicates readily in cell cultures from many species and tissues, including cat, dog, cattle, badger, coyote, deer, buzzard, chicken, and goose.

Host–Virus Relationship

Distribution, Reservoir, and Transmission

Pseudorabies has been recognized as a severe, highly fatal disease of newborn pigs in Europe and the United States, and has been reported in other parts of the world, such as Brazil, China, and possibly Africa. The principal reservoir of PRV appears to be the pig and transmission is frequently pig to pig. The virus is transmitted by ingestion and inhalation, and during coitus the virus can be transmitted from boar to sow or vice versa. Transmission can occur in a contaminated environment under crowded conditions.

Feral swine can transmit the virus to domestic swine and among wild animals, among which the raccoon has been the most studied. Infected racoons may transmit by close contact with swine and swine may be exposed by consuming infected raccoon carcasses. The pig is the primary source of viral spread to other species. Cases in dogs have been linked to consumption of feral swine tissues. The cat appears to be more sensitive, and infection in cats was observed in 51% of PRV-infected farms where cats were present.

Pathogenesis and Pathology

The virus replicates primarily in the upper respiratory epithelium including the tonsillar tissue. Virus can be isolated from the brain 24 hours following infection, which suggests that the route of infection is via the axoplasm. Viremia is difficult to demonstrate; however, viral shedding may last in nasal secretions for up to 14 days. Lower airway infection often results, and cardiac and splanchnic ganglia become involved.

The virus produces a nonsuppurative meningoencephalomyelitis with extensive damage to neurons, widespread perivascular cuffs, and gliosis. The brain stem is particularly affected, but lesions also occur throughout the cerebral cortex and cerebellum. There may be intranuclear inclusion bodies in all types of cells. In the respiratory form of the disease, a necrotizing tracheitis and pneumonia are produced that result in loss of epithelium in airways and necrosis of alveolar cells.

Microscopic lesions in aborted fetuses include necrosis of many organs, but primarily liver, spleen, visceral lymph nodes, and adrenal glands. Intranuclear inclusion bodies have been observed in degenerating hepatic cells, the cortical cells of the adrenal glands, and occasionally the reticuloendothelial cells of the spleen and lymph nodes. The placental lesions were characterized by degeneration and necrosis of the trophoblasts and mesenchymal cells of the chorionic fossae.

Host Response to Infection

IgM antibodies are first detectable about the fifth day after infection followed by measurable IgG antibodies about the seventh day, reaching maximum levels by the twelfth to fourteenth day.

LABORATORY DIAGNOSIS

Because symptoms of the disease in swine vary widely with the age of the animal, the dose of virus received, the strain of virus, and the route of exposure, clinical diagnosis is often difficult.

In the laboratory, a definitive diagnosis of pseudorabies can be made by viral isolation. Immunofluorescent staining of frozen tonsil or brain tissue can provide a rapid diagnosis. It is essential that proper controls be used in the interpretation of tonsillar fluorescence. Serologic tests for pseudorabies antibodies include solid-phase radioimmunoassay, immunodiffusion tests, enzyme-linked immunosorbent assay (ELISA), complement-fixation test, serum virus-neutralizing test (SVN), counterneuronal immunoelectrophoresis, and indirect hemagglutination. ELISA tests are used to differentiate antibody response to gene-deleted vaccines and field

infection. In an acute outbreak, serology may not be helpful because of the time needed for antibodies to develop. In the United States, the most commonly used tests are latex agglutination (LAT), ELISA, and SVN. In eradication efforts, the sensitive LAT, which is quick and easy to perform, is commonly used as a screening assay. For confirmation, the SVN and ELISA are used with specific ELISA tests, which are especially useful in detecting animals vaccinated with gene-deleted vaccines.

PREVENTION AND CONTROL

In an effort to avoid the disease in a breeding herd, a producer should 1) purchase animals from sources free of the disease, 2) require testing prior to purchase, 3) isolate new arrivals and test for antibodies a minimum of 12 days after receipt and isolation, 4) restrict human traffic among the swine and practice hygienic measures, and 5) make efforts to restrict contact of the swine with other animals. Feed is a potential source of virus and appropriate measures should be used.

In infected herds, quarantine is the most urgent obligation and it is recommended that the movement of swine be limited for slaughter only. Porcine origin antiserum with titers of at least 1:256 has proven effective in reducing death losses if administered to neonatal pigs. However, none is commercially available.

Attenuated live vaccines are available and have been successful in reducing death losses in endemic areas. These vaccines do not prevent reinfection with virulent field virus or the release of virulent virus for variable periods. Latently infected and vaccinated animals may shed the virus for indeterminate periods while asymptomatic.

Inactivated vaccines are commercially available. Their principal use has been in susceptible sows in endemic areas to provide antibodies to colostrum for protection of newborn pigs during the first few weeks of life. Genetically engineered gene-deletion vaccines are currently used in designated states since control programs utilize differential serology as part of a federal eradication program.

CANINE HERPESVIRUS

DISEASE

Canine herpesvirus (CHV) causes neonatal deaths, abortions, and mummification as well as fatal systemic infection in newborn pups and relatively mild infections in older dogs. The virus induces a generalized, often lethal infection within the first 2 weeks of life. Pups are either stillborn or die after a short illness.

CHV has been isolated from dogs with respiratory diseases, and, with other viruses and bacteria, may be involved in the "kennel cough" syndrome.

CHV can induce genital lesions in male and female dogs. Affected animals appear healthy but often present a history of infertility.

ETIOLOGIC AGENT

Physical, Chemical, and Antigenic Properties

Canine herpesvirus is a typical herpesvirus. There is no cross-neutralization between CHV and the viruses of herpes simplex, herpes simiae, pseudorabies, or infectious bovine rhinotracheitis. However, CHV appears to be antigenically related to herpes simplex virus.

Infectivity for Other Species and Culture Systems

A coyote herpesvirus, shown to be antigenically related to CHV, was found in coyote pups believed to be infected by indirect contact with dogs. No other animals have been reported to show susceptibility to CHV. Limited growth occurs in human lung cells and calf, monkey, pig, rabbit, and hamster kidney cells.

HOST–VIRUS RELATIONSHIP

Distribution, Reservoir, and Transmission

Canine herpesvirus has been isolated in Europe, Japan, Australia, New Zealand, and the United States. The only known reservoir of CHV in all geographic areas is the dog, with the possible exception of coyotes in the United States.

Modes of transmission of CHV may include transplacental, congenital, oral, and airborne transmission. There is also some evidence of transmission by indirect contact via an animal handler.

Pathogenesis and Pathology

Canine herpesvirus has been associated with respiratory disease in adult dogs, but the severe acute necrotizing and hemorrhagic disease occurs only in puppies infected at less than approximately 2 weeks of age. The virus can be isolated from the nose and pharynx of young dogs exposed intranasally. It can multiply in the respiratory and female genital tracts of older dogs and can be isolated for up to 7 days from the vagina of bitches inoculated intravaginally. It has also been isolated from pharyngeal mucosa. Through a necrotizing vasculitis, the virus is disseminated hematogenously, resulting in lesions in many organs. Grossly, the kidneys may appear mottled and there may be pulmonary congestion and edema, splenomegaly, lymphadenitis, and nonsuppurative meningoencephalitis.

Widespread foci of necrosis and hemorrhages with a slight inflammatory response characterize the lesions seen in most affected organs, that is, kidneys, liver, and lung. Intranuclear inclusions may be present in areas adjacent to necrotic lesions.

Host Response to Infection

Neutralizing antibodies develop in dogs inoculated with CHV, but the duration of immunity is not known. CHV induces serum-neutralizing antibodies in infected puppies. Reactivation of CHV in experimentally infected pups and dogs has been demonstrated with administration of corticosteroids.

LABORATORY DIAGNOSIS

Clinical signs and histopathology can be useful in diagnosis. Definitive diagnosis is by viral isolation and more rapidly by immunofluorescent staining of affected tissues.

PREVENTION AND CONTROL

Commercial CHV vaccines are not available. Hyperimmune globulin may be useful but difficult to obtain because the virus is poorly immunogenic. Removal or separation of infected animals should be considered.

FELINE HERPESVIRUS-1 (FELINE VIRAL RHINOTRACHEITIS)

DISEASE

Feline herpesvirus-1 (FHV-1) is the cause of feline viral rhinotracheitis (FVR). Along with upper respiratory disease, the virus is also associated with conjunctivitis, ulcerative keratitis, ulcerative stomatitis, abortions, and pneumonia.

ETIOLOGIC AGENT

Physical, Chemical, and Antigenic Properties

Feline herpesvirus has both "naked" (nonenveloped) particles, 108 nm in diameter, and enveloped particles, approximately 180 nm in diameter. Serologic comparisons have been made between various isolates of FHV from many parts of the world, and all have shown a homogeneity with the prototype strain designated (−27); however, differences in the clinical manifestations caused by various isolates have been observed. Serum neutralization has been most often used in comparing these viruses to other feline viruses, and recently immunoblot analysis of restriction enzyme patterns has been suggested for epidemiological studies.

Sensitivity to Physical and Chemical Agents

The infectivity is reduced or eliminated by ether, chloroform deoxycholate, and sodium hypochlorite. Virus in cell culture fluid loses 90% of its viability within 6 hours at 37°C, 6 days at 25°C, and 1 month at 4°C. The virus is most stable at pH 6, and complete activity is lost in 3 hours at pH 3 and pH 9. FHV can be recovered for up to

18 hours in a moist environment at 15°C, but for less than 12 hours in a dry room.

Infectivity for Other Species and Culture Systems

Natural infections with FVR virus have been observed only in the cat family. FHV-1 in vitro growth is limited mainly to cells of feline origin. The virus propagates to high titers with demonstrated cytopathic effect in primary cell cultures of feline testicle, lung, and renal cells.

Host–Virus Relationships

Distribution, Reservoir, and Transmission

Natural cases of the disease have been reported throughout the United States, Canada, Europe, Australia, and New Zealand. Cats serve as reservoirs. Healthy cats latently infected may shed virus when stressed, for example, by corticosteroid administration, and viral transcripts have been detected in trigeminal ganglia of latently infected cats.

The major avenue for spread of FHV-1 is by direct cat-to-cat contact through infectious discharges and aerosolized microdroplets. Indirect or fomite transmission via a contaminated environment, personnel, or feeding and cleaning utensils appears important only in catteries.

Pathogenesis and Pathology

The pathogenesis of the infection differs with the route of inoculation. As FHV-1 infection is often manifested in the upper respiratory tract, experimental studies have been done by nasal and ocular routes. When introduced intranasally, the virus produces rapid, cytolytic infection of epithelial cells of the nasal passages. The virus generally persists in the upper respiratory tract for 2 weeks. Although many cats develop conjunctivitis during the primary disease, very few develop corneal disease. Experimentally, suppression of local immune responses permitted viral access to the cornea. The resulting keratitis appears to be due to the immune response to the virus.

In the respiratory tract, changes occur in both stratified squamous and pseudostratified columnar epithelial cells. Lung changes consist of interstitial pneumonitis with focal necrotic lesions in the bronchi, bronchioles, and alveolar septa with alveolar accumulations of inflammatory cells and fibrinous exudate.

Intranuclear inclusion bodies are numerous in the stratified squamous epithelium of the conjunctiva with conjunctival and corneal lesions. Histologically, corneal ulcers reveal disorientation and degeneration of the epithelial cells, some of which contain nuclear inclusions.

Host Response to Infection

The primary immune response of cats to intranasal infection as measured by serum neutralizing antibodies is not impressive. Antibodies usually persist for 1 to 3 months, although titers have been observed to fluctuate in a cat between 1:48 and 1:256 over a 12-month period. Correlation between presence of antibodies and resistance to infection is not absolute.

Laboratory Diagnosis

Immunofluorescent staining can demonstrate viral antigens in the tissues of experimentally infected cats. Early in the course of FVR, the conjunctival and nasal mucosa contain sufficient numbers of infected cells for antigen detection.

Feline herpesvirus is isolated from tissue samples and from swabs of the ocular, nasal, or oropharyngeal mucosa. The virus can be cultured from nasal or pharyngeal swabbings for 14 to 21 days after infection, but most consistently during the first week.

Virus-neutralizing antibodies can be detected in the serum of convalescent cats. Paired samples, the first collected during acute illness, the other collected 2 or 3 weeks later, can be used for the serologic diagnosis of FVR.

Prevention and Control

All husbandry measures to ensure an adequate diet and to protect against unnecessary stresses help minimize risks of infection. Care should be taken to avoid introducing cats with either developing or subclinical disease to a colony.

A modified live feline viral rhinotracheitis vaccine is available. Protective immunity appears to be relatively short, and revaccination every 6 to 12 months is recommended. An intranasal vaccine is also available. A recombinant vaccine is reported experimentally to result in a reduced latency load.

Simian Herpesvirus B (Cercopithecine Herpesvirus-1)

Herpesvirus B causes a natural infection in Old World monkeys, that is, rhesus and cynomolgus species. The infection in monkeys is characterized by oral vesicular lesions similar to the cold sores in humans caused by herpes simplex virus. The disease in monkeys is not fatal and the virus may remain latent in infected animals. Direct contact is the most common means of viral spread in monkeys, since virus can be recovered from saliva and from the central nervous tissues of clinically asymptomatic, persistently infected animals.

The virus can cause fatal central nervous infection in humans and laboratory animals such as rabbits and unweaned mice. Most human infections are caused by a bite from a monkey secreting infectious virus, although handling virus-infected primary monkey kidney cell cultures can also lead to infection. The incubation period in humans is 10 to 20 days. Usually there is local inflammation at the bite site followed by vesicle formation and necrosis of the area. Virus reaches the central nervous system by peripheral nerves, and death may occur due to acute encephalitis or encephalomyelitis.

Herpesvirus B is morphologically similar to other alphaherpesviruses in the group. It can be readily inactivated by detergents. The virus can be cultivated on the chorioallantoic membrane of embryonated chick eggs and in rabbit, monkey, and human cell cultures that produce intranuclear inclusion bodies and syncytia formation. Strong cross-reactivity exists between human herpes simplex viruses and herpesvirus B.

Herpes simiae virus infection can be diagnosed by isolating virus from the central nervous tissues of fatal human cases. A PCR has been developed for viral identification; however, diagnostic detection of herpes B specific antibodies is difficult. There is no treatment for herpesvirus B infection in humans, nor has an effective vaccine been developed. Human gamma globulin, especially that which contains viral antibodies, should be used immediately after exposure to monkey bites. Caution and wearing of protective gear for handling monkeys remain the best way to avoid infection.

MAREK'S DISEASE

DISEASE

Marek's disease (MD) is a lymphoproliferative disease of chickens that may involve numerous tissues. Most frequently peripheral nerves are affected. Prior to vaccine development, MD was responsible for heavy losses, and increased losses to MD in vaccinated flocks have suggested an evolution toward greater virulence. There are three serotypes of Marek's disease virus (MDV). Serotype 1 (gallid herpesvirus-2 [GaHV-2]) includes isolates that cause mild to severe signs of disease. Serotype 2 (gallid herpesvirus-3 [GaHV-3]) isolates are nononcogenic. Serotype 3 consists of turkey isolates (HVT, meleagrid herpesvirus-1, [MeHV-1]). The three are classified as alphaherpesviruses.

Progressive paralysis of one or more extremities, incoordination, drooping wings, and lowered head position are the most common signs of MD. Mortality varies from 10% with mild MD to over 50% in unvaccinated birds.

ETIOLOGIC AGENT

Physical, Chemical, and Antigenic Properties

Noninfectious virus, which is associated with nuclear vesicles or the nuclear membranes of infected cell cultures, commonly measures 150 nm to 180 nm in diameter. The fully infectious particle observed in the cytoplasm of feather follicle epithelial cells measures 250 nm to 400 nm in diameter. The viral DNA has a

molecular weight of 1×10^8 and a buoyant density of 1.706 mg/cm^3. At least eight MDV structural proteins have been identified, and numerous virus-specific polypeptides have been demonstrated.

Resistance to Physical and Chemical Agents

Cell-free virus is readily inactivated at temperatures greater than 37°C and is only relatively stable at 25°C (4 days) and 4°C (2 weeks). Both MDV and HVT can be maintained for long periods at −70°C. Virus is inactivated by pH 3 and pH 11. Infectivity of dried MDV-infected feathers is destroyed by chlorine, organic iodine, a quaternary ammonium compound, cresylic acid, synthetic phenol, and sodium hydroxide.

Infectivity for Other Species and Culture Systems

The chicken is the primary natural host for the MDV, and disease is rare in other species except for quail. Marek's disease virus has not been shown to affect any nonavian animals. No etiologic link has been demonstrated between MDV and human cancer. The virus is most often cultivated on chicken or duck embryo fibroblast cells. Chicken kidney cells have also been used.

HOST–VIRUS RELATIONSHIPS

Distribution, Reservoir, and Transmission

Marek's disease is a major disease of domestic chicken flocks worldwide. The virus can persist in excreta, litter, and poultry house dust, and horizontal infection via aerosols of chickens appears to be the main method of transmission. Egg transmission is doubtful. Marek's disease virus matures to its enveloped infectious form only in the feather follicles and can then be spread to the environment via desquamated cells. Whole live cells from blood or tumor material, or infected whole cell cultures, are infectious experimentally. Cell-free fluid does not appear to be infectious. Certain chicken lines are genetically resistant to MDV, and resistance in most birds is associated with the development of serum-neutralizing antibody.

Pathogenesis and Pathology

The incidence of MD is variable depending on the strain of the virus and the strain and age of the chicken. It usually occurs in chickens between 2 and 5 months old and is commonly felt not to be seen in birds older than 22 weeks; however, disease has been observed in birds as young as 3 to 4 weeks and in 60-week-old laying hens. The virus primarily affects the nervous system although visceral organs and other tissues may be involved. Lesions are present in the nervous system and involve peripheral nerves and spinal roots. The principal nerve trunk involved shows gross lesions consisting of a grayish-white swelling, which histologically are characterized by extensive lymphocytic infiltrations. Edema may be present and myelin degeneration of nerve sheaths may be apparent.

Ocular lymphomatosis is another possible outcome of MDV infection, with blindness resulting due to iris involvement. Histologically, a similar infiltration of lymphocytes is present, which can also occur in the optic nerve.

In the visceral form, lymphoid tumors of varying degrees of severity infiltrate the gonads, liver, lung, and skin. Affected chickens have enlarged visceral organs with white nodular or miliary foci. Oclusive atherosclerosis has been observed experimentally.

Host Response to Infection

The immune response to MDV is complex, in that both humoral and cell-mediated immunity (CMI) develop in normal birds. MDV infection can be immunosuppressive. In addition, the immune response may be involved in tumor formation. Bursectomized birds survive experimental infection, suggesting that CMI is important. In chicks, passively acquired antibody is thought to limit the extent of infection rather than prevent it or clear the virus. Viral-specific antibodies appear within 1 to 3 weeks following infection and neutralizing antibodies persist for the life of the bird. Following infection, transient CMI suppression is common; it may persist in birds that develop neoplasms. Both B and T cells have been identified in tumors, and thymectomy has been shown to reduce the level of lymphomas in affected birds. It has been suggested that MD might have an autoimmune component based on antibody responses to myelin and peripheral nerves.

LABORATORY DIAGNOSIS

On necropsy, gross lesions are common in peripheral nerves, root ganglia, and the spinal roots. Lymphomatous lesions are characteristically composed of small lymphocytes, lymphoblasts, and reticulum cells. Arterial lesions of atherosclerosis are often present. Confirmatory diagnosis is made by viral isolation or by antigen detection using fluorescent antibody, immunoperoxidase, or ELISA on feather follicle cells. Antibodies can be detected by AGID agar gel immunodiffusion, indirect immunofluorescence, and viral neutralization and ELISA assays.

PREVENTION AND CONTROL

Experimentally, MDV-free flocks can be maintained by strict isolation, constant surveillance, and frequent monitoring for virus and antibody, but these techniques have been of limited commercial use. Commercial vaccines are available and have been effective in reducing the incidence of MD. The three live virus serotypes have been used for vaccines resulting in more vaccines becoming available. HVT vaccine (serotype 3) is the most economical to produce and is most effective when exposure is not heavy. Vaccination does not prevent infection or shedding of virulent MDV, but it does prevent tumor formation. Bivalent and polyvalent vaccines have been used successfully where monovalent vaccines have been ineffective. Embryo vaccination is currently used in at least 55% of broiler embryos. Genetically resistant lines of chickens have been maintained experimentally.

INFECTIOUS LARYNGOTRACHEITIS VIRUS (GALLID HERPESVIRUS-1)

DISEASE

Infectious laryngotracheitis virus (ILTV) usually occurs as an acute disease in chickens and represents a serious problem in areas of intense poultry husbandry. The virus produces signs of respiratory distress and coughing that often produce a bloody discharge. Mild enzootic forms of ILTV infection may result in reduced egg production, conjunctivitis, and persistent nasal discharge.

ETIOLOGIC AGENT

Physical, Chemical, and Antigenic Properties

ILTV is a characteristic alphaherpesvirus, 195 nm to 250 nm in diameter, with a DNA buoyant density of 1.704 g/cm^3. All strains have been demonstrated to be antigenically homogeneous.

Sensitivity to Physical and Chemical Agents

ILTV is inactivated by 3% cresol, 1% sodium hydroxide, and 1% lye, 24 hours' exposure to ether, and 10 to 15 minutes at 55°C. The virus can be stored for lengthy periods by lyophilization and freezing at −20°C to −60°C.

Infectivity for Other Species and Culture Systems

ILTV is primarily a disease of chickens, but the disease has also been reported in pheasants and peafowl. Young turkeys have been infected experimentally, and the virus replicates in embryonated turkey eggs. Starlings, sparrows, crows, doves, ducks, pigeons, and guinea fowl have been found to be resistant to ILTV.

Chicken kidney monolayer cell cultures, embryonated chicken eggs, and chicken embryo (kidney, liver, lung) cell cultures have been used to culture ILTV.

HOST−VIRUS RELATIONSHIP

Distribution, Reservoir, and Transmission

ILTV has been identified in almost every country in the world; it occurs primarily in areas with high concentrations of chickens and occasionally occurs in pheasants. Chickens are assumed to be the primary reservoir and mode of transmission, which occurs by direct contact through droplet infection of the ocular and respiratory secretions. Mechanical transmission can occur via contaminated equipment and litter. Egg transmission of ILTV has not been demonstrated. A carrier state can develop in birds with sublethal disease, and ILTV has been isolated from chickens 2 years after infection. Unvaccinated birds are susceptible to infection from vaccinated birds, and vaccinated birds may become carriers. Acutely infected birds represent a greater source of virus than clinically recovered carrier birds.

Pathogenesis and Pathology

ILTV in natural conditions enters through the upper respiratory tract and ocular tract. In the natural disease, the greatest concentration of ILTV is found in the trachea, since the virus replicates only in the nasal cavity, trachea, and lower respiratory tract. Latent virus has been demonstrated in the trigeminal ganglion. Viremia has not been reported.

In lethal infections of ILTV, thickening of tracheal mucosa, hemorrhage, congestive heart failure, and severe congestion of all internal organs have been found. Histopathology demonstrates fibrinous tracheobronchitis, with detachment of the tracheal epithelium and large intranuclear inclusion bodies in detached cells that are the basis for a strong presumptive diagnosis.

Host Response to Infection

The first signs of ILTV infection usually appear 6 to 12 days following natural exposure. Resistance to disease following the infection or vaccination usually persists for approximately 1 year. Infected birds develop precipitating and serum-neutralizing antibodies; however, the cell-mediated response appears to be important in resistance. Full immunity can be demonstrated in bursectomized chickens in the absence of a humoral response.

LABORATORY DIAGNOSIS

Virus can be isolated from tracheal and lung tissue in embryonated chicken eggs, cell culture, and ILTV DNA can be demonstrated by PCR. Immunofluorescent staining of trachea can demonstrate presence of viral antigen up to 14 days postinfection. ELISA-based serology is widely used.

PREVENTION AND CONTROL

Use of live ILTV vaccine results in carriers, which can shed to nonvaccinated susceptible birds. Since the virus can survive for 10 days at temperatures of 13°C to 23°C, the cleaning of infected premises is very important. Complete

depopulation and disinfection of premises has been used to control the disease.

Vaccination has been successful via the cloaca, infraorbital sinuses, intranasal instillation, feather follicles, and drinking water. Birds younger than 2 weeks of age do not respond as well as older birds. Water administration of ILTV vaccination does not give as complete or long-lasting immunity as other methods. For water vaccine to be effective, the virus has to penetrate into the nasal cavity or trachea. Cloacal administration of the vaccine leads to rapid absorption of the virus into the bursa of Fabricius and results in an immune response. This route is undesirable, however, since ILTV damages the bursa of young birds. Adequate ILTV vaccination occurs via aerosol procedures. Modified live ILTV vaccines have been associated with disease and chicken embryo origin vaccines have been demonstrated to increase in virulence after in vivo passage. The development of genetically engineered vaccines holds promise for improved control strategies.

SELECTED REFERENCES

Agius CT, Studdert MJ. Equine herpesvirus 2 and 5: comparisons with other members of the subfamily gammaherpesvirinae. Adv Virus Res 1994;44:357.

Belknap EB, Collins JK, Ayers VK, Schultheiss PC. Experimental infection of neonatal calves with neurovirulent bovine herpesvirus type 1.3. Vet Pathol 1994;31:358.

Bouchey D, Evermann J, Jacob RJ. Molecular pathogenesis of equine coital exanthema (ECE): temperature sensitivity (TS) and restriction endonuclease (RE) fragment profiles of several field isolates. Arch Virol 1987;92:293.

Calnek BW. Pathogenesis of Marek's disease — a review. In: Calnek BW, Spencer JL, eds. Proceedings of the International Symposium on Marek's Disease. Kennett Square, PA: American Association of Avian Pathologists, 1985:374–390.

Crabb BS, Studdert MJ. Equine herpesvirus 4 (equine rhinopneumonitis virus) and 1 (equine abortion virus). Adv Virus Res 1995;45:153.

Eberle R, Hilliard J. The simian herpesviruses. Infect Agents Dis 1995;4:55.

Engels M, Ackermann M. Pathogenesis of ruminant herpesvirus infections. Vet Microbiol 1995;53:3.

Hickman MA, Reubel GH, Hoffman DE, et al. An epizootic of feline herpesvirus type 1 in a large specific pathogen-free cat colony and attempts to eradicate the infection by identification and culling of carriers. Lab Anim 1994;28:320.

Hughes CS, Williams RA, Gaskell RM, et al. Latency and reactivation of infectious laryngotracheitis vaccine virus. Arch Virol 1991;21:213.

Kopotopoulos G. Goat herpesvirus 1 infection: a review. Vet Bull 1992;62:77.

Li H, Shen DT, O'Toole D, et al. Malignant catarrhal fever virus. Characterization of a United States isolate and development of diagnostic assays. Ann NY Acad Sci 1996;791:198.

Metzler AE. The malignant catarrhal fever complex. Comp Immun Microbial Infect Dis 1991;14:107.

Metzler AE, Schudel AA, Engels M. Bovine herpesvirus 1: molecular and antigenic characteristics of variant viruses isolated from calves with neurological disease. Arch Virol 1986;87:205.

Moore S, Gunn M, Walls D. The detection of bovine herpesvirus 1 in routine diagnostic submissions using PCR. Biochem Soc Trans 1995;23:355.

Naisse MP, Guy JS, Stevens JB, et al. Clinical and laboratory findings in chronic conjunctivitis in cats; 91 cases (1983–1991). J Am Vet Med Assoc 1993;203:834.

O'Toole D, Li H, Miller D, et al. Chronic and recovered cases of sheep associated malignant catarrhal fever in cattle. Vet Rec 1997;140:519.

Roizman B, Desrosiers RC, Fleckenstein B, et al. Family herpesviridae. In: Murphy FA, Fauquet CM, Bishop DHL, eds. Virus taxonomy. 6th Report of the International Committee on Taxonomy of Virus. Arch Virol 1995;10(suppl):114.

Sussman MD, Maes RK, Kruger JM. Vaccination of cats for feline rhinotracheitis results in a quantitative reduction of virulent feline herpesvirus-1 latency load after challenge. Virology 1997;22:379.

Tikoo SK, Campos M, Babiuk LA. Bovine herpesvirus 1 (BHV 1): biology, pathogenesis and control. Adv Virus Res 1995; 45:191.

Van Drunen Little-van den Hurk S, Tikoo SK, van den Hurk JV, et al. Protective immunity in cattle following vaccination with conventional and marker bovine herpesvirus-1 (BHV-1) vaccines. Vaccine 1997;15:36.

Van Oirschot JT. Pseudorabies: the virus, its hosts and the environment. Vet Med 1994;89:72.

Wilson WD. Equine herpesvirus 1 myeloencephalopathy. Vet Clin North Am (Equine Pract) 1997;3:53.

Witter RL. Increased virulence of Marek's disease virus field isolates. Avian Dis 1997;41:149.

64 — *Poxviridae*

Jeffrey L. Stott

Poxviruses infect many vertebrate and invertebrate species. Associated diseases typically affect the skin. Generalized clinical signs may or may not be apparent. The diseases associated with birds differ somewhat from those in mammals in that proliferative lesions tend to predominate over pustular lesions.

Poxviruses are large and complex and replicate in the cell cytoplasm. Of two subfamilies, *Chorodopoxviridae* infect vertebrates and *Entomopoxviridae* infect insects. The six genera of *Chorodopoxviridae* and their members are shown in Table 64.1.

Chorodopoxviridae have more than 30 structural proteins and several viral-specified enzymes, including a DNA-dependent transcriptase. Over 100 viral-associated polypeptides have been identified in vaccinia virus by two-dimensional electrophoresis, and 20 proteins have been identified by agar gel immunodiffusion. Virions are brick-shaped, with dimensions ranging from 300 to 450mm × 170 to 260mm. The external coat, composed of lipid and globular or tubular protein structures, encloses two lateral bodies and the core. Two forms of mature virions, extracellular and intracellular, have been described, with the extracellular form having an additional lipoprotein envelope. The genome is enclosed in the core and consists of a single molecule of double-stranded DNA (dsDNA). Of the multiple proteins encoded by the viral genome, a protein of 58,000 molecular weight (MW) forms the surface tubules and elicits neutralizing antibody and antibody that inhibits cellular fusion. Eight proteins, including the hemagglutinin, have been identified in the outer envelope of extracellular virus and at least four proteins are complexed with the genomic DNA.

ORTHOPOXVIRUS

DISEASE

Orthopoxvirus infection results in vesicular disease. Lesion development may be confined to specific areas of the skin or the infection may be of a generalized nature. Skin lesions often appear first as a rash or papule followed by pustule formation and eventual scabbing.

ETIOLOGIC AGENT

Orthopoxviruses include vaccinia, cowpox (Fig 64.1), buffalopox, camelpox, horsepox, monkeypox, ectromelia, and variola (smallpox in humans). They are morphologically indistinguishable. Both enveloped and nonenveloped forms have been described that are antigenically distinct and infective. A viral-specified hemagglutinin is produced and is associated with the virion. All orthopoxviruses produce cytoplasmic inclusion bodies. The viruses are antigenically related, and one virus induces protective immunity to the others. They can be distinguished by gel electrophoresis of proteins, serology, pock formation on chick embryo chorioallantoic membranes (by pock appearance and the ceiling temperature at which they develop), cytopathic effect in cell cultures, and genetic characterization techniques.

HOST–VIRUS RELATIONSHIP

The reservoirs of various orthopoxviruses are not well defined but probably include rodents. Transmission is by contact, by air, or by exposure to viral-contaminated fomites.

Immune responses to orthopoxviruses are both cellular and humoral. A cell-mediated immune response facilitates destruction of infected cells and is important in confining the virus to a localized area. Defects in cellular immunity permit widespread distribution of virus, resulting in generalized disease. Neutralizing antibodies are important in recovery from infection. Immunity appears to be of long duration.

LABORATORY DIAGNOSIS

Diagnosis of orthopoxvirus infection can be made by electron microscopy of virus extracted from lesions or by viral isolation. Isolation may be achieved by inoculation (scarification) of laboratory animals (especially rabbits), of cell cultures, or of the chorioallantoic membrane of

Table 64.1.   Genera (Subfamily: Chorodopoxviridae) of Significance to Veterinary Medicine

Genus	Members
Orthopoxvirus	Vaccinia
	Cowpox
	Buffalopox
	Camelpox
	Horsepox
Parapoxvirus	Bovine papular stomatitis (bovine pustular dermatitis)
	Orf (contagious ecthyma)
	Milker's node (pseudocowpox, paravaccinia)
Avipoxvirus	Fowlpox
	Turkeypox
	Junopox (peacocks)
	Quailpox
	Sparrowpox
	Starlingpox
Capripoxvirus	Sheeppox
	Goatpox
	Lumpy skin disease (Neethling virus)
Suipoxvirus	Swinepox
Leporipoxvirus	Myxoma, rabbit and squirrel fibroma

embryonated chicken eggs. The latter procedure has been widely used and may differentiate viral types.

VACCINIA

Vaccinia may infect cattle via handling (milking) by infected personnel; infected cattle can also infect personnel. Lesions occur on the teats and udder and appear as small papules that progress to pustules, which dry up and scab. Lesions may be ruptured by physical trauma such as milking, and secondary bacterial infections may lead to mastitis.

Vaccinia virus is the genus prototype and was used to vaccinate humans for smallpox (variola). The use of vaccinia has eliminated smallpox from the world. Vaccinia was originally believed to be a cowpox, but its origin is uncertain since it is quite distinct from its purported ancestor.

COWPOX

The general features and associated disease of cowpox virus is closely related to vaccinia, yet it is distinct antigenically. Severe dermal or pulmonary cowpox infections of exotic and domestic cats have been noted. The infection appears to be limited to Britain and western Europe. It has been suggested that rodents may serve as a reservoir of cowpox and closely related viruses.

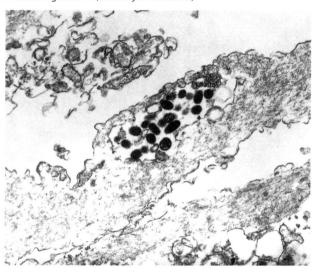

FIGURE 64.1.   *Cowpox virus in skin lesions under thin sectioning. 8000×. (Courtesy of A. Castro.)*

BUFFALOPOX

Buffalopox resembles vaccinia and cowpox and can occur as either a localized (inner thighs, teats, and udder) or generalized infection. The disease is of economic importance and commonly occurs in epidemic form. It has been reported in India, Indonesia, Russia, Pakistan, and Egypt. Buffalopox has been reported to infect humans.

CAMELPOX

Camelpox produces a generalized pustular disease and is of economic importance in countries with an indigenous camel population. It is primarily associated with younger animals and is characterized by fever, generalized rash, and sequential development of vesicular, pustular, and scabbing stages. Lesions most often develop on the limbs, neck, and head. Mammary glands, genitalia, and anal areas may also be affected. A few reports of humans contracting the virus from camels have been recorded. The virus has been documented in the Middle East, northeastern Africa, and parts of Asia.

HORSEPOX

Horsepox may take one of two forms: 1) a localized infection of the pastern with vesicular lesions and 2) a form of the disease involving multiple lesions on the oral mucous membranes.

PARAPOXVIRUS

Three parapoxviruses affecting animals include bovine pustular dermatitis virus (bovine papular stomatitis virus), orf virus (contagious ecthyma), and milker's node virus (pseudocowpox, paravaccinia).

Parapoxvirus lesions tend to be proliferative. Proliferating keratinocytes may undergo ballooning degeneration with development of cytoplasmic inclusion bodies. Lymphoid cells infiltrate the dermis and infected endothelial cells proliferate.

Parapoxviruses are morphologically unique in that an organized tubular, threadlike structure forms a crisscross pattern on the virion surface. The viruses are all antigenically related at the level of the inner coat. The outer envelopes, however, contain antigenically distinct epitopes. The viruses are resistant to ether and chloroform and are stable for long periods of time at ambient temperatures.

BOVINE PAPULAR STOMATITIS

DISEASE

This disease is of minor importance except under adverse husbandry conditions when infection can result in economic loss. The clinical disease is characterized by development of lesions on the muzzle, nostrils, lips, buccal papillae, dental pad, hard and soft palates, and tongue. Hyperemic papules, with central necrosis and concentric colored rings, are characteristic lesions.

HOST–VIRUS RELATIONSHIP

Bovine papular stomatitis has a worldwide distribution and appears to be limited to cattle, although humans can be infected. It is believed to persist in a latent state in cattle. Virus is present in oral and nasal secretions and transmission may occur by direct contact.

LABORATORY DIAGNOSIS AND CONTROL

Bovine papular stomatitis must be differentiated from other vesicular diseases. Virus may be isolated on cell cultures or directly visualized in skin scrapings or biopsy material by electron microscopy. Vaccines have not been developed, and proper management is the best control for the disease.

CONTAGIOUS ECTHYMA

DISEASE

Orf virus (Fig 64.2) is the etiologic agent of contagious ecthyma of sheep and goats (synonyms include scabby mouth, contagious pustular dermatitis of sheep, contagious pustular stomatitis, infectious labial dermatitis, and orf). The disease is characterized by lesions on the lips, mouth, interdigital areas, genitalia, and udder. Papules

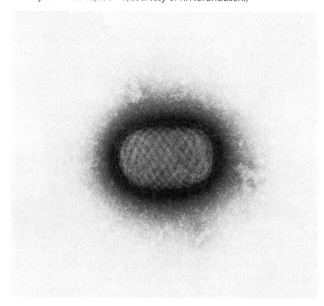

FIGURE 64.2. *Negatively stained preparations of contagious ecthyma virus. 40,000×. (Courtesy of R. Nordhausen.)*

and vesicles rapidly progress to pustules, followed by scab formation. Lesions on the lips result in reduced suckling or grazing, causing emaciation. Complications and losses can occur if secondary bacterial infections or screwworm infestations develop.

HOST–VIRUS RELATIONSHIP

In addition to sheep and goats, orf virus may infect related species and sometimes dogs and humans. The virus has a worldwide distribution and is maintained in nature by persistent infections and survival in dried scabs. Abrasive viral-contaminated forage results in extensive infection.

LABORATORY DIAGNOSIS AND CONTROL

Presumptive diagnosis is based upon clinical observations and pathology (e.g., epithelial lesions with characteristic ballooning cells and Type B cytoplasmic inclusion bodies). Virus can be identified by electron microscopy and isolated in embryonic sheep skin or testicular cells.

Vaccination in endemic areas is advisable and immunity is considered long term. Virulent virus is used in vaccination by scarification of the skin in areas not subject to clinical manifestations.

PSEUDOCOWPOX

Pseudocowpox is a mild disease of cattle that particularly affects lactating animals. Teat lesions develop as papules with an umbilicated center and undergo scabbing and desquamation. This results in a pathognomonic scab with a ring or horseshoe appearance. The virus often infects humans via direct contact, resulting in so-called milker's nodules.

Pseudocowpox occurs in most countries but has little economic significance. Immunity is of short duration and recurrent infections are common. Cattle occasionally develop chronic infections.

AVIPOXVIRUS

Avipoxviruses infect many avian species (see Table 64.1). Fowlpox virus is the genus prototype.

DISEASE

The industries for the raising of chickens, turkeys, and squab may experience variable economic losses due to avipoxvirus infections. The lesions are wartlike nodules of hyperplastic epithelium. Several forms of disease, which may occur in combinations, have been described. A cutaneous form involves primarily the skin of the head (comb, wattles, corners of the mouth, nostrils, and eyes). The cutaneous lesions have an inflamed and hemorrhagic base. A diphtheritic form is characterized by proliferative lesions on the mucous membranes and may extend into the sinuses; involvement of the larynx and trachea may result in dyspnea and rales. The lesions are characterized by inflammation, epidermal hyperplasia, and development of eosinophilic Type A inclusion bodies.

Economic losses in chickens may be due to emaciation and reduced egg production. Blindness and starvation cause the major losses in turkeys. Complications are most commonly responsible for significant losses and mortality rates up to 50%. Infection in canaries is almost always fatal.

ETIOLOGIC AGENT

Avipoxviruses average 258 nm × 354 nm in diameter and contain a DNA genome. Hemagglutinin is absent. Species within the genus are antigenically related. Avian poxviruses are differentiated by host range, serologic tests, plaque formation in cell cultures, and pock formation on the chorioallantoic membrane of embryonated chicken eggs. The viruses are insensitive to ether and highly resistant to desiccation.

HOST–VIRUS RELATIONSHIP

Avipoxviruses have a worldwide distribution. Viral transmission can occur by direct contact or via insects such as mosquitoes and culicoides. Mosquitos can harbor virus for up to 210 days. Virus can survive for long periods in scabs, and latent infections may contribute to viral persistence on a given premise.

Humoral and cellular immune responses develop following infection and apparently confer long-term immunity. Maternal antibody does not confer protection to hatched chicks.

LABORATORY DIAGNOSIS

Diagnosis of avian poxvirus infections are based on clinical signs and histopathology and electron microscopy. Virus can be isolated by inoculating susceptible birds, the chorioallantoic membrane of embryonated chicken eggs, and cell cultures (chicken and duck embryo fibroblasts).

TREATMENT AND CONTROL

Control of avian poxvirus infections can be aided by providing adequate nutrition, housing, and insect control among birds. Antibiotic treatment reduces secondary infections in affected flocks. Vaccination of chickens with virulent fowlpox virus is often successful. Vaccination by the feather follicle method or scarification of the wing-web or leg are common practices. Pigeonpox virus provides some protection against fowlpox but the degree and duration of immunity may be less than that obtained from homologous virus.

CAPRIPOXVIRUS

The genus Capripoxvirus includes sheeppox, goatpox, and lumpy skin disease (Neethling) viruses; sheeppox virus serves as the genus prototype. The viruses are more elongated than other poxviruses and measure about 115 nm × 194 nm; hemagglutinin is absent. The viruses are closely related but differ antigenically. Infection with any virus produces cross-protection to heterologous virus, with the exception of certain strains of goatpox virus. The viruses are predominantly host-specific, though some strains produce lesions in sheep, goats, and/or humans.

SHEEPPOX AND GOATPOX

DISEASE

Sheeppox and goatpox are the most important poxvirus diseases affecting domestic mammals. Disease will range in severity from inapparent to a severe generalized condition. All ages are susceptible but younger animals, especially in endemic areas, are most severely affected. Breed and immune status also affect disease severity. Upon infection, a viremia develops and virus is disseminated to the skin, lymph nodes, and multiple organs including the spleen, kidneys, and lungs. Affected animals stand with an arched back and stop eating. The first clinical signs of disease include pyrexia, rhinitis, and conjunctivitis followed by varying degrees of lesion development on external nares, lips, tongue, gums, and skin (especially where wool or hair is minimal). Skin lesions develop from small vacuoles through papular, vesicular, pustular, and necrotic stages with eventual scab formation. Infected cells in lesions contain eosinophilic cytoplasmic inclusion bodies. Lesions may also develop in the respiratory and alimentary tracts, liver, kidneys, and other organs. A nodular form of the disease has been referred to as *stone pox*. Increased mortality rates are associated with secondary bacterial infections and disseminated internal lesions.

HOST–VIRUS RELATIONSHIP

Infections occur predominantly in the Middle East and parts of Europe, North Africa, and the Indian subcontinent. Viral transmission is by aerosol, direct contact, and possibly arthropod vectors. Viral persistence is probably due to the survival of virus in scabs and its transmission to susceptible animals within an endemic area.

Antibodies, including those with viral-neutralizing activity, develop within 1 week of lesion development. Immunity is considered to be lifelong.

LABORATORY DIAGNOSIS

Histopathology, fluorescent antibody staining, electron microscopy, and serology can help confirm clinical diagnosis. Virus can be isolated in cell cultures of ovine, bovine, and caprine origin. The virus grows relatively poorly in embryonated chicken eggs as compared to orthopoxviruses and parapoxviruses.

TREATMENT AND CONTROL

Preventative measures such as import restrictions are practiced by countries free of the virus. Attenuated and inactivated viral vaccines are used in endemic areas.

LUMPY SKIN DISEASE

DISEASE

Lumpy skin disease of cattle (and buffalo) is caused by a virus (Neethling virus) closely related immunologically to sheeppox and goatpox viruses. Upon infection, a viremia and febrile response develop, followed by formation of nodular lesions on the skin (predominantly on the neck, face, muzzle, brisket, flank, legs, perineum, and scrotum) and internally in the respiratory, digestive, and reproductive tracts. A lymphadenitis is common and may result in lymph stasis, producing edema of limbs, dewlap, udder, vulva, scrotum, and prepuce. Other sequelae include decreased lactation, mastitis, abortion, and temporary sterility of bulls.

HOST–VIRUS RELATIONSHIP

Neethling virus appears to be confined to the African continent. Viral transmission probably occurs by direct contact and aerosol and insect vectors. Virus has been detected in semen, however, which may be an additional mechanism of transfer. Persistence of virus in nature is probably similar to that described for sheeppox and goatpox. It has been suggested that buffalo may serve as viral reservoirs.

LABORATORY DIAGNOSIS

Definitive diagnosis requires fluorescent antibody staining or electron microscopy of tissues, viral isolation in cell cultures (lamb and calf kidney) or embryonated chicken eggs (development of pocks on the chorioallantoic membrane), or serology.

TREATMENT AND CONTROL

Treatment is confined to supportive therapy. Vaccination results in long-term immunity. Countries free of lumpy skin disease have imposed import restrictions on stock from infected countries.

SUIPOXVIRUS

Swinepox virus is the only member of the genus Suipoxvirus and measures 220 to 260 nm × 150 to 180 nm.

DISEASE

The disease, which is essentially indistinguishable from that caused by vaccinia virus, is observed in pigs of all ages, although younger animals are more commonly affected. Lesions typically develop on the abdomen and inner thighs and sometimes on other areas of the skin. Lesion development progresses from papular through pustular and scabbing stages. Concurrent skin infections with other agents can cause a more severe clinical picture. Microscopically, hydropic degeneration, hyperplasia of epidermal cells, eosinophilic inclusion bodies, and nuclear vacuolation are observed. Inflammatory cells are found in the dermis. In utero infections have been described with lesions occurring all over the skin, tongue, and buccal mucosa of newborn piglets.

HOST–VIRUS RELATIONSHIP

Swinepox has a worldwide distribution. Virus may be spread by direct contact or mechanically by lice. Transplacental transmission may also occur. Upon introduction into a swine herd, virus persists by surviving in dried scabs and infecting susceptible animals.

Swine develop immunity in the absence of detectable neutralizing antibody, suggesting that local humoral immunity or cell-mediated immunity is important in viral clearance and protection against reinfection.

LABORATORY DIAGNOSIS

Although the skin lesions, associated with lice infestation, are highly suggestive, laboratory confirmation is often required to rule out other important vesicular diseases. Definitive diagnosis can be obtained by fluorescent antibody staining, electron microscopy of lesions, or virus isolation in porcine cell cultures.

CONTROL

Control of swinepox is best realized by elimination of external parasites. Vaccination is not common.

SELECTED REFERENCES

Buller RML, Palumbo GT. Poxvirus pathogenesis. Microbiol Rev 1991;55:80.

Dales S, Pogo BGT. Biology of poxviruses. In: Kingsbury DW, Zur Hausen H, eds. Virology monographs. Vol. 18. New York: Springer-Verlag, 1981.

Fenner F. Poxviral zoonoses. In: Beran GW, ed. Handbook of zoonoses. 2nd ed. Boca Raton, FL: CRC, 1994:503.

Fenner F. Poxvirus. In: Fields B, Knipe DM, Howley PM, et al., eds. Fields virology. 3rd ed. Philadelphia: Lippincott-Raven, 1995:2673.

Fenner F, Wittek R, Dumbell KR. The orthopoxviruses. San Diego: Academic, 1989.

Kitching RP, Bhat PP, Black DN. The characterization of African strains of capripoxviruses. Epidemiol Infect 1989;102: 335.

Kriz B. A study of camelpox in Somalia. J Comp Pathol 1982; 92:1.

Moss B. Molecular biology of poxviruses. In: Binns MM, Smith GL, eds. Recombinant poxviruses. Boca Raton, FL: CRC, 1992: 45.

Turner PC, Moyer RW. Poxviruses. Curr Top Microbiol Immunol 1990;163:125.

65 *Picornaviridae*

Jeffrey L. Stott

Picornaviruses comprise a large family of small RNA viruses that have great significance in human and veterinary medicine, most visibly with poliomyelitis in humans and foot-and-mouth disease in cattle. Five genera have been recognized including Aphthovirus, Enterovirus, Cardiovirus, Rhinovirus, and Hepatovirus. Members of four genera have veterinary importance (Table 65.1). Equine rhinoviruses are not yet included in an established genus but are genetically closest to aphthoviruses. The hepatovirus genus that contains human hepatitis A will not be further mentioned due to the lack of veterinary significance.

GENERAL FAMILY CHARACTERISTICS

Picornavirus genera are sufficiently similar to warrant a general description of the family. The viruses exhibit a cubic symmetry with diameters ranging from 22 nm to 30 nm and densities in cesium chloride of 1.33 to 1.45 g/cm^3. The capsid, which is icosahedral, is composed of 60 subunits, each consisting of four major structural proteins (VP1, VP2, VP3, and VP4). Each of these proteins is derived by systematic cleavage of a single precursor protein. Three structural proteins (VP1, VP2, and VP3) are exposed on the virion surface, while VP4 is internal and in close association with genomic RNA. The receptor responsible for viral adsorption to cell membranes is considered to reside in VP1. Furthermore, the major epitope or epitopes for inducing and binding neutralizing antibodies reside in VP1 and thus identify the multiple serotypes of the various genera.

The viral genome consists of a single piece of single-stranded RNA (SSRNA) that serves as messenger RNA. Consequently, the RNA genome is infectious. The genomic RNA possesses a poly A tract at the 3′ terminus, and the 5′ terminus is not capped. A small viral-specified protein, VPg, is associated with the 5′ terminus of the genome and may play a role in initiating RNA synthesis and in viral maturation (RNA packaging).

APHTHOVIRUS

Aphthovirus, commonly referred to as *foot-and-mouth disease (FMD) virus,* is economically one of the most important diseases of food animals. The economic significance of this disease is due to a combination of disease-associated losses and interference with international movement of animals. The virus infects wild and domestic cloven-hooved animals. Disease is most dramatic in cattle and swine; sheep and goats are usually not as severely affected. Economic loss due to FMD can be enormous, as demonstrated in 1997 by the outbreak among pigs in Taiwan that cost the government hundreds of millions of dollars.

DISEASE

Foot-and-mouth disease in cattle is characterized by fever, depression, excessive salivation, lameness, and formation of vesicular-type lesions on the mucous membranes of the mouth (tongue, dental pad, and gums) and the skin of the muzzle, interdigital spaces, udder, teats, and coronary band. Lesions may also develop in the epithelium of the pharynx, larynx, trachea, esophagus, rumen, and musculature of the heart. Lesions in the mouth result in reduced food consumption, weight loss, and emaciation. Secondary bacterial infections are responsible for a large part of FMD-associated damage by complicating foot, respiratory, and udder infections. While mortality is generally less than 3%, morbidity is extensive with losses due to decreased productivity and protracted convalescence. Mortality is notably increased in young pigs and sometimes calves.

ETIOLOGIC AGENT

Physical, Chemical, and Antigenic Properties

Aphthoviruses have a diameter of 23 nm (Fig 65.1). Seven serotypes of FMD include O, A, C, SAT1, SAT2, SAT3, and Asia 1. Serotypes O and A serve as genus prototypes. Analysis of genomic RNAs of various viral types using hybridization techniques indicates the presence of two distinct groups of FMD with homologies in the range of 25% to 40%; homologies within each group are in the vicinity of 65%. Extensive heterogeneity exists within serotypes and more than 60 subtypes have been designated by the World Reference Laboratory for FMD.

Resistance to Physical and Chemical Agents

Foot-and-mouth disease virus (FMDV) can survive for extended periods in animal secretions and products. The

Table 65.1. Picornaviridae of Veterinary Significance

Genus	Disease	Member	Serotypes
Aphthovirus	Vesicular	Foot-and-mouth	7
	Cardiac	disease virus	
Enterovirus	Enteric	Porcine enterovirus	11
	Vesicular		
	Reproductive		
	Poliomyelitis		
	Respiratory		
	Pulmonary (heart)		
	Questionable	Bovine enterovirus	7
	Hepatitis	Duck hepatitis	3
		(probable enterovirus)	
	Encephalomyelitis	Avian encephalomyelitis	1
		(probable enterovirus)	
Cardiovirus	Myocarditis	Encephalomyocarditis virus	1
Rhinovirus	Respiratory	Bovine rhinovirus	3
	Respiratory	Equine rhinovirus	3

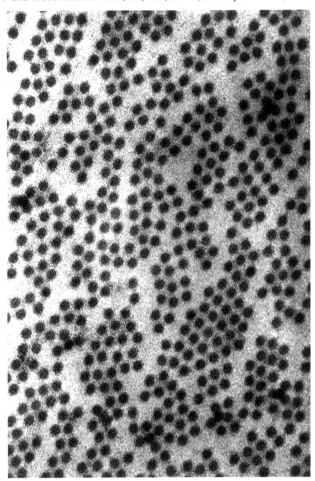

FIGURE 65.1. *Negatively stained preparation of foot-and-mouth disease virus (A12). 108,000×. (Courtesy of B. Baxt.)*

virus is inactivated by heating above 50°C and is acid sensitive (pH less than 6.5) and alkaline sensitive (pH greater than 11.0). FMDV resists inactivation by lipid solvents. Sodium hydroxide (1%) is recommended for disinfecting premises following FMD outbreaks.

Infectivity for Other Species and Culture Systems

Animals susceptible to infection and disease include cattle, domestic and wild pigs, sheep, goats, wild ruminants, buffalo, hedgehogs, armadillos, rats, nutria, grizzly bears, elephants, and capybara. Experimental infections of dogs, cats, rabbits, and chinchillas have been reported. Susceptible laboratory animals include guinea pigs, suckling mice, rats, rabbits, and hamsters. Some viral strains have been propagated in chick embryos, day-old chicks, and several other avian species. Virus replicates in a variety of cell cultures of bovine and ovine origin, baby hamster kidney (BHK) cells, and rabbit and murine cells.

HOST–VIRUS RELATIONSHIP

Distribution, Reservoir, and Transmission

Foot-and-mouth disease is endemic in Africa, South America, and parts of Europe and Asia. North and Central America, England, Ireland, Japan, Australia, New Zealand, Scandinavia, and the Caribbean region are currently considered free of FMD, although many of these countries have previously suffered outbreaks.

The epizootiology of FMD is complex; viral strain, animal host, and the environment interplay in this relationship. The relative importance of carrier animals (cattle, sheep, and buffalo) in viral dissemination is poorly defined. Inapparent infections, especially in vaccinated animals, contribute to viral maintenance. Virus can persist in cats, dogs, rodents, and other small animals. Wild game animals, through their migratory habits, facilitate long-range movement of the virus.

Virus may be transmitted by direct contact, aerosol, fomites, and possibly arthropod vectors (mechanical and possibly biologic). Virus may be recovered from tears, nasal discharge, saliva, urine, feces, milk, vaginal discharge, semen, and membranes of aborted fetuses. The survival of virus in such excretions depends upon temperature, pH, and humidity.

FMD can be transported over long distances via infected animals or their products. Virus remains viable for up to 3 months in frozen meat and up to 2 months in ham, bacon, and certain sausages. Virus persists for longer periods in lymph nodes and bone marrow, and when discarded as garbage, can constitute a mechanism for infection of dogs, cats, and swine. Animal hides can serve as a source of virus for extended periods of time. Humans may disseminate virus mechanically (fomites) or biologically by becoming infected. Airborne spread of virus is also considered important. The role of birds in viral dissemination is uncertain but may provide mechanical transmission by fecal excretion of ingested virus.

Pathogenesis and Pathology

The predominant route of FMDV infection is considered to be the respiratory tract with initial replication in the pharynx. A viremic stage precedes development of lesions and overt disease. The virus may be isolated from the vagina, rectum, pharynx, blood, and milk during this phase. Virus is produced by alveolar secretory cells of the bovine mammary gland. Viral transportation, from the vascular system to the epithelium where lesions develop, occurs via the papillae, since lesions appear to begin as single cell infections in the stratum spinosum adjacent to papillae. Virus can be detected by in situ hybridization in all epidermal tissues of pigs in the absence of cellular pathology.

Epithelial FMD lesions comprise 1) vesicle formation due to lysis of infected swollen cells with release of intracellular fluid, 2) intercellular edema, and 3) desiccated lesions produced by leakage of edema fluid without vesicle development. In a malignant form of FMD, virus infects the heart musculature causing degenerative changes and necrosis. In this instance, death often occurs early in infection, most commonly in young animals. Much of the damage caused by FMD outbreaks is due to secondary bacterial infections, including mastitis, lameness, and pneumonia.

Upon necropsy, vesicular lesions may be observed deep in the oral cavity and on the rumen pillars. Microscopically, such lesions typically exhibit inflammatory cellular infiltrates in the stratum spinosum. Lesions in skeletal and heart musculature, characterized by longitudinal yellow-whitish streaks representing myocardial necrosis, have been referred to as *tiger heart*.

Host Response to Infection

Serum IgG develops about 2 weeks postinfection and is type-specific. Colostral antibody in newborn calves has been reported to interfere with vaccination. The relative importance of local secretory, systemic, and cell-mediated immunity is not well defined. Duration of immunity is longer in cattle than in swine but apparently persists for only about a year. Serum-neutralizing antibody, actively or passively acquired, appears to correlate with protection in pigs.

LABORATORY DIAGNOSIS

Due to the economic and political significance of FMD and its similarity to other vesicular diseases — vesicular stomatitis (VSV), swine vesicular disease (SVD), and vesicular exanthema of swine (VES) — a rapid definitive diagnosis is essential. Virus from clinical samples (vesicular fluid and others) can be propagated in cell cultures or laboratory animals followed by physicochemical characterization and serology using complement fixation (CF), viral neutralization, enzyme-linked immunosorbent assay (ELISA), fluorescent antibody (FA), and agar gel immunodiffusion (AGID). Viral antigen can often be identified directly from tissues via CF, AGID, FA, and ELISA. Elec-

tron microscopy (EM) and immuno-EM microscopy can be used for rapid diagnosis. Polymerase chain reaction (PCR) techniques can be used for identification of genomic material.

Serologic diagnosis can be made by CF, ELISA, AGID, and viral neutralization (either in cell cultures or suckling mice). The AGID test can be used to identify antibody to group-reactive antigen (viral infection-associated antigen); such antibody is typically found only in animals that have experienced an active infection and not in animals vaccinated with inactivated virus. Recombinant FMDV nonstructural proteins (2C and 3AB1) can also be used in serology to distinguish vaccinated from naturally infected animals as vaccinates do not make antibody to these proteins.

TREATMENT AND CONTROL

No specific treatment exists for FMD. However, proper animal husbandry practices and treatment of secondary bacterial infections reduce losses.

Control of FMD is difficult due to its highly contagious nature, multiple hosts, viral stability, multiple antigenic types and subtypes, and short-term immunity. Countries free of FMD impose strict import regulations on animals, animal products, and potential viral-contaminated fomites from FMD countries. In the past, some countries experiencing FMD as a result of importation have utilized slaughter and quarantine in affected areas to eradicate an outbreak. Following cleanup measures, sentinel animals are employed to confirm absence of virus prior to restocking.

When a slaughter program is not economically feasible, quarantine and vaccination programs are used in concert. Countries with endemic FMD rely on vaccines exclusively; however, steps should still be taken to avoid importing additional viral strains since cross-protective immunity between strains is not guaranteed.

In countries using vaccination, inactivated vaccines of tissue culture origin, administered in adjuvant, are most common. The safety of live attenuated vaccines is questionable, so their use is not widespread. Vaccination is conducted one to three times a year since immunity is short-term. Vaccines must be of appropriate types and subtypes. Current research is directed at developing subunit, synthetic peptide, and recombinant-type vaccines. The latter two approaches have been directed at VP1 with encouraging results. In addition, molecular biologic techniques have successfully produced nonpathogenic variants that have successfully protected cattle against virulent viral challenge.

ENTEROVIRUS

The enterovirus genus encompasses many species-specific viruses including human and murine poliovirus, human coxsackie, echovirus and enterovirus, vilyuisk virus, and simian, bovine, and porcine enteroviruses. Additional members probably include avian encephalomyelitis virus and duck and turkey hepatitis virus. Enteroviruses are thermolabile (infectivity destroyed quickly at 50°C), insensitive to detergent treatment, and stable at low pH (can survive pH of 3).

PORCINE ENTEROVIRUSES

DISEASE

Eleven serotypes (possibly 13) of porcine enteroviruses associated with various disease syndromes have been described. Serotype 1 (Teschen and Talfan disease viruses), the swine enterovirus prototype, and swine vesicular disease virus (serotype 9) are discussed separately below. The disease syndromes associated with swine enteroviruses include poliomyelitis, vesicular disease, diarrhea, pneumonia, and heart disease. Some enteroviruses affecting reproductive functions of pigs are called *SMEDI* (stillbirth, *m*ummification, *e*mbryonic *d*eath, and *i*nfertility).

Three serotypes have been associated with polioencephalomyelitis in pigs following intranasal inoculation; strain variability has been observed relative to virulence, with Teschen disease and T80 (serotype 2) viruses being most severe. Pneumonia has been associated with several serotypes, including 2, 3, and 8. Myocarditis and pericarditis have been experimentally reproduced with serotype 2 and mulberry heart disease has been associated with serotype 3. Diarrhea is associated with porcine enterovirus infection, and six SMEDI groups (A to F) have been identified.

HOST–VIRUS RELATIONSHIP

Porcine enteroviruses are present in most swine-raising areas. Viral persistence is probably facilitated by the continued introduction of susceptible pigs and the presence of inapparent infections and carrier animals. Transmission occurs by direct contact, transplacental infection, and exposure to viral-contaminated feces.

Porcine enteroviruses typically infect the host via ingestion, inhalation, or both. The process of initial infection and subsequent dissemination is not clearly defined. Soon after infection, virus can be isolated from the respiratory system, blood, and intestines. The virus either directly passes to the intestinal area and initiates infection, or infection may be initiated in the respiratory tract with subsequent dissemination via the digestive tract or blood to the intestines. The virus has a tropism for intestinal tissues (spiral colon and ileum) and may also be isolated from mesenteric lymph nodes, liver, spleen, kidney, tonsils, turbinates, lung, diaphragm, central nervous system (brain and cord), and fetus, depending upon the viral strain.

Porcine polioencephalomyelitis is characterized by central nervous system disturbances such as paralysis,

paresis, and convulsions. SMEDI infections result in fetal mummification, stillbirths, and reduced litter size. The sequela to SMEDI infection depends on gestational age at the time of infection. Early infection often results in fetal adsorption and rebreeding or small litter size, while infection later in gestation results in fetal mummification and birth of dead piglets.

Immunity typically develops in pigs prior to sexual maturity due to early exposure to multiple endemic strains and serotypes. Breakdown of immunity is usually due to introduction of a new viral strain. Pigs suckling immune sows are not necessarily immune to infection. Virus introduced via the respiratory route may elude colostrum-derived antibody. Cell-mediated immunity to porcine enteroviruses has not been demonstrated.

LABORATORY DIAGNOSIS

Definitive diagnosis requires fluorescent antibody staining of necropsy tissues, viral isolation, PCR, or serology. Viral isolation can be attempted on primary pig kidney cell cultures; serology is conducted by standard procedures using paired serum samples to demonstrate seroconversion or increase in titer.

CONTROL

Control of porcine enterovirus infection is difficult due to the multiplicity of serotypes and their widespread distribution. Managerial procedures are the only control available and consist of controlled exposure of animals to viral-contaminated feces.

TESCHEN DISEASE VIRUS

DISEASE

Teschen disease may be expressed as a mild or severe form of polioencephalomyelitis. Mild forms, such as occur in several countries, are often referred to as *Talfan disease*, *benign enzootic paresis*, or *polioencephalomyelitis*. Acute disease is characterized by fever, anorexia, weakness, and variable degrees of central nervous system disorders (loss of rear limb coordination). As the disease progresses, animals may have trouble standing or walking and experience tremors, convulsions, and nystagmus with eventual development of paralysis. Such acute cases usually culminate in death within 3 to 4 days following onset of clinical signs.

The disease typically affects populations of susceptible animals as a simultaneous infection or as successive waves of disease. Populations of swine with endemic infections experience sporadic outbreaks of disease with young animals being most susceptible.

HOST–VIRUS RELATIONSHIP

Teschen disease, first described in the Teschen region of Czechoslovakia, is endemic in Central Europe and parts of Africa. Milder forms have been described in most parts of the world.

Gross lesions are typically absent in acute Teschen disease. If the disease process is prolonged, however, muscular atrophy may be apparent. Microscopically, polioencephalomyelitis is most evident in the spinal cord and cerebellum. Lesions are characterized by neuronal degeneration with subsequent formation of cellular aggregations (cell nodules). The cellular aggregation may be of glial, mesenchymal, or lymphocytic origin. Lymphocytic cuffing, while not pathognomonic, is typically observed around small blood vessels in the vicinity of the lesions.

LABORATORY DIAGNOSIS

The clinical signs described and the histopathologic observation of neuronal necrosis and cellular aggregations are indicative of the disease. Definitive diagnosis requires detection of viral antigen in tissues (FA), viral isolation, or serology.

TREATMENT AND CONTROL

Treatment of acute disease is futile, since 90% to 100% of affected pigs die. Inactivated vaccines have been used in Europe with variable success. Control measures vary with the country. The United States employs strict embargos to prevent introduction of the pathogenic forms of the virus, while Europe minimizes spread of disease by quarantine and vaccination.

SWINE VESICULAR DISEASE

DISEASE

Swine vesicular disease (SVD) resembles foot-and-mouth disease (FMD), vesicular stomatitis (VS), and vesicular exanthema of swine (VES). The disease is characterized by fever, weight loss, lameness, and development of vesicular lesions on the feet (coronary bands, soles, and interdigital areas), tongue, nares, lips, and skin. Ulceration may occur in the metacarpal and metatarsal areas, and sometimes the hoof may be shed.

HOST–VIRUS RELATIONSHIP

Swine vesicular disease is recognized in continental Europe, the Far East, and England. It is highly contagious and affects a wide host range that includes mice, humans, and sheep. The virus is closely related to human coxsackie virus B5.

The primary site of infection in pigs is believed to be the intestinal tract following viral ingestion. Following initial replication, virus is disseminated throughout the body and can be isolated from tissues and feces.

Upon necropsy, microscopic examination of the brain may reveal a diffuse encephalitis characterized by vascular cuffing and neuroglial cell clusters. Morbidity is moderate and mortality usually low. Secondary bacterial infections of lesions can extend the recovery phase.

LABORATORY DIAGNOSIS

Diagnosis of SVD should be based upon 1) identification of virus or viral antigens in lesions by fluorescent antibody staining or electron microscopy, 2) viral isolation on primary porcine cell cultures or in suckling mice, or 3) serology, for example, complement fixation, ELISA, viral neutralization, or counterimmunoelectrophoresis. A nested RT-PCR has also been described that can detect viral RNA in clinical specimens and is more sensitive than viral isolation on cell cultures; this assay is also able to distinguish SVD from the above mentioned porcine enteroviruses.

TREATMENT AND CONTROL

No specific treatment for SVD is available, and only experimental vaccines have been described. Control requires strict quarantine and import restrictions in countries free of disease. Upon introduction of virus into a SVD-free country, quarantine and animal depopulation are practiced.

BOVINE ENTEROVIRUS

Seven serotypes of bovine enteroviruses have been described. Viral isolations have been made from both healthy and diseased cattle. The role of these viruses in disease is uncertain. Virus can be isolated using standard virologic techniques and identified by viral neutralization, complement fixation techniques, and antigen-capture ELISA. Serology can be performed by viral neutralization or ELISA.

DUCK HEPATITIS

DISEASE

Duck hepatitis is a contagious and highly fatal disease of young ducklings. The first clinical sign is an abrupt reduction in activity by the ducklings. Birds squat down with eyes partially closed and subsequently fall with spasmodic thrashing of legs. Death occurs within a few hours of the onset of clinical signs. Morbidity is variable and mortality may approach 90%.

ETIOLOGIC AGENT

Duck hepatitis virus (DHV) is an enterovirus. It has a diameter of 20 nm to 40 nm and is resistant to lipid solvents, acidic pH, and trypsin. It is relatively thermostable and survives for long periods in fecal material. Three serotypes of DHV have been recognized based upon cross-protection studies.

While ducklings are the only naturally affected avian species, experimental infection of young chickens, pigeons, turkeys, geese, pheasants, and guinea fowl have been reported; high mortality is often observed in the latter three hosts.

Allantoic inoculation of chicken and goose embryonated eggs (ECEs) has been used to propagate virus. Infected chick embryos die 5 to 6 days postinoculation and appear stunted and edematous. Various chick, duck, and goose embryonic cell lines support viral replication. Development of cytopathic effect is variable.

HOST–VIRUS RELATIONSHIP

Duck hepatitis virus appears to have a worldwide distribution. Viral reservoirs are unknown, although brown rats are potential carriers. Transmission of virus occurs by direct and indirect contact (contaminated feces). The virus does not appear to be vertically transmitted.

Duck hepatitis pathogenesis is not well defined. Aerosol infections have been reported, and it has been suggested that initial viral replication occurs in the upper respiratory tract based upon the inability to infect ducklings following ingestion of encapsulated virus.

Primary gross lesions consist of an enlarged and hemorrhagic liver. Additional lesions may include an enlarged and mottled spleen and congested, swollen kidneys. Microscopic examination reveals hepatic cell necrosis, bile duct hyperplasia, and inflammatory responses in various organs.

Immunity develops following infection, and maternal transfer of antibody protects ducklings for several weeks.

LABORATORY DIAGNOSIS

Diagnosis of DHV may be suggested by the rapid spread and peracute nature of the disease. Hemorrhagic lesions in the liver of ducklings are essentially pathognomonic. Definitive diagnosis may be made by direct fluorescent antibody staining of necropsy tissues or of inoculated avian embryos. Serology has not been useful in DHV diagnosis. Viral neutralization in ducklings or chick and duck embryos has been used primarily to characterize and serotype viral isolates, the latter being useful in selecting proper vaccine strains.

TREATMENT AND CONTROL

No treatment for clinically affected ducklings exists. Proper sanitation reduces the incidence of infection, and administering immune serum to birds in the face of an outbreak reduces losses. Two vaccination procedures using attenuated or inactivated DHV vaccines have been used. Immunization of breeders facilitates maternal transfer of antibody. Ducklings may also be immunized directly. Success of the latter procedure requires that ducklings be free of maternal antibody.

AVIAN ENCEPHALOMYELITIS

DISEASE

Avian encephalomyelitis virus (AEV) is predominantly associated with a disease of young chickens (1 to 2 weeks of age) characterized by a dull expression in the eyes and progressive ataxia and tremors. Death typically occurs due to lack of food and water consumption or to being trampled by other birds. Offspring of some surviving birds may develop enlarged eyeballs, lens opacity, and blindness. Infection of mature birds results in decreased egg production, decreased hatchability, and production of diseased chicks. Morbidity rates average about 50 percent and mortality 5 to 25 percent or greater, depending upon viral virulence and the immune status of the flock.

ETIOLOGIC AGENT

Avian encephalomyelitis virus probably belongs to the genus enterovirus. Final classification awaits full characterization of the genome. The virus has a diameter of 24 nm to 32 nm with a density of 1.31 to 1.32 g/cm^3 in cesium chloride. The virus exhibits physicochemical characteristics similar to other enteroviruses. Only one serotype of AEV has been identified.

Besides chickens and turkeys, Japanese quail and pheasants are susceptible to AEV infection. Ducks, pigeons, and guinea fowl can be experimentally infected. Chick embryos can be infected (the yolk sac route is the most common), but rapid passage of field isolates is required before clinical signs (muscular dystrophy) are observed in the embryo. Cell culture systems for viral propagation include chicken neuroglial cells, embryo fibroblasts, brain cells, and pancreatic cells.

HOST–VIRUS RELATIONSHIP

Avian encephalomyelitis occurs wherever poultry is raised commercially. Persistence of AEV in nature is poorly understood and the existence of carrier birds is conjectural. Inapparent infections probably play a major role in viral perpetuation. Transmission occurs both horizontally and vertically. Horizontal transmission can occur by direct contact or via viral-contaminated feces. Young chicks typically excrete virus for up to 3 weeks. Vertical transmission from hen to embryo is common and eggs that hatch provide a source of infection for other birds.

The incubation period ranges from 11 days to 4 weeks. Chicks infected by vertical transmission express disease from 1 to 7 days following hatching. Oral administration of AEV results in primary viral replication in the duodenum. A viremia follows with infection of the pancreas, other visceral organs, and the central nervous system. Age-related susceptibility is associated with immunocompetence since development of humoral immunity correlates with loss of susceptibility.

Gross lesions are inconspicuous. Microscopically, the brain and spinal cord reveal a typical viral encephalomyelitis characterized by neuronal degeneration, perivascular cuffing, and gliosis. Visceral lesions, characterized by hyperplasia of lymphoid follicles, occur in the proventriculus, pancreas, and myocardium.

Humoral immune responses are considered to be responsible for viral clearance and protection. Neutralizing antibodies develop within 2 weeks of infection. Immunity is apparently of long duration as exposed flocks rarely have recurrent outbreaks. Maternal antibody protects young chicks for up to 10 weeks. Flock susceptibility is determined by embryo susceptibility testing.

LABORATORY DIAGNOSIS

Newcastle disease, ricketts, and various nutritional deficiencies can mimic AEV clinically. Histopathology can provide a presumptive diagnosis based upon observation of an axonal type of neuronal degeneration in the central nervous system and gliosis, lymphocytic perivascular infiltration, and lymphoid hyperplasia in visceral tissues.

Virus may be demonstrated by chick embryo inoculation with brain tissue homogenates; the embryo is permitted to hatch and AEV infection produces clinical disease within 10 days. Identification of viral antigen in necropsy tissues by fluorescent antibody staining or agar gel immunodiffusion provides definitive diagnosis. Serologic diagnosis can be performed by viral neutralization, AGID, and ELISA.

TREATMENT AND CONTROL

No treatment is available for AEV-affected birds other than supportive care in the form of proper husbandry. Attenuated and inactivated vaccines have been successfully used to control the disease. Birds in high AEV incidence areas may be vaccinated prior to reaching breeding age with live viral vaccine strains. Only part of the flock need be vaccinated since the virus will spread throughout the flock. Inactivated vaccines should be used if breeding flocks are to be immunized.

CARDIOVIRUS

DISEASE

Encephalomyocarditis (EMC) virus is a natural disease of rodents. Young pigs are the only domestic species affected, and the disease is predominantly a myocarditis. The disease in swine is typically manifested by sudden death with few, if any, preceding clinical signs. Mortality can be high, especially in young pigs.

ETIOLOGIC AGENT

Cardiovirus contains one viral serotype — the EMC virus. Viral strains belonging to the genus include mengovirus, Maus Elberfeld virus, Columbia SK virus, and MM virus.

HOST–VIRUS RELATIONSHIP

Encephalomyocarditis virus can be considered a murine virus, although it can infect nonhuman primates, humans, elephants, squirrels, calves, horses, and pigs. Lack of pig-to-pig transmission following experimental infections suggests that infection is initiated from rodent sources. However, pregnant sows experimentally inoculated with virus at 60 to 90 days' gestation can transmit the virus to the offspring; virus could be isolated from these piglets for up to 30 days. Vaccination may be feasible based upon the report that a genetically engineered avirulent mengovirus protected pigs against challenge.

The only gross lesions observed may be a spleen devoid of blood and myocardial lesions characterized by white longitudinal tracts of necrosis with zones of lymphocyte infiltration and calcification.

LABORATORY DIAGNOSIS

Viral isolation is advised since immune responses require about 5 days and may not develop prior to death. PCR techniques have also been successfully used for diagnosis of infection.

RHINOVIRUS

As a genus, rhinoviruses are characterized by acid sensitivity (pH of less than 5 to 6), resistance to ether, thermostability, densities in the range of 1.38 to 1.41g/cm^3

in cesium chloride, diameters in the range of 20 nm to 30 nm, and an RNA genome of 2.4 to 2.8 × 10⁶ daltons. The genus includes human, bovine, and probably equine rhinoviruses, all of which have demonstrated a tropism for the respiratory tract. Extensive serotype heterogeneity has been documented with more than 110 human serotypes and up to three bovine and three equine serotypes.

BOVINE RHINOVIRUS

Bovine rhinoviruses infect the upper respiratory tract. Clinical signs include serous nasal discharge, fever, coughing, anorexia, hyperpnea, dyspnea, or possibly pneumonia. Morbidity is high, as determined by serologic studies. The significance of rhinovirus as a pathogen is uncertain, and may depend on such factors as viral strain, concomitant bacterial infection, and environmental stress factors.

Transmission of the virus is probably by direct contact, aerosol, and contaminated materials.

Immune responses to bovine rhinovirus infection are poorly defined, but protective immunity is related to neutralizing antibody. Titers increase with age, probably due to reinfection with homologous and heterologous viral strains.

Diagnosis of clinical rhinovirus infection is difficult due to the multiplicity of viruses associated with respiratory disease. Viral isolation is possible only on bovine kidney cell cultures; a sandwich ELISA has been described for confirmation of bovine rhinovirus identity. Demonstration of a rising neutralizing titer on paired serum samples is useful.

EQUINE RHINOVIRUSES

Equine rhinoviruses are associated with inapparent and clinical respiratory infections of horses. The disease is similar to that in cattle with bacterial infections and stress serving as complicating factors.

Unlike human and bovine rhinoviruses, equine serotypes can infect multiple species, including guinea pigs, rabbits, monkeys, and humans. The viruses replicate in a variety of cell cultures derived from several animal species.

Transmission of equine rhinovirus is probably similar to that described for the bovine viruses. Horses can carry virus in pharyngeal tissues for up to 1 month.

Neutralizing antibodies develop about 7 days following infection and transfer of protective immunity to foals via colostrum has been indirectly suggested.

Diagnosis can be made by viral isolation on cell cultures or by serologic demonstration of rising antibody titers. RT-PCR has also been used on nasopharyngeal swabs to identify the presence of equine rhinovirus when virus isolation techniques failed.

SELECTED REFERENCES

Brown CC, Olander HJ, Meyer RF. Pathogenesis of foot-and-mouth disease in swine, studied by in situ hybridization. J Comp Pathol 1995;113:51.

Calneck BW, Luginbuhl RE, Helmboldt CF. Avian encephalomyelitis (epidemic tremor). In: Calneck BW, ed. Diseases of poultry. 9th ed. Ames, IA: Iowa State University, 1991:520.

Derbyshire JB. Enteroviruses. In: Leman AD, Straw BE, Mengeling WL, et al., eds. Diseases of swine. 7th ed. Ames, IA: Iowa State University, 1992:263.

Kitching RP. The application of biotechnology to the control of foot-and-mouth disease virus. Br Vet J 1992;148:375.

Li F, Drummer HE, Ficorilli N, et al. Identification of noncytopathic equine rhinovirus 1 as a cause of acute febrile respiratory disease in horses. J Clin Microbiol 1997;35:937.

McKenna TS, Rieder E, Lubroth J, et al. Strategy for producing new foot-and-mouth disease vaccines that display complex epitopes. J Biotech 1996;44:83.

Morgan DO, Moore DM. Protection of cattle and swine against foot-and-mouth disease, using biosynthetic peptide vaccines. Am J Vet Rec 1990;51:40.

Rueckert RR. Picornaviridae: the viruses and their replication. In: Fields BN, Knipe DM, Howley PM, et al., eds. Fields virology. 3rd ed. Philadelphia: Lippincott-Raven, 1996:609.

Woodbury EL. A review of the possible mechanisms for the persistence of foot-and-mouth disease virus. Epidemiol Infect 1995;114:1.

Woodcock PR, Fabricant J. Duck virus hepatitis. In: Calneck BW, ed. Diseases of poultry. 9th ed. Ames, IA: Iowa State University, 1991:597.

66 Caliciviridae

Yuan Chung Zee

Caliciviruses are small (36 ± 2 nm in diameter), nonenveloped, single-stranded RNA viruses (Fig 66.1). The name *calicivirus* is derived from the chalice-shaped spheres on the surface of negatively stained viral particles. Four members of this group, vesicular exanthema of swine virus, San Miguel sea lion virus, feline calicivirus, and rabbit hemorrhagic disease virus, are pathogens for animals. A few caliciviruses (human hepatitis E virus and Norwalk virus) are recently known to produce diseases in humans.

VESICULAR EXANTHEMA OF SWINE

DISEASE

Vesicular exanthema of swine (VES) is an acute viral disease characterized by the formation of vesicles most frequently on the mouth, lips, tongue, oral cavity, interdigital spaces, and coronary band of the foot. Clinically, vesicular exanthema of swine is indistinguishable from foot-and-mouth disease, swine vesicular disease, and vesicular stomatitis. The incubation period of the disease is approximately 24 to 72 hours and the course is about 1 to 2 weeks. Infected swine have a rise in temperature (41.5°C) lasting 6 days. The disease has a high morbidity but a low mortality. It is of great economic importance because the disease causes serious weight loss in fat pigs, slow gains in feeder stocks, death in suckling pigs, and abortion in pregnant sows. The last occurrence of this disease took place in the United States in 1956. Subsequently, the U.S. Department of Agriculture in 1959 declared VES an exotic disease and confined the study of this disease to a few laboratories with special permits.

ETIOLOGIC AGENT

Physical, Chemical, and Antigenic Properties

Vesicular exanthema of swine virus (VESV) is 34 ± 2 nm in diameter and has cup-shaped spheres on its surface. In swine cells infected with VESV, viral particles are seen associated with cytoplasmic cisternae (Fig 66.2) and, in crystalline arrays, in cytoplasm (Fig 66.3). The virus has a buoyant density of 1.36 to 1.39 g/cm^3 in cesium chloride (CsCl). The viral RNA, which is single-stranded, serves as

mRNA and is infectious. The VESV has one major polypeptide with a molecular weight of 6.0×10^4 to 6.5×10^4. The virus has no essential lipids, as it is resistant to ether, chloroform, and phospholipase C. Vesicular exanthema of swine virus differs from enterovirus in being stable at low pH (pH 5) and in being rapidly inactivated at 50°C in high concentrations of magnesium salts.

During the 27 years in which VES disease has run the full cycle from appearance to official extinction, 13 antigenic types of VESV have been identified. These distinct antigenic types can be differentiated by complement fixation and serum neutralization tests. The earlier serotypes (A to E) are more virulent than later isolates (F to J).

Resistance to Physical and Chemical Agents

Vesicular exanthema of swine virus can persist in the environment for long periods. In contaminated meat products, for example, virus can remain infectious for 4 weeks when stored at 7°C and for 18 years when stored at −70°C. The virus is completely inactivated by 2% sodium hydroxide or 0.1% sodium hypochlorite.

Infectivity for Other Species or Culture Systems

The naturally occurring VES disease is confined only to swine of all ages and breeds. Experimentally, VESV causes plaque-like lesions at inoculated sites of otarid and phosid seals. Vesicles are also produced at the sites of inoculation in horses and hamsters. Virus is isolated in low titers from some sites of inoculation and draining lymph nodes. Vesicular exanthema of swine virus can be propagated in cell lines of swine kidney or Vero monkey kidney.

HOST–VIRUS RELATIONSHIP

Distribution, Reservoir, and Transmission

Vesicular exanthema of swine made its first appearance in California in 1932. Outbreaks were reported every year in California between 1932 and 1951, with the exception of a two-year period, 1937–1938, when no cases were reported. The disease first appeared outside of California in 1951, and from 1952 to 1953 it spread to a total of 42 states in the United States. The disease had never been reported elsewhere in the world except Iceland and Hawaii. These two incidents resulted from shipping contaminated pork products from California and were quickly eradicated.

There is good evidence that marine mammals may serve as reservoirs for VESV infection of terrestrial

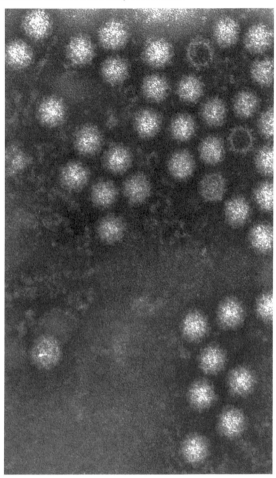

FIGURE 66.1. *Negatively stained preparations of feline calicivirus. 240,000×. (Courtesy of A. Castro.)*

animals. In 1972, isolation of a calicivirus was made from California sea lions on San Miguel Island off the coast of southern California. This calicivirus was named *San Miguel sea lion virus (SMSV)*, which was indistinguishable from VESV by morphologic, biophysical, and biochemical criteria. In addition, SMSV, when experimentally inoculated into swine, produces a disease clinically resembling VES. There are currently more than 13 serotypes of SMSV, and they are serologically distinct from VESV. Three serotypes of SMSV are known to produce a clinical disease in swine indistinguishable from VES. A new serotype of calicivirus recently isolated from California sea lions also produced vesicular lesions similar to that of VESV when inoculated into pigs. Isolates of SMSV have also been identified from a number of marine pinnipeds including elephant seals and northern fur seals, as well as from opaleye fish and a liver fluke of the sea lion.

More recently, SMSV has been isolated from asymptomatic domestic swine. Serum-neutralizing antibodies to several serotypes of SMSV and VESV have been demonstrated in marine mammals and domestic swine populations. Earlier epidemiologic studies during the outbreaks of vesicular exanthema in swine herds showed a close correlation between feeding of raw garbage and outbreaks of the disease. Sea lion parts are known to have been utilized as food source for swine, and raw garbage feeding was practiced at that time. Therefore, it is likely that vesicular exanthema in California could originate from feeding SMSV-infected marine animal parts to swine herds. The disease can spread among swine herds by either direct contact or feeding on contaminated raw garbage. Isolation of caliciviruses from skunks that are antigenically and genotypically related to SMSV indicate that skunks may be infected by consuming SMSV-infected marine mammal parts.

Pathogenesis and Pathology

Primary lesions are mainly of fluid-filled vesicles at the sites of inoculation in the snout, coronary band, and tongue in swine inoculated intradermally with VESV and

FIGURE 66.2. *Parallel rows of VESV particles in cytoplasmic cisternae. 72,000×. (Reproduced with permission from Zee YC, Hackett AJ, Talens LT. Electron microscopic studies on the vesicular exanthema of swine virus. II. Morphogenesis of VESV Type H54 in pig kidney cells. Virology 1968;34:596.)*

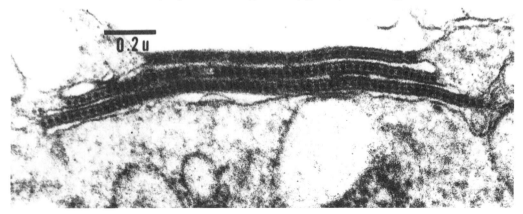

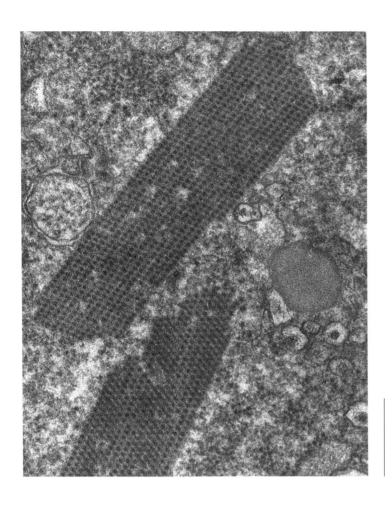

FIGURE 66.3. *Section of a viral crystal in VESV-infected cells. 64,000×. (Reproduced with permission from Zee YC, Hackett AJ, Talens LT. Electron microscopic studies on the vesicular exanthema of swine virus. II. Morphogenesis of VESV Type H54 in pig kidney cells. Virology 1968;34:596.)*

SMSV. Fever is seen in most infected animals. Virus replicates in the malpighian layer of the epidermis. Viremia is observed in some animals infected with SMSV 5 days after inoculation. Virus is recovered from nasal–oral passages for up to 5 days after infection in swine inoculated with VESV or SMSV. Formation of secondary vesicles takes place on the coronary band and interdigital space of the feet 3 to 4 days after exposure to the virus. Within 5 to 6 days after infection, the vesicles rupture and healing takes place unless complicated by secondary bacterial infection of the ruptured vesicles. Vesicle fluid contains a high amount of virus, which can infect secondary sites on the animal or contaminate the environment.

Vesicle formation in the epithelium of the skin is the major pathologic lesion observed in this viral infection. Lesions are usually limited to nonhaired portions of the integument and tongue. In serious cases, lesions in lymph nodes consisting of distribution of lymphocytes and edema of the node are noted. A mild encephalitis is seen in swine infected with VESV and virus is recovered from brain tissue of swine infected with SMSV.

Host Response to Infection

Neutralizing antibodies to VESV and SMSV appear in the sera of animals infected with viruses 3 days after inoculation. The titers reach a peak within 7 to 10 days after

infection.

LABORATORY DIAGNOSIS

It is impossible to differentiate vesicular exanthema of swine from other vesicular diseases of swine (swine vesicular disease, foot-and-mouth disease, vesicular stomatitis) on the basis of clinical signs. Because this disease resembles foot-and-mouth disease, prompt laboratory diagnosis must be carried out in suspected cases.

The susceptibility of animal species to virus-induced vesicular lesions in domestic animals is summarized in Table 66.1. The classical test of differentiating vesicular disease by inoculating several species of susceptible testing animals is no longer a desirable alternative. The weaknesses of this method of diagnosis are the need to use infectious virus, a long waiting period, high expense, and testing variability.

Reliable procedures such as immune electron microscopy, fluorescent antibody technique, complement fixation, and viral neutralization test can be used to diagnose this disease. In the laboratories authorized to study this disease, the use of an enzyme-linked immunosorbent assay (ELISA) for rapid diagnosis of this disease should be explored. A gene probe to detect cali-

Table 66.1.   Susceptibility of Domestic Animals to Four Viruses Producing Vesicular Lesions in Swine

| | Virus | | | |
Test Animals	SVD	VESV	FMD	VSV
Cattle	−	−	++	++
Swine	++	++	+	+
Sheep	−	−	+	−*
Horse	−	−*	−	++
Guinea pig	−	−*	+	+
Suckling mice	+	−	+	+
Humans	+	−	−*	+

* Occasional lesions produced with specific strains of the virus.

civirus from tissue samples has been developed.

TREATMENT AND CONTROL

There is no treatment for VES. There are no vaccines for control of the disease, in part because the disease is now considered to be eradicated in the United States. Enforcement of laws requiring cooking of garbage before feeding it to swine was the most important factor in eliminating the disease.

FELINE CALICIVIRUS

DISEASE

Feline calicivirus (FCV) primarily causes an upper-respiratory infection in cats characterized by fever (40°C to 49°C), sneezing, and nasal and ocular discharges. Clinical symptoms include rhinitis, conjunctivitis, oral ulcerations, and in severe cases, pneumonia. More recently, joint or muscle soreness, hyperaesthesia, and limping have been reported in kittens infected with FCV. The incubation period of the disease is 2 to 3 days and infected cats usually recover in 7 to 10 days in the absence of secondary bacterial infections. Experimentally, FCV caused a more severe disease in cats chronically infected with feline immunodeficiency virus (FIV) than in non-FIV infected cats.

ETIOLOGIC AGENT

Physical, Chemical, and Antigenic Properties

Feline calicivirus is 36 ± 2 nm in diameter and shows a characteristic calicivirus morphology by electron microscopy. It has a buoyant density of 1.39 g/cm³ in

CsCl. The virus is nonenveloped and contains a single-stranded RNA molecule. The virus has one major capsid polypeptide. Neutralization tests carried out with various isolates of FCV showed considerable cross-reactivity, indicating that all isolates are probably variants of a single serotype.

Resistance to Physical and Chemical Agents

Feline calicivirus is resistant to many common disinfectants. It is readily inactivated by a 0.175% sodium hypochlorite solution (Clorox), which is the disinfectant of choice. The virus is stable at a pH of 4 to 5 and is inactivated at 50°C within 30 minutes.

Infectivity for Other Species and Culture Systems

Feline calicivirus has been isolated from cats all over the world and is probably a common pathogen among cats. Infection of cheetahs with FCV has been reported. There is no evidence that FCV produces disease in laboratory animals.

Feline calicivirus can be propagated in cell lines of cat kidney and lion kidney. Some strains have been grown in Vero monkey kidney and dolphin kidney cells.

HOST–VIRUS RELATIONSHIP

Distribution, Reservoir, and Transmission

The disease occurs worldwide. Infected cats recovered from the disease carry virus in the oropharyngeal region for as long as 2 years and serve as the reservoirs of infection. Viral aerosol from an infected animal is the major mode of transmission of this disease.

Pathogenesis and Pathology

Cats probably acquire the infection with FCV via the respiratory route. The primary sites of viral replication are epithelial cells of the tonsillar crypt, tongue, oral cavity, conjunctiva, and alveoli. A viremia is present during the acute phase of the infection.

Macroscopic lesions mainly comprise vesicles on the tongue, hard palate, and external nares, leading to ulceration in a few days. In severe cases of natural disease or experimental infection with heavy doses of virus, an acute to subacute interstitial pneumonia is present. Microscopic lesions consist of foci of necrotic epithelial cells on the tongue and in the oral cavity with vesicle formation. Erosion of the vesicles with subsequent ulceration occurs in the mucosa. Regeneration of the oral mucosa takes place in 10 to 12 days unless complicated by secondary bacterial infection. In cases of interstitial pneumonia, initial necrosis of alveolar Type 1 epithelial cells occurs, followed by replacement of denuded alveolar walls with alveolar Type II cells and mononuclear cells.

Host Response to Infection

Cats infected with FCV or vaccinated with inactivated or live modified FCV vaccines develop serum-neutralizing antibodies. Kittens born to cats that are immune to FCV acquire maternal serum-neutralizing antibody to FCV from the colostrum. Titers of natural antibody are highest at one week of age and disappear by 10 to 14 weeks of age.

LABORATORY DIAGNOSIS

Clinical diagnosis of FCV infection is difficult because a variety of agents will produce similar respiratory symptoms in the cat. Laboratory tests must be utilized for definitive diagnosis. They include the isolation of FCV in feline cell cultures from nasal secretions, throat swabs, or conjunctival scrapings, and the identification of FCV antigen in conjunctival scrapings of tonsillar biopsies by the immunofluorescence technique.

TREATMENT AND CONTROL

Treatment for FCV infection in cats is mainly supportive and symptomatic. Broad-spectrum antibiotics help prevent secondary bacterial infections, and fluid therapy is useful in the event of dehydration. Nose drops containing antihistamines and antibiotics may be beneficial during early stages of infection.

All isolates of FCV are considered variants of one serotype, since there is considerable serologic cross-reactivity between these isolates. Furthermore, cats immunized with one variant of FCV are protected against many other variants. Both inactivated and modified live FCV vaccines are commercially available and afford reasonable protection against FCV infection. The FCV vaccines are usually combined with feline rhinotracheitis (a herpesvirus) and feline panleukopenia (a parvovirus), and administered either intranasally or intramuscularly.

FCV infection is controlled primarily by isolating cats that show respiratory symptoms and disinfecting cages and premises with Clorox before susceptible animals are introduced.

RABBIT HEMORRHAGIC DISEASE

DISEASE

Rabbit hemorrhagic disease (RHD) is an acute infectious disease of the European rabbit, *Oryctolagus cunniculus*, with a very high mortality rate. It is caused by a calicivirus and is characterized by a febrile response and hemorrhagic lesions in the lungs and liver. The disease has an incubation period of 24 to 48 hours. Rabbit hemorrhagic fever was first reported in China in 1984 and in the next several years the disease spread to Europe, northern

Africa, and Mexico City. A unique feature of RHD is that the disease is only fatal to rabbits over 2 months of age.

ETIOLOGIC AGENT

Physical, Chemical and Antigenic Properties

Rabbit hemorrhagic disease virus (RHDV) is approximately 40 nm in diameter and has a characteristic calicivirus morphology in negatively stained electron micrographs. It has a single-stranded RNA genome.

Infectivity for Other Species and Culture Systems

Rabbit hemorrhagic disease virus has not been grown in cell culture successfully. Studies conducted on RHDV and RHD have utilized virus prepared from liver homogenates. The virus does not infect other species of mammals except the European rabbit.

HOST–VIRUS RELATIONSHIP

Distribution, Reservoir, and Transmission

Although RHD was first reported in China, a similar disease in the European brown hare, *Lepus europaeus*, caused by a different calicivirus, had been recognized earlier in Europe. It is possible that a mutation of the European brown hare calicivirus led to the emergence of RHDV causing the lethal pandemic of rabbits. The disease is transmitted by the oral–fecal route.

Pathogenesis and Pathology

Gross pathologic findings show an enlarged spleen, swollen liver, and the presence of clotted blood in blood vessels in the lungs and liver. The disseminated intravascular coagulopathy induced by RHDV is a unique feature not observed in other calicivirus infections but is present in diseases caused by members of the Flaviviridae such as yellow fever and dengue in humans.

LABORATORY DIAGNOSIS

Immunofluorescence and ELISA tests have been developed for the diagnosis of RHD. The genome of RHDV has been completely sequenced so the utilization of polymerase chain reaction (PCR) would be a logical choice.

TREATMENT AND CONTROL

There is no treatment for the acute disease. Inactivated vaccine by formalin is effective against the disease in rabbits. Prevention of transporting RHDV-contaminated materials into commercial rabbitries is the key factor. It is interesting to note that although most countries have focused on the control and prevention of RHD, Australia is considering using RHDV as a biologic weapon to control its rabbit problem.

SELECTED REFERENCES

Berry ES, Skilling DE, Barlough JE, et al. New marine calicivirus serotype, infective for swine. Am J Vet Res 1990;51:1184.

Gelberg HB, Lewis RM. The pathogenesis of vesicular exanthema of swine virus and San Miguel sea lion virus in swine. Vet Pathol 1992;19:424.

House JA, House CA. Vesicular diseases. In: Lemans AD, Straw BE, Mengeling WL, et al., eds. Diseases of swine. 7th ed. Ames, IA: Iowa State University, 1992:387.

Meyers G, Wirblich C, Thiel HJ. Rabbit hemorrhagic fever virus — molecular cloning and nucleotide sequencing of a calicivirus genome. Virology 1991;184:664.

Povey RC, Hale CJ. Experimental infections with feline caliciviruses (picornaviruses) in specific-pathogen-free kittens. J Comp Pathol 1974;84:245.

Povey RC, Koonse H, Hays MB. Immunogenicity and safety of an inactivated vaccine for the prevention of rhinotracheitis, caliciviral disease, and panleukopenia in cats. J Am Vet Med Assoc 1980;177:347.

Ohlinger VF, Haas B, Meyers G, et al. Identification and characterization of the virus causing rabbit hemorrhagic disease. J Virol 1990;64:3331.

Schaffer FL. Caliciviruses. In: Fraenkel-Connat H, Wagner RR, eds. Comprehensive virology. Vol 14. New York: Plenum, 1979:249–278.

Studdent MJ. Caliciviruses. Arch Virol 1978;58:157.

67 *Togaviridae and Flaviviridae*

JEFFREY L. STOTT

TOGAVIRIDAE

The family Togaviridae contains a large number of viruses with diverse properties. "Toga" comes from the Latin word for gown or cloak, which refers to the envelope possessed by all members of the family. Currently the family consists of two genera, alphavirus and rubivirus (rubella). Rubivirus will not be mentioned further here as humans are the only natural host. Viruses of the alphavirus genera are arthropod-borne, while those of the other genera are often referred to as *nonarbo* togaviruses.

ALPHAVIRUS

Alphaviruses represent a major genus of the Togaviridae family, with Sindbis virus serving as the genus prototype. The genus was originally designated as Group A arboviruses based upon antigenic relatedness as determined by hemagglutination inhibition. All members of the genus are arthropod-borne, mosquitoes serving as the primary biologic vector. Relative to veterinary medicine, eastern equine encephalitis (EEE), western equine encephalitis (WEE), Venezuelan equine encephalitis (VEE) viruses, and Getah virus are of major importance; the three encephalitis viruses also pose a serious threat to human health.

DISEASE

As their names suggest, eastern, western, and Venezuelan equine encephalitis viruses cause an encephalitis in horses. Infection may result in an inapparent or mild infection (febrile response and mild depression) with no obvious signs of disease. Such infections are more common with WEE, while EEE and VEE are typically more virulent. Viral invasion of the nervous system is associated with clinical disease; however, death from VEE may occur in the absence of neurologic signs. Horses experiencing central nervous system (CNS) involvement often move about aimlessly and may walk into obstacles. Later, there is severe depression associated with unusual stances. Varying degrees of muscular paralysis may be observed prior to death, which typically occurs 2 to 4 days after onset of clinical signs. Horses that recover may have permanent CNS damage. Mortality may reach up to 50%

with WEE, in contrast to mortalities as high as 80% for VEE and 100% for EEE.

Significant disease in domestic birds may also be caused by EEE and WEE; EEE is more common and mortality may reach 50% to 70%. Reports of clinical disease in pheasants are common, and disease has also been described in ducks, chukar, chickens, and turkeys. The clinical disease is primarily one of encephalitis with clinical signs including leg paralysis, torticollis, and tremors. Wild birds may also be infected but rarely experience disease. Getah virus appears to be predominantly an equine pathogen. Infection of horses may result in severe clinical disease characterized by fever, rash, and edema of the limbs.

ETIOLOGIC AGENT

Physical, Chemical, and Antigenic Properties

Alphaviruses, formerly Group A arboviruses, represent a major genus within the Togaviridae family. The viral particles (60 nm to 64 nm in diameter) consist of a single-stranded positive-sense RNA genome enclosed within an icosahedral nucleocapsid (30 nm to 35 nm in diameter) that is in turn enclosed within a host cell–derived plasma membrane envelope. The virion core is composed of a single core protein, while the envelope exhibits peplomers that consist of two glycoproteins (E1 and E2). A third glycoprotein (E3) has been described in Semliki Forest virus. Glycoprotein E2 appears to carry the major neutralization and hemagglutination epitopes. E1 also has some (probably minor) neutralizing and hemagglutinating epitopes. It has been suggested that extensive diversity of E1 may be responsible for generating strain diversity. All members of the genus are antigenically related as determined by hemagglutination inhibition (HI). While HI does demonstrate cross-reactions within the genus, it is capable of defining three major virus complexes (VEE, Semliki Forest, and WEE complexes) and several individual viruses such as EEE that do not group into complexes. Getah virus is included within the Semliki Forest virus complex. In addition to the many members within the genus, subtypes or variants have been identified to exist within the equine encephalitis viruses. Through viral neutralization and modified HI techniques, two antigenic variants of EEE and several subtypes of WEE have been defined. Six subtypes (I to VI) have been identified within the VEE complex and six

385

variants (A to F) have been described within subtype 1. Multiple subtypes are also associated with Getah virus. Such extensive variation within genus members is probably a reflection of the high frequency of RNA replication error due to absence of RNA replicase proofreading. In addition to extensive genetic and antigenic variation, various subtypes and variants often exhibit differences in virulence, biochemical characteristics such as electrophoretic mobility of protein and RNA digests, physicochemical characteristics, host range, geographic distribution, and transmissibility by vector.

Resistance to Physical and Chemical Agents

Alphaviruses are sensitive to lipid solvents, chlorine, phenol, and heating to 60°C for 30 minutes. They are relatively insensitive to trypsin and are stabilized in buffer (pH 7.6) in 50% glycerine. Virus can be held indefinitely at 4°C in the lyophilized state.

Infectivity for Other Species and Culture Systems

The equine encephalitis viruses enjoy a wide host range that includes humans, horses, rodents, reptiles, amphibians, monkeys, dogs, cats, foxes, skunks, cattle, pigs, birds, and mosquitoes. Getah virus appears to be primarily an infection of horses and mosquitoes, although pigs are also naturally infected. Alphaviruses can be propagated in a variety of cell cultures including chick and duck fibroblasts, VERO, L cells, and mosquito cells; cytopathology is often absent in the latter. A variety of laboratory animals can be experimentally infected, suckling mice being the most common. Embryonated chicken eggs and young chicks may also be susceptible to infection.

HOST–VIRUS RELATIONSHIP

Distribution, Reservoir, and Transmission

The equine encephalitis viruses appear to be confined to the Western Hemisphere. EEE was classically associated with the eastern United States but has since been identified in the Caribbean region and Central and South America. WEE was classically associated with the western United States but has since been described throughout the United States (although it is rare on the eastern seaboard) and South America. VEE is essentially confined to South and Central America, although incursions into the United States have been documented; the United States considers VEE to be a foreign animal disease. Getah virus appears to be confined to Southeast Asia and Australia.

Of prime importance in the epidemiology of alphaviruses is the biologic vector — the mosquito. Peak times of disease are routinely recorded in late summer, with an abrupt halt when the vector is diminished due to adverse conditions, such as cold or drought. As is characteristic of an arthropod-borne virus, the vector must ingest an infective blood meal. The alphaviruses are biologically transmitted. This method involves actual infec-

tion of the vector, in contrast to mechanical vector-mediated transmission, in which the insect transmits virus in the same manner as a contaminated needle. For a biological vector to become infected it must obtain a blood meal from a host that is sufficiently viremic. The level of viremia required to infect the vector is dictated primarily by viral strain, the feeding insect, or both. Upon ingestion, the virus initiates infection in the gut with eventual distribution to the salivary gland, where replication provides a ready source of virus to infect additional hosts upon feeding. The time required for this process is the extrinsic incubation period. Once infected, the vector remains infected for life. Certain viruses may be transmitted from one life stage to the next (as in ticks) or via the egg; such transmission has not been demonstrated in alphaviruses.

The life cycles of the various alphaviruses differ somewhat. EEE virus infection associated with clinical disease is primarily confined to humans, equine species, and birds, especially ring-necked pheasants. Natural EEE infections have also been documented in other species, including pigs, dogs, cats, pet hamsters and guinea pigs, squirrels, mice, foxes, skunks, and wild birds. Antibodies have been identified in reptiles and amphibians and they can be experimentally infected. The primary transmission cycle appears to involve swamp mosquitoes and birds, with occasional spillover into adjacent pheasant farms, horses, and humans. Horses and humans are not a major source of virus due to minimal viremia. On pheasant farms, transmission may also occur by birds pecking each other. The overwintering reservoir of EEE is probably wild swamp birds, although other mammalian and reptilian hosts may also play a role since virus has been isolated during winter months from cats, dogs, mice, foxes, and skunks.

The host–virus relationship of WEE is similar to that of EEE with the primary transmission cycle being between mosquitoes and birds, with spillover into humans, horses, and domestic birds. Virus has also been isolated from wild birds, bats, dogs, cats, hamsters, mice, squirrels, amphibians, and reptiles. The overwintering hosts include birds and possibly reptiles and amphibians.

The primary transmission cycle of VEE appears to involve mosquitoes, birds, and wild rodents. When spillover into equine species occurs, the horse may also serve as a major source of virus because, unlike EEE and WEE, VEE replicates to high titers. While human infection is probably a dead-end event, inapparently infected cattle and pigs may also potentially serve as an infective source for mosquitoes. Vampire bats may also be infected. The reservoir of VEE is uncertain and may involve low-level transmission between mammalian and avian hosts and mosquitoes.

The life cycle of Getah virus is probably similar to the encephalitis viruses with the primary cycle of transmission being between horses, pigs, and mosquitoes.

Pathogenesis and Pathology

Alphavirus infections can range from inapparent to severe, fatal disease. Infection typically occurs following the bite of an infected insect, with primary viral replication occurring locally and in adjacent lymph nodes. The primary viremia, which persists for several days, serves to infect various target organs throughout the body; it is followed by the secondary viremia. The encephalitis viruses may gain entry into the CNS if the viremia is of sufficient level. Virus appears to enter the nervous tissue via exposed nerve endings or neuromuscular junctions, resulting in a necrotizing encephalitis in 1 to 3 weeks. Lesions often develop throughout the gray matter of the brain and include neuronal degeneration, vascular cuffing, infiltration of neutrophils and vascular cuffing, infiltration of neutrophils and later lymphocytes, microglial proliferation, and hemorrhage. It has been suggested that much of the pathology may be due to an immunologic mechanism. Macroscopic lesions in the CNS may be absent or consist of necrosis and hemorrhage. Microscopically, a necrotizing encephalitis is characterized by perivascular cuffing and infiltration of cells, gliosis, hemorrhage, neuronal necrosis, and swollen endothelial cells. Additional necrotic lesions may be found in nonneural tissues, including lymphoid tissues (with myeloid depletion of bone marrow, spleen, and nodes), pancreas, adrenal cortex, liver, myocardium, and small blood vessels.

Getah virus infection may result in a rash and edema of the limbs, which is thought to be the result of vascular damage. The pathology in horses does not typically involve the CNS. Principal lesions may include maculae in the dermis, subcutaneous tissue edema, and lymphoid hyperplasia (nodes and spleen). Skin lesions are characterized by perivascular cuffing and infiltration of lymphocytes and polymorphonuclear neutrophils (PMNs).

Host Response to Infection

Upon infection, an inflammatory response ensues within 4 to 5 days. Antibody production begins, as does production of interferon and activation of natural killer cells. The latter two may play a role in limiting early viral replication and dissemination. The development of antibody appears to be important in limiting viral replication and spread, as well as in preventing reinfection. Antibodies develop to all viral proteins and exhibit such activities as neutralization, inhibition of hemagglutination, and complement fixation. Peak antibody titers typically develop within 2 weeks. This antibody may be effective in neutralizing virus, enhancing viral clearance, lysing virus in the presence of complement, or lysing infected cells via complement or killer cells. In addition to systemic production, there may also be local antibody production in the CNS. Cell-mediated immunity also appears to play a role in viral clearance and protective immunity. Cytotoxic T cells can be identified as early as 3 to 4 days postinfection. While most studies are of an indirect nature (in vitro studies and T cell transfer in mice), cytotoxic T cells probably contribute to both recovery and protective immunity.

LABORATORY DIAGNOSIS

Diagnosis of alphavirus infection may be based on signs of encephalitis associated with past history and appropriate seasonal conditions. Such diagnosis can only be speculative, however, and laboratory diagnosis via viral isolation or serology is required. Viral isolation is carried out using blood or CNS tissue, the latter being preferable due to the uncertainty of viremia when signs of encephalitis are observed. Virus may be isolated in a variety of systems, including cell cultures, chick embryos, and suckling mice. Virus is subsequently identified via viral neutralization or HI. Serologic diagnosis is best performed using paired serum samples in an HI test. However, care must be taken in interpreting results because animals that have undergone previous alphavirus infections may respond to later infections with broadly cross-reactive antibodies. In addition, previous vaccination history should be noted, since this can also affect interpretation of single-sample serology.

TREATMENT AND CONTROL

No treatment for clinically ill animals is available. Control of alphavirus infections can be achieved through vaccination and pest management programs. Vector control can be approached through eliminating mosquito breeding sites by water control or spraying programs. In the case of domestic bird farms, the use of tightly screened (insect-proof) rearing pens and locating such pens away from freshwater swamps is also advisable. The practice of trimming the birds' beaks can also minimize mechanical (pecking) transmission from bird to bird.

Vaccines have been developed for the equine encephalitis virus via attenuation (VEE) or inactivation (EEE and WEE). These vaccines are safe and efficacious and may also be used by bird farms if diluted.

FLAVIVIRIDAE

The Flaviviridae family contains a large number of viruses within three genera, flavivirus, pestivirus, and hepatitis C virus. No serologic cross-reactions have been identified between the three genera. Only those viruses associated with disease entities in veterinary medicine are discussed here.

FLAVIVIRUS

Included in the flavivirus genus are three viruses that have as their primary sequela encephalitis (Japanese encephalitis virus, louping-ill virus, and turkey meningoencephalitis virus) and a virus (Wesselsbron virus) characterized by a hemorrhagic-type pathogenesis somewhat similar to that of dengue virus and yellow fever virus. Additional members of the family include dengue, yellow fever, St. Louis encephalitis, tick-borne encephalitis, Murray Valley encephalitis, and Powassan. While these viruses may infect animals, and thus are important to human health from an epidemiologic viewpoint (e.g., tick-borne encephalitis and Powassan disease viruses may be present in ruminant milk and provide a source of infection for humans), they are not associated with overt animal disease.

ETIOLOGIC AGENT

Physical, Chemical, and Antigenic Properties

The name *Flavivirus* is derived from the Latin word, *flavus,* meaning yellow, since yellow fever virus is the family prototype. Until their reclassification in 1984, the Flaviviruses were considered a genus within the Togaviridae family, and before that were classified as Group B arboviruses. Members of the genus consist of small (45 nm), spherical, enveloped particles with small surface projection. Viral density is 1.19 to 1.20 g/cm^3 in sucrose. The virion is composed of three structural proteins, including a single envelope glycoprotein (E), a membrane-like protein (M), and a core protein (C); at least six nonstructural proteins have been identified. The viral genome is a single linear strand of positive-sense RNA. The various species within the Flavivirus genus are antigenically classified by complement fixation (CF), HI, and viral neutralization. The latter two assays define epitopes on the envelope protein.

Resistance to Physical and Chemical Agents

The genus is stable at a pH of 7 to 9 and is inactivated by heating to 50°C, lipid solvents, ultraviolet light, ionic and nonionic detergents, and trypsin.

HOST–VIRUS RELATIONSHIP

Distribution, Reservoir, and Transmission

Most flaviviruses are considered biologically to be arboviruses based upon their transmission between vertebrate host and hematophagous arthropods, both of which support viral replication. Additional means of transmission may exist, however, and some flaviviruses have not been demonstrated to be arthropod-transmitted.

Pathogenesis and Pathology

Flavivirus infection can range from being inapparent to frank clinical disease. Viruses that cause encephalitis have a similar pathogenesis. Following penetration of the host, virus replicates locally and in adjacent lymph nodes with subsequent distribution into the blood via the thoracic duct (primary viremia). Via the blood, virus is disseminated throughout the body, with additional replication occurring in extraneural tissues including muscle, myocardium, vascular endothelium, lymphatic, and glandular tissue. This second round of viral replication results in additional viremia at which time virus may enter the CNS, possibly via exposed olfactory nerve endings. General neuropathologic changes often include an inflammatory response and neuronal damage.

Some members of the family, including Wesselsbron, are associated with a hemorrhagic fever, although encephalitis may also occur; dengue and yellow fever viruses are also associated with this type of disease syndrome. Infection is similar to that of the encephalitis viruses, but extensive extraneural pathology is observed, including hemorrhagic diathesis, increased capillary permeability and shock, lymphoid necrosis, myocarditis, and hepatic necrosis and jaundice (hepatitis).

Host Response to Infection

Both humoral and cell-mediated immune responses have been studied following flavivirus infection. Antibodies (HI and viral-neutralizing) typically develop within 4 to 6 days postinfection. In addition to neutralizing virus (predominantly specific for the envelope protein, E), antibody to viral-specified proteins expressed on the surface of infected cells (NSI would appear to be important) is probably capable of participating in cell lysis via complement and/or antibody-dependent cell-mediated cytotoxicity (ADCC). Cytotoxic T cell responses are predominantly directed at the nonstructural proteins. Antibody titers in cerebrospinal fluid usually develop about 4 days after serum titers. Humoral responses appear to play an important role in both recovery and long-term protection. Cell-mediated immune responses (cytotoxic T cells) appear to develop at the same time as, or soon after, development of antibody. Such immune responses also appear to contribute to viral clearance. Following infection, immunity is probably lifelong.

JAPANESE ENCEPHALITIS

Japanese encephalitis virus (JEV) is the prototype of the JE antigenic complex within the genus. JEV infection is typically inapparent but can cause clinical disease in humans, horses, and swine and abortions and neonatal deaths in swine. The clinical disease in horses resembles eastern equine encephalitis (EEE) and has a mortality of about 5%. Infection of pregnant sows can result in significant losses due to abortion and stillbirths, depending upon viral strain. Affected fetuses exhibit typical encephalitic lesions. Infection of boars may also result in sterility due to a reduction in spermatogenesis and histopathologic changes in the epididymis and tunica testis.

In geographic distribution, JEV is confined to temperate and tropical areas of Asia. Serologic surveys have demonstrated a high prevalence of infection in horses, cattle, and swine, with most infections being inapparent or mild. Infection of horses and humans is considered to be an epidemiologic dead end due to low-level viremias. In contrast, infected swine and birds serve as amplifying hosts for the virus because of a high viremia. The biological vector of JEV is the mosquito, with *Culex* species being of prime importance. In swine, virus may also be transmitted from the infected dam to the fetus and from boar to sow via insemination of viral-contaminated semen. Maintenance of JEV in temperate climates has not been totally elucidated, but probable mechanisms would include transovarial transmission in mosquitoes, hibernating adult female mosquitoes, and persistent infections in birds and possibly snakes or lizards. Maintenance of virus in tropical regions probably involves continual transmission between insects, birds, and swine.

Diagnosis of JEV is accomplished by isolating virus from cerebrospinal fluid or from blood if the sample is obtained during the viremic period. Inoculation of cell cultures (vertebrate and insect) or suckling mice is appropriate for viral propagation. Viral antigen may also be demonstrated directly in brain tissue sections by means of immunologic probes. Serologic diagnosis is possible by demonstrating a fourfold rise in antibody titer with hemagglutination inhibition (HI), complement fixation (CF), radio immunoassay (RIA), ELISA, and viral neutralization. RIA and ELISA are well suited to demonstrate an early infection via titration of antiviral IgM. Such an assay is often desirable since preexisting IgG, induced by related flaviviruses, will not complicate interpretation.

Control of JEV has been approached through vaccination programs. Both attenuated and killed vaccines with reported efficacy are available. Extensive antigenic variation has been described for JEV, but its potential for complicating vaccine programs has not been fully determined. Use of vector control measures, such as water management and spraying programs, has been reported to be marginally successful.

Louping-Ill

Louping-ill virus is a member of the tick-borne encephalitis virus complex. The virus naturally infects many animal species, including humans, sheep, horses, deer, goats, pigs, and wild birds. The disease is primarily associated with sheep, and a mortality of 4% may be observed in enzootic areas. Higher mortality may occur if susceptible sheep are brought into an endemic area. Louping-ill is biphasic, with initial fever and weakness followed by development of neurologic signs such as hyperexcitability, cerebellar ataxia, and progressive paralysis. The disease gets its name from the leaping gait sometimes observed in ataxic animals. As in sheep, infection of humans, cattle, swine, goats, and horses may result in neurologic disease. Experimental infection of certain species of grouse has been reported to result in neurologic disease as well. While deer are susceptible to infection, clinical disease has not been described.

Louping-ill appears to be confined to the British Isles, Norway, and possibly Bulgaria and Turkey. The seasonal nature of the disease (spring and summer) is a reflection of vector activity. The primary biologic vector appears to be the tick, *Ixodes rincinus*. However, the virus may also be transmitted by aerosol, and experimentally infected goats have shed virus in milk with subsequent infection of suckling kids. Thus, contaminated milk could be a potential human health hazard.

Diagnosis of louping-ill is carried out by viral isolation, fluorescent antibody (FA) staining of CNS tissue sections, or serology. Virus can be isolated using vertebrate or insect cell cultures and intracerebral inoculation of suckling mice with CNS tissue or blood. Propagated virus can be definitively identified by viral neutralization. Serologic diagnosis can be conducted by CF, HI, or viral neutralization.

Louping-ill can be controlled by tick control measures, such as dipping and spraying of sheep. A formalin-inactivated cell culture-origin vaccine is available and effective. Lambs born to immune dams are protected by colostral antibody for approximately 4 months.

Wesselsbron

Wesselsbron virus is associated primarily with disease in sheep, although cattle, goats, humans, wild rodents, and wild fowl may also be infected. Infection of sheep may result in death of pregnant ewes and newborn lambs; abortion may also occur, with neurologic defects being a common finding. Clinical disease in the newborn and pregnant ewe is characterized by hepatic necrosis and jaundice, subcutaneous edema, gastrointestinal hemorrhage, and fever; mortality in lambs can approach 30%. Cattle, horses, and swine typically experience inapparent infections; humans may experience fever and muscular pain.

Wesselsbron virus is transmitted in the summer and fall months by mosquitoes, *Aedes* species being the primary vectors. The disease appears to be confined to southern Africa, although the virus has been isolated from mosquitoes in Thailand.

Diagnosis may be based upon viral isolation or serology. Viral isolation may be conducted using a variety of cell cultures (BHK and lamb kidney), chick embryos, or suckling mice. Serology may be conducted by viral neutralization, HI, or CF; however, prior exposure to other flaviviruses may make interpretation difficult. Control of Wesselsbron is attempted via immunization of lambs with an attenuated vaccine.

Israel Turkey Meningoencephalitis

Israel turkey meningoencephalitis was first described in Israeli turkeys as a progressive paralysis associated with nonpurulent meningoencephalitis; mortality may reach 50%. Natural disease appears to be confined to turkeys (10 weeks of age or older) in northern Israel, and transmission by mosquitoes is suggested by the seasonal nature of disease (late summer and fall) and the ability of mosquitoes to support viral replication.

Viral isolation is the preferred diagnostic technique by inoculation of chick embryos, suckling mice, or chick embryo fibroblast cell cultures. Development of an effective attenuated vaccine has been reported.

PESTIVIRUS

The pestivirus genus includes the etiologic agents of bovine viral diarrhea (BVDV), border disease (BDV), and hog cholera (also referred to as classical swine fever [CSFV]), all of which are important pathogens of livestock. In contrast to the flavivirus genus, pestiviruses are not arthropod-borne. They are readily inactivated by low pH, heat, organic solvents, and detergents. Virions range from 40 nm to 60 nm in diameter and are composed of up to four structural proteins, including three envelope glycoproteins and a capsid protein. The genome is of positive polarity and contains a single, large open reading frame. All three viruses are important food-animal pathogens and will be described sequentially. They are very closely related and can only be distinguished by application of monoclonal antibodies and/or molecular biology techniques.

BOVINE VIRUS DIARRHEA VIRUS

DISEASE

Bovine virus diarrhea virus (BVDV) is responsible for a disease complex classically referred to as *bovine virus diarrhea-mucosal disease (BVD-MD)*. Signs of illness include depression, anorexia, scouring, excessive salivation, recumbency, dehydration, reduced lactation, cessation of rumination, conjunctivitis, congestion, ulcerations in the mucous membrane of the oral cavity, and reproductive problems (abortion, teratogenesis) in pregnant cows. Severely affected cattle have a high temperature (40°C to 41.5°C) and a leukopenia. As a herd disease, BVD-MD varies from one with a high morbidity and a low mortality to one with a low morbidity and a high mortality. The disease affects cattle of all ages, but young stock are more likely to show signs of illness. Upon emergence of a cytopathic BVDV strain, cattle with persistent noncytopathic BVDV infections develop mucosal disease. A relatively more severe BVDV-associated disease in calves has been recently recognized, characterized by severe thrombocytopenia and hemorrhage of mucosal surfaces and internal organs.

ETIOLOGIC AGENT

Physical, Chemical, and Antigenic Properties

Size estimates for the BVDV purified by various procedures, and representing different strains, range from less than 50 nm up to 120 nm. Recent studies on BVDV morphology (NADL strain) indicate that the infectious virus purified on potassium tartrate gradients is oval to pleomorphic in shape with a diameter of approximately 120 nm (±30 nm). The virus is composed of a unit membrane-like envelope that surrounds an internal core-like structure (Fig 67.1).

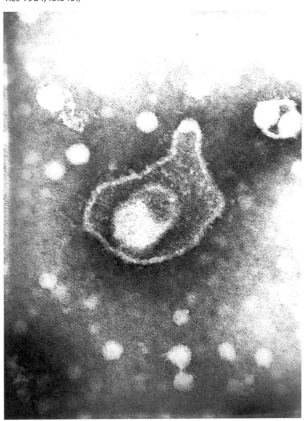

FIGURE 67.1. *Negatively stained preparations of bovine virus diarrhea virus. 250,000×. (Reproduced with permission from Chu HJ, Zee YC. Morphology of bovine viral diarrhea virus. Am J Vet Res 1984;45:845.)*

The density of BVDV in sucrose is 1.12 g/cm³. The genome of BVDV is RNA, which is infectious. The virus is composed of four structural proteins.

BVDV is the type species of the pestivirus genus. It is serologically related to hog cholera and border disease virus (BDV) of sheep. In fact, observations on the physical and biologic similarities between BVDV and BDV, and their antigenic relationship as determined by viral neutralization using polyclonal serum, made these agents indistinguishable in vitro. More recently, the application of monoclonal antibodies and nucleotide sequencing has permitted differentiation of these closely related viruses.

Multiple strains of BVDV have been described; however, the differences are subtle and until recently did not warrant a serologic subdivision of the genus. Two biotypes have been described with one being cytopathogenic for cell cultures and the other not. The cytopathic strains apparently arise by mutational events in noncytopathic strains. In addition, with the recent identification and characterization of some highly pathogenic BVD viruses, two groups (I and II) have been proposed with Group I including the classic BVD viruses and Group II comprising the recently characterized highly pathogenic strains and those associated with severe thrombocytopenia and hemorrhagic disease. An alternative classification has also been suggested, however, that would divide the pestiviruses into four groups (pestivirus Types 1 to 4): Type 1 would include classic BVDV, Type 2 would comprise CSFV, Type 3 would include classic BDV, and Type 4 would comprise the pestivirus-like viruses and pathogenic BVDV.

Resistance to Physical and Chemical Agents

BVDV is sensitive to lipid solvents such as ether and chloroform and is inactivated by treatment with trypsin. The virus is most stable in the pH range from 5.7 to 9.3, with maximum stability at pH 7.4. The virus is readily maintained in a lyophilized or frozen ($-70°C$) state for many years.

Infectivity for Other Species and Culture Systems

In addition to cattle, sheep, goats, and pigs are susceptible to infection with BVDV. As with border disease virus (see below), parenteral inoculation of pregnant sheep with BVDV usually results in an inapparent infection. With certain strains of BVDV, however, a febrile response may occur. Experimental infection of pregnant ewes with the NADL strain of BVDV has produced placental lesions, abortions, mummified fetuses, and congenital malformations. In utero infection of sheep with BVDV or BDV can result in prenatal dysmorphogenesis, early postnatal death, or the birth of clinically affected or apparently healthy progeny. The outcome depends on the gestational stage at which infection takes place.

Isolates of BVDV, whether cytopathogenic or noncytopathogenic, can be grown in cell culture systems. The cells that are most susceptible include bovine embryonic skin-muscle cells and embryonic bovine kidney cells. Immunofluorescence is usually used to detect noncytopathogenic strains. Cytopathogenic strains produce plaques and can be used for accurate viral titrations. Other cell cultures of bovine origin that support BVDV replication include bovine fetal lung, fetal endometrium, and tracheal ring organ cultures and blood macrophages.

HOST–VIRUS RELATIONSHIP

Distribution, Reservoir, and Transmission

BVDV has a worldwide distribution. Serologic surveys have been conducted in various parts of the United States and abroad. Prevalence rates vary from 59% to 73% in surveys of states where 100 or more cattle were tested. Similar incidence rates were found in Europe. Sheep, goats, and possibly pigs serve as reservoir host for BVDV.

BVDV does not produce signs of illness in rabbits, mice, or pigs. Serologic studies conducted in the wildlife of nine African countries recorded neutralizing antibody titers to BVDV in 17 species. Such results indicate that infection is widespread and suggest that some free-living species may be reservoirs of infection in the wild.

Transmission is by contact and by contaminated feed, water, or litter.

Pathogenesis and Pathology

The consequences of infection of cattle with BVDV vary from an inapparent infection to severe fatal disease. Infection of the bovine fetus with BVDV causes a viremia in the fetus that can persist into adult life. Viral persistence into neonatal life is associated with specific immunotolerance in which antibodies are lacking but virus is present in blood. Experimental infection of pregnant heifers before 180 days of gestation, the age at which the fetus becomes immunocompetent to BVDV, produces a number of persistently infected calves. BVDV displays an affinity for cells of the immune system. Peripheral lymphocytes from calves infected with BVDV may be unresponsive to stimulation with phytohemagglutinin, indicating immune suppression.

BVDV is capable of crossing the placenta and is teratogenic. Fetopathogenicity of the virus can lead to death of the fetus or developmental abnormalities, including intrauterine growth retardation and deformities of the CNS. Ocular lesions and congenital cerebellar lesions have been described in fetuses as a result of BVDV inoculation into susceptible pregnant animals.

Lesions similar to those produced by rinderpest virus occur primarily in the alimentary tract, lymphatic system, and upper respiratory tract. They consist of congestion, hemorrhage, edema, and erosion of mucosal membranes. The oral lesions, which are often small, shallow, and irregular, may be found on the muzzle, tongue, dental pad, esophagus, and pharynx. Hemorrhages and erosions are occasionally seen in the rumen. The abomasum is inflamed and edematous. Edema and congestion with extensive erosions may be seen in the intestine. Lymphoid depletion or damage to immunocompetent cells is consistently observed. Peyer's patches are enlarged and may be completely devoid of lymphoid tissues. Lymph nodes throughout the alimentary tract may be enlarged. Cerebellar hyperplasia, cataracts, retinal degeneration and hypoplasia, and neuritis of optic nerves are found in congenitally infected calves. Immune complexes consisting of BVDV, antiviral antibody, and complement have been found in the renal glomeruli of diseased cattle.

Host Responses to Infection

BVDV usually induces high serum neutralization (SN) antibody titers. Cattle that recover from infection have long-lasting immunity. After experimental inoculation SN antibodies are detectable in 2 weeks. High titers of IgG are present in the serum and follicular fluid. IgG, IgM, and IgA concentrations are low in uterine and vaginal secretions.

BVDV may persist, especially in animals infected in utero, without circulating antibodies, presumably owing to immunologic tolerance or to destruction of immunocompetent cells. Immunologic tolerance to BVDV has been demonstrated.

LABORATORY DIAGNOSIS

Clinical diagnosis may be difficult. BVD-MD must be differentiated from other diseases such as malignant catarrhal fever or rinderpest, which can present with similar clinical signs and pathologic changes.

Rapid diagnosis of cytopathogenic and noncytopathogenic strains can be made by immunofluorescent (IF) staining of cells collected by nasopharyngeal brush swabbings of diseased animals. A definitive diagnosis is made by viral isolation followed by identification by SN or IF. Viral isolation may be attempted from nasal secretions, feces, blood, lymph nodes, turbinates, and intestines. If cytopathogenic changes are not observed after three passages in cell cultures, noncytopathogenic strains can be identified by IF or by the ability of the noncytopathogenic strain to interfere with a cytopathogenic strain (cellular resistance test). Serum neutralization test to demonstrate a fourfold increase in antibody titer in paired serum samples may also be used for diagnosis. Recent development of polymerase chain reaction (PCR) to certain serotypes of BVDV has been achieved.

TREATMENT AND CONTROL

BVDV infection is considered one of the most important causes of economic loss to the cattle industry. Therefore, there is a need for safe and efficient vaccines. Safety continues to be a problem with live vaccines. Most available live-virus vaccines have been developed by serial passage of virus in cell culture. At least one vaccine has been developed using a temperature-sensitive mutant. One problem with such vaccines is inadvertent contamination of bovine cell cultures used for vaccine production with virulent but noncytopathogenic BVDV strains. Virus has even been detected in the irradiated or heat-inactivated serum used for propagation of cell cultures.

The parenteral administration of live attenuated vaccines against BVDV, either alone or combined with infectious bovine rhinotracheitis (IBR) virus and parainfluenza virus (PI3), in general provides satisfactory immunity. Postvaccinal reactions may occur, however, and compromise the reputation of vaccination. Some vaccination breaks may be due to vaccination (live virus) of cattle harboring a noncytopathogenic strain of the BVDV. The vaccine virus, although attenuated, is derived from a cytopathogenic strain and may be capable of unlimited growth in immunotolerant, persistently infected cattle. Also, live vaccines should not be used in pregnant animals.

Since colostral antibodies persist for 4 to 6 months in calves, vaccination prior to this time is not effective. If they are vaccinated prior to 4 to 6 months of age, revaccination is necessary.

Immunization of calves with an ethanol saponin vaccine (killed-virus vaccine) against BVDV results in the production of neutralizing antibodies in high titers and the vaccinated animals are resistant to challenge with virulent virus. The duration of immunity is unknown.

BORDER DISEASE VIRUS

DISEASE

Border disease (BD) is a congenital pestivirus infection classically associated with sheep. However, congenital infection of cattle and goats may also result in fetal disease that has many similarities to BD of sheep. Expression of fetal disease is variable and the clinical outcome is dependent upon multiple factors, including gestational age, infecting viral strain, the host, and probably other unrecognized factors. Infection of the developing fetus may result in fetal death, mummification, abortion, stillbirth, or birth of lambs exhibiting weakness, poor viability, anatomic anomalies, CNS disturbances (tremors), abnormal hairy birth coats, or some combination of these characteristics. In certain countries, lambs expressing the latter two conditions have been referred to as "hairy shakers." Infection of the neonate or adult animal is typically inapparent; however, the infected neonate may have a reduced growth rate.

ETIOLOGIC AGENT

Physical, Chemical, and Antigenic Properties

Border disease virus (BDV) is classified as a pestivirus and its morphologic, physicochemical, and antigenic properties are very similar to those of bovine virus diarrhea virus (BVDV). The density of BDV in sucrose is $1.115\,gm/cm^3$. Extensive molecular characterization of the virus has not been conducted. However, based upon its close antigenic relationship with BVDV and similar host range, it may be appropriate to consider BDV as representing strains of BVDV.

Multiple strains of BDV have been isolated, most of which are noncytopathic in cell cultures. The virus is closely related to hog cholera virus (HCV) and BVDV as determined by multiple serologic techniques. In fact, serologic differences between BDV and BVDV are no more pronounced than those observed between strains of BDV.

Resistance to Physical and Chemical Agents

Border disease virus exhibits physicochemical properties similar to BVDV. The virus is inactivated by chloroform, ether, trypsin, and heating to 56°C for 20 minutes.

Infectivity for Host Species and Culture Systems

While BDV is classically associated with infection of sheep, its host range includes cattle and goats. Furthermore, pregnant sows have been experimentally infected with some viral strains with subsequent development of fetal cerebellar hypoplasia. The virus can be propagated in primary and secondary cell cultures of bovine and ovine origin, and in established cell lines including pig kidney, fetal lamb muscle, and bovine turbinate.

HOST–VIRUS RELATIONSHIP

Distribution, Reservoir, and Transmission

Border disease was initially described in the late 1940s as a congenital disease of sheep in England and Wales. The disease has since been recognized in many European countries, Australia, New Zealand, Canada, and the United States.

The epizootiology of BD is poorly defined, due in part to the broad spectrum of clinical signs and the inability to adequately differentiate BDV from BVDV using in vitro techniques.

Viral persistence in nature is probably due to the presence of persistently infected ruminant species. Congenitally infected sheep may experience lifelong viremia and shed virus in multiple excretions, including those of respiratory, digestive (feces and urine), and reproductive origin. Persistently infected cattle and goats may also potentially serve as viral reservoirs. Cattle persistently infected with BDV can transmit virus to sheep, and BDV-infected sheep can transmit virus to cattle.

Transmission of BDV is probably most common by the oral and intranasal routes. Additional mechanisms could include transfer of virus during routine immunizations when needles are not changed between inoculations, cell culture source (bovine and ovine cells) vaccines contaminated with virus, and insemination of females with vial-contaminated semen.

Pathogenesis and Pathology

Following infection of the dam, virus is disseminated to the placenta via a viremia, with subsequent infection of the fetus; a placentitis may accompany viral replication. If the placenta is sufficiently damaged, fetal nutrition may be compromised with resulting growth retardation. Upon infection, the fetus experiences generalized viral dissemination, the resulting damage being influenced by fetal age. Infection in the first trimester is relatively more severe than infection later in gestation. Infection after 80 days' gestation often results in viral clearance or control of the disease process.

The effect of infection on various organs is related to their developmental stage. Organs that are actively developing are most severely affected. Relative to the CNS, viral-induced lesions are apparently due to reduced or altered myelination and demyelinization, leading to congenital tremor of the newborn lamb. Degeneration and necrosis of the CNS germinal layers and inflammatory cell infiltration are associated with development of hydranencephaly, porencephaly, and cerebellar dysplasia. The skin and fleece abnormalities are due to alterations in the growth and development of the epidermis and primary follicles.

Histologically, dysmyelination of the CNS is considered the most characteristic feature of BD. Hypercellularity of the white matter, mild meningoencephalitis, and perivascular infiltration of mononuclear cells may also be apparent. The predominant skin lesion is characterized by the presence of enlarged primary follicles and reduction in the number of secondary follicles.

Host Response to Infection

Infection of an adult animal with BDV typically results in a humoral immune response at 3 to 5 weeks and includes neutralizing antibody that persists for more than a year. Such postnatal infections are typically resolved by the immune response. The fetal immune response is closely tied to gestational age at the time of infection. Generally speaking, infection during the first half of gestation results in a persistent viremia and failure to generate an immune response. Such animals may remain immunologically tolerant to the virus for their entire prenatal and postnatal life. Infection during the second half of gestation, at a time when the fetus is gaining immunologic competence, can result in both a humoral and cellular immune response; the development of such an immune response may resolve the infection. However, antibody formation, neonatal ingestion of high-titer colostrum, or both may not eliminate the virus.

LABORATORY DIAGNOSIS

Variability in clinical signs expressed by congenitally infected lambs can make clinical diagnosis of BD difficult. Definitive diagnosis can be achieved by immunofluorescent antibody staining of infected tissues. Serologic demonstration of BDV-specific antibody in precolostral serum is also of diagnostic value, but it must be kept in mind that congenitally infected animals may be immunologically unresponsive.

TREATMENT AND CONTROL

To date, effective treatment of congenital BD has not been described. Safe and effective vaccines are not available. An ideal vaccine should be noninfectious, because attenuated viruses may initiate persistent infections.

Alternative control measures include animal depopulation and culling of affected and suspect animals.

HOG CHOLERA VIRUS

DISEASE

Hog cholera (swine fever) is first manifested by fever (104°F or higher) and loss of appetite. The affected animals appear dull and drowsy. They crowd together in corners or under haystacks, as if chilled. Vomiting and diarrhea are common. A mucopurulent discharge from the eyes is frequently observed. Nervous signs such as grinding of the teeth, local paralysis, locomotor disturbances, and occasionally convulsions are observed. Congenital infections of the dam result in small litters, fetal death, premature births, stillbirths, cerebellar ataxic piglets, and tremors. Typical cases may be complicated by secondary bacterial invasion, which is principally in the form of pneumonia and ulcerative enteritis. The morbidity is 95% to 100% and the mortality is almost as high. In Europe the disease is usually less severe. This milder chronic form of the disease is difficult to detect and to eradicate.

ETIOLOGIC AGENT

Physical, Chemical, and Antigenic Properties

Hog cholera virus (HCV) is a member of the pestivirus genus of the family Togavirus. HC virions concentrated on glycerol gradients are spherical in shape with a diameter of 53 ± 14 nm. The virion envelope measures 6 nm in width.

The HCV genome is single-stranded RNA with a single open reading frame (ORF). The virion is composed of three major structural proteins.

Serologic cross-reaction with BVDV and BDV has been observed, although the proteins involved have not been identified.

Resistance to Physical and Chemical Agents

HCV is chloroform- and ether-labile. It is fairly stable in response to pH changes; a pH of less than 1 to 4 or greater than 13 is necessary to inactivate the virus within an hour. Virions inactivate quickly when allowed to dry in the air but persist for up to several months in pork or garbage. The virus is completely inactivated in canned hams when an internal temperature of 65°C is maintained for 90 minutes. The virus survives for 3 days at 50°C in defibrinated blood.

Infectivity for Other Species and Culture Systems

Domestic swine and wild hogs are the only naturally susceptible species.

HCV replicates in cultures of porcine cells such as spleen, kidney, testicle, and peripheral blood leukocytes. Most strains of the virus are noncytopathogenic and may persist in culture for many cell passages. The presence of HCV in infected cell cultures is demonstrated by immunofluorescent techniques. Some cytopathogenic strains have been reported. Viral antigen has been detected by immunofluorescence as soon as 4 hours after infection of pig kidney cells.

Noncytopathogenic strains of HCV have been found to interfere with the replication of both vesicular stomatitis virus and western equine encephalomyelitis.

HOST–VIRUS RELATIONSHIP

Distribution, Reservoir, and Transmission

HCV has a virtually worldwide distribution; however, some countries, including the United States and Canada, have eradicated the disease.

Infected domestic swine and wild hogs serve as the reservoir host. Wild hogs may act as inapparent carriers. Swine lungworms have been reported to serve as a reservoir and intermediate host for HCV. Lungworms in affected pigs may acquire HCV, which is transmitted through their ova to succeeding generations of worms.

Transmission is by droplet, fomites, and ingestion of infected materials, particularly uncooked garbage. Birds may act as mechanical carriers.

Pathogenesis and Pathology

Hog cholera is an acute, highly contagious disease characterized by degeneration in the walls of the smaller blood vessels, resulting in multiple hemorrhages, necrosis, and infarctions in internal organs. The incubation period is usually 3 to 8 days. Initially the virus replicates in the lymphoid tissues of the upper respiratory tract or in the tonsils. The virus has an affinity for mesodermal tissues, particularly hemopoietic and vascular tissues. Damage to these cells produces enlarged lymph nodes and generalized hemorrhages. The course of disease is 5 to 16 days.

Secondary bacterial pneumonia and enteritis often accompany the viral disease. Historically, hog cholera was erroneously believed to be caused by *Salmonella choleraesuis*. It was later shown that the disease was of viral etiology and that the bacterium played only a secondary role in the disease.

The principal lesions involve petechial hemorrhages on all serous surfaces. Hemorrhagic lymphadenitis, petechial hemorrhages in the kidney, and infarction in the spleen are also observed. Microscopic lesions of nonsuppurative encephalitis may be seen.

Host Response to Infection

Animals that recover from hog cholera have a long-lasting immunity. Neutralizing antibody titers correlate with resistance to HCV infection.

Suckling pigs acquire colostral antibodies from the immune dam. The half-life of this colostral antibody is 13 days. Pigs that have maternal antibody titers of 1 : 1000 or above still have some antibody at 4 months.

LABORATORY DIAGNOSIS

Diagnosis of hog cholera can be confirmed by isolating and identifying HCV from the spleen, tonsils, lymph nodes, and blood. Since many strains are noncytopathogenic in cell culture, the fluorescent antibody method is preferred for the detection of HCV.

TREATMENT AND CONTROL

Over the years, three methods of vaccination have been employed. Killed-viral vaccines such as the crystal violet killed vaccine are safe but not fully effective. In general, it takes longer to produce an adequate immunity with inactivated viral vaccine, more injections are required, and a dependable immunity does not persist longer than 8 months. Simultaneous vaccination with virulent HCV and high-titered antiserum has caused severe reactions and death of some pigs. This is not an acceptable method of vaccination. Attenuated vaccines made by serial passage of virus in rabbits or cell culture elicit a strong immune response but are not safe. Heterotypic vaccines using BVDV have also been investigated but have not provided adequate protection against hog cholera.

Hog cholera virus is spread through fresh pork, the trimmings of which often find their way back to swine in the form of garbage. Laws requiring the cooking of all garbage fed to swine have long been in effect in many European countries, the United States, and Canada.

Hog cholera can be eradicated by strict quarantine and slaughter measures. These procedures are extremely expensive but the benefits are thought to outweigh the cost.

SELECTED REFERENCES

Brownlie T. Pathogenesis of mucosal disease and molecular aspects of bovine virus diarrhoea virus. Vet Microbiol 1990;23:371.

Calisher CH, Monath TP. The alphaviruses and flaviviruses. In: Lennette EH, Halonen P, Murphy FA, eds. Laboratory diagnosis of infectious diseases: principles and practices. Vol. 2. New York: Springer-Verlag, 1988:414.

Duffel SJ, Harkness JW. Bovine virus diarrhea–mucosal disease infection in cattle. Vet Rec 1985;117:240.

Harkness JW. Classical swine fever and its diagnosis: a current review. Vet Rec 1985;116:288.

Johnston RE, Peters CJ. Alphaviruses. In: Fields B, Knipe DM, Howley PM, et al., eds. Fields virology. 3rd ed. Philadelphia: Lippincott-Raven, 1995:843.

Moening V. Pestiviruses: a review. Vet Microbiol 1990;23:35.

Monath TP, Heinz FX. Flaviviruses. In: Fields B, Knipe DM, Howley PM, et al., eds. Fields virology. 3rd ed. Philadelphia: Lippincott-Raven, 1995:961.

Schlesinger SA, Schlesinger M, eds. The togaviridae and flaviviridae. New York: Plenum, 1986.

Terpstra C. Border disease: a congenital infection of small ruminants. Prog Vet Microbiol Immunol 1985;1:175.

Walton TE. Venezuelan, eastern and western encephalomyelitis. In: Gibbs ERJ, ed. Virus diseases of food animals. Vol. II. New York: Academic, 1981:585–625.

68 *Orthomyxoviridae*

Alex A. Ardans

Influenza viruses are designated as the orthomyxoviruses. They are divided into Types A, B, and C based on the antigenic differences between their nucleoprotein (NP) and matrix (M) proteins. Type A influenza viruses naturally occur in humans, horses, swine, and birds. Types B and C are found only in humans. Influenza A viruses are further divided into subtypes. The nomenclature system includes the host of origin, geographic origin, strain number, and year of isolation. A description of the two major surface antigens, the hemagglutinin and the neuraminidase, is given in parentheses — for example, A/swine/New Jersey/8/76 (H1 N1). By convention, the host of origin for human strains is now omitted.

MORPHOLOGY

When examined by electron microscopy, influenza viruses are irregularly shaped spherical particles approximately 120 nm in diameter (Figs 68.1 and 68.2). Of two distinct types of surface spikes, one is rod-shaped and corresponds to the hemagglutinin (HA), while the other is mushroom-shaped and possesses neuraminidase (NA) activity. Both the HA and the NA are glycoproteins that attach to the viral envelope by short sequences of hydrophobic amino acids. The viral envelope, a lipid bilayer derived from the host cell plasma membrane, surrounds a matrix protein (M) shell, which in turn surrounds eight single-stranded RNA molecules along with the nucleoprotein (NP) and three large proteins (PB1, PB2, and PA) responsible for RNA replication and transcription. Each of the eight genomic RNA species encodes for one, or sometimes two, polypeptides. This independent nature of the viral genes is thought to be responsible for the characteristic phenomena of high recombination frequencies in mixed infections as well as multiplicity reactivation of ultraviolet-irradiated virus, and is the basis for one theory explaining the origin of new pandemic strains.

VIRAL PROTEINS

Hemagglutinin

All strains of influenza are capable of agglutinating erythrocytes from humans, guinea pigs, and chickens as well as many other species. Antibodies to the HA prevent infection of host cells. The HA together with the neuraminidase act as the two major strain-specific surface antigens and are very important with regard to host immunity. In fact, it is the variation of these molecules that is primarily responsible for the recurrent outbreaks of influenza and the failure to control them by vaccination. The hemagglutination functions in the initial virus attachment to its cellular reception. Its later cleavage allows fusion of the viral envelope with an intercellular membrane allowing transfer of virion nucleocapsid into the cell cytoplasm. There are now 15 recognized hemagglutinins.

Neuraminidase

The neuraminidase is responsible for the cleavage of the sialic acid–containing receptor and the elution of the viral particle from the host cell. This phenomenon prevents self-aggregation and promotes release of the virus from the infected cell. Antibody against the NA does not protect against infection but does confer protection against disease and reduces transmissibility. There are nine recognized NA subtypes.

Nucleoprotein

The nucleoprotein (NP) was originally designated the soluble, or S, antigen and is the innermost component of the influenza virion. It is coiled into a double helix 50 nm to 60 nm in diameter and is intimately associated with the RNA segments and the three different polymerases.

The NP is one of the type-specific antigens used to categorize the influenza virus into Types A and B, and can be identified by enzyme-linked immunosorbent assay (ELISA), double immunodiffusion, complement fixation, single radial diffusion, agar-gel precipitation, and the hemagglutination inhibition tests.

Matrix Protein

The nonglycosylated matrix protein is also a type-specific antigen of influenza viruses. However, antibodies against M provide little, if any, protection against infection. This structural protein surrounds the nucleoprotein to form the inner part of the viral envelope.

Nonstructural Proteins

There are at least two nonstructural proteins, NS1 and NS2. Their function is at this time unknown.

FIGURE 68.1.   *Negatively stained preparation of influenza A virus. 150,000×. (Reproduced with permission from Air GU, Laver WG. The molecular basis of antigenic variation in influenza virus. Adv Virus Res 1986;31:53.)*

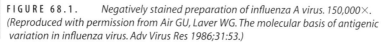

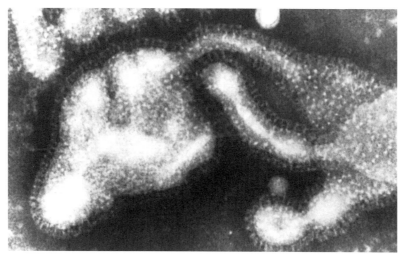

FIGURE 68.2.   *Diagram of influenza virus. The diagram illustrates the main structural features of the virion. The surface of the particle contains three kinds of spike proteins — the hemagglutinin (HA), neuraminidase (NA), and matrix (M2) protein — embedded in a lipid bilayer derived from the host cell and covers the matrix (M1) protein that surrounds the viral core. The ribonucleoprotein complex making up the core consists of at least one of each of the eight single-stranded RNA segments associated with the nucleoprotein (NP) and the three polymerase proteins (PB2, PB1, PA). RNA segments have base pairing between their 3' and 5' ends forming a panhandle. Their organization and the role of NS2 in the virion remain unresolved. (Reproduced with permission from Murphy B, Weneter RG. Orthomyxoviruses. In: Fields B, Knipe DM, Howley PM, et al., eds. Fields virology. 3rd ed. New York: Lippincott-Raven, 1996:1401.)*

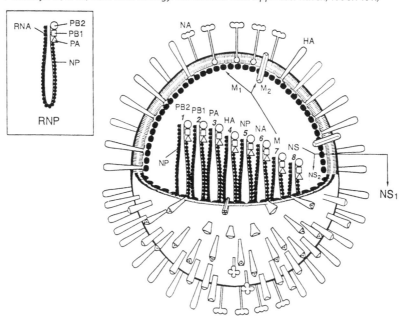

Polymerase Proteins

The polymerase proteins (PB1, PB2, PA) are found in association with their NP and viral RNA. They are the largest of the viral proteins and are responsible for RNA polymerization of the viral genome. PB2 and PB1 are necessary for complementary RNA synthesis, while PA and NP are required for viral RNA synthesis.

Viral Genome

The influenza A genome has 10 genes along 8 RNA segments of negative sense. Because of this segmented arrangement, reassortant is possible resulting in the production of new strains. Influenza viral variation is frequent and occurs in two ways, drift and shift. Antigenic drift is due to point mutations resulting in amino acid replacement mainly in HA epitopes. Antigenic shift occurs with reassortment among the segmented RNA when a cell is infected with two different influenza viruses. This mechanism is postulated for those new viruses that result in human pandemics.

EQUINE INFLUENZA

DISEASE

Equine influenza is an acute disease affecting both the upper and lower respiratory tracts of horses. While horses of all ages are affected, those between 2 and 6 months are at greatest risk. The mortality rate for equine influenza is low to moderate while the morbidity rate can approach 100%. The incubation period lasts from 1 to 3 days. Disease is manifested by a high fever, 103°F to 106°F, which lasts about 3 days. Other clinical signs include a frequent, strong, dry cough lasting 1 to 3 weeks, a nasal discharge that is originally serous in character but that later becomes mucoid, anorexia, depression, photophobia, lacrimation along with a mucopurulent ocular discharge, corneal opacity, and occasionally the loss of eyesight. Limb edema and muscle soreness can occur and, in some severe outbreaks, acute deaths due to fulminant pneumonia have occurred. Enteritis was observed in a 1989 outbreak in Northern China due to a new equine virus, A/equine/2/Jilin.

Equine influenza viruses are designated as Type A influenza. They have been divided into two subtypes, A/equine/1 (H7N7) and A/equine/2 (H3N8), based on antigenic differences in their HA. A/equine/1 has one prototype, A/equine/1/Prague. Antigenic drift has occurred among A/equine/1 viruses with the subsequent designation of two subgroups that do not appear significant in vaccinal immunity. Significant drift has occurred among A/equine/2 viruses from the original prototype A/equine/2/Miami/63 first isolated from a severe 1963 outbreak in Florida horses. Additional prototypes A/equine/2/Fountainblue, A/equine/2/Kentucky, along with other variants including a 1989 Chinese virus,

demonstrated the considerable drift occurring in the A/equine/2 viruses that have vaccine implications. The disease is worldwide in occurrence and is a common and troublesome problem at shows, sales, stables, and racetracks.

ETIOLOGIC AGENT

Resistance to Physical and Chemical Agents

Equine influenza virus is usually inactivated at 56°C in 30 minutes. Like other members of the orthomyxovirus group, the virus is inactivated by phenol, lipid solvents, detergent, formalin, and oxidizing agents such as ozone.

Infectivity for Other Species and Culture Systems

Equine influenza virus infects horses, asses, and mules. It can be experimentally adapted to infect mice when introduced intranasally.

All orthomyxoviruses, including equine influenza virus, can be propagated in the amniotic cavity of embryonated chicken eggs. Equine influenza virus can also be grown in chick embryo kidney, bovine kidney, rhesus monkey kidney, and human embryo kidney cells.

HOST–VIRUS RELATIONSHIP

Pathogenesis and Pathology

Equine influenza virus infects both the upper and lower respiratory tracts. There is an early lymphopenia and frequently enlargement of the lymph nodes of the head. Initially there may only be a slight serous nasal discharge, which later becomes mucoid. Fatal pneumonia can occur in foals and on occasion in older animals. Occasionally there is ventral edema of the trunk and lower limbs. A/equine/2 has been known to cause a postinfection encephalopathy in foals. Catarrhal and even hemorrhagic enteritis as well as kidney damage may occur. The most typical pathologic lesions are characteristic of bronchiolitis, in which the bronchioles are successively consolidated. Severe necrotizing myositis with elevated serum enzyme levels has been observed with A2 infections. Most animals recover within 2 to 3 weeks; those that do not may develop chronic obstructive pulmonary disease (COPD). Prolonged recovery and severity of disease appear to be related to the level of stress an affected horse undergoes. Adequate rest is an important consideration in an influenza outbreak.

The disease is most commonly transmitted via aerosol infection and can spread extremely rapidly due to the frequent, violent cough. Infected animals continue to shed virus for about 5 days after the first signs appear.

LABORATORY DIAGNOSIS

A tentative clinical diagnosis of equine influenza can be made from the characteristic rapid spread and the frequent dry cough. A definitive diagnosis requires either the isolation of the virus, demonstration of viral antigen, or the demonstration of rising antibody titers between acute and convalescent sera by complement fixation (CF) and hemagglutination inhibition (HI) tests. During an initial outbreak, it is critical for the success of future vaccination programs to isolate and type the virus. If a new type is involved, serology alone could be misleading, and while the antigen capture enzyme-linked immunosorbent assay (ELISA) is a rapid test for antigen detection, it does not recognize an antigenic drift that may be occurring.

TREATMENT AND CONTROL

Vaccination is effective against equine influenza infection in horses. Protection, however, is dependent on the manner of vaccination and the quality of the vaccine, with particular emphasis placed on proper selection of vaccine strains. Available vaccines contain inactivated virus of both A/equine/1 and A/equine/2 subtypes. Classically, A/equine/Prague/56 (H7N7) and A/equine/Miami/63 (H3N8) have been used as the prototype A/equine/1 and A/equine/2 strains, respectively. There is increasing evidence of antigenic diversity among contemporary equine influenzas in nature, suggesting that the effectiveness of the conventional vaccine strains in providing protection will become limited with time. For this reason, current vaccines include some of the newer variant A/equi/2 viruses. The various inactivated vaccines available are incorporated with adjuvants that have proved to significantly augment their immunogenic potential. Initial immunization requires two doses of vaccine 2 to 4 weeks apart. These should be followed by a single booster when the horse is 1 year of age and then repeated every 6 months until the horse is about 3 years of age, at which time the booster interval may be increased to not more than 1 year.

In horses, a relationship between nasal antibody and resistance to challenge has been demonstrated. Moreover, it is believed that antibody on the respiratory mucosal surface confers protection. The presence of prechallenge serum antibody has been shown to shorten the duration of viral excretion and febrile response.

In addition to vaccination, isolation and quarantine measures are advised during outbreaks to reduce the spread of disease. Human antiviral drugs, amantadine and rimantadine, have been evaluated for their action in the horse. Oral dosage did not produce effective plasma concentrations and care must be exercised to not exceed the seizure threshold when administered intravenously. Continuous surveillance of the antigenicity of equine influenza strains is essential in order to monitor viral change.

SWINE INFLUENZA

DISEASE

Swine influenza is an acute disease of pigs involving the upper respiratory system. The natural disease commonly affects large numbers of animals in the herd almost simultaneously. Swine influenza occurs more frequently during colder months. Disease caused by swine influenza alone is usually mild; however, disease may be severe when secondary infection occurs.

The incubation period is short, requiring at most several days. Disease symptoms include fever, anorexia, leukopenia, extreme weakness, and prostration. Respiratory symptoms also occur, including hyperpnea, dyspnea, sneezing, painful coughing, and a nasal discharge. Some cases develop edema of the lungs and bronchopneumonia. A conjunctivitis may also be observed. Most animals recover uneventfully in 2 to 6 days but with considerable weight loss.

Swine influenza was first recognized during the human influenza pandemic in 1918. These viruses had similar antigenic properties and there is speculation about whether the same virus was involved with both humans and swine. It is known that the swine influenza virus can spread from pigs to humans causing illness, and there is concern that swine influenza may be a reservoir for human epidemics. Veterinarians, pork producers, and swine abattoir employees face risk from exposure.

Swine influenza is found in many parts of the world, including European countries such as Britain, Czechoslovakia, and Poland; it is also found in Russia and other countries of the former Soviet Union, Hong Kong, and Kenya. In the United States, swine influenza is a common infection of pigs primarily in the midwestern and central states, where the H1N1 virus is most commonly responsible for disease outbreaks. Disease has occurred due to H3N2 viruses in other parts of the world.

Antigenic differences among swine influenza viral strains have not been great enough to justify the designation of subtypes.

HOST–VIRUS RELATIONSHIP

Pathogenesis and Pathology

On postmortem examination, the mucosa of the upper respiratory tract is congested and the cervical and mediastinal lymph nodes are edematous. Affected lung lobes may be atelectatic and emphysematous. There may be pneumonia with consolidation. The spleen is often moderately enlarged, and the gastric mucosa is often hyperemic.

Transmission of the disease is by droplet infection. Viral maintenance and swine exposure were previously thought to depend on earthworms containing viral-infected larvae of the pig lungworm (*Metastrongylus* spp.).

Pigs fed such earthworms and simultaneously exposed to *Haemophilus* (para) *suis* often developed typical swine influenza. A less elaborate explanation assumed that recovered animals acted as viral carriers. Previous evidence of transplacental infection has been disputed by recent studies. Transmission of influenza viruses between pigs and birds has been suggested by the isolation of an influenza from sick turkeys of an H1N1 virus strain antigenically and genetically identical to viruses isolated from pigs.

LABORATORY DIAGNOSIS

Swine influenza is suspected whenever there is an explosive appearance of upper respiratory disease involving many pigs, particularly during the fall or winter months. A definitive diagnosis requires either viral isolation from nasal secretions or the lung or demonstration of a rising titer between acute and convalescent sera. Swine influenza virus can be cultivated in 10- to 12-day-old embryonated chicken eggs and various tissue culture monolayer systems involving primary or stable cell cultures.

TREATMENT AND CONTROL

Swine that have recovered from influenza develop H1, serum neutralizing (SN), complement fixation (CF), precipitating, and neuraminidase inhibiting antibodies. There is a controversy as to whether recovered animals are immune. Some researchers believe they are and that subsequent respiratory outbreaks in a herd in a given season must be caused by another agent. Others have demonstrated that pigs with neutralizing antibody may still succumb to challenge with swine influenza virus and *H. suis* combined. Pigs born to immune sows are protected for as long as 13 to 18 weeks by passive transfer of maternal antibodies.

Immunization using various viral preparations has been attempted with little success. In the United States, there are no immunizing agents commercially available.

Treatment for swine influenza entails supportive measures including a draft-free environment with clean, dry, and dust-free bedding, fresh clean water, and a good source of feed. Antibiotics given on a herd basis may help prevent secondary bacterial infection. Recovery often occurs as suddenly as the onset of disease.

AVIAN INFLUENZA

DISEASE

Avian influenza affects the respiratory, enteric, or nervous systems of many species of birds. Viruses of relatively low virulence may cause few signs while others may cause high mortality. Most outbreaks produce respiratory signs such as sneezing, coughing, rales, sinusitis, and lacrimation. Other signs include depression, diarrhea, and a decline in egg production or fertility. The disease caused by a highly pathogenic virus was once called *fowl plague.* Viruses that cause virulent disease should be classified as highly pathogenic avian influenza (HPAI) viruses. Domestic turkeys, in particular, have often been infected by influenza, which has caused substantial losses over the years. There is wide genetic diversity among avian viruses and at least 15 hemagglutinins and 9 neuraminidases have been identified. Thus, a large number of viral subtypes are possible. Evidence exists that all HA subtypes are maintained in aquatic bird populations, including ducks, gulls, and shorebirds. Most infections in aquatic birds produce no clinical signs. In wild ducks, influenza virus replicates in intestinal mucosal cells and is excreted in high concentrations. Virus has been isolated from lake and pond water and surveys have demonstrated that as many as 60% of juvenile birds may be infected as they congregate prior to migration.

HOST–VIRUS RELATIONSHIP

Geographic Distribution, Reservoir, and Mode of Transmission

Highly virulent avian influenza is a major threat to the world's poultry industry. To date, it has been found in Asia and South and North America, and historically has been associated with HA subtypes H5 and H7. In both the Pennsylvania outbreak of 1983–1984 and the recent outbreak in Mexico involving H5N2 virus, early isolations yielded virus of low pathogenicity. It appears that the HA gene is important in pathogenicity in that highly pathogenic viruses possess HAs that are readily cleaved. Early Pennsylvania isolates had a glycosylation site in the cleavage region that may have blocked cleavage. It appears that a single mutation removed that glycosylation site, which resulted in a highly pathogenic virus. Similarly, in the Mexican outbreaks differences were observed in low- and high-pathogenicity H5N2 viruses involving the cleavage site. As a result, it is recommended that the HA cleavage site sequence also be determined in evaluating pathogenicity of isolates.

The disease is transmitted through poultry flocks mainly through ingestion of virus, but it may also be transmitted by inhalation and by mechanical means involving movement of personnel throughout flocks or between premises. Furthermore, some believe that for waterfowl, a fecal–water–cloacal route of transmission may be important in addition to the fecal–water–oral route. Outbreaks of highly virulent avian influenza may be self-limiting because few birds survive the disease to serve as carriers.

Waterfowl have been implicated as the major natural reservoir for influenza. Infected ducks can shed virus for prolonged periods without showing clinical signs or producing a detectable antibody response. There is evidence that influenza can persist in some birds for several months after infection. In the past, although avian influenza has frequently been isolated from imported exotic birds, prompting strict quarantine measures on newly imported birds, there is no evidence for spread in this manner as has been demonstrated with Newcastle disease virus. Furthermore, avian influenza may be transmitted on such objects as shoes, clothing, and crates that come in contact with infected birds or premises. While the possibility of vertical transmission of avian influenza through infected eggs exists, no evidence exists for its spread by this means.

Avian influenza viruses have been found to be capable of infecting a wide range of mammalian species in addition to birds. In fact, avian strains have been implicated in the deaths of mink during an epidemic in Sweden and in the disease of seals as well as the emergence of new strains in northern China affecting horses. Avian influenza virus can be propagated in cell cultures of human, bovine, canine, chicken, and rabbit origin.

Pathogenesis and Pathology

The pathogenesis of avian influenza varies widely depending on strain of virus, age and species infected, concurrent infections, and husbandry. At necropsy, lesions include foci of necrosis of various sites including the skin, comb, wattles, spleen, liver, lung, kidney, intestine, and pancreas. There may be fibrinous exudates in the air sacs, oviduct, pericardial sac, or peritoneum. Other lesions include petechiation of the heart muscle, abdominal fat, and the mucosa of the proventriculus, a nonsuppurative encephalitis, and a serofibrinous pericarditis.

LABORATORY DIAGNOSIS

A definitive diagnosis requires viral isolation and identification or the demonstration of rising antibody titer by H1, viral neutralization tests, soluble antigen fluorescent antibody test, agar gel precipitation, or ELISA technique. Avian influenza can be cultivated in chick embryos; duckling, calf, and monkey kidney cell cultures; and from samples of trachea, lung, air sac, sinus exudate, or cloacal swabs. Antigen capture ELISA tests have been used for rapid viral detection.

TREATMENT AND CONTROL

Recovered birds remain immune to subsequent challenge by a homologous strain for at least several months. Birds immunized parenterally with inactivated vaccines are completely protected against challenge by a heterologous strain with the same HA and are partially protected against heterologous strains possessing the same neuraminidase. Following immunization, chickens remain immune for at least 84 days, approximately twice as long as turkeys remain immune. It has been demonstrated that anti-HA antibody is important for protection against

infection while antineuraminidase antibody protects against disease and reduces virus shedding but does not prevent infection.

In practice, however, appropriate vaccines are rarely available to the poultry industry owing to great genetic and antigenic diversity among avian viruses. In several states, such as Minnesota and California, the rapid isolation of virus during outbreaks has permitted the development of inactivated vaccines felt to be effective in limiting the severity of an outbreak. There is hope that a polyvalent vaccine with a broader protective range may be developed.

For the most part, control of avian influenza is through the prevention of exposure. Careful husbandry to prevent the introduction of the virus into the flock is important. New birds should not be introduced into a started flock, and careful precautions should be taken to prevent either direct or indirect contact with wild, migratory, or exotic birds. Since turkeys have been found also to be susceptible to a strain of influenza typically associated with pigs, it is a good management practice not to have pigs on the same farm as turkeys. Eggs for hatching should come from flocks demonstrated to be free of the virus. Virus has been demonstrated to persist for 105 days in liquid manure following depopulation. Strict measures should be employed to eliminate movement of personnel and equipment, potentially contaminated by manure, between flocks and premises. During an outbreak, isolation of a flock along with orderly marketing of the flock should be considered.

Drugs such as amantadine, used for human influenza prevention, have not been cleared for use in birds for consumption and to date there is no satisfactory treatment for avian influenza. Treatment of infected flocks with broad-spectrum antibiotics is useful in controlling secondary invaders, and proper nutrition and husbandry may help reduce mortality.

ZOONOTIC SIGNIFICANCE OF ANIMAL INFLUENZAS

A growing body of evidence suggests that pandemic strains of human influenza often arise as a result of recombination between human and animal strains. Waterfowl appear to be of particular significance in the origin of new human isolates. It appears that ducks may act as a "melting pot" where various strains of influenza can come together and undergo genetic reassortment, resulting in new strains of influenza. Swine have also been implicated as mixing vessels as "avian-like" and "human-like" influenza viruses can be frequently isolated. Since the internal genes are critical for host range, and the HA and NA are important with regard to host immunity, a recombination event could result in the formation of a new strain containing the same or similar internal genes while having new or very different HA and NA. This new virus might still be infective to humans, but it could possess surface antigens very different from those previously experienced by the human population. The result could be an influenza pandemic as the new strain rapidly spreads through a susceptible population.

In the past, major antigenic shifts have taken place among human influenza viruses leading to pandemics in the human population. Each of the last three shifts had its origin traced to China. The role of China in the emergence of these pandemic strains has not been completely resolved; however, China is known to contain a large reservoir of different influenza A viruses among wild and domestic species, particularly ducks. Furthermore, the mass production of ducks and the proximity of human habitations to the farms, also in close association with swine, has been implicated by some as an ideal situation for establishing new antigenic strains and introducing these viruses to the human population.

Among animal strains, only swine influenza has been proven to have zoonotic potential. There is evidence that the agent responsible for the great human pandemic of 1918 was either very similar or identical to the agent producing swine influenza, which is speculated to have been an avian virus that passed to swine.

SELECTED REFERENCES

Abraham A, Siranandan V, Halvorson DA, Newman A. Standardization of enzyme-linked immunosorbent assay for avian influenza virus antibodies in turkeys. Am J Vet Res 1986; 47:561.

Air GM, Laver WG. The molecular basis of antigenic variation in influenza virus. Adv Virus Res 1986;31:53.

Alexander DJ. The epidemiology and control of avian influenza and Newcastle disease. J Comp Pathol 1995;112:105.

Austin FJ, Webster RG. Antigenic mapping of an avian H1 influenza virus haemagglutinin and interrelationships of H1 viruses from humans, pigs and birds. J Gen Virol 1986;67:983.

Burrows R, Spooner RR, Goodridge D. A three-year evaluation of four commercial equine influenza vaccines in ponies maintained in isolation. Dev Biol Stand 1977;39:341.

Garcia M, Crawford JM, Latimer JW, et al. Heterogenicity in the hemagglutinin gene and emergence of the highly pathogenic phenotype among H5N2 avian influenza viruses from Mexico. J Gen Virol 1996;77:1493.

Garin B, Plateau E, Gillet-Forin S. Serological diagnosis of influenza A infections in the horse by enzyme immunoassay. Comparison with the complement fixation test. Vet Immunol Immunopathol 1986;13:357.

Hinshaw VS, Webster RG, Turner B. The perpetuation of orthomyxoviruses and paramyxoviruses in Canadian waterfowl. Can J Microbiol 1980;26:622.

Karunakaran D, Newman JA, Halvorson DA, Abraham A. Evaluation of inactivated influenza vaccines in market turkeys. Avian Dis 1987;31:498.

Kawaoka Y, Bean WJ, Webster RG. Evolution of the hemagglutinin of equine H3 influenza viruses. Virology 1989;169:283.

Kida H, Shortridge KE, Webster RG. Origin of the hemagglutinin gene of H3N2 influenza viruses from pigs in China. Virology 1988;162:160.

Kodikalli S, Siranandan V, Nagaraja KV, et al. Antigen capture enzyme immunoassay for detection of avian influenza virus in turkeys. Am J Vet Res 1993;54:1385.

Mumford JA. The diagnosis and control of equine influenza. Proc Am Assoc Eq Pract 1990;36:377.

Rees WA. Amantadine and equine influenza: pharmacology, pharmacokinetics and neurological effects in the horse. Eq Vet J 1997;29:104.

Scholtissek C. Molecular evolution of influenza viruses. Virus Genes 1995;11:209.

Scholtissek C. Source for influenza pandemics. Eur J Epidemiol 1994;10:455.

Taylor HR, Armstrong SJ, Dimmock NJ. Quantitative relationships between an influenza virus and neutralizing antibody. Virology 1987;159:288.

Webster RG, Wright SM, Castrucci MRS, et al. Influenza — a model of an emerging virus disease. Intervirology 1993;35:16.

Webster RG, Sharp GB, Claas ECJ. Interspecies transmission of influenza viruses. Am J Resp Crit Care Med 1995;152: 525.

Webster RG, Bean WJ, Gorman OT. Evolution and ecology of influenza A viruses. Microbiol Rev 1992;56:152.

Wilson WD. Equine influenza. Vet Clin North Am 1993;9:257.

69

Paramyxoviridae

YUAN CHUNG ZEE

Viruses in Paramyxoviridae are enveloped, pleomorphic particles (150 nm in diameter) containing a linear single-stranded RNA genome (molecular weight 7.0×10^6). Its nucleocapsid has helical symmetry (Fig 69.1). Members of Paramyxoviridae are divided into three genera based mainly on size of nucleocapsid, presence or absence of neuraminidase, and antigenic relationship (Table 69.1). Some members of this group cause serious respiratory or systemic diseases in mammalian and avian species.

MORBILLIVIRUSES

CANINE DISTEMPER

DISEASE

Canine distemper (CD) is the most serious viral disease of dogs. The classic textbook description of the disease is of an acute viral infection characterized by diphasic fever, ocular and nasal discharges, anorexia, depression, vomiting, diarrhea, dehydration, leukopenia, thrombocytopenia, respiratory distress, skin rash, hyperkeratosis of the foot pads and nose, muscle spasms, and signs of central nervous system (CNS) involvement. The most frequent symptoms are diarrhea, respiratory signs, fever, catarrhal ocular or nasal discharges, hyperkeratosis of foot pads, and nervous signs. It is important to recognize that canine distemper infection in dogs can produce a variety of clinical signs that range from no visible disease to several symptoms in the infected animals. The disease has an incubation period of 3 to 5 days. The mortality rate of the disease depends largely on the immune status of the infected dogs. Mortality is highest among puppies and in cases where there are complications such as pneumonia and encephalitis.

ETIOLOGIC AGENT

Physical, Chemical, and Antigenic Properties

Canine distemper virus (CDV) is variable in shape and size. Viral particles are spherical and vary in diameter from 150 nm to 300 nm. The viral nucleocapsid is helical in symmetry and is enclosed by a lipoprotein envelope (5 nm to 8 nm in thickness) that contains spikes 9 nm to 13 nm in length. The virus has a buoyant density of 1.23 g/cm^3 in cesium chloride. The viral nucleic acid is a linear single-stranded RNA and the viral capsid is composed of six major polypeptides.

The large glycosylated H polypeptide is responsible for the adsorption of CDV to receptor sites of susceptible cells. The other glycosylated polypeptide (F) causes fusion of cells infected by CDV.

All members of the morbilliviruses are closely related antigenically since they all share the six major polypeptides. However, differences in the major polypeptides of different members of morbilliviruses could be distinguished by peptide mapping. Canine distemper virus has only one antigenic type.

Resistance to Physical and Chemical Agents

Canine distemper virus is labile to environmental factors, such as extremes of temperature, pH, and several disinfectants. It is inactivated by visible light, ultraviolet light, and heating at 60°C for 30 minutes. The virus can survive in tissues for 48 hours at 25°C and for 14 days at 5°C. The optimal pH stability for CD virus is 7.0. Viral infectivity is lost above pH 10.4 or below pH 4.4. Canine distemper virus is readily inactivated by disinfectants, such as 0.2% Roccal (a quaternary ammonium compound) and 0.75% phenol solution. It should be kept in mind that most viral inactivation studies are carried out in laboratory conditions. Labile viruses, such as the CD virus, can persist longer in cool, shady environments or in serum or tissue debris.

Infectivity for Other Species and Culture Systems

Canine distemper virus infects a wide range of animals. In addition to dogs, other members of the Canidae (e.g., fox, coyote, wolf), the Mustelidae (e.g., ferret, mink, skunk, badger), and the Procyonidae (e.g., raccoon, panda) are susceptible to CD viral infection. Canine distemper in some members of the Felidae (lion, tiger) has been reported. Ferrets are especially susceptible to CD infection and are frequently employed as laboratory animals in the study of this disease. In recent years, African wild dogs have been endangered by a canine distemper epizootic among domestic dogs near Masai Mara National Reserve. There is no evidence that CD virus produces an infection in humans.

FIGURE 69.1. *Negatively stained preparations of bovine parainfluenza Type 3 virus. 120,000×. (Courtesy of A. Castro.)*

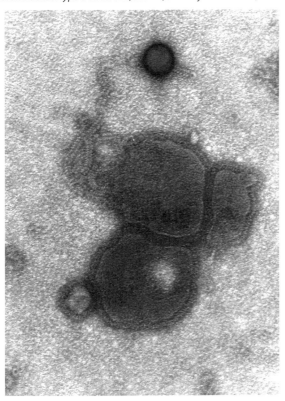

Canine distemper virus can be isolated and propagated in primary canine and ferret kidney cell cultures. The virus has been successfully adapted to embryonated chicken eggs and various cell cultures including bovine kidney, Vero monkey kidney, and human amnion or fibroblast continuous cultures. The virus can also be adapted to newborn Swiss mice and weanling hamsters.

HOST–VIRUS RELATIONSHIP

Distribution, Reservoir, Transmission

Canine distemper is found worldwide. The dog is the main reservoir for the disease. Infected dogs secrete virus in their nasal and ocular secretions during the course of the disease. Virus is present in the urine of experimentally infected dogs 6 to 22 days after exposure to CD virus. Feces of infected dogs also contain virus. It is likely that the disease is transmitted by droplet infection or by direct contact.

Pathogenesis and Pathology

In dogs experimentally infected with CD virus by the aerosol route, virus can be detected in bronchial lymph nodes and in tonsils 2 days after viral exposure. Leukocyte-associated viremia appears on the second and third day postinfection, and on the fourth day the virus

Table 69.1. Major Subgroups of Paramyxoviridae

Subgroup	Vernacular Name	Neuraminidase	Hemagglutinin	Natural Host
Paramyxovirus	Newcastle disease virus (Paramyxovirus Type 1)	+	+	Avian
	Avian paramyxoviruses (Types 2–9)	+	+	Avian
	Mumps	+	+	Human
	Parainfluenza 1 (Sendai)	+	+	Human, murine, avian
	Parainfluenza 2	+	+	Human, canine, simian
	Parainfluenza 3	+	+	Human, bovine, ovine, equine
	Parainfluenza 4	+	+	Human
	Parainfluenza 5	+	+	Human, canine, simian, avian
	Nariva	+	+	Murine
Morbillivirus	Measles	−	+	Human
	Canine distemper virus	−	−	Canine
	Phocine distemper virus	−	−	Seals
	Rinderpest	−	−	Bovine
	Peste des petits ruminants virus	−	−	Ovine, caprine
Pneumovirus	Respiratory syncytial virus	−	−	Human, bovine, feline, caprine
	Pneumonia virus of mice	−	−	Murine

may be detected in mononuclear cells of the lymphatic system, the alimentary tract, and the respiratory tract. From about the seventh to the ninth day onward, widespread viral invasion of the epithelial cells of the conjunctiva, the lymphatic system, the respiratory tract, the alimentary tract, the urogenital tract, the endocrine system, and the foot pad occurs, resulting in characteristic clinical symptoms of the disease. Viral antigen first appears in the meningeal macrophages on the ninth day and later in ependymal cells, glial cells, and neurons. Damage to these cells in the brain gives rise to the central nervous disorders seen in canine distemper. A subacute, delayed, demyelinating encephalomyelitis is seen in dogs with persistent infection by CD virus. Available evidence, such as isolation of infectious virus from brain tissue, high levels of antibody to CDV polypeptides, and interferon in cerebrospinal fluid of infected dogs, indicates that CDV undergoes complete replication in the brain, giving rise to chronic neurologic symptoms.

Pathologic lesions in CD are a reflection of organ systems in which viral replication has occurred. A depletion of lymphocytes in the tissues of the lymphatic system is frequently observed, followed by regenerative hyperplasia during the recovery stage. Degenerative changes and intracytoplasmic, and to a lesser extent, intranuclear eosinophilic inclusion bodies are found in the epithelial cells of the alimentary tract, the urogenital tract, and the endocrine system. There is often a diffuse interstitial pneumonia with desquamation of alveolar epithelial cells and macrophages along with thickening of alveolar walls. Hyperkeratosis of footpads and nose may be seen. Central nervous system lesions are those observed with diffuse demyelinating meningoencephalomyelitis comprised of infiltration of mononuclear cells; swelling and desquamation of meningeal cells, glial cells, and neurons; perivascular cuffing; dilation of blood vessels; and extensive breakdown of myelin and axis cylinders.

Host Response to Infection

Canine distemper produces a long-lasting immunity in dogs who recover from the viral infection. Neutralizing antibodies first appear in serum of infected dogs 8 to 9 days after viral exposure, reaching a peak in 4 to 5 weeks. Neutralizing antibody persists at a significant level in most animals for at least 1 year after infection. In dogs experimentally infected with CDV, viral-specific IgA is not detected in the serum. The antiviral IgM levels are equivalent in both persistently infected dogs and recovered animals, while high levels of IgG are seen only in animals recovered from disease. A lymphocyte-mediated immune response is also generated by dogs infected with CDV and is partially responsible for the recovery from the disease.

Acute canine distemper infection causes immune depression. Fatal infection of CDV in dogs is associated with systemic depletion of T and B lymphocyte-dependent areas in lymphoid tissues, whereas in persis-

tently infected or convalescent dogs, repopulation of lymphoid tissues with associated germinal center formation occurs 2 to 3 weeks after viral infection.

LABORATORY DIAGNOSIS

Since the clinical signs that accompany canine distemper infection are nonspecific and variable in dogs, definitive diagnosis of the disease must rely on laboratory tests, which include 1) the isolation and identification of CDV by inoculating susceptible dog or ferret cell cultures with secretions or tissue suspensions from dogs, 2) the demonstration of canine distemper viral antigen in mononuclear cells in the blood or conjunctival smears by the immunofluorescent technique or the peroxidase technique, and 3) the demonstration of rising IgG titers in paired sera by enzyme-linked immunosorbent assay (ELISA).

TREATMENT AND CONTROL

Treatment for CD is supportive in nature. Antibiotics are used to prevent secondary bacterial infections and electrolyte solutions are important in restoring the fluid balance. Anticonvulsants can be used for the symptomatic relief of nervous disorders. Despite intensive supportive care, some dogs infected with CDV fail to make a satisfactory recovery. Animals that recover from CDV infection develop a long-lasting immunity.

Vaccination against CD is the best means of controlling the disease. Both modified live and inactivated CD viral vaccines are commercially available. Modified live viral vaccines induce a higher antibody titer, a longer duration of immunity, and in general afford better protection against the disease. The use of these biologic products by veterinarians around the world has greatly reduced the incidence of this disease in dogs, and in many countries vaccination for CD has become an important aspect of any canine health program. Recent commercial development of distemper viral vaccine in canarypox viral vector has proven to protect ferrets against canine distemper viral challenge.

Maternally derived antibody to CDV interferes with the successful vaccination of puppies against canine distemper. Ideally, puppies should be vaccinated for CD at an age when maternally derived antibody has declined to a level that allows the replication of vaccine virus to induce an active immunity. Since it is not possible to test the serum of every puppy for neutralizing antibody prior to vaccination, one of the following two alternatives has been recommended for CD vaccination in puppies. If early vaccination of puppies is required, a second booster CD vaccine should be administered at 12 to 14 weeks of age regardless of the time the first CD vaccine is given. The second alternative is to give the puppy a measles viral vaccine followed by a canine distemper viral vaccine some weeks later. Measles virus is antigenically related to canine distemper virus and confers protection to CDV infection in puppies. Measles virus is not neutralized by antibodies to canine distemper virus, and this heterotypic (measles) virus is able to sensitize antibody-producing cells to produce a rapid and pronounced CD-neutralizing antibody titer following exposure to canine distemper virus. The precise mechanisms of heterotypic vaccination are not fully comprehended at present.

Caution should be exercised when vaccination for wild and exotic animals against CD is required. Inactivated canine distemper viral vaccine has been shown to be effective in immunizing foxes, ferrets, mink, bush dogs, and maned wolves. Although modified live CDV vaccine is proven to be safe and immunogenic in bush dogs, maned wolves, and fennec foxes, there have been reports of CD in kinkajous and lesser pandas following vaccination with a modified live CDV vaccine. It is always advisable to vaccinate exotic species with an inactivated viral vaccine, especially when information regarding live viral vaccines on those species is not available.

PHOCINE DISTEMPER

Phocine distemper is an infectious disease of seals similar to canine distemper. The disease has a high mortality rate and is caused by phocine distemper virus (PDV), a morbillivirus. The virus is antigenically related to canine distemper virus. Studies on the detection of phocine distemper viral RNA in seal tissues using hybridization and the polymerase chain reaction (PCR) amplification assay indicate that PDV is genetically distinct from the canine distemper virus. There is also evidence that dolphin and porpoise morbilliviruses are genetically distinct from PDV. The pathogenesis and epidemiology of phocine distemper are not well understood at the present time.

RINDERPEST

DISEASE

Rinderpest is an acute or subacute viral disease of ruminants, particularly cattle, characterized by fever, lymphopenia, nasal and lacrimal discharges, diarrhea, and necrotic stomatitis. The disease has an incubation period of 3 to 8 days. The mortality rate is high in animals that have had no previous exposure to the virus, such as European cattle. Because it does not exist in North America, rinderpest is considered an exotic disease in the United States. The disease has been largely eradicated from many parts of the world, but it is enzootic in parts of Asia and Africa. The reemergence of rinderpest in East Africa since 1979 poses a serious threat to the susceptible cattle populations in many countries that do not have this disease. Strict caution should be exercised to quarantine animals or animal products from East Africa.

ETIOLOGIC AGENT

Physical, Chemical, and Antigenic Properties

Rinderpest viral particles are pleomorphic with an average diameter of 120 nm to 300 nm. The viral nucleocapsid has a helical symmetry and is enclosed by a lipoprotein envelope, which contains spikes. The viral nucleic acid is RNA. The virus contains six major polypeptides, which are antigenically related to those of other members of the morbilliviruses. Rinderpest virus has only one antigenic type.

Resistance to Physical and Chemical Agents

Rinderpest virus is inactivated by sunlight within 2 hours and is rapidly inactivated by ultraviolet light. The virus is inactivated by heat exponentially, but small amounts of virus may survive heating at 56°C for 50 to 60 minutes or at 60°C for 30 minutes. Rinderpest virus is relatively stable between pH 4.0 to 10.2. It is inactivated by lipid solvents or disinfectants, such as phenol or strong alkaline compounds.

Infectivity for Other Species and Culture Systems

Rinderpest virus infects all species of the order *Artiodactyla*, which includes cattle, water buffalo, pigs, warthogs, sheep, and many species of African antelope. The virus can be adapted to grow in laboratory animals, such as rabbits, mice, and guinea pigs, and in embryonated chicken eggs. Rinderpest virus can be cultivated in primary or continuous cell cultures of bovine, ovine, and porcine origin.

HOST–VIRUS RELATIONSHIP

Distribution, Reservoir, and Transmission

Rinderpest is presently enzootic in certain regions of Asia (India, Pakistan, Afghanistan, Cambodia) and Africa (equatorial and northeast). East Africa was, in general, free from rinderpest in domestic and wild animals from 1966 to 1979. Introduction of infected cattle into East Africa (Uganda, Kenya, Tanzania) and West Africa (Niger, Nigeria, Chad, Cameroon) in recent years has led to a recrudescence of rinderpest in those regions. Outbreaks of rinderpest in Europe through the introduction of infected animals have been successfully eradicated.

Domestic and wild animals infected with rinderpest virus serve as reservoirs for the disease, especially in species that have a high innate resistance to the disease. These species, including certain breeds of indigenous cattle, Thompson's gazelle, and others, do not show clinical signs of the disease but can shed virus for long periods of time. Rinderpest virus is found in high titers in the nasal discharges and feces of infected animals. Virus is also detected in the saliva, conjunctival secretions, and urine of animals infected with rinderpest. Transmission of the disease requires direct contact of susceptible animals with secretions and excretions of infected animals.

Pathogenesis and Pathology

The primary site of viral entry in natural rinderpest infection is the upper respiratory tract, although cattle can be experimentally infected by any parenteral route of inoculation. During the incubation period, which is the time between the infection and the first sign of fever, virus initially replicates in the tonsils and regional lymph nodes. Primary viral multiplication does not take place in the mucosa of the respiratory tract. Leukocyte-associated viremia is present from the second to third day after infection. Dissemination of virus takes place throughout the body, and virus replicates in spleen, bone marrow, lymphoid tissue, and mucosa of the respiratory tract and the alimentary tract by the end of the incubation period. The second, or prodromal, phase of rinderpest is the time between the onset of fever (105°F to 107°F) and the appearance of mucosal lesions in the mouth. This phase usually lasts 2 to 5 days and is characterized by high titers of virus in lymphoid tissues and gastrointestinal mucosa. During the next, or mucosal, phase of the disease, mouth lesions appear, followed by diarrhea. High titers of virus are found in lymphoid tissues, gastrointestinal mucosa, respiratory tract tissues, and blood. Mortality is high in cases with severe diarrhea. With the appearance of antibody, the amount of virus starts to decline. The convalescent phase begins with the healing of mouth lesions, and complete recovery from the disease may take 4 to 5 weeks.

Lesions of rinderpest reflect sites of viral replication. Depletion of lymphocytes in germinal centers of lymphoid tissues and infiltration of mononuclear cells in these areas are common histologic lesions. Necrosis of epithelial cells of the respiratory and alimentary tracts leading to erosion and ulceration of the mucosa also occurs.

Host Response to Infection

Animals recovered from rinderpest infection develop a long-lasting immunity. Neutralizing antibody appears in the serum of infected cattle. In cattle vaccinated with modified live rinderpest viral vaccine, both IgM and IgG$_2$ serum antibodies appear 2 weeks after vaccination. The antibody levels reach a peak by the fourth week postvaccination and maintain a plateau for 2 weeks before declining. No serum IgA antibody response to rinderpest vaccine is detected.

LABORATORY DIAGNOSIS

Clinical symptoms, pathologic lesions, and herd history may be helpful in presumptive diagnosis. Laboratory diagnosis must be applied to differentiate rinderpest from many other infectious diseases, such as bovine viral diarrhea, infectious bovine rhinotracheitis, malignant catarrhal fever, foot-and-mouth disease, bluetongue, salmonellosis, and coccidiosis. The most reliable laboratory diagnostic tests are 1) the demonstration of specific antigen in tissues by the fluorescent antibody technique or the direct immunoperoxidase test, 2) the isolation and identification of rinderpest virus in susceptible cell cultures, and 3) the demonstration of significant titer rise of rinderpest serum antibodies by the ELISA method.

TREATMENT AND CONTROL

There is no effective treatment for rinderpest. It is important to note that reported outbreaks of rinderpest in areas free of disease are always associated with the introduction of infected animals. Contaminated meat, utensils, or vehicles are not important in transmitting rinderpest because the virus is labile to environmental factors. Therefore, restricting live animal importation from rinderpest enzootic areas and slaughtering affected herds remain the best measures for preventing the disease from being introduced into areas free of rinderpest.

Vaccination of domestic animals is practiced in enzootic areas to control rinderpest. Inactivated rinderpest viral vaccine has been used in the past to immunize cattle with good success, but it has been replaced in recent years by modified live vaccines, which induce a longer-lasting immunity. The live viral vaccines are attenuated by passage in goats (caprinized), rabbits (lapinized), chick embryos (avianized), or in calf kidney cell cultures. Among the modified live rinderpest viral vaccines, the high passage cell culture vaccine is the most desirable, because this vaccine does not induce severe clinical reactions or death in different breeds of cattle. Efforts are now being made to develop a vaccinia recombinant vector vaccine for rinderpest that is currently being tested on cattle in Africa. Modified live rinderpest viral vaccine has also been used effectively to protect goats against peste des petits ruminants virus, a member of the morbillivirus group that produces a rinderpest-like disease in goats and sheep.

PARAMYXOVIRUSES

NEWCASTLE DISEASE

DISEASE

The majority of avian paramyxovirus isolates from domestic and wild birds can be divided into nine serologic groups (see Table 69.1). Newcastle disease virus (NDV) is the prototype virus of the avian paramyxovirus serotype 1 and is the most serious disease-causing avian paramyxovirus. Newcastle disease is a highly infectious disease in chickens and is characterized by respiratory distress, diarrhea, and neural signs. The severity of the disease is dependent upon the virulence of the strain that is responsible for the infection. The most virulent strains (GB, Milano, Herts, Ca-1083, Largo) are referred to as *velogenic* and produce mortality rates in affected birds as high as 90% or more. The disease caused by *mesogenic* strains (Roakin, Mukteswan, Haifa) is less severe and the mortality rate is often less than 25%. The *lentogenic* strains (B1, LaSota, Ulster, F, V4) are almost avirulent and are frequently employed as vaccines. The incubation period of Newcastle disease varies from 4 to 11 days.

ETIOLOGIC AGENT

Physical, Chemical, and Antigenic Properties

Newcastle disease virus is pleomorphic. Its diameter varies from 100 nm to 300 nm and consists of an envelope and internal component. The envelope contains spikes (8 nm in length) that are the antigenic components involved in hemagglutination and neuraminidase activities. The internal component or nucleocapsid is about 17 nm to 18 nm in diameter. The molecular weight of the RNA of NDV is estimated to be 5.5×10^6 which codes for six major polypeptides of which two are glycosylated. The glycoprotein HN is responsible for hemagglutination and neuraminidase activities and the glycoprotein F causes fusion among infected cells.

Resistance to Physical and Chemical Agents

Newcastle disease virus can be inactivated in varying degrees by such physical and chemical agents as heat, ultraviolet light, pH, oxidation processes, and chemical compounds (lysol, phenol, detergents, and butylated hydroxytoluene). It is important to keep in mind that the rate of viral inactivation varies with the strain of NDV, quantity of virus initially exposed, time of exposure, and presence of organic matter in the environment. Infectious virus has been recovered from contaminated areas and eggshells several weeks following an outbreak of Newcastle disease. It can survive in fresh eggs for many months and in frozen carcasses for a few years.

Infectivity for Other Species and Culture Systems

Newcastle disease virus infects chickens, guinea fowls, turkeys, and a large number of species of domestic and wild birds. Sea birds are less susceptible but may act as carriers. Humans accidentally infected with NDV when exposed to infected birds or live viral vaccines may develop a self-limiting conjunctivitis.

Newcastle disease virus can be propagated in the chorioallantoic cavities of 10- to 12-day-old embryonated chicken eggs. The most commonly used cell cultures for the cultivation of NDV are primary chick embryo kidney, primary chick fibroblast, and baby hamster kidney (BHK) cells.

HOST–VIRUS RELATIONSHIP

Distribution, Reservoir, and Transmission

Newcastle disease is worldwide in distribution and domestic birds are the major reservoir for the disease. Although NDV has been isolated from a large number of wild birds such as sparrows, crows, ducks, and geese, they play a minimal role in transmitting this disease. The epizootic outbreak of the exotic velogenic strain of NDV in California in 1971 has been attributed to the introduction of caged birds.

Aerosol via the respiratory tract is the most common route for transmission of NDV. Infected birds begin to shed virus 2 to 3 days after exposure from their respiratory tracts. Investigations following NDV outbreaks suggest that flies and wind-borne forces may be the responsible factors in some instances.

Pathogenesis and Pathology

In natural or experimental infection of chickens with NDV, viral replication occurs at the site of initial exposure, followed by primary viremia. Widespread multiplication of virus in cells of parenchymal organs leads to a secondary viremia, which in some instances leads to the infection of the cells of the CNS. Disease takes several different forms in chickens, depending on the virulence of the strains involved. The very virulent velogenic strains cause very rapidly fatal infections involving the visceral organs (Doyle's form) or the CNS (Beach's form). Mesogenic strains of NDV cause a disease represented by respiratory and, occasionally, nervous symptoms in infected chickens with low mortality (Beaudette's form), while lentogenic strains produce a mild or often inapparent disease (Hitchner's form).

Lesions in ND vary greatly. In chickens with inapparent infections, lesions are rarely observed. In more severe forms of the disease, hemorrhagic necrosis is seen in the intestinal tract, respiratory tract, and visceral organs. In chickens with CNS involvement, necrosis of the glial cells, neuronal degeneration, perivascular cuffing, and hypertrophy of endothelial cells are observed.

HOST RESPONSE TO INFECTION

Chickens infected with NDV produce antibodies 6 to 10 days after viral exposure, reaching a peak in 3 to 4 weeks. Antibodies to the envelope glycoprotein, HN, exhibit viral neutralizing and hemagglutination inhibition activities and are responsible for host immunity to the disease. Humoral antibodies (IgM and IgG), secretory antibody (IgA), and cell-mediated immunity all appear to play a role in immunity to ND.

LABORATORY DIAGNOSIS

As the clinical symptoms and pathologic lesions of ND are variable and nonspecific, definitive diagnosis of the disease must depend on laboratory methods. These include the following:

1. Isolating and identifying the virus by inoculating embryonated eggs or cell cultures with respiratory exudate or tissue suspensions (spleen, lung, or brain). Due to the widespread use of live vaccine strains of NDV, in the field it is necessary to reproduce the disease in chickens with the viral isolate.
2. Demonstrating NDV antigen in affected tissues or cell cultures by the immunofluorescence technique.
3. Demonstrating rising NDV antibody titers by the hemagglutination inhibition, neutralization, or ELISA method.

TREATMENT AND CONTROL

Sanitary management to prevent exposure of susceptible chickens to NDV is an important aspect of control against the disease.

Since there is only one serotype of NDV, vaccination is another major step in preventing ND. Minor antigenic differences among strains of NDV are not sufficient to prevent gross immunity. The majority of live vaccines used are lentogenic strains of NDV administered in drinking water or applied as aerosols. Occasionally, mesogenic strains are employed as vaccines and are inoculated by wing-web, feather-follicle, or intramuscularly to chickens 4 weeks old or older. Inactivated oil-emulsion NDV vaccines by formalin and betapropiolactone are available and are administered by the parenteral route. Live NDV vaccine is effective in protecting market turkeys when it is administered 2 to 3 times by spray.

PARAINFLUENZA

The parainfluenza viruses are members of the paramyxovirus subgroup. Parainfluenza viruses are antigenically distinct and five serotypes, designated 1 to 5, have been recognized (see Table 69.1). They are frequently associated with upper respiratory infections in humans and animals. Parainfluenza virus Type 2 has been implicated as one of the causative agents of acute tracheobronchitis in dogs (kennel cough) and Type 3 for acute respiratory disease in cattle (shipping fever). The etiology of upper respiratory infection is complex. Although routine isolation of parainfluenza viruses from animals exhibiting signs of upper respiratory infection is common, the inoculation of parainfluenza virus alone into susceptible animals can rarely produce the severe clinical symptoms observed in field cases. Other agents, viral or bacterial, play an important part in the pathogenesis of upper respiratory infections.

PARAINFLUENZA TYPE 2

DISEASE

Infectious tracheobronchitis or kennel cough in dogs is characterized by sudden onset, mild fever, slight to copious nasal discharge, and a harsh, nonproductive cough. Although parainfluenza Type 2 virus alone is capable of producing clinical signs similar to those of kennel cough experimentally in dogs, a more severe clinical disease results when dogs are dually infected with *Bordetella bronchiseptica*. Experimental infection of dogs with *B. bronchiseptica* also induces clinical signs of kennel cough.

ETIOLOGIC AGENT

The morphology of parainfluenza Type 2 virus is similar to that of the paramyxovirus group. It has a helical nucleocapsid surrounded by an envelope. Its nucleic acid is RNA. The virus is relatively unstable and is rapidly inactivated at pH 3.0 and at temperatures of 37°C and above. The virus hemagglutinates chicken and guinea pig red blood cells. Parainfluenza Type 2 virus is antigenically related to SV-5 virus of monkeys, a member of parainfluenza Type 2 group.

Parainfluenza Type 2 virus can be propagated in embryonated chicken eggs and in kidney cell cultures of human, dog, and monkey; intracytoplasmic eosinophilic inclusion bodies and syncytial formations are present in cells infected with parainfluenza Type 2 virus. Infected cells also exhibit hemadsorption of guinea pig red blood cells. The virus can infect guinea pigs and hamsters experimentally and a strain of parainfluenza Type 2 virus causes acute laryngotracheobronchitis in children.

HOST–VIRUS RELATIONSHIP

The major route of parainfluenza Type 2 viral infection in dogs is via the respiratory tract. Infectious aerosols from infected dogs are responsible for transmitting disease to susceptible animals. The virus replicates in the epithelial cells of the upper respiratory tract, causing cellular necrosis and a loss of ciliary action. Virus is isolated from nasal secretions from the first to eighth day after exposure. No virus has been found in blood or internal organs. The infection tends to localize in the upper respiratory tract.

LABORATORY DIAGNOSIS

Case history of close confinement and clinical signs such as dry cough are useful in the presumptive diagnosis of kennel cough in dogs. Definitive diagnosis must be based on laboratory procedures such as the isolation and identification of parainfluenza Type 2 virus from clinical specimens or the rise in the serum hemagglutination inhibition or neutralizing antibody titers.

TREATMENT AND CONTROL

Antibiotics may help reduce the severity of this disease. Expectorants containing codeine can be used for cough and upper respiratory congestion.

Because of the highly contagious nature of the disease, it is important to isolate infected dogs from others in the hospital or to treat infected animals as outpatients. Live modified parainfluenza Type 2 viral vaccines are commercially available. They are either combined with other canine viral vaccines such as canine distemper and canine hepatitis or with a *Bordetella bronchiseptica* vaccine. Challenge studies have shown that none of the vaccinated dogs had clinical signs of disease after exposure with aerosols of parainfluenza Type 2 virus, while unvaccinated dogs showed clinical signs of upper respiratory infection 5 days after challenge exposure.

PARAINFLUENZA TYPE 3

DISEASE

Parainfluenza Type 3 virus (PI-3) is an agent implicated in "shipping fever" in cattle, one of the clinical disease syndromes in the bovine respiratory disease complex. The disease is characterized by high fever (107°F or above), conjunctivitis, respiratory distress, mucopurulent rhinitis, and pneumonia. The disease is widespread in the United States and remains one of the major causes of economic losses in the cattle industry. A number of viruses (parainfluenza Type 3, bovine diarrhea virus, infectious bovine rhinotracheitis, bovine respiratory syncytial virus) and bacteria (*Pasteurella multocida*, *Pasteurella haemolytica*, *Mycoplasma* spp.) contribute to the pathogenesis for "shipping fever." Other strains of parainfluenza Type 3 viruses have been isolated from upper respiratory infections of humans, sheep, horses, and water buffaloes.

ETIOLOGIC AGENT

The diameter of the parainfluenza Type 3 virus particles varies from 100 nm to 300 nm. The bovine strain of PI-3 virus has a buoyant density of $1.197 \, g/cm^3$ in cesium chloride. Its RNA is single-stranded. The virus has six structural polypeptides, two of which are glycosylated.

Parainfluenza Type 3 virus is inactivated at pH 3.0 and at 55°C in 30 minutes. It is also destroyed by lipid solvents. The virus hemagglutinates red blood cells of humans, guinea pigs, and birds. The human, bovine, and ovine strains of PI-3 virus are antigenically related but can be differentiated serologically by neutralization and hemagglutination inhibition tests.

The bovine strains of PI-3 can be propagated in cell cultures of bovine, porcine, equine, and human origin. Infected cells show syncytial formation and contain intracytoplasmic and intranuclear inclusion bodies. Experimentally, guinea pigs and hamsters can be infected with PI-3 virus with no apparent symptoms.

HOST–VIRUS RELATIONSHIP

Strains of PI-3 virus have been isolated from cattle with respiratory diseases in various parts of the world. It is estimated that over 50% of the cattle in the United States carry circulating antibody against the virus. Experimental production of pneumonia in calves has been accomplished by intranasal inoculation of high doses of PI-3 virus. However, inoculation of PI-3 virus alone rarely produces the severe clinical symptoms observed in field outbreaks of "shipping fever." Since PI-3 virus is frequently present in cattle with no apparent signs of disease, its pathogenic role in "shipping fever" of cattle can only be assumed in the presence of other viruses and bacteria.

The natural route of transmission is via the respiratory tract by infected aerosols. Epithelial cells of the respiratory tract and the Type 2 alveolar cells are the targets of parainfluenza Type 3 viral infection. Virus can be recovered from nasal secretions in animals 5 to 10 days after exposure, and infected cattle are the major reservoir of infection.

LABORATORY DIAGNOSIS

The diagnosis of parainfluenza Type 3 viral infection must rely on laboratory techniques such as the isolation and identification of PI-3 virus in susceptible cell cultures or the demonstration of rising hemagglutination inhibition titers in paired sera.

TREATMENT AND CONTROL

An antiprostaglandin compound such as flunixin meglumine is beneficial in treating pneumonia in calves induced by experimental inoculation of parainfluenza Type 3 virus.

Inactivated and modified live parainfluenza Type 3 viral vaccines are commercially available. The PI-3 viral vaccine is usually combined with other viral vaccines (BVDV, IBRV, etc.), with bacterins (*Pasteurella* sp., etc.), or with both. Protein subunit vaccines prepared from glycoproteins of parainfluenza Type 3 virus are found to be immunogenic in lambs and mice. The PI-3 vaccines induce high antibody titers in cattle and protect calves against PI-3 viral infection. Opinion is divided, however, on the effectiveness of PI-3 viral vaccines in preventing "shipping fever" in cattle. Isolation of animals showing clinical signs of bovine respiratory disease and good management practice are key factors in preventing this disease in cattle.

PNEUMOVIRUSES

PNEUMOVIRUS

Respiratory syncytial virus and pneumonia virus of mice are two members of the pneumovirus genus. The members of this group lack neuraminidase and the nucleocapsid has a diameter of 12 nm, which is smaller than the nucleocapsid of the paramyxovirus (18 nm). All members of the pneumovirus are antigenically related but are antigenically distinct from other paramyxoviruses. Respiratory syncytial viruses comprise several serotypes that cause upper and lower respiratory tract infections in humans, chimpanzees, cattle, cats, and lambs. Bovine respiratory syncytial virus has recently assumed a more important role in causing bronchiopneumonia in calves.

BOVINE RESPIRATORY SYNCYTIAL VIRUS

Bovine respiratory syncytial virus (BRSV) causes an acute pneumonia in calves, which show such clinical symptoms as coughing, fever, anorexia, nasal discharge, and respiratory distress. The pneumonia is characterized by bronchitis and alveolitis with multinucleated syncytia and alveolar epithelial hyperplasia. The disease has been reported in North America, Japan, Europe, and Australia.

Not all cattle infected with BRSV show clinical signs of the disease. Infected animals serve as the reservoir of the disease. The virus can be recovered from nasal secretions of infected calves and, in experimental infections, viral antigens can be detected by immunofluorescence in nasopharyngeal cells, in epithelial cells of bronchioli and alveoli, and in cells of mesenteric lymph nodes.

BRSV infection can be diagnosed by direct staining of nasopharyngeal smears with immunofluorescent antibody to BRSV or by ELISA of serum antibody to BRSV.

Cattle infected with BRSV develop serum-neutralizing antibody 3 days after viral exposure, reaching a peak after 3 to 4 weeks. There is also evidence of a cell-mediated immune response in cattle to BRSV. An attenuated live bovine respiratory syncytial viral vaccine is available, and field trials of this vaccine show some promise of reducing economic losses from the disease. Chemotherapeutic treatment of daily intravenous injection of 2-deoxy-D-glucose did not alter gross and histologic changes produced by the virus in the lungs. The drug is also ineffective when given after clinical respiratory tract signs had developed.

FELINE RESPIRATORY SYNCYTIAL VIRUS

Feline respiratory syncytial viral isolates have been identified in cats with mild respiratory symptoms, urolithiasis, and neoplasms. However, experimental infection in cats with various isolates failed to produce clinical disease. Feline respiratory syncytial virus (FRSV) can be isolated from clinically healthy cats by means of oropharyngeal swabs on feline kidney and liver cell cultures. The virus causes a cytopathic effect in these cells, characterized by vacuolation and multinucleated giant cell formation. The virus is approximately 115 nm in diameter and has a buoyant density of 1.19 g/cm^3 in sucrose. The role of FRSV in disease is unknown at present. It is only of particular importance to investigators studying feline leukemia-sarcoma viruses and vaccine manufacturers who use cats and feline cell cultures.

SELECTED REFERENCES

Alexander DJ. Newcastle disease and other paramyxovirus infections. In: Calnek BW, ed. Diseases of poultry. 9th ed. Ames, IA: Iowa State University, 1991:496–519.

Barrett T, Blixenkrone-Moller M, Domingo M, et al. Round table on morbilliviruses in marine mammals. Vet Microbiol 1992;33:287.

Chalmers WSK, Baxendale W. A comparison of canine distemper vaccine and measles vaccine for the prevention of canine distemper in young puppies. Vet Rec 1994;135:349.

Hall WW, Imagawa DT, Choppin PW. Immunological evidence for the synthesis of all canine distemper virus polypeptides in chronic neurological diseases in dogs. Chronic distemper and old dog encephalitis differ from SSPE in man. Virology 1979;98:283.

Krakowka S, Higgins RJ, Koestner A. Canine distemper virus: review of structural and functional modulations in lymphoid tissues. Am J Vet Res 1980;41:284.

McNulty MS, Bryson DG, Allan GM. Experimental respiratory syncytial virus pneumonia in young calves: microbiologic and immunofluorescent findings. Am J Vet Res 1983;44:1656.

Plowright W. Rinderpest virus. In: Gard S, Hallover G, Meyer KF, eds. Virology monographs. Vol 3. New York: Springer-Verlag, 1968:27–110.

Sheshberadaran H, Norrby E, McCullough KC, et al. The antigenic relationship between measles, canine distemper and rinderpest viruses studied with monoclonal antibodies. J Gen Virol 1986;67:1381.

Stephensen CB, Welter J, Thaker SR, et al. Canine distemper virus (CDV) infection of ferrets as a model for testing morbillivirus vaccine strategies: NYVAC- and ALVAC-based CDV recombinants protect against symptomatic infection. J Virol 1997; 71:1506.

Wagener JS, Sobonya R, Minnich L, Taussig LM. Role of canine parainfluenza virus and *Bordetella bronchiseptica* in kennel cough. Am J Vet Res 1984;45:1862.

70 *Rhabdoviridae*

Yuan Chung Zee

Rhabdoviruses (the Greek word *rhabdo* means rod) are bullet-shaped, enveloped, single-stranded RNA viruses that have a very wide host range. Members of the family Rhabdoviridae infect vertebrates, invertebrates, and plants (Table 70.1). Rhabdoviruses of the genus vesiculovirus and the genus lyssavirus cause diseases in animals and humans. Rhabdoviruses share a common morphology, require a viral RNA polymerase for replication, and have mature virions that bud off from plasma membrane or into intracytoplasmic vacuoles (Figs 70.1, 70.2). Rhabdoviruses contain lipids and carbohydrates of host cell origin.

RABIES

DISEASE

Rabies virus infects all warm-blooded animals, including humans, causing a severe and usually fatal disease of the central nervous system. The incubation period is very long, varying from 2 to 3 weeks to 6 months. Clinical signs involve the central nervous system (CNS) but vary somewhat depending on the host species. The early symptoms of human rabies are headache, extreme thirst, vomiting, and anorexia. More advanced symptoms include painful spasms of the pharyngeal muscles when drinking (hydrophobia), excitement to sensory stimulation, and general paralysis. With one or two reported exceptions, death is usually the outcome once clinical signs develop. The course of rabies in dogs generally lasts 3 to 8 days. Displays of behavior change are common during the early phase of disease; sometimes fever, dilation of the pupils, and photophobia are present. During the advanced stage, the furious form is frequently observed. The affected dog becomes nervous and irritable. It has a tendency to hide and bites without provocation. Clinical signs include profuse salivation and frothing at the mouth, difficulty in swallowing and drinking, convulsions, and muscular incoordination. Sometimes dogs affected with rabies enter a paralytic or dumb stage without going through a furious phase. Characteristic clinical symptoms of this form of rabies are paralysis of pharyngeal muscles, paralysis of the lower jaw, and complete incoordination resulting in coma and death of the animal.

The clinical signs of rabies in cats are similar to those in dogs. Rabid cats have a greater tendency to hide in secluded places and are often more vicious. Clinical signs of rabies in horses resemble those of tetanus or yellow star thistle poisoning in California. Difficulties in swallowing, progressive paralysis, and ataxia are often observed. Cattle affected with rabies are usually excitable and restless. Frequent clinical signs are salivation, choking, absence of rumination, rectal straining, and paralysis of hindquarters.

ETIOLOGIC AGENT

Physical, Chemical, and Antigenic Properties

The morphology of rabies virus is very similar to vesicular stomatitis virus. The virus is bullet-shaped, measuring 180nm in length and 80nm in width. It contains an envelope with short spikes (6nm to 7nm in length). A central cylindrical core of ribonucleoprotein runs throughout the longitudinal axis. The virus has a buoyant density of $1.20\,\text{g/cm}^3$ in cesium chloride. The viral RNA is single-stranded. Five major proteins designated as L, G, N, M_1, and M_2 are identified with the rabies virus. The major surface glycoprotein G can be separated into two components, G_1 and G_2, and is associated with pathogenicity.

Strains of rabies virus isolated from naturally occurring cases are referred to as "street virus," and attenuated laboratory strains are referred to as "fixed virus." These strains may differ in their biologic properties in laboratory animals; for example, virulence, length of incubation period, histopathology, and the antigenic variations between these strains can be distinguished by the utilization of monoclonal antibodies. It has been shown that vaccinated mice were protected against challenge with the field strain that was more closely related to the vaccine strain than the more antigenically distant strains. In certain geographic locations, the choice of proper strain for vaccine production is an important consideration.

Resistance to Physical and Chemical Agents

Rabies virus is inactivated by heating at 56°C for 30 minutes and by chemical agents such as formalin (1%), cresol (3%), and beta-propiolactone (0.1%). The virus may persist in infected brain tissue for up to 10 days at room temperature and for several weeks at 4°C.

Infectivity for Other Species or Culture Systems

Rabies virus infects and replicates in all warm-blooded animals. The virus can be readily propagated in chicken embryo or duck embryo as well as in a number of cell cultures, especially in baby hamster kidney cells (BHK21) and human diploid cells (WI-26).

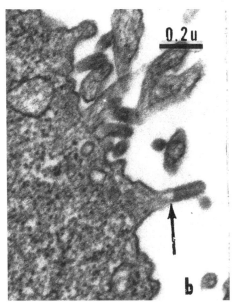

FIGURE 70.1.   *Vesicular stomatitis virus budding from plasma membrane of an infected L cell. 40,000×. (Reproduced with permission from Zee YC, Hackett AJ, Talen L. Vesicular stomatitis virus maturation sites in six different host cells. J Gen Virol 1970;7:95.)*

HOST–VIRUS RELATIONSHIP

Distribution, Reservoir, and Transmission

Rabies is worldwide in distribution. At present, rabies occurs in most parts of the world except Australia, the British Isles, Cyprus, Japan, New Zealand, and Scandinavia. The disease is endemic in many countries in Africa, Asia, North and South America, and Western Europe. Severe epizootics of rabies are frequently reported in certain countries, such as India, Ethiopia, and the Philippines.

Of the many animals that are susceptible to rabies, several species, including foxes, skunks, wolves, raccoons, mongooses, coyotes, and bats, are important reservoirs for the disease. A particular species usually serves as the important reservoir for a certain geographic region, for example, foxes for Western Europe, skunks and raccoons for North America, and mongooses for Africa and Asia. The domestic dog, however, remains the most important source of rabies in humans. In recent years, awareness of the role of cats in human rabies exposures has increased.

Due to the continuing rise in travel since the 1980s to certain risk countries (e.g., Morocco, India, Thailand), it has been strongly suggested by the World Health Organization that travelers to these countries be vaccinated against rabies.

Most rabies cases are caused by the bite of a rabid animal — the saliva of most infected animals contains infectious virus. In exceptional circumstances, rabies may be acquired by inhaling aerosol containing rabies virus in infected bat caves or by virus passing through intact mucous membranes. Recently, a few human rabies cases have been reported from recipients of cornea transplants from infected donors.

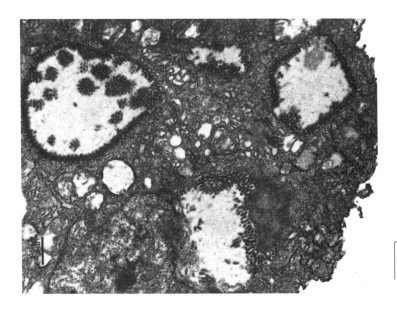

FIGURE 70.2.   *Vesicular stomatitis virus budding into the lumen of cytoplasmic vacuole in an infected chick fibroblast. 17,000×.*

Table 70.1.   Major Subgroups of Rhabdoviruses

Subgroup	Vernacular Name	Natural Host	Disease
Vesiculoviruses	Vesicular stomatitis	Horses, cattle, swine	Vesicular lesions
Lyssavirus	Rabies	All warm-blooded animals	Rabies
	Lagos bat	Bat	CNS
	Makola	Shrews	CNS
	Bovine ephemeral	Cattle	Systemic infection; fever
Fish rhabdo	Egtved (viral hemorrhagic septicemia)	Trout	Systemic; NS
	Salmonid	Salmon	Necrosis of organ
	Spring viremia	Carp	Abdominal dropsy
Insect rhabdo	Sigma	Drosophila	Carbon dioxide sensitivity
Plant rhabdo	Lettuce necrotic yellow	Lettuce	Necrosis

Pathogenesis and Pathology

The primary route of infection in rabies is through the bite of a rabid animal that contains infectious virus in its saliva. Several factors, including the virulence of the strain, the quantity of infectious virus in the saliva, and the susceptibility of the species, play a role in establishing rabies in the recipient animal. Foxes, cattle, hamsters, and coyotes are particularly susceptible to rabies. Dogs and cats are more susceptible than humans and rodents. The length of the incubation period after viral exposure varies greatly and depends on the anatomic distance between the bite site and the CNS, the severity of the bite, and the amount of infectious virus in the saliva.

Following viral exposure, the rabies virus persists in the local muscle tissues for hours or days, and viral replication takes place in striated muscle cells near the inoculation site. The presence of rabies virus at the neuromuscular junction suggests that the nicotinic acetylcholine receptor is responsible for the attachment of the virus to muscle cells. There is no evidence that a viremia is present for the dissemination of rabies virus to the CNS. Experimental infections show uptake of rabies virus at motor and sensory nerve endings, and the virus spreads within the axons of nerve cells to the ventral horn cells of the spinal cord at a rate of 12 mm to 24 mm per day. At this stage antibodies are inefficient to inhibit viral transport. Viral replication occurs in the spinal cord cells and spreads to the brain. Direct transneuronal transfer of virus from neuronal perikarya and dendrites to adjacent axon terminals is a mechanism of dissemination of rabies in the CNS. Brain stem, cerebral cortex, and hippocampus are particularly susceptible to rabies infection and the destruction of brain cells in these regions gives rise to clinical symptoms of rabies. It should be pointed out, however, that the virus can persist in the brain of infected skunks, rats, raccoons, bats, and foxes for many months without producing overt clinical signs. It has been shown experimentally in rodents that rabies virus after peripheral inoculation can be found in the spinal cord 24 to 72 hours postinoculation and in the brain 96 to 192 hours postinoculation. Recent studies employing a polymerase chain reaction (PCR) assay to detect viral-specific RNAs demonstrated rabies viral RNAs in the trigeminal ganglia at 18 hours and in the brain stem at 24 hours postinoculation.

Rabies virus can spread from the CNS to other organs, such as salivary glands, cornea, and tonsils, via the peripheral nerves. Viral replication in salivary glands occurs rapidly and infected saliva is the major source of infection. Low levels of rabies virus have been found in the excrement of infected bats.

A nonpurulent polioencephalomyelitis with perivascular cuffing is the most prominent pathologic lesion in rabies. Nonspecific inflammatory lesions such as neuronal degeneration and glial proliferation appear in the brain stem, cerebral cortex, and thalamus — areas in the CNS where rabies virus replicates extensively. The presence of acidophilic intracytoplasmic inclusion bodies (Negri bodies) in the infected neurons from hippocampus or Ammon's horn used to be regarded as the pathognomonic lesion for rabies diagnosis that differentiates rabies from all other CNS infections.

Host Response to Infection

Animals and humans vaccinated with rabies vaccine develop circulating neutralizing antibodies to the virus 3 weeks after primary vaccination. High neutralizing antibody titers may be detected in clinically infected hosts. Humoral immune response is generally considered important prior to or at the time of rabies exposure. There is evidence that susceptibility to infection is inversely correlated with the capacity to produce a high level of neutralizing antibodies. Both T and B lymphocytes are necessary for optimum clearance of rabies virus from the CNS. Interferon and interferon-mediated enzymes (pppA [2'p 5'A]n synthetase, poly[rI] poly[rC] protein kinase) are found in the brains of rabies virus-infected rats. The cellular and humoral immune responses are important in preventing rabies by vaccination but so far have not been found to function in recovery from rabies infections.

LABORATORY DIAGNOSIS

In the diagnosis of human rabies, clinical history of animal bite is very important. Every effort should be taken to locate the suspected animal and quarantine it. Definitive laboratory tests for rabies can be performed on the animal if it dies in quarantine. Clinical signs of rabies resemble those of poliomyelitis, other viral infections of the CNS, and tetanus. If there is no history of exposure, serologic tests such as the modified counterimmunoelectrophoresis test and the indirect fluorescent antibody test for detecting rabies antibody in the serum of a patient during clinical illness can be employed. Definitive laboratory diagnosis can only be obtained by isolating rabies virus from the saliva or from nervous tissues at autopsy. In cases of animal bites, different protocols must be adopted for different circumstances. If the biting animal can be located, it must be put under observation in quarantine. If the animal is rabid, it usually develops clinical signs within 1 week and death will follow shortly. If the animal dies in quarantine, its head and neck should be sent for laboratory diagnosis. If the biting animal cannot be located, antirabies treatment of bitten persons may be initiated.

Clinical diagnosis of rabies in animals requires differentiation from other infectious or noninfectious diseases of the CNS. Rabies is suspected in endemic or epizootic areas when an animal exhibits 1) abnormal behavior, 2) changes in its voice pattern, 3) increased excitability or sexual desire, and 4) paralysis of legs and lower jaw leading to death. Laboratory diagnosis is required for definitive diagnosis of rabies. The demonstration of Negri bodies in neurons by histologic methods used to be the routine diagnostic procedure for rabies. Drawbacks of this method are the difficulty of differentiating some Negri bodies from other nonspecific inclusion bodies in the neurons and that Negri bodies are not always located in neurons during the course of the disease. Finding Negri bodies constitutes a positive diagnosis but failure to find them does not exclude rabies definitively. A confirming rabies diagnosis can be obtained by intracerebral inoculation of young mice with brain suspension from suspected animals. Inoculated mice usually develop clinical signs within 17 days of inoculation and Negri bodies are found in mouse brains 24 hours before death. The demonstration of rabies antigen in infected tissues by immunofluorescence is at present the most widely used test for rabies diagnosis. This test is highly reliable and as sensitive as the mouse inoculation test. Its major advantage is that it can be completed within hours.

Early diagnosis is very important in the control and treatment of rabies. Recent utilization of monoclonal antibodies directed against glycoprotein antigen of rabies virus has provided a more sophisticated method for diagnosing rabies viral infection and for differentiating rabies from rabies-related viruses of the lyssavirus group (Duvenhage, Lagos bat, and Mokola). Monoclonal antibodies to rabies glycoprotein antigen can also be used to confirm vaccine-induced rabies in dogs, cats, and foxes.

TREATMENT AND CONTROL

In the event of possible human exposure to rabies, every case must be individually evaluated. Specific antirabies treatment is initiated only after the following factors are taken into consideration:

1. Species of biting animal — dogs, cats, skunks, foxes, coyotes, raccoons, and bats are more likely to be infected with rabies, whereas squirrels, hamsters, and chipmunks have never induced human rabies in the United States.
2. Circumstance of biting incident — an unprovoked attack is more likely to implicate rabies.
3. Type of exposure — depth and extent of wound and the area of the bite (near head region or not).
4. Presence of rabies in the region.
5. The vaccination status of the biting animal — a properly immunized dog is less likely to have rabies.

Treatment of potential human rabies should be under the direction of a physician. Immediate and thorough cleaning of the local wound with soap and water can help to reduce the incidence of rabies. Due to the prolonged incubation period of rabies postexposure, vaccination is often effective. A combination of passive and active immunization is considered the best postexposure prophylaxis for treatment of bites from rabid animals and from animals suspected of being rabid. One dose (40 IU/kg) of the heterologous antibodies serum is administered only once, at the time when the first dose of the rabies vaccine is being given. Currently a beta-propiolactone or tri-n-butyl phosphate-inactivated rabies vaccine propagated in human diploid cells (WI-38) is used for humans. The complete course of vaccination requires six doses given subcutaneously on days 0, 5, 7, 14, 30, and 90. This human diploid cell rabies vaccine contains a high titer of rabies virus, evokes a high immunologic response, and causes less severe side reactions. It is superior to the duck embryo rabies vaccine. Preexposure vaccination, usually three doses of the human diploid rabies vaccine, is recommended for those in the high-risk group for rabies such as veterinarians or animal handlers.

Rabies in animals can be controlled by eliminating wild animal reservoirs and vaccinating susceptible animals. Strict quarantine of imported wild and domestic animals for up to 6 months from rabies regions has kept some regions, such as Australia and Hawaii, free of rabies. Once rabies is introduced into a region, however, eliminating reservoirs is difficult.

Various types of inactivated and live attenuated rabies vaccines are commercially available for vaccinating dogs and cats. Routine vaccination of dogs and cats every 2 to 3 years is the most effective method of increasing the proportion of immunized pets in rabies control programs. The reported 12 cases from 1974 to 1978 of vaccine-origin canine rabies associated with the use of the attenuated live rabies Flury strain vaccine in low egg passage has led to the cancellation of approval for this rabies vaccine in the state of California. Caution should be exercised when live vaccines are used, especially in a different species. Live attenuated rabies vaccines produced for dogs should not be used for animals such as cattle and skunks because the vaccines may cause rabies in these species. Most states in the United States prohibit vaccination of wild animals with rabies vaccines. A genetically engineered vaccinia vaccine containing a single rabies virus gene has been approved for limited field trials in wild animals in the United States. The recombinant rabies vaccinia vaccine can be given orally with bait to wild animals. The vaccine is also being tested in cattle in Argentina. There is no evidence that accidental human inoculation with a licensed, attenuated live rabies vaccine has resulted in human rabies.

There is no effective treatment of rabies in animals.

VESICULAR STOMATITIS

DISEASE

Vesicular stomatitis virus (VSV) causes an acute febrile disease in horses, cattle, and swine. The disease is characterized by the formation of vesicles in the mucosal lining of the mouth and tongue. Lesions range from mild punctate erosions on the dental pad to severe ulcers on the tongue. Formation of vesicles is also observed on the teats, on the skin of the coronary band, and in the interdigital spaces of the foot. The clinical symptoms of VSV are often similar to those of foot-and-mouth disease and vesicular exanthema of swine. Vesicular stomatitis infection is seldom lethal, and the infected animals return to normal appetite and weight within several weeks after infection. The disease is sporadic in California and New Mexico; as of July, 1997, there have been seven positive cases, six equine and one bovine, reported in California. The virus produces an acute, influenza-like illness in humans, and accidental inoculation of VSV into human eye can cause a severe conjunctivitis. Experimental infection of mice with VSV can produce a fatal encephalitis, and the susceptibility of VSV in mice is age-dependent.

ETIOLOGIC AGENT

Physical, Chemical, and Antigenic Properties

Vesicular stomatitis virus is a bullet-shaped virus with one end rounded and the other end flat. VSV is approximately 175 nm in length and 70 nm in width. It has a cylindrical nucleocapsid that is about 50 nm in diameter and has a helical symmetry. The nucleocapsid is surrounded by an envelope containing spikes measuring 10 nm in length. The genome of VSV consists of a single-stranded RNA, which has inverted terminal repetitions. There are five major proteins. The virus has a buoyant density of 1.18 g/cm^3 in cesium chloride. Based on serologic tests, five antigenic types of VSV have been identified: New Jersey, Indiana, Cocal, Argentina, and Brazil.

Resistance to Physical and Chemical Agents

Vesicular stomatitis virus is inactivated by high temperatures (50°C to 60°C for 30 minutes) and by light, ultraviolet light, and lipid solvents. It is also sensitive to common disinfectants such as Clorox, roccal, phenol, and formalin. The virus is more resistant to lye (NaOH); 2% to 3% lye fails to inactivate VSV after an exposure of 2 hours. The virus can be preserved for years at −70°C and by freeze-drying under vacuum.

Infectivity for Other Species or Culture Systems

Vesicular stomatitis virus infects and causes diseases in horses, mules, cattle, swine, deer, and humans. Most mammalian species can be infected with VSV, and the virus can be propagated in laboratory animals such as mice and guinea pigs and in embryonated chick eggs. Vesicular stomatitis virus can grow in almost every cell culture in use and produces a cytopathic effect and visible plaques. The virus can also replicate in mosquitoes when it is experimentally inoculated into the thorax.

HOST–VIRUS RELATIONSHIP

Distribution, Reservoir, and Transmission

Vesicular stomatitis is a disease of North, Central, and South America. It is mostly endemic in nature and the reservoir for the virus is still not known. Insects such as the four-spotted leafhopper have been implicated, but definitive proof is lacking.

Direct contact is the most important mode of transmission of VSV. Since large quantities of virus are present in the vesicles in the mouth, contamination with infected saliva can transmit the infection to healthy animals. Cattle can be experimentally infected by the aerosol route. Several insects (stable fly, tabanids, mosquitoes) were demonstrated to be mechanical carriers of VSV and presumably can transmit the disease. Vesicular stomatitis virus (Indiana type) has been isolated from *Phlebotomus* sand flies on several occasions in Panama.

Pathogenesis and Pathology

In cattle experimentally infected with VSV (New Jersey field isolate) internasally, intralingually, or both, lesions range from mild punctate erosions on the dental pad to severe ulcers involving the tongue and oral mucosa 4 to 6 days postinfection. Fever (103°F to 104°F) is present in all infected animals. In severe cases, sloughing of the mucous membrane on the surface of the tongue causes extensive salivation and anorexia. High titers of virus are found in the vesicle fluid and saliva but not in the blood. The absence of viremia in all infected animals at any time after infection indicates that virus does not disseminate to other parts of the body. The lesions disappear in some animals in 1 week while in some animals new lesions appear 10 to 20 days following the initial lesions. Chronic ulcerative oral lesions can persist 48 days after infection.

In milking cows, vesicles on the teat can lead to the complete sloughing of the teat.

The pathology of VSV, like other vesicular diseases, is characterized by the formation of vesicles in the mouth and on the teats and feet. The vesicles, which are slightly elevated and are filled with clear serous fluid, rupture in a few days, exposing the underlying surfaces. The ulcerative lesion may heal, but in more advanced cases extensive sloughing of the tissue occurs. Histologically the lesions are characterized by necrosis of epithelial cells, intercellular edema, and inflammatory cellular infiltration.

Host Response to Infection

Infected or vaccinated animals develop high neutralizing antibody titers (>32,000; 80% plaque reduction assay) 10 days after exposure. Serologic response can also be measured by the complement fixation test and enzyme-linked immunosorbent assay (ELISA).

LABORATORY DIAGNOSIS

Diagnosis of VSV is important because its lesions resemble those caused by foot-and-mouth disease. Laboratory diagnosis is required for the definitive identification of VSV infection. The animal inoculation test was once the only one available for the differential diagnosis of vesicular diseases, but now the following laboratory tests are used to detect VSV: 1) electron microscopy or immuno-electron microscopy on vesicle fluid, 2) immunofluorescence antibody staining of vesicle tissues, 3) isolation of VSV using susceptible cell cultures, and 4) demonstration of a rise in antibody titer by the ELISA method.

TREATMENT AND CONTROL

Attenuated live and inactivated VSV vaccines are commercially available. The primary practice of VSV vaccination has been in dairy herds in epidemic areas to prevent economic losses from interruption of milk production. There is no effective treatment for the disease other than providing good nursing care for the affected animals. Sick animals should be separated from clinically healthy ones.

BOVINE EPHEMERAL FEVER

Bovine ephemeral fever (BEF) is primarily a disease of cattle characterized by fever, lameness, and nasal discharge. The mortality of the disease is very low. Economic loss is associated with loss of milk production in infected cows. Bovine ephemeral fever virus (BEFV) can infect other species of animals, including water buffalo, sheep, waterbuck, and wildebeest. The virus can be propagated in suckling mice, mammalian cell cultures such as BHK-21, VERO cells, and insect cell cultures such as *Aedes albopictus* cells.

Bovine ephemeral fever viruses are bullet-shaped or cone-shaped particles with a length of 120 nm to 170 nm and a diameter of 60 nm to 80 nm. The virus is enveloped and contains a single-stranded RNA. It has a buoyant density of 1.19 g/cm³ in cesium chloride and has six proteins. The virus is inactivated by heat (10 minutes at 56°C) and by high pH (12.0) or low pH (2.5) within 10 minutes.

Bovine ephemeral fever is enzootic in Africa, Australia, and Asia. It has never been reported in North and South America. The disease is not transmitted by direct contact. There is some evidence that BEF may be transmitted by insect vectors, since BEFV has been isolated from mosquitoes and biting midges (*Culicoides*).

Pathologic changes in BEF are not distinctive, usually consisting of edema in the pericardial, peritoneal, and pleural cavities, congestion of lymph nodes, and perivascular neutrophilic infiltration.

Diagnosis is accomplished by the isolation of BEFV by intracerebral inoculation of suckling mice with blood of infected animals, by fluorescent antibody technique, or by the detection of a rise in neutralizing antibody titer in paired serum samples. Animals infected with BEFV are immune for several years. Experimental attenuated live and inactivated vaccines have been developed, but commercial ones are not yet available.

SELECTED REFERENCES

Bahmanyar M, Fayag A, Nour-Salehi S, et al. Successful protection of humans exposed to rabies infection. JAMA 1976;235:2751.

Bishop DHL, ed. Rhabdoviruses. Vol. 3. Boca Raton, FL: CRC, 1980.

California Department of Health Services, Veterinary Public Health. California compendium of rabies control, 1996. Calif Vet 1996;50:13.

Fishbein DB, Robinson LE. Rabies. New Engl J Med 1993;329:1632.

Fogelman V, Fischman HR, Horman JT, Grigor JK. Epidemiologic and clinical characteristics of rabies in cats. J Am Vet Med Assoc 1993;202:1829.

Koprowski H, Wiktor T. Monoclonal antibodies against rabies virus. In: Kennett RH, McKearn TJ, Bechtal KB, eds. Monoclonal antibodies. New York: Plenum, 1981:335–351.

MacFarlan RI, Dietzschold B, Wiktor TJ, et al. T cell responses to cleaned rabies virus glycoprotein and to synthetic peptides. J Immunol 1984;133:2748.

National Association of State Public Health Veterinarians. Compendium of animal rabies vaccines. Part I: Recommendations for immunization procedures. MMWR 1985;33:714.

Robinson LE, Fishbein DB. Rabies. Small Anim 1991;6:203.

St. George TD. Ephemeral fever. In: Gibbs EPH, ed. Virus diseases of food animals. New York: Academic, 1981:541–564.

Tsiang H. Pathophysiology of rabies virus infection of the nervous system. Adv Virus Res 1993;42:375.

Wagner RR, ed. The Rhabdoviruses. New York: Plenum, 1987.

71 *Coronaviridae*

Jeffrey L. Stott

The Coronaviridae family consists of two genera — coronavirus and torovirus — and a possible third, arterivirus. The toroviruses infect humans and animals and are predominantly associated with enteric disease. Toroviruses have been associated with enteric disease of horses (Berne virus), cattle (Breda virus), pigs, and cats. The virions have a typical pleomorphic morphology and virion organization is characteristic of the Coronaviridae family. This genus will not be further discussed here as the members are not well studied. The coronavirus genus contains many important pathogens of veterinary significance and is described below: the arterivirus genus, which has tentatively, and probably only temporarily, been placed in this family will be discussed separately.

CORONAVIRUS

Coronaviruses infect a wide range of mammals (including humans) and birds. They exhibit a marked tropism for epithelial cells of the respiratory and enteric tracts. In addition to such infections, other diseases caused by coronaviruses include hepatitis, neurologic disease, infectious peritonitis, nephritis, pancreatitis, runting, and adenitis (Table 71.1). These viruses are divided into three antigenic groups: porcine transmissible gastroenteritis virus, canine and feline coronavirus, and feline infectious peritonitis virus constitute Group I; porcine hemagglutinating encephalomyelitis virus, bovine coronavirus, and turkey coronavirus make up Group II; and infectious bronchitis virus is comprised by Group III.

Coronavirus has a unique morphologic appearance characterized by large club-shaped surface projections (peplomers) extending out of a somewhat pleomorphic lipid-containing envelope that encloses a coiled helical nucleocapsid structure (Fig 71.1). Virion size ranges from 75 nm to 160 nm in diameter, and the genome consists of a single molecule of ssRNA (positive sense).

Two viral-specified structural glycoproteins (S and M) are found in the envelope. Glycoprotein S is largely external to the membrane perimeter and gives rise to the typical club-shaped projections (approximately 20 nm in length) of the virion membrane. The glycoprotein contains epitopes to which neutralizing antibodies and cell-mediated cytotoxicity are directed and is responsible for virion binding to host cell membranes. Glycoprotein M is a transmembrane molecule and is more deeply embedded in the envelope. Antibodies directed against M may

neutralize the virus in the presence of complement. The third major structural protein is a basic phosphoprotein (N) that forms a long, flexible, helical nucleocapsid enclosing the genomic RNA.

TRANSMISSIBLE GASTROENTERITIS VIRUS

DISEASE

Transmissible gastroenteritis (TGE) is a highly contagious enteric disease of swine caused by a coronavirus. The disease is characterized by severe diarrhea and vomiting and by high mortality in young piglets (less than 2 weeks of age). Mortality in older pigs (greater than 5 weeks) is usually low.

ETIOLOGIC AGENT

Physical, Chemical, and Antigenic Properties

Transmissible gastroenteritis virus (TGEV) is pleomorphic. Diameters of the virion (including surface projections of 12 nm to 20 nm) have been reported in the range of 94 nm to 168 nm. Transmissible gastroenteritis virus is antigenically related to human coronavirus (HCV 299E), canine coronavirus (CCV), feline coronavirus (FECV), and feline infectious peritonitis virus (FIPV).

Resistance to Physical and Chemical Agents

Transmissible gastroenteritis virus is inactivated by lipid solvents (ether and chloroform), heating at 56°C for 45 minutes, and exposure to sunlight. The virus is stable when frozen, resists inactivation by trypsin and acidic pH (pH of 3), and is relatively stable in pig bile.

Infectivity for Other Species and Culture Systems

Transmissible gastroenteritis has only been described in swine; however, experimental infections of cats, dogs, foxes, and starlings (*Sturnus vulgaris*) have resulted in viral isolation from their feces for up to 20 days following infection. Serologic studies have also suggested natural infection of skunks, opossums, muskrats, and humans. Virus has also been demonstrated in house flies (*Musca*

Table 71.1. Coronaviruses of Significance to Veterinary Medicine

Virus	Primary Host	Disease
TGEV[a]	Swine	Enteric; respiratory
FIPV[a]	Feline	Peritonitis; pleuritis; CNS; ocular; fetal; enteric; respiratory; kidney; hepatitis; pancreatitis
FECV[a]	Feline	Enteric
CCV[a]	Canine	Enteric
HEV[b]	Swine	Enteric; respiratory; CNS
BCV[b]	Bovine	Enteric
IBV	Avian (chicken)	Respiratory tract; reproductive tract; kidney
TCV	Avian (turkey)	Enteric
PCV	Swine	Enteric
ECV	Equine	Enteric

TGEV = transmissible gastroenteritis virus; FIPV = feline infectious peritonitis virus; FECV = feline coronavirus; CCV = canine coronavirus; HEV = hemagglutinating encephalomyelitis virus; BCV = bovine coronavirus; IBV = infectious bronchitis virus; TCV = turkey coronavirus; PCV = porcine coronavirus; ECV = equine coronavirus.
[a] These viruses are antigenically related.
[b] These viruses are antigenically related.
All other viruses are apparently distinct antigenically. However, ECV has not been studied.

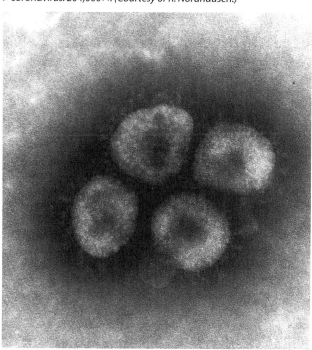

FIGURE 71.1. *Negatively stained preparation of bovine coronavirus. 204,000×. (Courtesy of R. Nordhausen.)*

domestica Linneaus) following experimental and natural infection.

The virus has been propagated in various cell culture systems, including pig kidney, testis, salivary gland, and thyroid; organ cultures of esophagus, ileum, cecum, colon, and nasal epithelium; canine kidney cell cultures; and embryonated chicken eggs (amniotic cavity). Development of cytopathic effect may require multiple passages in cell culture systems.

HOST–VIRUS RELATIONSHIP

Distribution, Reservoir, and Transmission

The incidence of TGEV has been documented in much of the northern hemisphere including the United States, Canada, Mexico, Colombia (South America), Europe, Asia, Japan, and Taiwan.

The primary mode of TGEV persistence in nature is the fecal carrier state in recovered swine. Maintenance of TGEV, in an enzootic sense, probably requires a continual source of susceptible pigs. The role of starlings, dogs, and house flies in viral maintenance has yet to be determined.

The primary mode of TGEV transmission appears to be ingestion of feces-contaminated feed. Virus can replicate in the respiratory tract; however, its role in natural transmission has not been established.

In the midwestern United States, TGE occurs predominantly during the colder winter months. This seasonality is probably due in part to the fact that the virus resists freezing but is relatively unstable in warm temperatures and sunlight. A bird role in the epizootiology of TGE has been suggested. Experimentally infected starlings excrete virus for up to 32 hours. The massive concentrations of starlings in the winter months in the midwestern states and their close association with livestock feeding operations could be a significant factor in TGEV transmission. Virus has also been demonstrated to replicate in house flies. Humans can spread virus via fecal contamination on their boots.

Pathogenesis and Pathology

Following ingestion, the virus is transported to the small intestine. Viral resistance to low pH and trypsin permits passage through the stomach without inactivation. Six to twelve hours following intragastric inoculation, viral replication occurs in villus epithelial cells of the jejunum, mid-intestine, and ileum; the highest viral titer is found in the jejunum. The infected columnar epithelial cells on the villi are destroyed, resulting in atrophy of the villi. Villus blunting and increased crypt depth are observed 24 to 40 hours postinfection and coincide with the peak of diarrhea. The villi do remain covered with cells due to the migration of new epithelial cells from the crypt. However, these cells are morphologically and functionally abnormal due to immaturity, as reflected by impaired ability to produce certain digestive enzymes (lactase, alkaline and acid phosphatase, adenosine triphos-phatase, succinic dehydrogenase, and nonspecific esterase) and by a deficiency in (Na+, K+) ATPase activity. The presence of undigested lactose in the intestinal lumen and altered ion transport contribute to the diarrhea and dehydration.

Principal lesions consist of thinning of the intestinal wall, villus atrophy, and gastrointestinal distension with yellow fluid containing curds of undigested milk. Degenerative changes may also be observed in the kidney with accumulation of urates in the renal pelvis.

Host Response to Infection

Following infection with TGEV, neutralizing antibodies develop in about 7 days. The presence of secretory IgA probably plays a major role in protective immunity and viral clearance. Intramuscular immunization of pigs with TGEV results in development of a humoral IgG response but no protective immunity. Conversely, pigs immunized orally develop IgA titers in mucosal secretions that appear to protect the intestinal lamina propria. Infection of sows with TGEV results in production of IgA-producing B cells, which migrate to the mammary gland, resulting in secretion of protective IgA in colostrum. The duration of antibody production in the mammary gland is 9 to 12 months. Cell-mediated immunity also plays a role in protective immunity. Passive transfer of mononuclear leukocytes from immune donor pigs to susceptible histocompatible piglets results in reduced disease expression. These transferred cells "home" to epithelium of the small intestine. In vitro studies have demonstrated lymphocytes to be capable of killing viral-infected target by ADCC-like or NK-like phenomena. High levels of Type I interferon are produced by infected intestinal cell populations and may play a role in controlling viral replication.

LABORATORY DIAGNOSIS

Definitive diagnosis of TGEV is possible by viral isolation through inoculation of animals (pigs 2 to 7 days old) or cell cultures (pig kidney, testis, or thyroid), and immunofluorescence staining of cell cultures or epithelial cells of the intestine. Electron microscopy (EM) or immuno-EM can also be conducted on fecal contents or intestine for diagnostic purposes.

Serologic diagnosis is employed when acute and convalescent sera are available. Several quantitative assays are available, of which neutralization and enzyme-linked immunosorbent assay (ELISA) would be appropriate.

TREATMENT AND CONTROL

Treatment of infected pigs is generally considered to be of little use. Helpful management practices include replacement of fluids, providing a warm, dry, and clean environment, and administering antibacterial drugs to reduce complications associated with enteropathogenic *Escherichia coli.*

Vaccination of pigs can potentially be conducted by immunization of newborn piglets, immunization of sows, or both. Vaccination of pregnant sows probably holds the most promise; subsequently protective immunity is passively transferred via colostrum to the susceptible newborn. Use of vaccines, attenuated or inactivated, has given variable results. Current knowledge of TGE immunity suggests that the oral route is best for maximal stimulation of local immunity (secretory IgA) at the surface of the intestinal mucosa. Intramammary immunization of sows has given variable results and is of questionable practicality.

The practice of infecting sows with virulent TGEV at least 3 weeks prior to farrowing to induce an immune response by providing colostral immunity to piglets can spread infection to susceptible young.

HEMAGGLUTINATING ENCEPHALOMYELITIS VIRUS

DISEASE

Hemagglutinating encephalomyelitis virus (HEV) is associated with an encephalomyelitis and "vomiting and wasting disease" (VWD) in young piglets. The two diseases appear to be caused by different strains of the same virus.

Encephalomyelitis typically occurs in piglets less than 2 weeks of age and is characterized by anorexia, lethargy, vomiting, constipation, and signs of central nervous system (CNS) disturbance. Mortality is high, up to 100%; pigs that survive appear to recover completely. Vomiting and wasting disease also occurs soon after birth and is characterized by retching and vomiting, constipation, rapid weight loss, and depression. Some pigs die soon after appearance of clinical signs, but most develop chronic infections with eventual death from starvation or secondary infections. Surviving pigs are unthrifty.

ETIOLOGIC AGENT

Physical, Chemical, and Antigenic Properties

Hemagglutinating encephalomyelitis virus is antigenically related to the bovine coronavirus. Virion diameters range from 100 nm to 150 nm with a core of 70 nm to 130 nm. Peplomers are about 20 nm to 30 nm in length. The virus is capable of hemagglutination (HA) and hemadsorption (HAd) with chicken, rat, mouse, hamster, and turkey erythrocytes.

Resistance to Physical and Chemical Agents

Hemagglutinating encephalomyelitis virus is sensitive to lipid solvents, including sodium deoxycholate; it is also heat labile and relatively stable under freezing conditions.

Infectivity for Other Species and Culture Systems

Hemagglutinating encephalomyelitis virus can be propagated in primary pig kidney (PK) or pig thyroid (PT) cells with formation of characteristic syncytia.

HOST–VIRUS RELATIONSHIP

Distribution, Reservoir, and Transmission

Hemagglutinating encephalomyelitis virus was first isolated and associated with disease (encephalomyelitis and VWD) in Canada in the late 1950s. Subsequently, the virus has been isolated from pigs in the United Kingdom, United States, western Europe, Australia, and Japan.

Pigs are the only known host of HEV, and subclinical or inapparent carrier states may exist. Nasal secretions contain virus (viral replication occurs in the respiratory tract) and airborne virus and direct animal contact are mechanisms of transmission.

Pathogenesis and Pathology

The pathogenesis of HEV infection has been studied under experimental conditions on colostrum-deprived day-old pigs. Following oronasal inoculation, primary viral replication occurs in the epithelial cells of the nasal mucosa, tonsils, lungs, and small intestine. Virus subsequently spreads along peripheral nerves to the CNS. Prior to disease expression, viral antigen is present in the trigeminal, inferior vagal, and superior cervical ganglia, solar and dorsal root ganglia of the lower thoracic region, and the intestinal nerve plexuses. Infection in the brain stem is initiated in the trigeminal and vagal sensory nuclei and subsequently spreads to other nuclei and the rostral portion of the brain stem. Later stages of the infection may be characterized by viral replication in the cerebrum, cerebellum, and spinal cord; virus is typically found in nervous plexuses of the stomach late in infection. The pathologic basis for the vomiting syndrome is unknown and may be a result of viral-induced injury in either the brain stem or peripheral nervous tissues.

Gross pathologic changes in natural HEV infections are minimal; a mild catarrhal rhinitis is sometimes evident in encephalomyelitis, and gastroenteritis is sometimes observed in VWD.

Lesions in the CNS are of a nonsuppurative encephalomyelitis characterized by perivascular cuffs of mononuclear cells, formation of glial nodes, neuronal degeneration, and meningitis. Respiratory tract lesions consist of focal or diffuse interstitial peribronchiolar pneumonia with cellular infiltrates composed of monocytes, lymphocytes, and neutrophils.

Host Response to Infection

Humoral immune responses may be determined by viral neutralization, hemagglutination inhibition (HI), and agar gel immunodiffusion (AGID). The clinical disease is self-limiting in pig populations and is due to the rapid development of maternal antibodies and transfer via colostrum.

LABORATORY DIAGNOSIS

Diagnosis of HEV encephalomyelitis or VWD in piglets requires viral isolation or demonstration of an ascending antibody titer. Brain and upper cord tissues are typically obtained for histopathology and viral isolation. Viral antigen may be visualized directly by fluorescent antibody staining on necropsy tissue sections, or virus may be isolated on primary pig kidney or thyroid cell cultures. Serologic diagnosis of HEV infection using paired serum samples can be performed by virus neutralization or HI.

TREATMENT AND CONTROL

No effective treatment has been described for HEV-induced encephalomyelitis or VWD. No vaccines are available. Clinical outbreaks are self-limiting.

BOVINE CORONAVIRUS

DISEASE

Bovine coronavirus (BCV) is an enteric pathogen responsible for diarrhea in calves 1 day to 3 weeks of age. The clinical disease is characterized by anorexia and a yellow-liquid diarrhea, the volume being dependent upon milk consumption. Bovine coronavirus strains antigenically indistinguishable from enteropathogenic BCV have been isolated from the tracheal organ cultures of young calves with respiratory disease. Intranasal and intratracheal inoculation of these isolates into newborn calves results in upper respiratory tract infection.

ETIOLOGIC AGENT

Physical, Chemical, and Antigenic Properties

Bovine coronavirus is antigenically related to HEV of swine and a human coronavirus, OC43. The virus has a mean diameter of 120 nm and a density of 1.18 g/ml in sucrose. The virus exhibits hemagglutination and hemadsorption with erythrocytes of hamsters, mice, and rats.

Resistance to Physical and Chemical Agents

Bovine coronavirus is acid stable (pH of 3.0). The virus is inactivated by ether, chloroform, and sodium deoxycholate. It is sensitive to high temperatures.

Infectivity for Other Species and Culture Systems

Infection with BCV is limited to bovine species, the disease being expressed primarily in neonates. The virus has been propagated in suckling mice, and following such passage will infect suckling rats and hamsters by both intracerebral and subcutaneous routes. It has been propagated in Madin-Darby bovine kidney (MDBK), African green monkey kidney (VERO), bovine fetal thyroid (BFTy) cells, and bovine fetal brain (BFB) cells. Trypsin treatment of the latter two fetal cell cultures enhances plaque formation and cell fusion. Certain isolates are difficult to propagate in vitro and may require passage in the natural host.

HOST–VIRUS RELATIONSHIP

Distribution, Reservoir, and Transmission

The distribution of BCV is worldwide wherever a sufficient number of animals can support its maintenance in the population. Little is known about viral reservoirs. Transmission is primarily by ingestion of virus from feces-contaminated feed, teats, and fomites.

Pathogenesis and Pathology

Following oral infection of calves with enteropathogenic BCV, diarrhea develops within 24 to 30 hours. Four hours after onset of diarrhea, viral antigen is detectable in the epithelium of the small intestine and colonic crypts. Initiation of infection is facilitated by proteolytic enzymes in the intestinal tract since trypsin treatment of coronaviruses in cell culture results in enhanced viral growth. Infection of mesenteric lymph nodes is also suggested by lymphoid depletion, karyorrhexis in cortical reticuloendothelial cells, and presence of viral antigen. Villous atrophy occurs in the small intestine and is characterized by replacement of columnar with cuboidal cells.

Host Response to Infection

Infection of animals with BCV results in a humoral immune response that is identifiable by viral neutralization, hemagglutination inhibition (HI), hemadsorption inhibition (HAI), and ELISA tests. Local immune responses play an important role as circulating antibodies do not protect calves from infection. Neonatal ingestion of colostral IgA protects the intestinal lumen for a limited time.

LABORATORY DIAGNOSIS

Diagnosis of BCV-induced neonatal diarrhea requires identification of the virus in fecal samples or intestinal sections. This can be achieved by viral isolation, electron microscopy, fluorescent antibody staining, or counterimmunoelectrophoresis.

TREATMENT AND CONTROL

Treatment is dictated by the severity of the disease. In addition to providing animals with a warm, dry environment, electrolyte solution should be administered for dehydration and antibiotic therapy should be used to control secondary infections.

Control of BCV infection can be facilitated by good management practices that minimize exposure, such as avoiding introducing new animals into an intensive calving operation and maintaining sanitary conditions. Oral vaccines induce local antibody and protection within 72 hours.

Vaccine efficacy can be reduced by the presence of colostral antibody.

CANINE CORONAVIRUS

DISEASE

Canine coronavirus (CCV) infection of dogs is highly contagious and can range clinically from inapparent to a fatal gastroenteritis. Neonatal animals are most susceptible to CCV-induced enteritis. Signs include anorexia, lethargy, vomiting, and diarrhea.

ETIOLOGIC AGENT

Physical, Chemical, and Antigenic Properties

Canine coronavirus is antigenically related to transmissible gastroenteritis virus, feline coronavirus, and feline infectious peritonitis virus. The virus is pleomorphic, with reported dimensions of 75 nm to 80 nm in width and 180 nm to 200 nm in length. Multiple antigenic variants of CCV have been recognized.

Resistance to Physical and Chemical Agents

Canine coronaviruses are inactivated by lipid solvents and are heat-labile. The viruses are acid-stable (pH of 3.0) and retain infectivity under cool conditions.

Infectivity for Other Species and Culture Systems

Canine coronavirus infects domestic and wild canine species; several primary and continuous canine cell cultures, including primary kidney and thymus; and continuous lines of thymus, embryo, synovium, and kidney. The canine kidney cell line, A-72, appears to be more consistently susceptible to CCV. The virus also infects feline kidney and embryo fibroblast cell lines.

HOST–VIRUS RELATIONSHIP

Distribution, Reservoir, and Transmission

Canine coronavirus was first isolated from an epidemic of diarrhea in dogs in Germany. Areas in which the virus has since been documented include the United States, Canada, parts of mainland Europe, England, Australia, and Thailand.

Inapparent or persistent infections (or both) of CCV contribute to viral maintenance. Infected dogs excrete virus in their feces for about 2 weeks. The stability of CCV under cool temperatures is important in viral survival in feces and would account for the increased incidence of disease in the winter months. The mode of transmission is through the ingestion of feces-contaminated materials.

Pathogenesis and Pathology

Following an incubation period of 1 to 4 days, virus infects cells of the upper duodenum and subsequently proceeds caudally throughout the small intestine. Diarrhea occurs 1 to 7 days postinfection, virus being present in feces within 1 to 2 days following the appearance of clinical signs. Virus spreads to regional mesenteric lymph nodes and occasionally to the liver and spleen. Viral replication in the intestinal epithelium results in desquamation and shortening of the villi. The diarrhea associated with CCV infection appears to be due to a loss of digestive enzymes and reduced adsorptive capacity. Fluid loss may be extensive and death occurs in neonates that have become dehydrated, stressed, or have concurrent bacterial infection. Intestinal healing usually occurs within a week.

While CCV infection is widespread, mortality is typically low, especially in older animals. Thus, necropsy of CCV-infected dogs is unusual. Gross observation of the gut reveals dilated intestinal loops showing watery diarrhea, hemorrhage, and mucosal congestion of the bowel. Mesenteric lymph nodes may be enlarged.

Histologically, intestinal villi are shortened, goblet cells are abundant, and the lamina propria shows increased cellularity.

Host Response to Infection

Neutralizing antibodies to CCV are generally low in titer because a viremic stage does not occur. Mucosal immunity appears to be protective as dogs orally infected with CCV become immune while those immunized parenterally do not.

LABORATORY DIAGNOSIS

Virus or viral antigens can be visualized by electron microscopy (EM) or fluorescent antibody (FA) staining of feces or necropsy tissues. Antiserum, specific for CCV, is commonly used to aggregate virus prior to negative staining for EM. Virus can be isolated from feces or intestinal tissue in staining for EM.

TREATMENT AND CONTROL

Treatment of CCV-associated gastroenteritis is limited to relief of dehydration and electrolyte loss in severe cases.

Antigenic diversity of CCV makes vaccine development difficult. Parenteral vaccines are available on a limited basis in certain regions. Their use is questionable due to the apparent importance of local immunity at the level of the intestinal mucosa.

PORCINE CORONAVIRUS

Coronavirus-like viruses have been isolated from swine exhibiting epizootic diarrhea. One such isolate, CV777, is antigenically distinct from the two established porcine viruses, TGEV and HEV. Experimental infection of pigs with the CV777 isolate results in diarrhea, vomiting, and dehydration. Pathogenesis studies have demonstrated viral replication in both the small and large intestine.

FELINE INFECTIOUS PERITONITIS

DISEASE

Feline infectious peritonitis (FIP) is a contagious and highly fatal disease of domestic and some wild feline species. Fever, weight loss, dyspnea, and abdominal distension are common clinical signs. The disease is primarily observed in cats 6 months to 5 years and 14 to 15 years of age. In utero infections can result in stillbirths or birth of kittens that soon develop clinical disease.

Primary disease is a mild infection with a slight ocular or nasal discharge. Most exposed cats undergo a mild or inapparent infection but probably remain persistently infected; 1% to 5% develop overt clinical FIP.

Two distinct forms of FIP are recognized: 1) an effusive (wet) and 2) a noneffusive (dry) form. The effusive form, which is two to three times as common as the dry form, is characterized by inflammation of visceral peritoneum, pleura, and omentum and results in fluid accumulation. The noneffusive form is generally characterized by lesions in internal organs, CNS, and eyes. Mortality rates can be high.

ETIOLOGIC AGENT

Physical, Chemical, and Antigenic Properties

Feline infectious peritonitis virus (FIPV) is antigenically related to transmissible gastroenteritis virus (TGEV), canine coronavirus (CCV), human coronavirus 229E, and feline enteric coronaviruses (FECV) that do not produce FIP. It has been suggested that FECV represents variant strains of FIPV with reduced virulence. Multiple strains of FIPV have been identified with differing levels of replication in cell cultures. The virus is 100 nm in diameter, with the peplomers extending 15 nm from the envelope. The virus is resistant to acid and trypsin but is readily inactivated by most disinfectants, including lipid solvents.

Infectivity for Other Species and Culture Systems

In addition to infecting domestic cats, FIPV has been associated with disease in wild *Felidae* such as lions, mountain lions, leopards, jaguar, lynx, caracal, sand cats, and pallas's cats. Young pigs can be experimentally infected with FIPV, resulting in development of lesions similar to those induced by TGEV. Suckling mice are susceptible to infection, with virus replicating in the brain. The virus can be propagated in vitro in feline organ cultures, cell lines, and mononuclear phagocytes.

HOST–VIRUS RELATIONSHIP

Distribution, Reservoir, and Transmission

Feline infectious peritonitis has been identified in the United States, Great Britain, South Africa, Canada, the Netherlands, Japan, Switzerland, Australia, Belgium, Germany, and France.

The primary reservoir of FIPV is persistently infected cats. Transplacental transmission of virus from dam to fetus is assumed to occur as a result of pregnancy-induced immunosuppression with subsequent activation of latent virus. Postnatal infection of cats by ingestion of virus has been demonstrated experimentally and is probably the most common in nature.

Pathogenesis and Pathology

The pathogenesis of FIP is complex, and much remains to be resolved. Virus apparently initiates infection in the upper respiratory tract or intestinal epithelium and regional lymph nodes followed by phagocyte-mediated dissemination of virus to various target organs. Development of clinical disease is associated with viral dissemination and development of antibody, and its form — effusive or noneffusive — is apparently influenced by the immune response. The development of antibody, elicited by FIPV, facilitates virus uptake by phagocytes. It has been suggested that absence of a cell-mediated immune response results in the effusive form of the disease, and partial cell-mediated immune response results in the noneffusive form. The effusive form is characterized by pyogranulomatous vasculitis around small venules in the visceral peritoneum, pleura, and omentum. These lesions are considered to be induced by antigen-antibody-complement complexes. The noneffusive form is characterized by granulomatous lesions of a more localized nature. Tissues involved include the mesenteric lymph nodes, kidneys, meninges, and the ependyma of the brain and spinal cord. Fluids do not accumulate to any large extent in the body cavities.

Host Response to Infection

The basis of immunity to FIPV is poorly understood. Following infection, cats may develop serum antibody titers, as determined by viral neutralization and indirect fluorescent antibody techniques. Altered or deficient immunologic mechanisms play a role in permitting viral dissemination. Stress and concurrent infections may facilitate immune suppression. Serum antibody to FIPV or cross-reactive antibodies previously induced by an FIPV-related virus may cause disease expression rather than protection. Current knowledge suggests that this antibody facilitates viral uptake by phagocytic cells where the virus effectively replicates. Furthermore, viral antigens complexing with antibodies and subsequent fixation of complement play a role in lesion development.

LABORATORY DIAGNOSIS

Feline infectious peritonitis can often be diagnosed based upon clinical observation in association with serology and hematology. Fluid accumulation in the peritoneal or pleural cavity, as determined by paracentesis, in association with a positive serum or fluid antibody titer, is indicative of effusive FIP. Noneffusive FIP is more difficult to diagnose and must be differentiated from other infectious, granulomatous, and neoplastic conditions. Histologic examination for pyogranulomatous or fibronecrotic inflammatory lesions and vasculitis, in association with serology, facilitates diagnosis. Polymerase chain reaction (PCR) techniques have been developed for identification of FIPV sequences in clinical material.

Serologic diagnosis may be determined by viral neutralization, ELISA, or indirect fluorescent antibody techniques. A serum titer of greater than 1:3200 would support a diagnosis of FIP. In certain instances, however, titers in cats with FIP may be low. In addition, the antibodies detected may be due to an infection with an antigenically related non-FIP coronavirus; titers in cats that have experienced FECV infections may range from 1:25 to 1:3200.

TREATMENT AND CONTROL

No treatment for FIP has been described that consistently reverses the disease process. Use of immunosuppressive drugs has been described for treatment of FIP in animals that are not debilitated. In the case of cats with effusive FIP, abdominocentesis or thoracocentesis is beneficial.

Control of FIP is best realized by decontaminating (with quaternary ammonium compounds) infected premises, isolating serologically positive cats from those with no titer, and screening newly acquired cats for serum antibody. Vaccines are currently available.

FELINE ENTERIC CORONAVIRUS

Feline enteric coronaviruses (FECV) cause a mild to inapparent diarrhea in young kittens 4 to 12 weeks old. Following experimental infection of cats with FECV, clinical disease may occur at 2 to 7 days and be characterized by vomiting followed by a transient diarrhea.

Multiple isolates of FECV have been reported and probably represent variants of a common prototype that infects swine, dogs, and cats. The virus is ubiquitous in cats and antigenically related to FIPV, TGEV, and CCV.

Upon infection, the virus replicates within the cells of the small intestine, tonsils, mesenteric lymph nodes, and upper respiratory tract. The primary target tissue is the small intestine. Clinical disease is observed when sufficient numbers of columnar epithelial cells have been infected and destroyed. Persistent FECV infections in cats are common and virus is shed in feces.

Immunity to FECV infection appears to be conferred to kittens by ingestion of maternal antibodies until they are 4 to 12 weeks of age.

Diagnosis of FECV can be aided by electron microscopy of stool specimens or PCR techniques. An increase in serum antibody titer also suggests infection.

Treatment of infected kittens is uncommon, since the disease is usually not severe enough to require clinical treatment. In severe cases, administration of electrolyte solutions is indicated.

No vaccines for FECV are available or warranted.

AVIAN INFECTIOUS BRONCHITIS VIRUS

DISEASE

Avian infectious bronchitis virus (IBV) is associated with respiratory disease in young chicks 10 days to 4 weeks of age; however, all ages, sexes, and breeds are susceptible to infection. The virus also causes disease of the reproductive tract and kidneys. The respiratory disease is characterized by respiratory distress, rales, coughing, nasal discharge, and depression. The clinical course lasts 6 to 18 days. Morbidity is 100% and mortality may exceed 25%. Chicks with no maternal antibody may experience permanent oviduct damage and fail to lay eggs when reaching maturity. Birds over 6 weeks of age also experience high morbidity but mortality is usually low.

Infection of laying flocks results in a drop of egg production, an increase in unsettable eggs, and a decrease in hatchability of eggs set. Pullets in good condition return to normal production within a few weeks.

Infectious bronchitis virus-associated renal disease is dependent upon viral strain. Many viral strains with an affinity for the kidneys cause only mild or inapparent respiratory signs. Mortality due to renal involvement is commonly 10% to 15%, with deaths occurring over 10 to 14 days.

ETIOLOGIC AGENT

Physical, Chemical, and Antigenic Properties

Avian infectious bronchitis virus is antigenically distinct from other coronaviruses. The virus is 80 nm to 120 nm in diameter, including surface projections. Four major structural proteins of IBV have been described; these include spike (S) proteins (composed of two glycopolypeptides), a membrane glycoprotein, and a nucleocapsid protein. Multiple strains of IBV have been identified and grouped by serologic techniques, polypeptide patterns in polyacrylamide gel electrophoresis (PAGE), and oligonucleotide fingerprinting. Strain-specific epitopes for viral neutralization and hemagglutination have been identified on the S1 protein with monoclonal antibodies. Group determinants have been identified on the membrane protein by a similar manner.

Resistance to Physical and Chemical Agents

Most strains of IBV are inactivated within 15 minutes at 56°C. The virus is quite stable at cold temperatures and has survived cool conditions for up to 56 days in winter. Stability at acidic pH is strain-variable, with some strains surviving at pH 3 for 3 hours at 4°C. Lipid solvents inactivate the virus.

Infectivity for Other Species and Culture Systems

The chicken is the only known natural host of IBV. However, quail and sea gulls have been experimentally infected. Suckling mice can be infected by intracerebral inoculation. The virus can be cultivated in developing avian embryos, cell cultures, and organ cultures. Turkey embryos have also been successfully infected with IBV, but less efficiently.

Avian infectious bronchitis virus can be grown in chick embryo cells (kidney, lung, and liver), embryonic turkey kidney cells, and monkey kidney (VERO) cells. Organ cultures have been used to propagate IBV including tracheal and oviduct cultures.

HOST-VIRUS RELATIONSHIP

Distribution, Reservoir, and Transmission

Avian infectious bronchitis virus has a worldwide distribution. The mechanism (or mechanisms) whereby IBV persists in nature is uncertain. Possible reservoirs include persistently infected birds, perpetual cycles of transmission, or both. Virus has been recovered for up to 49 days from infected chickens held in isolation and for even longer periods under natural conditions.

Viral transmission occurs by inhalation, the respiratory tract being the primary site of infection. Virus is shed in respiratory and fecal materials, with subsequent spread by contaminated fomites and aerosol.

Pathogenesis and Pathology

The incubation period of IBV infection is 18 to 36 hours. Virus gains entry via the respiratory tract. Primary infection occurs in the mucosa; the respiratory form of IBV results primarily in a tracheitis and bronchitis. Mortality may be as high as 25% in young chicks. Strains exhibiting an affinity for the kidneys damage the tubules, resulting in renal failure and terminal uricemia.

Infection produces primarily a serous, catarrhal, or caseous exudate in the trachea, nasal passages, and sinuses. The air sacs may contain a caseous exudate, and small areas of bronchopneumonia may be apparent. Young chicks may experience a more severe infection, with lesions developing in the oviduct. Chickens in production may experience a reduction in oviduct length and weight. Chickens infected with nephrotropic viral strains experience a nephrosis characterized by swollen and pale kidneys with uric acid crystals causing distension of the tubules and ureters.

Microscopically, the respiratory tract is most often the site of pathology, including cellular infiltration and edema of the mucosa and submucosa, vascular congestion, hemorrhage in the submucosa, vacuolation of the epithelium, and hyperplasia.

Host Response to Infection

Infectious bronchitis virus elicits humoral and cellular immune responses. Humoral responses can be measured by viral neutralization, complement fixation (CF), and hemagglutination inhibition (HI) tests. Local immune responses have been demonstrated in tracheal organ cultures and nasal washings. Cell-mediated immune responses have also been demonstrated. Passively transferred maternal antibody titers decrease to negligible levels within 4 weeks of hatching.

Chickens recovered from natural infection appear to be resistant to homologous viral challenge. The duration of immunity is variable and difficult to determine due to the multiplicity of IBV strains. Passive transfer of maternal antibody does not confer total protection to the chick but tends to reduce disease severity and mortality.

Local tracheal immunity appears to play a major role in resistance to IBV. The relative importance of humoral versus cellular immunity is unclear. The observation that chickens may be protected in the absence of demonstrable antibody would suggest an important role for cell-mediated immunity.

LABORATORY DIAGNOSIS

Diagnosis of infectious bronchitis may be based upon direct visualization of viral antigen in tracheal smears by fluorescent antibody staining, viral isolation, or serology. Infectious bronchitis must be differentiated from other acute respiratory diseases such as Newcastle disease (ND), laryngotracheitis (LT), and infectious coryza (IC).

Viral isolation is conducted by inoculation of the chorioallantoic sac of 10- to 11-day-old embryonated chicken eggs. Inoculum consists of tracheal exudates. Serial passage in ECEs may be required before embryo dwarfing or mortality is observed.

Serologic diagnosis of IBV can be conducted on paired serum samples using viral neutralization, hemagglutina-tion inhibition (HI), agar gel immunodiffusion (AGID), complement fixation (CF), fluorescent antibody (FA), and ELISA assay.

TREATMENT AND CONTROL

No specific treatment for infectious bronchitis is available but proper husbandry practices that reduce environmental stress are advised. In addition, replacing drinking water with electrolyte solution may be advisable as soon as respiratory signs appear.

Control of infectious bronchitis may be approached through management procedures and vaccination. Spread of the virus may be reduced by strict isolation of an affected flock. Replacement stock should be only day-old chicks reared in isolation. Ventilating poultry houses with filtered air under positive pressure has also been reported to prevent airborne diseases.

Attenuated and inactivated vaccines have been developed for the control of IB. Inactivated vaccines induce neutralizing antibodies, but their efficacy has been questioned. Live viral vaccines attenuated by serial passage in embryonated chicken eggs have reduced pathogenicity but also decreased immunogenicity.

Vaccines may be administered via aerosol or in drinking water. High passage vaccine viruses apparently have a reduced invasiveness and generally require aerosol administration.

The multiplicity of IBV strains and serotypes has made it difficult to develop efficacious vaccines. No single strain has been identified as capable of inducing more than limited protection to heterologous viruses. Multivalent vaccines are available, but in certain instances prolonged reactions to vaccination and some interference between vaccine strains has been reported.

CORONAVIRUS ENTERITIS OF TURKEYS

DISEASE

Coronavirus enteritis (CE) is an acute and highly contagious disease of turkeys. Synonyms of the disease include bluecomb disease, mud fever, transmissible enteritis, and infectious enteritis. It is of major economic importance to the turkey industry and affects turkeys of all ages. The disease affects primarily the alimentary tract and is characterized by depression, subnormal body temperature, anorexia, inappetence, loss of body weight, and wet droppings. Darkening of the head and skin and tucking of the skin over the crop are characteristics of infected growing turkeys. A rapid drop in egg production with eggshells being chalky is seen in producing breeder hens. Morbidity is essentially 100%, and mortality varies with age and environmental conditions.

ETIOLOGIC AGENT

Physical, Chemical, and Antigenic Properties

Turkey coronavirus (TCV) is apparently unrelated antigenically to other coronaviruses. The virus has a density of 1.16 to 1.24 g/ml in sucrose and an average diameter of 135 nm. The virus is inactivated by chloroform treatment and is resistant to acidic pH (pH of 3 at 20°C for 30 minutes).

Infectivity for Other Species and Culture Systems

Natural and experimental turkey coronavirus infection is confined to turkeys. Laboratory propagation of the virus has been limited to turkey and chicken embryos. Attempts to grow TCV in cell cultures have been unsuccessful.

HOST–VIRUS RELATIONSHIP

Distribution, Reservoir, and Transmission

Coronaviral enteritis has been reported in the United States, Canada, and Australia. The virus persists in turkeys for life following recovery from the disease. It is stable in frozen feces and survives throughout the winter months in infected droppings. Transmission of TCV is primarily by infected feces from carrier birds. Introduction of virus onto a premise may occur via carrier turkeys, feces-contaminated fomites such as personnel and equipment, and possibly mechanical transmission by free-flying birds.

Pathogenesis and Pathology

The incubation period of coronaviral enteritis may vary from 1 to 5 days. Gross lesions are predominantly confined to the intestinal tract, with petechial hemorrhages sometimes apparent on the mucosal surface. Lesions are most distinct in the jejunum but may also occur in the duodenum, ileum, and cecum. Watery and gaseous contents are present in the duodenum, jejunum, and ceca; ceca are often distended with fluid. The breast muscles are typically dehydrated and the carcass generally appears emaciated.

Microscopic studies have demonstrated viral replication to occur within 24 hours in cells over the shortened villi. Epithelial cells, which have become shortened, tend to lose their microvilli, and mononuclear cells infiltrate the lamina propria.

Host Response to Infection

Turkeys respond to TCV infection with a humoral and cellular immune response. Serum antibodies (IgM, IgA, and IgG) develop following infection but by 21 days only IgG is present. Local IgA antibody is found in intestinal secretions and bile for at least 6 months. In addition, a cell-mediated immune response has been reported following exposure of intestinal surfaces to viral antigen. Passive transfer of maternal immunity has not been observed and administration of antiserum to young poults does not afford protection.

LABORATORY DIAGNOSIS

Definitive diagnosis of coronaviral enteritis requires identification of viral antigen in intestinal tissue sections, viral isolation, or demonstration of antibody. Virus may be isolated by inoculation of embryonated turkey eggs or young poults and its presence confirmed by fluorescent antibody staining of infected tissues. Serologic diagnosis can be conducted on paired serum samples by viral neutralization or indirect FA tests.

TREATMENT AND CONTROL

No specific treatment is effective in reducing morbidity. Antibiotic therapy for secondary infections should include mycostatin for control of intestinal mycosis. Adding calf milk-replacer and potassium chloride to drinking water and providing additional heat in brooder houses may be helpful.

Turkey coronavirus vaccines are not available but prevention of infection is possible. The disease has been eliminated in some areas by depopulation and decontamination of premises. An alternative to viral elimination is exposing poults (5 to 6 weeks of age) to recovered carrier birds under ideal environmental conditions for the purpose of inducing protective immunity. Such a program is recommended only on farms with continued problems and when all other methods of control have failed.

EQUINE CORONAVIRUS

Coronavirus-like virions have been isolated from both mature horses and foals experiencing enteritis. The viruses found in mature horses were antigenically distinct from TGEV, BCV, and IBV.

ARTERIVIRUS

The arterivirus genus was previously in the Togaviridae family but is now considered a floating genus within the Coronaviridae family. The members of this genus include equine arteritis virus (EAV), porcine reproductive and respiratory syndrome virus (PRRSV), lactate dehydrogenase virus (LDV), and simian hemorrhagic fever virus (SHFV). EAV and PRRSV are of veterinary significance and will be discussed in detail. All members of the genus have positive-strand RNA genome enclosed within a nucleocapsid that is in turn enclosed within an envelope; viruses are readily inactivated in the presence of detergents.

EQUINE ARTERITIS

DISEASE

EAV was initially the only member of the arterivirus genus. Animals with equine arteritis (pink eye) develop fever (up to 42°C), stiffness of gait, edema of the limbs, and swelling around the eyes. Respiratory distress, excessive nasal discharge, and lacrimation are also observed. There is a leukopenia involving principally lymphocytes. Abortion occurs in 50% to 70% of infected pregnant mares. A high percentage of horses infected with EAV develop mild or inapparent disease, although foals can experience relatively severe disease. Horses may develop persistent infections, and in the case of stallions the virus may be shed in semen.

ETIOLOGIC AGENT

Physical, Chemical, and Antigenic Properties

EAV is an enveloped, single-stranded RNA virus. Purified EAV particles are spherical and have a diameter of 60 ± 13 nm. An inner core of 35 ± 9 nm can be observed. Estimates of the buoyant density of EAV range from 1.17 to 1.18 g/cm^3.

As many as nine viral-associated proteins have been resolved from radio-labeled, purified virus. Two proteins, VP7 and VP8, are major proteins. VP8 appears to be the major core component or nucleocapsid protein. Six of the proteins are glycoproteins. The virion lacks hemagglutinin. Only one antigenic type of EAV is known.

Resistance to Physical and Chemical Agents

EAV is readily inactivated by lipid solvents and by sodium deoxycholate. It survives 20 but not 30 minutes at 56°C. It is stable at low temperature (at or below −70°C). It is susceptible to common disinfectants and detergents.

Infectivity for Other Species and Culture Systems

Equine arteritis has not been reported in animals other than horses. In cell culture, EAV replicates in primary cultures of horse kidney, rabbit kidney, and hamster kidney. It also replicates in cell lines such as BHK-21, RK-13, and VERO. It produces plaques in overlay cultures.

HOST–VIRUS RELATIONSHIP

Distribution, Reservoir, and Transmission

EAV probably has a worldwide distribution. It is currently recognized in North America and Europe. The only reservoir is the infected horse. The virus is spread by semen and aerosol. Upon infection by insemination, mares shed large amounts of virus in respiratory secretion and urine, contributing to the vertical spread of virus.

Pathogenesis and Pathology

The incubation period for natural cases is 2 to 15 days. Following experimental infection, high levels of virus are found in practically all organs 3 days after exposure. The main replication sites are macrophages and endothelial cells. The basic lesions involve small arteries about 0.5 mm in diameter. The arterioles (less than 0.3 mm) and the large muscular and elastic arteries are free of specific lesions. Veins and lymphatics are often distended with blood or lymph, respectively, but are neither inflamed nor necrotic. Arterial lesions are found in every organ but more conspicuously in the cecum, colon, spleen, lymph nodes, and adrenal capsule. Natural infection of foals has been described as primarily an infection of the respiratory tract characterized by interstitial pneumonia, lymphocytic arteritis, and periarteritis with fibrinoid necrosis of the tunica media; renal tubular necrosis was also noted in some animals.

The specific microscopic lesion starts with necrosis of muscle cells in the arterial media. Edema and a few leukocytes then appear in the adventitia. In some horses, vascular changes result in edema of the ventral body wall and limbs, extending in geldings and stallions to the prepuce and in mares to the udder. Horses become dehydrated due to the extensive edema and reduced feed and water intake. Abortion is probably due to uterine lesions in the mare rather than fetal lesions.

Host Response to Infection

Infected horses develop neutralizing antibody within 2 weeks postinfection. Extensive immunologic studies have not been conducted.

LABORATORY DIAGNOSIS

Diagnosis may be tentatively based upon histopathologic observation with characteristic lesions (including necrotic foci with intranuclear inclusions) in lung, liver, and lymph node, and inflammatory lesions in small arteries; immunohistology techniques can be used to identify viral antigen in lesions. Viral isolation may be conducted on a variety of tissues and fluids, including lymph node, blood, and nasal swabs; additional tissues can also yield virus if it is highly virulent. Cell cultures of renal origin are commonly used for isolation. PCR has been used to identify viral genetic sequences in clinical samples, semen, and infected cell cultures. Serologic diagnosis can also be done using standard techniques such as ELISA.

TREATMENT AND CONTROL

No treatment for equine arteritis is available. An attenuated cell culture-source vaccine is available, and its use may be warranted in expensive equine breeding operations.

PORCINE REPRODUCTIVE AND RESPIRATORY SYNDROME VIRUS

Porcine reproductive and respiratory syndrome virus (PRRSV) was isolated in the United States in 1992, subsequent to the isolation of Lelystad virus (LV) in the Netherlands in 1991. The U.S. and European isolates of PRRSV represent genetically distinct groups of the same virus. The former are very closely related while genetic homology with Lelystad virus is different. Both viruses are associated with outbreaks of reproductive and respiratory disease in pigs. Relative to causing abortion in pregnant sows, strains of PRRSV vary greatly in virulence.

PRRSV infection is an economically important disease of swine and can cause significant losses due to late-term abortion (third trimester), stillbirths, birth of weak animals, and neonatal respiratory disease. Experimental infection of pregnant sows can result in abortion, depending upon viral strain. Experimental infection of neonatal pigs can result in fever, labored abdominal breathing, conjunctivitis, and lymph node enlargement. The virus targets multiple organs and at necropsy findings can include diffuse interstitial pneumonitis, myocarditis, vasculitis, encephalitis, and lymphadenopathy. Heart lesions develop late in the infection process. Clinical outbreaks of PRRSV can be complicated by bacterial pneumonia, septicemia, or enteritis. Based upon viral isolation and immunohistology, PRRSV appears to replicate extensively in pulmonary macrophages and macrophages/dendritic cells found in lymphoid tissue. The virus probably initiates infection via the aerosol route by initially infecting the tonsils followed by development of a viremia that can last for many weeks in the face of an antibody response.

Diagnosis of PRRSV is difficult due to many inapparent infections and similarity to other respiratory diseases. It can be identified by viral isolation or molecular biology techniques. The presence of PRRSV-specific antibody can be identified by ELISA. Vaccines have been developed for this viral infection.

SELECTED REFERENCES

Ahn K, Chae C, Kweon CH. Immunohistochemical identification of porcine respiratory coronavirus antigen in the lung of conventional pigs. Vet Pathol 1997;34:167.

Andries K. Hemagglutinating encephalomyelitis virus. In: Pensaert MB, ed. Virus infections of porcines. Amsterdam: Elsevier, 1990:177.

Appel M. Canine coronavirus. In: Appel M, ed. Virus infections of carnivores. Amsterdam: Elsevier, 1987:115.

Cavanagh D, Brown TDK, eds. Coronaviruses and their diseases. New York: Plenum, 1990.

Clark MA. Bovine coronavirus. Br Vet J 1993;149:51.

Del Piero F, Wilkinns PA, Lopez JW, et al. Equine viral arteritis in newborn foals: clinical, pathological, serological, microbiological and immunohistochemical observations. Equine Vet J 1997;29:178.

Done SH, Paton DJ, White ME. Porcine reproductive and respiratory syndrome (PRRS): a review, with emphasis on pathological, virological and diagnostic aspects. Br Vet J 1996;152:153.

Glaser AL, deVries AA, Rottier PJ, et al. Equine arteritis virus: a review of clinical features and management aspects. Vet Qrtly 1996;18:95.

Horzinek MC, Flewett TH, Saif LJ, et al. A new family of vertebrate viruses: Toroviridae. Intervirology 1987;27:17.

Kapur V, Elam MR, Pawlovich TM, Murtaugh MP. Genetic variation in porcine reproductive and respiratory syndrome virus isolates in the midwestern United States. J Gen Virol 1996;77:1271.

Koopmans M, Horzinek MC. Toroviruses of animals and humans: a review. Adv Virus Res 1994;43:233.

Lai MMC. Coronaviruses: organization, replication and expression of the genome. Annu Rev Microbiol 1990;44:303.

Laude H, Van Reeth K, Pensaert M. Porcine respiratory coronavirus: molecular features and virus-host interactions. Vet Res 1993;24:125.

McIntosh K. Coronaviruses. In: Fields B, Knipe DM, Howley PM, et al., eds. Fields virology. 3rd ed. Philadelphia: Lippincott-Raven, 1995:1095.

Mebus CA. Neonatal calf diarrhea virus. In: Dinter Z, Morein B, eds. Virus infections of ruminants. Amsterdam: Elsevier, 1990:295.

Olsen CW. A review of feline infectious peritonitis virus: molecular biology, immunopathogenesis, clinical aspects and vaccination. Vet Microbiol 1993;36:1.

Rossow KD, Collins JE, Goyal SM, et al. Pathogenesis of porcine reproductive and respiratory syndrome virus infection in gnotobiotic pigs. Vet Pathol 1995;32:361.

Saif LJ. Mucosal immunity; an overview and studies of enteric and respiratory coronavirus infections in a swine model for enteric disease. Vet Immunol Immunopathol 1996;54:163.

Sirinarumitr T, Paul PS, Halbur PG, Kluge JP. An overview of immunological and genetic methods for detecting swine coronaviruses, transmissible gastroenteritis virus, and porcine respiratory coronavirus in tissues. Adv Exp Med Biol 1997;412:37.

Snijder EJ, Horzinek MC. Toroviruses: replication, evolution and comparison with the members of the coronavirus-like superfamily. J Gen Virology 1993;74:2305.

Sparks AH, Gruffydd TJ, Harbour DA. Feline infectious bronchitis: a review of clinico-pathological changes in 65 cases, and a critical assessment of their diagnostic value. Vet Rec 1991;129:209.

72 Reoviridae

Jeffrey L. Stott

Viruses in the Reoviridae family infect a wide range of species, including mammals, fish and shellfish, insects, and plants. The family is grouped into nine genera: orthoreovirus, orbivirus, rotavirus, aquareovirus, coltivirus, oryzavirus, cypovirus, phytoreovirus, and fijivirus. The latter four genera are confined to insects, plants, or both. The coltivirus genera includes Colorado tick fever virus, which is arthropod-transmitted and a human pathogen. Orthoreoviruses (Fig 72.1) infect vertebrate species; the mammalian reovirus Type 1 serves as the species prototype. The orbivirus host range includes both vertebrate and invertebrate species, with bluetongue virus serving as the species prototype. Rotaviruses (Fig 72.2) infect vertebrate species with the human rotavirus serving as the species prototype. The aquareovirus host range includes fish and shellfish with golden shiner virus serving as the prototype. Table 72.1 includes a list of genera and species that are important in veterinary medicine.

MAMMALIAN ORTHOREOVIRUSES

DISEASE

Mammalian reoviruses have been recovered from most animal species of veterinary importance, including equine, bovine, ovine, porcine, feline, and canine species. Infections are most commonly associated with mild to moderate respiratory and enteric diseases. Infection of dogs with all three reovirus types (1, 2, and 3) has been documented and experimental infection results in respiratory disease characterized by development of a mucoid nasal discharge, fever, and mild cough. All three serotypes have been isolated from cats, many with diarrhea. The clinical disease has been described as mild and of short duration. Experimental infection of kittens with serotype 3 resulted in conjunctivitis, photophobia, gingivitis, serous lacrimation, and nasal discharge. All three serotypes of reovirus have been isolated from sheep, and experimental infections with serotype 1 have been reported to cause enteritis and pneumonia. Types 1, 2, and 3 have been isolated from swine and may cause a mild pneumonia and enteric disease. Orthoreoviruses appear to have minimal disease significance in cattle and horses.

ETIOLOGIC AGENT

Physical, Chemical, and Antigenic Properties

Mammalian reoviruses are represented by three serotypes, 1, 2, and 3; serotype 1 serves as the species prototype. The virus has a density of 1.36g/cm^3 in cesium chloride and exhibits an icosahedral symmetry with a diameter of approximately 96 nm. The viral particle possesses a double protein coat and contains a segmented (10 segments) dsRNA genome. The inner protein core is composed of six proteins (three major and three minor) and contains the viral transcriptase and replicase activity. One of the inner coat proteins, lambda 2, forms spikes that project outward and through the outer coat. The outer coat is composed of three proteins (two major and one minor). The 10 dsRNA segments exist in three general size classes (three large, three medium, and four small) which are in turn reflected in their translation into three size classes of proteins. The type-specific coat protein, sigma 1, functions in hemagglutination (HA) of human erythrocytes (Type 3 also agglutinates bovine erythrocytes); is responsible for induction of neutralizing antibody, T lymphocyte-mediated suppressor, and T lymphocyte cytotoxic activity; and is responsible for inhibiting host cell DNA synthesis, tissue tropism, and tissue injury. The outer coat protein, sigma 3, gives rise to type-specific hemagglutination-inhibition (HI) antibodies and partial type-specific viral neutralizing antibodies. An additional coat protein, 1C, a cleavage product of m1, is involved in pathogenesis and strain-dependent virulence within a given serotype. The core spike protein, lambda 2, induces antibodies with type specificity as determined by HI, induces group specificity by viral neutralization, is responsible for inhibiting host cell transcription and translation, and plays a role in initiating persistent infection.

Multiple strains of reovirus have been identified by variations in virulence and in genome segment migration in sodium dodecyl sulfate polyacrylamide gel electrophoresis (SDSPAGE).

Resistance to Physical and Chemical Agents

Reoviruses are stable at 70°C. The viruses are resistant to lipid solvents and stable over a wide pH range (pH 3 to 9).

Table 72.1.   Reoviridae Genera Considered to Be of Importance in Veterinary Medicine

Genus	Serogroup	Minimum Number of Serotypes
Orthoreoviruses	Mammalian	3
	Avian	11
Orbiviruses	Bluetongue	24
	Epizootic hemorrhagic disease	9
	African horsesickness	9
	Equine encephalosis	5
Rotaviruses	Not designated	Uncertain
Aquareoviruses	Not designated	Uncertain

FIGURE 72.2.   *Negatively stained preparations of bovine rotaviruses. 204,000×. (Courtesy of R. Nordhausen.)*

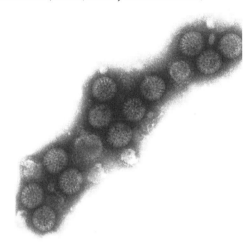

FIGURE 72.1.   *Negatively stained preparations of avian orthoreoviruses. 204,000×. (Courtesy of R. Nordhausen.)*

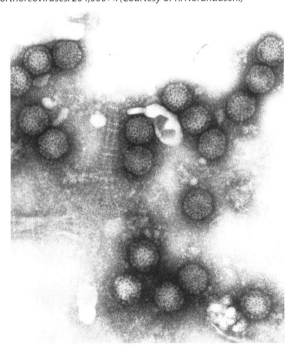

Infectivity for Other Species and Culture Systems

Reoviruses infect most mammals and many insects. They replicate in a wide range of cell cultures, monkey kidney, and mouse L cell fibroblasts.

HOST–VIRUS RELATIONSHIP

Distribution, Reservoir, and Transmission

Mammalian reoviruses have a wide geographic distribution. Persistence in nature is probably by multiple mechanisms, including perpetual transmission to susceptible hosts and persistent infections in certain animals. The mode of transmission is apparently by direct contact or exposure to materials contaminated by viral-infected feces and respiratory discharge.

Pathogenesis and Pathology

Studies in mice have demonstrated enteric strains of virus capable of infecting intestinal epithelial cells resulting in local inflammation and diarrhea. In some cases the virus gains entry to the systemic circulation and may produce lesions at a distant site. Strains capable of causing myocarditis in mice are able to infect cultured myocytes and cause cytopathic effect. Entry of virus by the respiratory route is poorly understood.

Host Response to Infection

Infection of mice with mammalian reoviruses can result in induction of interferon and type-specific antibody, delayed-type hypersensitivity, cytotoxic T lymphocytes, and suppressor T lymphocytes. These activities appear to be induced by the outer capsid protein, lambda 1. The relative importance of such immune responses in protective immunity to natural infections is not well defined. Local immunity at the level of mucosal surfaces may be important in protection against viruses that induce disease at such local sites.

LABORATORY DIAGNOSIS

Virus can be isolated from rectal, nasal, and throat swabs by cell culture techniques, although blind passage may be required before cytopathic effect (CPE) becomes visible. Identification of mammalian reoviruses is by HI, viral neutralization (VN), or complement fixation (CF) techniques. Serologic tests using paired sera can also be conducted by HI, VN, or CF.

TREATMENT AND CONTROL

Since reovirus infection in animals is usually mild, treatment is usually not required. No vaccines or control measures have been described and will receive little attention in the future unless such viruses are determined to be of importance.

AVIAN ORTHOREOVIRUSES

DISEASE

Avian reoviruses are of economic significance to the poultry industry. Reovirus infection of poultry involves multiple organs with overt clinical disease being most recognized in chickens as an arthritis (viral arthritis) and tendon synovitis; avian reoviruses are the major cause of avian arthritis. The disease is primarily associated with broiler chickens, and less prominently with layer birds and turkeys. Mortality, poor growth, poor food efficiency, and carcass condemnations are associated with acutely infected flocks. Avian reoviruses have also been associated with respiratory and enteric disease, myocarditis, hepatitis, hydropericardium, pericarditis, ruptured gastrocnemius tendons, and pasting (young chickens).

ETIOLOGIC AGENT

Physical, Chemical, and Antigenic Properties

The avian reoviruses possess a dsRNA genome of 10 segments. The avian reoviruses differ from their mammalian counterparts in that they produce cell fusion in cell cultures, lack hemagglutinating activity, and are typically unable to grow in mammalian cell lines. Avian and mammalian reoviruses exhibit varying degrees of antigenic relatedness. At least 11 serotypes exist. Strains of avian reoviruses exhibit a range in virulence. All share common antigens as determined by agar gel immunodiffusion (AGID) and complement fixation (CF). Avian and mammalian orthoreoviruses exhibit similar physicochemical properties.

Infectivity for Other Species and Culture Systems

Avian reovirus replicates in embryonated chicken eggs and primary cell cultures of chicken embryo, lung, kidney, liver, and testicle, as well as certain established mammalian cell lines, such as African Green monkey kidney (VERO) and baby hamster kidney (BHK).

HOST–VIRUS RELATIONSHIP

Distribution, Reservoir, and Transmission

Avian reoviruses are prevalent worldwide in chickens, turkeys, and other avian species. Perpetuation of avian reoviruses in nature is by continued transmission to susceptible birds and persistent infection. Transmission occurs both horizontally and vertically. Horizontal transmission occurs via direct and indirect contact. Vertical transmission has been demonstrated following oral, tracheal, and nasal inoculation of breeder chickens.

Pathogenesis and Pathology

Infection with avian reoviruses is usually inapparent. Acute avian arthritis is characterized by an initial inflammatory response in the joints that then progresses in many cases to pannus formation, erosion of underlying cartilage, and ultimately fibrosis. The route of infection influences the incubation period, with contact exposure resulting in approximately 13 days' incubation while footpad inoculation results in viremia within 3 days.

Gross lesions in chickens with reovirus-induced avian arthritis are extensive swelling of the digital flexor and metatarsal extensor tendons. Inflammation of the tendon areas often proceeds to a chronic hardening and fusion of the tendon sheaths.

Microscopic lesions of acute avian viral arthritis include edema, coagulation necrosis, and perivascular infiltration of lymphocytes and macrophages. Thickening of the tendon sheaths is caused by reticular cell proliferation, synovial cell hyperplasia and hypertrophy, infiltration of heterophils and macrophages, and periostitis. Synovial cavities are filled with sloughed synovial and inflammatory cells. The chronic disease is characterized by formation of villi on synovial membranes, increase in fibrous connective tissue, and infiltration or proliferation of reticular cells, lymphocytes, macrophages, and plasma cells. Lesions in other organs include heterophil infiltration between myocardial fibers and hepatic necrosis.

Host Response to Infection

Immunologic responses to avian reoviruses have been demonstrated by AGID, CF, and viral neutralization tests. The mechanism or mechanisms responsible for protective immunity are poorly defined, and variable degrees of cross-strain protection have been reported.

LABORATORY DIAGNOSIS

Reovirus-induced avian arthritis must be differentiated from similar diseases such as adenovirus infection and bacterial and mycoplasmal synovitis. A definitive diagnosis requires direct fluorescent antibody (FA) staining of tissues (tendon sheaths), viral isolation, or serology.

TREATMENT AND CONTROL

No treatment for avian viral arthritis has been described. The infection can best be controlled by proper management procedures and vaccination. Decontamination of a poultry house following total removal of infected birds apparently prevents infection of a new population. Attenuated and killed vaccines have been administered to breeder flocks, with the resulting immunity transferred to progeny. However, administration of attenuated vaccines to breeder chickens in production can result in egg transmission of the virus with subsequent decreased hatchability, increased young chick mortality, and increased incidence of early viral arthritis or tenosynovitis at 7 to 14 days of age. Attenuated virus has been used successfully to immunize young chicks, with no evidence of interference by maternal antibody. Despite in vitro cross-reactions between strains, vaccination ensures protection against the homologous virus only.

ORBIVIRUSES

Orbiviruses are important pathogens of livestock. Fourteen serogroups have been described and four are of veterinary significance: 1) bluetongue virus (BTV), 2) epizootic hemorrhagic disease virus (EHDV), 3) African horsesickness virus (AHSV), and 4) equine encephalosis virus (EEV).

Like other reoviruses, orbiviruses possess a segmented dsRNA genome (10 segments), have a double capsid, and replicate in the cytoplasm. The virus has a density of $1.38\,g/cm^3$ in cesium chloride and diameters of 65 nm to 80 nm. Unique properties of the orbiviruses, relative to the orthoreoviruses and rotaviruses, include the following:

1. Orbiviruses have a diffuse and poorly defined outer coat with no obvious symmetry.
2. Orbiviruses are acid-sensitive and exhibit a moderate loss of infectivity following treatment with lipid solvents.
3. Orbiviruses are not enteric pathogens but are arthropod-borne and thus infect insects as well as vertebrate species.

BLUETONGUE AND EPIZOOTIC HEMORRHAGIC DISEASE VIRUSES

DISEASE

Bluetongue (BT) and epizootic hemorrhagic disease (EHD) are arthropod-borne orbivirus diseases of domestic and wild ruminant species. Infection may result in acute to subclinical disease depending upon several factors, including viral strain; animal species, breed, and age; environmental conditions; and stress. Acute BT disease is classically associated with sheep (soremuzzle, catarrhal fever) and deer. Cattle are commonly infected but clinical disease is uncommon. Acute epizootic hemorrhagic disease is classically associated with deer but may also clinically affect cattle; Ibaraki virus, recently identified as being closely related to EHDV serotype 2, was initially recognized as causing clinical disease in cattle in Japan. The two viruses, BTV and EHDV, share similar infection and disease patterns. Acute disease is typically characterized by catarrhal inflammation of mucous membranes (mouth, nose, digestive tract) and the coronary band; cattle often exhibit a vesicular-type dermatitis. Degenerative changes in cardiac and skeletal musculature result in emaciation, weakness, lameness, and a protracted convalescence. Following an acute BTV infection in sheep, breaks in the wool fiber are apparent.

In addition to causing acute clinical disease, BTV and EHDV can cross the placenta and infect the developing fetus. The outcome depends upon gestational age. Infection in the first trimester may result in fetal death. As gestational age increases, infection may result in abortion, stillbirths, birth of dummy or deformed animals, or birth of asymptomatic and sometimes viremic animals. In addition to disease-associated losses, BTV causes significant economic loss by restricting animals and their germplasm from international movement.

BTV has more recently been recognized as a potential pathogen of carnivores. Inadvertent infection of pregnant dogs with BTV-contaminated vaccine has caused abortion and death. Serologic evidence of BTV infection has been demonstrated in African carnivores.

ETIOLOGIC AGENT

Physical, Chemical, and Antigenic Properties

The viruses are composed of seven structural proteins, two being in the outer coat and five making up the inner core. The outer capsid protein, VP2, contains the serotype-specific epitopes that can be recognized by viral-neutralizing and hemagglutination-inhibiting (HI) antibodies. The outer coat protein, VP5, has been suggested to play a role in adsorption to cell receptors. A minimum of four nonstructural (NS) proteins have been identified, with NS-1 being responsible for the cytoplasmic macrotubular structures characteristic of orbivirus-induced cytopathic effect (CPE). The core proteins, VP5, and nonstructural proteins contain group-specific determinants demonstrable by immune precipitation, AGID, CF, and enzyme-linked immunosorbent assay (ELISA). BTV and EHDV share limited common antigenic determinants.

Extensive heterogeneity within the BTV serogroup has been well documented. Up to 24 serotypes have been described; multiple variants exist within some serotypes, as determined by electrophoretic migration of genomic RNA (electrophorotype). Multiple isolates of EHDV have been reported, two serotypes being present in the United States; the number of EHDV serotypes worldwide is uncertain, but at least nine have been described. The potential for reassortment of genome segments to occur between viruses within the same serogroup has been demonstrated by in vitro coinfection studies. Such reassortment has recently been demonstrated to occur between strains and between serotypes of BTV in calves experimentally infected with multiple viruses. The significance of this phenomenon in nature relative to the evolution of orbivirus heterogeneity is uncertain.

Infectivity for Other Species and Culture Systems

Bluetongue and EHD viruses infect many domestic and wild ruminants including sheep, cattle, goats, deer, antelope, and elk. The viruses are arthropod-borne and multiply in the vector, *Culicoides* species. The viruses can be adapted to growth in suckling mice, suckling hamsters, embryonated chick eggs (ECEs), and a variety of mammalian and insect cell cultures. Viral adaptability to lab animals, ECEs, and cell cultures depends upon viral strain. Replication of BTV in ECEs is facilitated by an incubation temperature of 33.5°C.

HOST–VIRUS RELATIONSHIP

Distribution, Reservoir, and Transmission

Bluetongue virus, and probably EHDV, have a worldwide distribution that is only limited by the requirement for a susceptible ruminant population and competent vector. The latter is governed by climatic conditions. The more extreme lower and upper latitudes that do not support *Culicoides* populations are free of virus. While BTV and EHDV activity has been documented in many countries, serotype distribution varies. Furthermore, expression of clinical disease also varies between countries; for example, EHD in deer has only been described in the United States and Canada; Ibaraki virus (a member of the EHDV serogroup) has only been associated with disease in cattle in Japan; and both BTV and EHDV have been isolated from *Culicoides* in Australia, but no disease has been observed.

The reservoirs of BTV and EHDV are not well defined, and persistence of virus in nature depends upon multiple factors. In climates that permit insect (*Culicoides*) activity year-round, the virus can easily persist by a perpetual vector animal host cycle. Many geographic areas do not permit vector activity during certain seasons. In these areas, the virus may be reintroduced by infected animals or infected vectors. In addition, the virus may persist through undetected low-level *Culicoides* activity during winter months, in animals experiencing long-term viremias, or in the developing fetus.

Transmission of BTV and EHDV is primarily by *Culicoides* species that serve as biologic vectors. The primary species involved in transmission varies between countries. Vectors other than *Culicoides* may include ticks (mechanical or biologic transmission or both). Additional mechanisms of transmission include the vertical (dam to fetus) and the horizontal (sire to dam via infected semen).

Pathogenesis and Pathology

The pathogenesis and pathology of BT and EHD are very similar. Sheep and deer are most susceptible to clinical disease; cattle are more resistant.

In infected sheep, bluetongue virus multiplies initially in the lymph nodes draining the site of infection. Viremia may occur as early as 3 days postinfection with a subsequent febrile response. Upon systemic distribution, virus multiplies in the endothelium of small blood vessels, resulting in vascular occlusion, stasis, and exudation. These are especially evident in the mouth, skin, and coronet, where the epithelium suffers from hypoxia and is easily damaged by abrasion. Virus in the circulation is cell-associated, most being found in erythrocytes. Virus is also found in lymphocytes, and in vitro studies have demonstrated viral replication in monocytes, macrophages, and lymphocytes. Duration of viremia is variable but usually persists for 2 to 3 weeks in the presence of high titering viral-neutralizing antibody. Acutely affected animals may die due to pneumonia or heart failure.

The pathogenesis of BT disease in cattle is poorly defined, but it has been suggested that disease expression is related to a Type I hypersensitivity reaction such as might occur in animals previously sensitized by related orbiviruses. A similar phenomenon has been described following infection of sheep previously sensitized by poorly immunogenic virus. Compared to viremia in sheep, viremia in cattle is often extended in duration and may persist for months and possibly years in a latent state.

Gross lesions associated with BT disease include edema and hyperemia of the buccal and nasal mucosa, skin, and coronary band. Ulcerations and erosions may occur on the buccal mucosa. In the pulmonary artery there are vascular lesions consisting of hyperemia, edema, and congestion. Petechial hemorrhages may also be apparent in the heart muscle, pericardium, and skeletal musculature. A characteristic of acute BT in cattle is development of a dermatitis and thickening of the skin with prominent folds in the cervical areas.

Host Response to Infection

Upon infection, animals develop both a humoral and cellular immune response, the latter being poorly defined. Viral-neutralizing (type-specific) and nonneutralizing (group-specific) antibodies develop 7 to 14 days after infection. However, virus can coexist with high antibody titers for variable periods of time. Varying degrees of cross-serotype viral neutralization may be observed following a primary infection with a single viral type. Upon subsequent exposures to additional serotypes, serum antibodies develop broadly cross-reactive neutralizing activity, including recognition of serotypes not previously encountered. This cross-reactive nature of neutralizing antibody may be responsible for the varied degrees of protection observed in animal (sheep) cross-protection studies.

Cell-mediated immune (CMI) responses have been detected in sheep and cattle following immunization with killed virus or exposure to live virus.

Maternal immunity is transferred via colostrum and appears to protect offspring for up to 4 months against infection.

LABORATORY DIAGNOSIS

Diagnosis of BT in sheep, or BT and EHD in deer, can usually be based upon clinical signs in endemic areas. The seasonal nature of disease (late summer and fall months) also facilitates a field diagnosis. Bluetongue and EHD cannot be distinguished on a clinical basis in deer and cattle.

Diagnosis of BT in cattle or in sheep flocks in nonendemic areas requires virologic or serologic testing. Direct identification of BTV antigen in necropsy tissues is not often attempted, and viral isolation procedures are preferable. Isolation is performed by inoculation of susceptible sheep, ECEs, suckling mice, or cell cultures. The cell cultures most often used include VERO and BHK; multiple blind passages are often required before cytopathic effect is observed. Upon adaptation to cell culture, virus can be identified by fluorescent antibody staining or viral neutralization. Identification of BTV and EHDV RNA in infected tissues can be realized by a variety of PCR techniques.

Serologic diagnosis can be performed using tests for group-specific (AGID, CF, ELISA, IFA) or type-specific (viral neutralization, HI) antibodies. Paired serum samples are required to demonstrate seroconversion or an increase in titer. Differentiation of BTV and EHDV infections may prove difficult and a type-specific assay is advised.

TREATMENT AND CONTROL

No specific treatment for BT or EHD is available. Advisable husbandry practices to reduce animal stress include confining affected animals in sheltered and dry areas. Secondary infections can be treated with appropriate antibiotic therapy.

Control of BT is difficult because it is transmitted by insects. Exposure to biting gnats may be reduced in some instances by removal of animals from infected areas, treatment with insect repellents, and housing animals in sheds. Vaccination of sheep with attenuated BTV has been practiced for many years in South Africa; this vaccine employs many different serotypes. The use of attenuated vaccines in sheep in the United States is limited to serotype 10; this virus is responsible for very little of the infection that occurs. Texas and California have additional vaccine serotypes available for use within those respective states. Concern about the safety of attenuated viral vaccines is partially responsible for their limited availability in the United States. There is a fear of reversion to virulence in the primary host, vector, or secondary host. The need for multiple serotypes in the case of BTV raises concerns about the potential dangers of genomic reassortment between vaccine viruses. Vaccination of pregnant ewes may result in fetal infection, and vaccine virus may be transmitted to other pregnant ruminants with similar results.

The production cost of killed virus vaccines and recombinant baculovirus-expressed virus-like particles will probably limit their commercial development. Vaccination of cattle with an experimental inactivated vaccine resulted in hypersensitization; upon subsequent challenge with virulent virus, animals responded with exacerbated acute clinical disease.

No vaccines have been developed for EHDV.

AFRICAN HORSESICKNESS VIRUS

DISEASE

African horsesickness (AHS) is an arthropod-borne orbivirus disease affecting primarily horses. The disease varies in severity and may range from acute to subclinical. The clinical disease may be expressed primarily as a fever (horsesickness fever), an acute pulmonary disease, a chronic or cardiac form, or a combination of the latter two. The pulmonary form of acute disease is characterized by severe edema of the lungs, coughing, dyspnea, a febrile response, nasal discharge, accelerated respiration, and hyperemia of conjunctival and mucous membranes. A more chronic form of the disease is characterized by extensive tissue edema in the neck, head, and supraorbital fossae; bulging eyes; and lesions in the heart. The severity of the disease appears to be influenced by the viral strain and the immune status of the host.

ETIOLOGIC AGENT

Physical, Chemical, and Antigenic Properties

The causative agent belongs to a distinct serogroup, AHS virus (AHSV). Nine serotypes of the virus have been identified by cross-neutralization studies in mice. All types share common group-specific CF antigens.

Infectivity for Other Species and Culture Systems

African horsesickness viral infections have been documented in horses, donkeys, mules, zebras, Angora goats, and dogs. Horses appear to be the most susceptible to clinical disease. Virus can be propagated in suckling mice and adapted to grow in ECEs, adult mice, and cell cultures (VERO and BHK).

HOST–VIRUS RELATIONSHIP

Distribution, Reservoir, and Transmission

African horsesickness is predominantly confined to the African continent, although it has been active in the Middle East, the Mediterranean area, and parts of Asia. The reservoirs of AHSV are uncertain but may include the vector where climatic conditions permit and possibly mules, asses, zebras, and dogs.

Transmission of AHSV is predominantly, if not solely, by *Culicoides* species. Aedes mosquitoes have been experimentally infected with virus with a persistent infection resulting; their significance in AHSV epidemiology is unknown. Dogs may become infected with AHSV by eating infected horse meat. Subsequent dog-to-dog spread can occur by tick bite. As described for bluetongue virus, AHS is seasonal and its appearance correlates with vector activity. The virus probably moves from one area to another by transportation of infected animals or by infected *Culicoides* being carried on the wind.

Pathogenesis and Pathology

The incubation period of the disease is about 7 days. Mortality may range from 25% to 95%. Virus replicates in cells of the lymph nodes, spleen, thymus, and pharyngeal mucosa. Acute illness is characterized by fluid-distended lungs and a fluid-filled thorax. Additional lesions may include subendocardial hemorrhages, inflamed intestines, swollen liver, and excess fluid in the pericardial sac and abdominal cavity. The more chronic form is characterized by a hydropericardium and hydropic degeneration of the myocardium. The lungs are less edematous than in the acute pulmonary form.

Host Response to Infection

All serotypes share common group antigens and induce development of antibodies that may be recognized by CF, AGID, and indirect FA. Viral neutralizing antibodies also develop following infection; these are predominantly serotype-specific, but some cross-neutralization activity has been observed.

LABORATORY DIAGNOSIS

Field diagnosis of AHS, especially in nonendemic areas, should be supported by viral isolation or serology, since it must be differentiated from equine infectious arteritis, trypanosomiasis, and anthrax. Intracerebral inoculation of suckling mice with blood or tissue suspension is the preferred method of isolating virus. Serial passage may be required for viral adaptation. Cell cultures are not as efficient in isolating virus as mouse or horse inoculation. Virus can be identified by viral neutralization, HI, or FA.

Serologic diagnosis requires paired serum samples for demonstrating seroconversion or an increase in antibody titer. Assays routinely used for such purposes include CF, AGID, FA, viral neutralization, or HI. The latter two assays are type-specific and predominantly identify only a single type.

TREATMENT AND CONTROL

No specific treatment of AHS is available. Hyperimmune horse serum confers transient protection. Stabling of horses in insect-secure facilities at night is assumed to reduce exposure of animals to the *Culicoides* vector. Attenuated viral vaccine, including the nine recognized serotypes, are available in Africa. A yearly vaccination program is advised but the efficacy of the vaccine is questionable.

EQUINE ENCEPHALOSIS VIRUS

Equine encephalosis is a recently (1967) recognized orbivirus-induced disease of horses in South Africa. The acute disease is characterized by brain edema, catarrhal enteritis, venous congestion, and fatty liver degeneration. Virus has been isolated from aborted fetuses. Mortality is variable. Serologic studies have demonstrated widespread infection but sporadic and relatively low prevalence of acute disease. The five recognized serotypes of equine encephalosis virus (EEV) share unique common group antigens.

ROTAVIRUSES

DISEASE

Rotaviruses are a major cause of enteritis and diarrhea in many mammals (including humans) and birds. Disease is most often associated with neonates and can result in significant economic losses in species of veterinary significance. Clinical rotavirus infection is most often associated with neonatal (1 to 3 days of age) calf diarrhea. Pigs are also very susceptible. The virus primarily infects adsorptive cells of the intestinal villi with resulting diarrhea. The clinical severity of the infection depends on factors such as age, viral virulence, the presence of passive immunity, and secondary infection.

ETIOLOGIC AGENT

Physical, Chemical, and Antigenic Properties

Rotaviruses represent a distinct genus of the family Reoviridae. The viruses are nonenveloped, contain a segmented (11 segments) dsRNA genome, and exhibit a double-shelled capsid morphology with an overall diameter of approximately 70 nm (see Fig 72.2). The buoyant density of the virus is 1.36 g/cm^3 in cesium chloride. The outermost capsid has a well-defined, smooth, circular appearance and encloses an inner core structure. Up to 11 structural proteins of bovine rotavirus have been identified.

Multiple strains, serotypes, and groups (A–F) of rotavirus have been recognized based upon serologic characterization, electropherotype of genomic RNA segments in SDSPAGE, and genetic sequence data. Serotype specificity is based upon viral neutralization. Viral protein 7, a glycosylated coat protein, is the dominant protein responsible for serotype specificity. Viral protein 6, a major core protein, contains antigenic epitopes for group and subgroup specificity, and an additional coat protein, VP4, which induces neutralizing antibody, is the viral hemagglutinin and dictates species susceptibility.

Infectivity for Other Species and Culture Systems

Rotaviruses obtained from one species have been successfully used to infect other species, often with expression of clinical disease. The extent of experimental and natural cross-species infectivity is not established. At this point, it has been suggested that rotaviruses are predominantly species-specific.

A major advance in the propagation of rotaviruses was the discovery that low concentration of trypsin facilitated viral replication. The enzyme works directly on the virus by cleaving an outer coat protein, VP3, which subsequently facilitates viral uncoating within the cell. The most common cell lines used are kidney epithelial cells, especially the rhesus monkey kidney cell line, MA-104.

HOST–VIRUS RELATIONSHIP

Distribution, Reservoir, and Transmission

Rotaviruses are considered to be distributed worldwide in multiple species. Adults may become persistently infected with virus. High titers of virus are excreted in the feces of infected animals, and transmission to other animals is by ingestion of virus. Potential means of transmission include being borne by air and water and by ingestion of contaminated feed.

Pathogenesis and Pathology

Rotavirus pathogenesis is similar in most species. Upon ingestion, virus traverses the alimentary tract and infects the adsorptive columnar epithelial cells lining the apical halves of the intestinal villi. The infection progresses from the upper to the lower portions of the small intestine, and in some species, to the colon. Upon infection, damage to the adsorptive epithelial cells results in diarrhea. Villus atrophy ensues and the sloughed columnar epithelial cells are replaced by immature cuboidal-type cells from the crypts.

At necropsy, the intestinal contents are found to be liquid to semiliquid. The intestinal mucosa may appear normal or inflamed and hemorrhagic. Histopathology reveals villus atrophy, cuboidal cells covering the villi, and crypt cell hyperplasia.

Host Response to Infection

Animals infected with rotavirus develop local and systemic humoral immune responses demonstrable by various serologic techniques. Viral-neutralizing antibody is serotype-specific and directed at VP3 or VP7. Complement fixation (CF), immunoelectron microscopy (IEM), and ELISA all identify antibodies specific for group and subgroup determinants. Infection of animals with a given strain of rotavirus appears to elicit a humoral immune response to the homologous virus and boosts the titer to heterologous strains previously encountered. The presence of local immunity is variable.

LABORATORY DIAGNOSIS

Diagnosis of rotavirus-induced diarrhea requires identification of viral antigen in necropsy tissues, viral isolation, serology, or some combination of these. Electron microscopy (EM), IEM, or indirect fluorescent antibody (IFA) staining of intestinal tissue sections permits visualization of virus or viral antigens. Techniques for direct identification of rotavirus in feces include EM, ELISA, AGID, counterimmuno-electroosmophoresis, SDSPAGE of extracted viral genomic RNA, and dot-blot hybridization of viral genomic RNA using cloned-labeled complementary DNA (cDNA) probes.

Viral isolation is usually conducted on MA104 cells in the presence of low concentrations of trypsin. Avian rotaviruses are isolated on primary chicken embryo liver and kidney cells.

Serologic diagnosis utilizes CF, IFA, ELISA, IEM, HI, inhibition of reverse-phase hemagglutination, and viral neutralization. Serology must be interpreted with caution due to the widespread distribution of rotavirus infection.

TREATMENT AND CONTROL

Treatment of clinically ill animals is guided by disease severity. Common practices include administration of electrolyte solution, antibiotic therapy in case of secondary infection, and housing animals in a warm and dry atmosphere.

Attempts to control rotavirus infection have met with varied success. Proper sanitation practices can minimize exposure.

The efficacy of available inactivated bovine rotavirus vaccines has been variable. Multivalent vaccines will probably be required to achieve vaccine efficacy under field conditions.

AQUAREOVIRUSES

Aquareoviruses are morphologically and physicochemically similar to orthoreoviruses, though they have 11 segments of dsRNA. Seven of the 12 proteins (genome segment 11 encodes two proteins) are structural, with VP7 representing the major capsid protein. Six genotypes (A–F) have been suggested for aquareovirus. This genus is associated with infection of both fish and shellfish with the golden shiner virus (GSV) serving as the prototype species. Viral pathogenesis is not defined, although necrotic lesions in internal organs have been described in infected fish; high mortalities may occur in fish hatcheries. Aquareoviruses replicate in fish or shellfish cell lines at 16°C and can induce syncytia formation. Some correlation between geographic location and genogroup isolation might suggest that an infection can occur through a food source.

SELECTED REFERENCES

Barber TL, Jochim MM, eds. Progress in clinical and biological research. Vol. 178. Bluetongue and related orbiviruses. New York: Alan R. Liss, 1985.

Bellamy AR, Roth GM. Molecular biology of rotaviruses. Adv Virus Res 1990;38:1.

Bernard J, Bremont M. Molecular biology of fish viruses: a review. Vet Res 1995;26:341.

Dodet B, Heseltine E, Saliou P. Rotaviruses in human and veterinary medicine. Trends Microbiol 1997;5:176.

Gerdes GH, Pieterse LM. The isolation and identification of Potchefstroom virus: a new member of the equine encephalosis group of orbiviruses. J South Afr Vet Assoc 1993;64:131.

Gibbs EPJ, Geiner EC. Bluetongue and epizootic hemorrhagic disease. In: Monath TP, ed. The arboviruses: epidemiology and ecology. Vol 2. Boca Raton, FL: CRC, 1998:1.

Mellor PS, Boorman J. The transmission and geographical spread of African horse sickness and bluetongue viruses. Ann Trop Med Parasitol 1995;89:1.

Murray PK, Eaton BT. Vaccines for bluetongue. Aust Vet J 1996; 73:207.

Subramanian K, Hetrick FM, Samal SK. Identification of a new genogroup of aquareovirus by RNA–RNA hybridization. J Gen Virol 1997;78:1385.

Urbano P, Urbano FG. The Reoviridae family. Comp Immun Microbiol Infect Dis 1994;17:151.

Virus taxonomy. Sixth Report of the International Committee on Taxonomy of Viruses. Arch Virol 1995;10(suppl):1.

Walton TE, Osburn BI, eds. Bluetongue, African horse sickness and related orbiviruses. Boca Raton, FL: CRC, 1992.

73 *Birnaviridae*

Jeffrey L. Stott

The family Birnaviridae encompasses three genera including avibirnavirus (infects poultry), aquabirnavirus (infects fish), and entomobirnavirus (infects insects). Infectious bursal disease virus (genus avibirnavirus) is the best studied. Infectious pancreatic necrosis virus of fish (infects fresh and saltwater fish) is also of significance in veterinary medicine.

INFECTIOUS BURSAL DISEASE

DISEASE

Infectious bursal disease (IBD) is a viral-induced condition of young chickens and is associated with significant economic loss. The infection takes two forms and is dependent upon age. Chicks 3 to 6 weeks of age experience clinical disease with morbidity approaching 100% and mortality as high as 20% to 30%. Chicks less than 3 weeks of age infected with virus experience subclinical infections. Economic losses are attributable to impairment of immunologic responsiveness.

The clinical disease is characterized by soiled vent feathers (birds often peck at their own vents), diarrhea, depression, anorexia, trembling, severe prostration, dehydration, and eventual death. Economic losses are typically due not so much to bird death but rather to reduced weight gain and carcass condemnation due to hemorrhages in skeletal muscle.

Infection of birds less than 3 weeks of age results in more economically devastating inapparent infection. Such birds are extensively immunocompromised and exhibit increased susceptibility to many diseases. Furthermore, affected birds respond poorly to vaccination.

ETIOLOGIC AGENT

Physical, Chemical, and Antigenic Properties

Infectious bursal disease virus (IBDV) shares many features with the Reoviridae family in that the virus has a double capsid and a segmented (two segments) double-stranded RNA (dsRNA) genome. The virus exhibits an icosahedral symmetry with reported diameters ranging from 55 nm to 60 nm (Fig 73.1). Seven structural proteins, two major and five minor, have been identified. Two serotypes have been tentatively identified by viral neutralization test, and antigenic variation exists within types; VP_2 contributes significantly to induction of viral neutralizing antibody.

Resistance to Physical and Chemical Agents

Infectious bursal disease virus is extremely stable and resists inactivation following acid treatment (stable at pH of 2), lipid solvents, various disinfectants, and heat (survives 60°C for 30 minutes).

Infectivity for Other Species and Culture Systems

Infectious bursal disease virus is primarily associated with chickens. However, turkeys and ducks are naturally susceptible to infection. Viral replication occurs in embryonating chicken eggs with subsequent embryo mortality. Virus can also be propagated on chick embryo and other avian cell cultures and avian B lymphocyte cultures.

HOST–VIRUS RELATIONSHIP

Distribution, Reservoir, and Transmission

Infectious bursal disease occurs worldwide in poultry-raising areas with concentrated bird populations. Persistence of virus in nature is largely due to the environmental stability of the virus. Virus has reportedly persisted in poultry houses, following depopulation, for 122 days. Inapparent infections also contribute to viral perpetuation, but carrier birds have not been identified.

Transmission of IBDV is considered to occur via ingestion of virus from feces or feces-contaminated fomites, feed, and water.

Pathogenesis and Pathology

Following ingestion of virus, replication occurs in the primary target organ, the bursa of Fabricius (BF), within 24 hours postinfection. Viral replication occurs primarily in the lymphoid follicles, the susceptible cells probably being IgM-bearing lymphocytes. Microvilli on the BF are reduced in size and number with subsequent surface erosion. The infected follicles become depleted in cells and involute. Additional lymphatic tissues may also be

FIGURE 73.1. *Negatively stained preparations of infectious bursal disease virus. 250,000×. (Courtesy of R. Nordhausen.)*

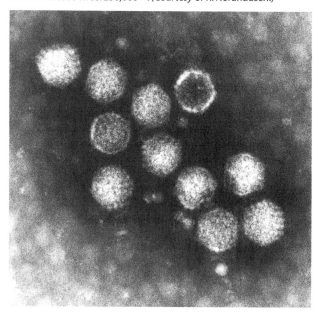

directly or indirectly affected (lymphoid depletion) including thymus, spleen, tonsils, and harderian gland.

The basis of impaired immunologic responsiveness in chicks infected early in life has been attributed to bursal injury, which results in failure to seed B lymphocytes to peripheral lymphoid organs. Such a phenomenon results in a decrease of humoral immunity. A certain degree of reduced cellular immunity has also been demonstrated in young chicks and is apparently due to viral-induced activation of macrophage-like suppressor cell activity.

Gross lesions observed in clinically affected birds may include darkened pectoral muscles and hemorrhages in the pectoral and leg muscles. Gross appearance of the BF will depend on the state of disease. The BF initially becomes enlarged due to edema and hyperemia and is followed in turn by progressive atrophy. In more progressed states, areas of bursal necrosis and hemorrhage are apparent.

Histologically, the epithelial surfaces of the BF have multiple erosions, and the medullary portion of lymphoid follicles becomes depleted of lymphocytes. Extensive edema and infiltration of heterophils occur, followed by formation of cystic cavities bound by columnar epithelial cells. Pathology in other lymphoid organs is less severe and recovery more rapid.

Host Response to Infection

Following infection, birds develop a humoral immune response that is measured by viral neutralization, agar gel immunodiffusion, and enzyme-linked immunosorbent assay (ELISA) tests. Adult birds transfer maternal antibody to developing embryos, and if present in sufficient titer, the antibody lends protection to the hatched chick for variable periods of time.

LABORATORY DIAGNOSIS

Field diagnosis can usually be made based upon clinical observation, high morbidity, and rapid recovery. Examination of the cloacal bursa for atrophy provides retrospective evidence of inapparent IBDV infection in young chicks. Definitive diagnosis of IBD can be carried out by applying direct fluorescent antibody (FA) staining to sectioned necropsy tissues or viral isolation from the bursa and spleen. Isolation can be made by inoculation of embryonated chicken eggs or cell cultures. Serology is also useful for diagnostic purposes.

TREATMENT AND CONTROL

No treatment has been described for affected birds. Control of the disease may be facilitated by proper sanitation practices. Vaccination programs are widely used to control IBD. Immunization of breeder flocks is conducted to facilitate passive transfer of immunity to chicks. Vaccination of chicks is also practiced, but to be effective, levels of maternal antibody must be low. Both attenuated and killed virus vaccines are available.

INFECTIOUS PANCREATIC NECROSIS

Infectious pancreatic necrosis virus (IPNV) is primarily associated with disease in salmonids that are less than 6 months old and mortality can approach 100%; older fish under stressed conditions may also express acute disease. Affected fingerlings appear dark in color and swim with a rotating action (whirling). Internally, petechial hemorrhages in the pyloric and pancreatic tissues can be observed, along with tissue necrosis. The virus also affects commercially raised yellowtails with similar high mortality and is classically referred to as *viral ascites* due to excessive ascites and associated abdominal distension. European and Japanese eels can also be infected with resulting clinical disease. Transmission in fish is horizontal and possibly vertical. Carrier fish exist and serve as a source of infection via infected feces, urine, and sex products, especially under hatchery conditions. Identification of the virus can be realized by inoculation of fish cell cultures and reverse-transcriptase-polymerase chain reaction (RT-PCR) techniques. Viral isolation may require blind passage. Up to 10 serotypes of IPNV have been described with the neutralizing epitopes being mapped to VP_2. While vaccines are not currently available, husbandry efforts that minimize animal stress and introduction of infected replacement stock and/or eggs can minimize losses. Experimental inactivated vaccines have been described but are not commercially available.

SELECTED REFERENCES

Blake SL, Schill WB, McAllister PE, et al. Detection and identification of aquatic birnaviruses by PCR assay. J Clin Microbiol 1995;33:835.

Lasher HN, Davis VS. History of infectious bursal disease in the USA — the first two decades. Avian Dis 1997;41:11.

Ley DH, Yamamoto R, Bickford AA. The pathogenesis of infectious bursal disease: serologic, histopathologic, and clinical observations. Avian Dis 1983;27:1060.

Lukert PD, Saif YM. Infectious bursal disease. In: Calnek BW, ed. Diseases of poultry. 9th ed. Ames, IA: Iowa State University, 1991:648.

McAllister PE. Salmonid fish viruses. In: Stoskopf MK, ed. Fish medicine. Philadelphia: WB Saunders/Harcourt Brace Jovanovich, 1993:384.

Nagarajan MM, Kibenge FS. Infectious bursal disease virus: a review of molecular basis for variations in antigenicity and virulence. Can J Vet Res 1997;61:81.

74 *Retroviridae*

RICHARD M. DONOVAN

INTRODUCTION

Retroviruses (family Retroviridae) are enveloped, single-stranded RNA viruses that replicate through a DNA intermediate using an RNA-dependent DNA polymerase (reverse transcriptase). This large and diverse family includes members that are oncogenic, are associated with a variety of immune system disorders, and cause degenerative and neurologic syndromes.

CLASSIFICATION

The family Retroviridae is classified into seven genera (Table 74.1). Classification is based on genome structure and nucleic acid sequence in addition to older classification criteria based on morphology, serology, biochemical features, and the species of animal from which the retrovirus was isolated.

The genus lentivirus (Latin *lenti*, meaning slow) includes the human immunodeficiency viruses (HIV) as well as many important animal retroviruses. Lentiviruses are most often associated with chronic immune dysfunction and neurologic diseases.

The genus spumavirus (Latin *spuma*, meaning foam) are nononcogenic viruses found in spontaneously degenerating cell cultures, causing the formation of multinucleated vacuolated (foamy) giant cells. No diseases have been associated with spumaviruses in humans or animals.

The remaining retrovirus genera are often termed the oncoviruses (Greek *onkos*, meaning tumor) or the RNA tumor viruses because of their ability to produce neoplasia, although they are now known to be associated with other kinds of diseases. These genera are the mammalian Type C retroviruses, mammalian Type B retroviruses, Type D retroviruses, avian Type C retroviruses, and BLV-HTLV retroviruses. All of these genera have members that cause diseases of veterinary significance, with the exception of the mammalian Type B retrovirus genus, which contains only one member that infects mice.

Several additional features need to be considered in the classification and description of the Retroviridae. Exogenous retroviruses spread horizontally (or vertically but nongenetically) from animal to animal, similar to the mechanism of transmission of other kinds of viruses. In contrast, endogenous retroviruses are transmitted genetically. These retroviruses persist as integrated DNA proviruses that are passed from generation to generation

through the DNA in the gametes of the host animal species. Thus, the endogenous proviral genome occurs in each cell of the animal. Many vertebrates possess such endogenous retroviral DNA sequences. These endogenous retroviruses are usually not pathogenic for their host animals and are often not expressed. When replication of endogenous viruses does occur in the host cell of origin, it is usually restricted. Cells from animal species other than the host species are sometimes unrestricted, however, and can support the replication of the retrovirus in an exogenous manner. The endogenous mode of transmission occurs in many of the oncoviruses, but is not known to occur in the lentiviruses or the spumaviruses.

Some members of the oncoviruses are also classified by their interaction with cells of different species. Ecotropic strains replicate only in cells from animal species of origin and xenotropic strains replicate only in cells of other species. Amphotropic strains replicate in both. Most of the endogenous retroviruses are also xenotropic.

Finally, the morphology of retroviruses in transmission electron micrograph is also useful in classification (Fig 74.1). The size range of retrovirus particles is from 80 nm to 130 nm. Type A particles occur only inside cells and consist of a ring-shaped nucleoid surrounded by a membrane. B-type virions have an eccentric core and C-type virions a central core. D-type virions have a morphology intermediate between B and C virions with an elongated, dense core. The core of lentiviruses has a shape that resembles an ice-cream cone.

GENERAL FEATURES OF RETROVIRUSES

Many of the features of retroviruses are known in great detail because of the extensive work done on the oncoviruses in cancer research and the lentiviruses in AIDS research. The members of the family Retroviridae share many common features in their composition, organization, and life cycle, although the details of individual retroviruses vary.

COMPONENTS OF RETROVIRUSES

A typical retrovirus virion is composed of 2% nucleic acid (RNA), 60% protein, 35% lipid, and 3% (or more) carbohydrate. Its buoyant density is 1.16 to 1.18 g/mL.

Table 74.1.   Genera and Selected Species of Retroviridae

Genus	Species
Mammalian Type B Retroviruses	Mouse Mammary Tumor Virus
Mammalian Type C Retroviruses	Murine Leukemia Virus
	Feline Leukemia Virus
Avian Type C Retroviruses	Avian Leukosis Virus
	Avian Erythroblastosis Virus
	Avian Myeloblastosis Virus
	Avian Myelocytomatosis Virus
	Rous Sarcoma Virus
Type D Retroviruses	Mason-Pfizer Monkey Virus
	Simian Type D Retrovirus
BLV-HTLV Retroviruses	Bovine Leukemia Virus
	Human T-lymphotropic Virus 1
	Human T-lymphotropic Virus 2
	Simian T-lymphotropic Virus
Lentivirus	Visna/Maedi Virus
	Caprine Arthritis Encephalitis Virus
	Equine Infectious Anemia Virus
	Bovine Immunodeficiency Virus
	Feline Immunodeficiency Virus
	Primate Lentiviruses (HIV-1, HIV-2, SIV)
Spumavirus	Human Spumavirus
	Simian Foamy Virus
	Bovine Syncytial Virus
	Feline Syncytial Virus

Retroviral Lipids

Retroviral lipids are mainly phospholipid and occur in the virion envelope. They form a bilayered structure similar to the outer cell membrane from which the retrovirus envelope is derived.

Retroviral Nucleic Acid

Retroviral RNA. Retroviral particles contain RNA as their genetic material. This genomic RNA is present in each retroviral particle as a dimer of two linear, single-stranded, positive sense copies that are noncovalently joined near their 5′ ends (Fig 74.2A). Hence, the virion is diploid. The genomic RNA has a sedimentation size of 60 to 70S in neutral sucrose gradients. Upon denaturation, each RNA copy has a sedimentation coefficient of 38S. The molecular weight of monomer RNA determined by electrophoresis in polyacrylamide gels is approximately 2 to 5×10^6 daltons, or about 7 to 11×10^3 bases. Host cell transfer RNA (tRNA) is associated with genomic RNA near the 3′ terminus and serves as a primer for the synthesis of DNA by the reverse polymerase. The type of tRNA packaged in the virion is useful in the classification of retroviruses. The 3′ terminus of each RNA monomer has a poly (A) tract. The 5′ terminus has a methylated nucleotide cap.

Proviral DNA. Within a cell, the retroviral RNA genome is reverse transcribed into a DNA copy, and it is the proviral DNA form that serves as the intracellular retroviral genome. The retroviral DNA is several hundred bases longer than the retroviral RNA genome due to duplication of repeated and unique terminal sequences present in the RNA genome during the reverse transcription process. These sequences form the long terminal repeats (LTR) that flank the genes in the retroviral DNA (Fig 74.2B). The proviral DNA is covalently integrated in the DNA of the infected host cell.

Retroviral Nucleic Acid Structure and Sequence. The sequence of structural genes of retroviruses, from the 5′ end to the 3′ end of genomic RNA, is Gag-Pol-Env. Some retroviruses, such as the lentiviruses and spumaviruses, have additional genes that regulate expression of the retroviral genome and other accessory functions. Highly oncogenic retroviruses often have an oncogene in place of a portion of the Pol and/or Env gene.

Retroviral Proteins

Retroviral Structural Proteins. Retroviral structural proteins are coded for by the Gag gene and the Env gene (Fig 74.3). Gag (group specific antigen) proteins form the core of the virus and consist of three major proteins. The nucleocapsid (NC) is a small protein (about 5 kd to 10 kd) that interacts with retroviral RNA. The capsid (CA) protein (about 25 kd) forms the major structural element of the retroviral core. The matrix (MA) protein (about 15 kd) serves to join the retroviral core with the retroviral envelope. In some retroviruses, there are additional small core proteins.

The Env (envelope) gene is responsible for the synthesis of two glycoproteins that are linked to form a dimer. The glycoprotein outside of the retrovirus (SU, surface) is a knob-like glycoprotein (about 100 kd) that is responsible for binding the retrovirus to its cellular receptor during infection. The other glycoprotein (TM, transmembrane) is a spike-like structure (about 50 kd) that attaches the SU protein to the retroviral envelope.

Retroviral Enzymes. The Pol gene codes for several proteins with enzymatic activities that are important for the replication of retroviruses. These enzymatic proteins are found within the retroviral particle, but in a much lower molar concentration than the retroviral structural proteins.

The reverse transcriptase (RT) enzyme is responsible for the production of the retroviral DNA genome from the retroviral RNA genome. To accomplish this, reverse transcriptase possesses several catalytic functions, including an RNA-dependent DNA polymerase and an RNase H activity. RT requires the presence of a divalent cation to function, and the type of divalent cation (magnesium or manganese) that a particular retrovirus requires is useful in retroviral classification. The measurement of reverse transcriptase activity is one of the principal laboratory methods for the detection and assay of retroviruses.

The Pol gene also codes for other enzymes. The retroviral protease (PR) mediates cleavage of Gag and Pol

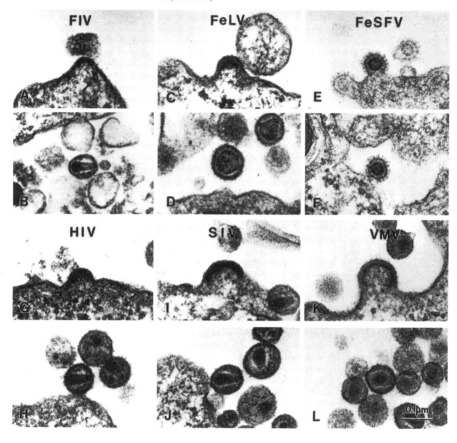

FIGURE 74.1.   *Transmission electron photomicrographs of budding and mature virions of feline immunodeficiency virus (A,B); feline leukemia virus (C,D); feline syncytium-forming virus (E,F); human immunodeficiency virus (G,H); simian immunodeficiency virus (I,J); and visna-maedi virus (K,L). Uranyl acetate and lead citrate stain. (Reproduced with permission from Yamamoto JK, Sparger E, Ho EW, et al. Pathogenesis of experimentally induced feline immunodeficiency virus infection in cats. Am J Vet Res 1988;49:1246.)*

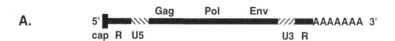

A.

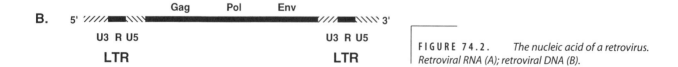

B.

FIGURE 74.2.   *The nucleic acid of a retrovirus. Retroviral RNA (A); retroviral DNA (B).*

polyproteins during retroviral assembly and maturation. The retroviral integrase (IN) functions to covalently link the retroviral DNA into the host cell's DNA as an integrated provirus.

Other Retroviral Proteins.   For many members of the Retroviridae, only the proteins coded by the Gag, Pol, and Env genes are present. Other retroviruses contain additional genes whose products serve functions such as controlling

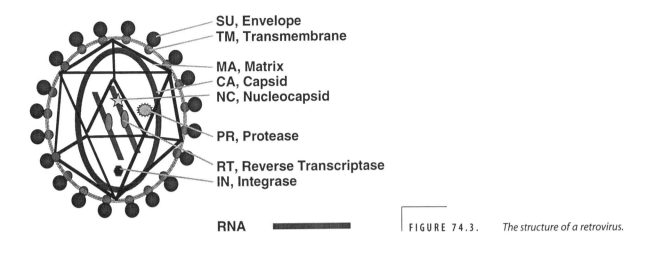

SU, Envelope
TM, Transmembrane

MA, Matrix
CA, Capsid
NC, Nucleocapsid

PR, Protease

RT, Reverse Transcriptase
IN, Integrase

RNA ▬▬▬

FIGURE 74.3.   *The structure of a retrovirus.*

FIGURE 74.4.   *The life cycle of a retrovirus.*

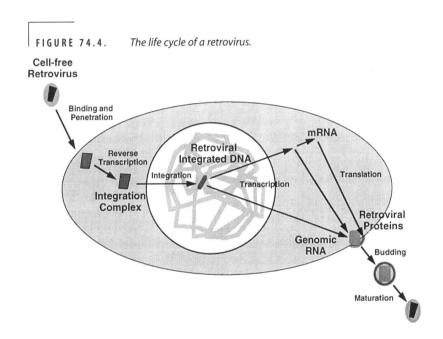

the level of provirus transcription, facilitating transport of retroviral mRNA, and enhancing retroviral replication in specific cell types.

RETROVIRAL REPLICATION

A general scheme of retroviral replication is shown in Figure 74.4. A retroviral particle binds to a specific receptor on the surface of a target cell via the SU protein. The retrovirus penetrates the cell and the retroviral core undergoes specific structural changes. The retroviral RNA within the modified core is reverse transcribed by RT using the associated tRNA primer, first to an RNA/DNA hybrid form, then to a linear double-stranded DNA form with long terminal repeats.

The newly made retroviral DNA is still associated with some viral core proteins and enzyme activities in a structure termed the *integration complex*. In some retroviruses, infection must occur within dividing cells so that the integration complex can access the host DNA, while in other retroviruses the integration complex is actively transported into the nucleus of the cell, allowing such retroviruses to replicate in nondividing or terminally differentiated cells.

The retroviral DNA is integrated into the host cell's DNA by the activity of the IN enzyme. The integration of retroviruses is not at a specific site within the cellular DNA, rather integration can occur at many sites.

The integrated DNA provirus behaves very much as a eukaryotic gene. It may be transcribed into mRNA and genomic RNA using host cell enzymes to produce more virus, or it may remain latent for long periods of time and replicate when the cellular DNA is replicated by the cell.

New retroviral particles are produced by budding from cellular membranes. Immature retroviral Gag polyprotein and genomic RNA assemble and acquire envelopes as they exit infected cells by budding through the plasma membranes into which retroviral SU and TM envelope proteins have been inserted.

In the final step, the retroviral protease (PR) cleaves the Gag polyprotein into the mature structural proteins of matrix, capsid, and nucleocapsid.

IMMUNOLOGIC CHARACTERISTICS OF RETROVIRUSES

Retroviral proteins possess various types of antigenic sites. Type-specific antigens that define the serologic subgroups are associated with the envelope glycoproteins. Group-specific antigens are shared by related viruses and, in general, are associated with the virion core proteins. There are also interspecies antigens that are shared by otherwise unrelated viruses derived from different host species. Reverse transcriptase (RT) is also antigenic and contains type-, group-, and interspecies-specific determinants.

ONCOGENIC VIRUSES AND ONCOGENES

Oncogenic viruses can produce tumors or cancers in a suitable host. Tumors are new and inappropriate cell growths or neoplasia. Cancers are malignant tumors that are characterized by loss of normal cellular controls that results in unregulated growth, lack of differentiation, and ability to invade local tissues and metastasize to other parts of the body. Cancers or malignant tumors are classified by their tissue of origin: sarcomas are malignant tumors of connective tissue; carcinomas are malignant tumors of epithelial origin; and leukemia, lymphoma, and leukosis are neoplasia of white blood cells.

The ability of oncogenic viruses to cause cancers under either natural or experimental conditions has been the subject of intense study for almost a century and this work has made tremendous contributions to the understanding of viruses, neoplastic disease, and cell biology. The fundamental discovery in the field is that oncogenic viruses cause cancer via genes they carry or activate. These genes are termed *oncogenes*.

| ONCOGENESIS BY RETROVIRUSES

There are several mechanisms by which retroviruses are associated with cancer. Highly oncogenic or acutely transforming retroviruses cause cancer rapidly and efficiently, often within days or weeks of infection. Such retroviruses are rare in natural animal populations, but are used extensively in the laboratory for the study of cancer. Rous sarcoma virus (RSV) of chickens, which was

discovered in 1910, is the prototype of highly oncogenic retroviruses.

In highly oncogenic retroviruses, all or part of an oncogene exists in the viral genome, usually in place of viral genes. This retroviral oncogene is responsible for the ability of a highly oncogenic retrovirus to cause oncogenic transformation of a cell. There are more than 20 different retroviral oncogenes known. Each of these has a corresponding gene that can be found in the genome of normal cells. The normal gene that corresponds to a viral oncogene is termed a *c-oncogene* or *proto-oncogene*, and the viral version is called a *v-oncogene*.

In a normal cellular environment, the gene products of proto-oncogenes usually have some function in growth regulatory pathways, such as protein kinases, growth factors or their receptors, GTP binding proteins, or transcriptional activation factors. When they are part of a retroviral genome, these proto-oncogenes are under the control of the retroviral LTR rather than being regulated by normal cellular mechanisms, and are often expressed at high levels. The v-oncogene may also be truncated, contain point mutations, or be fused with another retroviral gene. This aberrant expression of aberrant protein can lead to abnormal growth of the infected cell and the beginning of progression to neoplasia.

For example, in RSV the src oncogene is responsible for sarcomatous transformation. The v-src gene was originally acquired from the normal c-src cellular proto-oncogene when recombination occurred between retroviral and the cellular genomic sequences for c-src. The c-src gene product is a 60-kd protein that has protein kinase activity and is located near the inner surface of the plasma membrane. The kinase activity is part of an intricate cellular signal transduction pathway that mediates cell growth. Other examples of v-oncogenes with c-oncogene counterparts in normal cells are found in other acute transforming retroviruses, for example, myb (avian myeloblastosis virus), erb (avian erythroblastosis virus), myc (avian myelocytomatosis virus), and ras (mouse sarcoma virus).

Highly oncogenic retroviruses are usually defective. The reason they are defective is that they don't have their full complement of Gag-Pol-Env genes because the v-oncogene takes the place of a portion of the retroviral genome. In order to replicate, these defective retroviruses require a replication competent helper virus to supply the missing gene products. The helper retrovirus is usually a closely related retrovirus that is not defective and contains the usual Gag-Pol-Env complement of genes. Since the defective, highly oncogenic virus is packaged into a virion composed of the envelope proteins of the helper virus, the host range of the highly oncogenic virus is dependent upon the helper virus. The presence of the genome of one retrovirus with the protein components of another virus is termed a *pseudotype*.

Weakly oncogenic (nonacutely transforming) retroviruses cause cancer less rapidly and much less efficiently than do highly oncogenic retroviruses. Such viruses do exist in natural and domestic animal populations. Weakly oncogenic retroviruses do not carry a v-oncogene and do not require a helper virus. However, examination of the tumors produced by the weakly oncogenic viruses usually shows a clonal proliferation of cells with a retroviral genome near a cellular oncogene. For example, avian leukosis virus is often integrated near or in the c-myc gene.

The mechanism by which weakly oncogenic retroviruses cause cancer is known as *insertional oncogenesis*. During retroviral replication, proviral DNA is inserted into many random locations in the host genome. Occasionally the integration of the provirus occurs close to a cellular proto-oncogene. This can sometimes produce inappropriate transcription of the oncogene, either by read-through from the retroviral promoter, or by enhancer activity by the retroviral LTR. Integration of the provirus near a proto-oncogene tends to be a very rare event and therefore occurs much less frequently and at much lower efficiency than when the retrovirus carries its own oncogene. The tumors are clonal in origin because, although many cells are infected, only one rare cell has undergone insertional oncogenesis and progresses to a tumor. In addition, the inappropriate activation of a proto-oncogene is just one event in a multifactorial process that leads to cancer.

A third mechanism of retroviral oncogenesis occurs in the bovine leukemia virus–human T lymphotropic virus genus of Retroviridae. These viruses have a regulatory gene called Tax in addition to Gag, Pol, and Env. The protein product of Tax functions as a transactivator to upregulate retroviral transcription by binding to specific DNA sequences in the LTR of the retrovirus. Under some circumstances, the Tax protein can sometimes also bind to transcriptional activator sequences in cellular genes and may disrupt regulatory pathways of the infected cell. Unlike insertional oncogenesis, the integrated provirus is not necessarily adjacent to a proto-oncogene, since it is the Tax protein that produces the oncogene activation (in trans), rather than the retroviral DNA itself.

Finally, many retroviruses, particularly the lentiviruses, cause defects in the immune system. Profound immunodeficiency is often associated with opportunistic neoplastic disease.

Oncogenesis by DNA Viruses

Many of the DNA viruses, including the adenoviruses, papovaviruses (polyoma, papilloma), herpesviruses, hepadnaviruses, and poxviruses, have oncogenic potential. In contrast to highly oncogenic retroviruses, the v-oncogenes of DNA viruses are not cellular derivatives but are true viral genes. The normal function of these viral genes is to activate cellular pathways for DNA replication. This activation is required for DNA viruses in order to multiply in resting cells that lack the enzymes and materials the virus needs for its own DNA replication. The mechanism of neoplastic transformation by oncogenic DNA virus is that the viral genes that activate cellular DNA replication are functional, but the genes for viral production for some reason are not. This causes the infected cell to get inappropriate activation signals without the subsequent viral production that destroys the cell. The result is inappropriate cell activation and division, and is one of the initial steps that can lead to the development of a cancer.

Like the weakly oncogenic retroviruses, insertion and transactivation mechanisms are also known for DNA viruses.

FELINE LEUKEMIA/SARCOMA VIRUS

DISEASE

Feline leukemia virus (FeLV) causes one of the most important and dangerous infectious diseases of cats. The most significant consequence of persistent FeLV infection is severe immunosuppression that results in the development of secondary opportunistic infections and death. Clinical signs produced by FeLV can include any of the following: anemia, jaundice, depression, weight loss, decreased appetite, diarrhea or constipation, blood in the stool, enlarged lymph nodes, respiratory distress, decreased stamina, excessive drinking and urination, geophagia, fetal resorption, abortion, infertility, and a syndrome resembling panleukopenia. Other FeLV diseases include a neurologic syndrome and immune-complex glomerulonephritis.

Lymphosarcoma is the most important proliferative disease caused by FeLV. Approximately one-third of all cat tumors are hematopoietic tumors, and the majority of those are lymphosarcomas caused by FeLV. The tumor masses may cause such problems as respiratory distress; intestinal inflammation with diarrhea, vomiting, or constipation; liver or kidney disease; cloudy eyes; and neurologic abnormalities. Symptoms include pale gums, weakness, lethargy, vomiting, diarrhea, weight loss, anorexia, breathing difficulties, increased thirst, and neurologic abnormalities. FeLV can also produce proliferative disease of erythroid and myeloid cells.

Fibrosarcomas account for about 10% of all cat tumors. Feline sarcoma virus (FeSV) is believed to be responsible for only some of these fibrosarcomas and tends to produce the fibrosarcomas in young cats. The more common fibrosarcomas that occur in older cats are not associated with FeSV. The FeSV-induced fibrosarcomas are poorly differentiated and more invasive than non-FeSV-induced tumors.

ETIOLOGIC AGENT

Classification

Three subgroups of exogenous FeLV (A, B, and C) are distinguishable by viral interference tests and antibody neutralization tests. These two properties are associated with the envelope glycoprotein.

Feline sarcoma viruses (FeSV) are replication defective, highly oncogenic (acute transforming) viruses that have acquired an oncogene through recombination of the FeLV genome with one of several cellular oncogenes. FeSVs are thought to arise *de novo* in FeLV-infected cats and not to be naturally transmitted from cat to cat.

Cats also have endogenous feline retroviruses such as RD-114 that are transmitted genetically. Multiple copies of the RD-114 provirus are found in all cat cells. These endogenous viruses are not associated with any known feline disease.

Physical, Chemical, and Antigenic Properties

Morphologically, the feline retroviruses are typical mammalian Type C retroviruses. FeLV is composed of two envelope proteins, gp70 (SU) and p15E (TM), and three Gag proteins, p10 (NC), p15 (MA), and p27 (CA). The Gag proteins are produced in great excess in infected cells and are important in laboratory diagnosis.

Resistance to Physical and Chemical Agents

Like most enveloped viruses, FeLV is sensitive to inactivation by lipid solvents and detergents. FeLV is rapidly inactivated at 56°C, but only minimal inactivation occurs at 37°C for up to 48 hours in culture medium. The virus is rapidly inactivated by drying.

Infectivity for Other Species and Culture Systems

FeLV-A replicates exclusively in cat cells. FeLV-B and FeLV-C replicate in a variety of cell types, including human cells. The host range specificity of FeLV is associated with the envelope glycoprotein, gp70. No relationship has been shown between FeLV and human disease, and there is no evidence that FeLV disease is transmissible to humans.

Since the much rarer sarcoma virus, FeSV, is defective, the host range of this virus is dependent upon the helper leukemia virus that supplies the protein for its envelope. Most experimental studies have been conducted with the FeSV (FeLV-B) pseudotype. FeSV can transform fibroblasts from nonfeline species including dog, mouse, guinea pig, rat, mink, sheep, monkey, rabbit, and human. FeSV has been found to be oncogenic in many of the animal species tested. In general, sarcomas induced by FeSV in nonfeline species are regressor tumors and fetal or newborn animals are required to demonstrate oncogenesis.

HOST–VIRUS RELATIONSHIP

Distribution, Reservoir, and Transmission

Feline leukemia virus infection is worldwide in distribution. The only reservoir for FeLV is the infected cat. About 2% of the cats in the United States are seropositive, indicating either past or current infection. About half of the seropositive cats are positive for FeLV antigens by immunofluorescent antibody test (IFA) of their peripheral blood leukocytes, indicating current infection. FeLV-A occurs in infected cats either alone (50%) or in combination with FeLV-B or FeLV-C.

FeLV is excreted in saliva and tears and possibly the urine of infected cats. Transmission appears to occur during close contact via biting or licking (grooming). It is possible that infection may occur via contaminated feeding dishes. Prolonged, extensive cat-to-cat contact is required for efficient spread. In environments with multiple cats, the presence of one infected cat greatly increases the risk of infection for other cats. FeLV is also transmitted congenitally, and most kittens exposed in utero or before 8 weeks of age become persistently viremic.

Pathogenesis and Pathology

Upon penetrating the oral, ocular, or nasal membranes, the FeLV replicates in lymphocytes in the local lymph nodes of the head and neck. Acute FeLV disease, manifested by fever, lymphadenopathy, and malaise, develops 2 to 4 weeks after infection; however, these signs are seldom conspicuous. In about one-half of infected cats, the animals recover quickly and become FeLV antibody positive, FeLV antigen negative. Some of these cats have probably cleared the virus and in some the virus remains latent. The long-term significance of latent FeLV infection has not been determined, and FeLV-viremia may be reactivated under conditions of stress or corticosteroid therapy in some of these cats.

In cats that do not mount an adequate immune response, the FeLV replicates in the rapidly dividing cells of the bone marrow. These cats are persistently infected with FeLV and are positive for FeLV antigen by the IFA test in peripheral blood leukocytes. The cycle of infection is complete after viral replication in epithelial cells of the salivary glands, where infectious FeLV is shed in the saliva.

The time from the onset of viremia to the appearance of the later signs of FeLV infection is termed the *induction period*. This period ranges from 2 to 52 months, with an average of about 2 years. Most persistently viremic cats die within 3.5 years of infection.

Overall, the most frequent clinical manifestation of persistent FeLV infection is severe immune deficiency, with secondary opportunistic infections. It is characterized by a drastic reduction in the total number of lymphocytes and neutrophils. Immune cell dysfunction can be demonstrated as reduced T cell blastogenic responsiveness and impaired antibody production, and even FeLV-infected healthy cats have immune cell alterations when compared with uninfected cats. This manifestation of persistent FeLV infection has been termed *Feline Acquired Immune Deficiency Syndrome (FAIDS)*. Care must be taken with this terminology because the term *FAIDS* is also used for the syndrome caused by feline immunodeficiency virus (FIV), which is a different retrovirus.

Lymphoid tumors are relatively common in cats and are probably almost exclusively caused by FeLV. Most feline lymphosarcoma are T-cell tumors. Only a minority of cases of feline leukemia are true lymphoid leukemia characterized by absolute peripheral blood lymphocytosis. FeLV can also cause a variety of other myeloid proliferative disorders, in addition to myeloid blastopenic diseases.

Host Response to Infection

About half of FeLV-infected cats produce protective amounts of neutralizing antibodies to the major envelope glycoproteins while FeLV is confined to cells of the local lymph nodes, and the virus is eliminated or remains latent. These cats do not become persistently infected with FeLV, and usually live out a normal life span.

The response to FeLV infection depends on the age of the cat, the dose of virus received, and probably other genetic and virologic factors. Kittens tend to respond poorly and have a significantly increased incidence of chronic viremia and viral-induced proliferative disease compared to older cats.

LABORATORY DIAGNOSIS

Because some cats are able to clear a FeLV infection, and many cats have been vaccinated against FeLV, tests for antibody to FeLV are of limited utility. The most useful tests for FeLV diagnosis detect FeLV antigens. An enzyme-linked immunosorbent assay (ELISA) is available for FeLV antigens in serum or saliva and is especially useful as a rapid screening method. An immunofluorescence antibody test (IFA) is used to detect FeLV antigens inside of infected cells. This assay is more complex to perform; however, if a cat has become IFA-positive, it is stronger evidence that the virus is replicating in the bone marrow and that the cat is persistently viremic.

TREATMENT AND CONTROL

Vaccines against FeLV are available, although their efficacy under field conditions is controversial. Current FeLV vaccines either contain the inactivated ("killed") whole virus or a subunit protein preparation of the virus. Kittens should be vaccinated twice starting at 9 to 10 weeks of age, with the second dose of the vaccine given 3 to 4 weeks later, and with annual booster vaccinations.

FeLV infection in catteries can be controlled by test and removal procedures and can be combined with FeLV vaccination, since vaccination will not interfere with the laboratory detection of FeLV antigen in infected cats.

A diagnosis of FeLV infection does not necessarily dictate euthanasia, since an FeLV-positive healthy cat may live for years. Since the cat is probably shedding virus that could infect other cats, however, precautions to reduce the chance of spreading the virus and contact with opportunistic pathogens should be instituted. Chemotherapy can extend the life of a cat with lymphosarcoma. Various antiviral compounds including interferon have also been used to treat cats with FeLV infection.

SIMIAN TYPE D RETROVIRUS

DISEASE

Simian Type D retrovirus (Simian AIDS-related virus, SRV) produces a fatal immunosuppressive disease in monkeys. Infected animals show an initial generalized lymphadenopathy and splenomegaly accompanied by fever, weight loss, diarrhea, anemia, lymphopenia, granulocytopenia, and thrombocytopenia. Profoundly immunosuppressed animals subsequently become infected by opportunistic pathogens, the most common of which is disseminated cytomegalovirus (CMV).

ETIOLOGIC AGENT

Classification

Primate retroviruses can be found in four distinct genera: 1) the simian type D retrovirus (SRV), 2) the HTLV/BLV genus, which includes the simian T-lymphotropic viruses (STLV) and human T-lymphotropic viruses (HTLV), 3) the primate lentiviruses comprised of the human immunodeficiency viruses Types 1 and 2 (HIV-1 and HIV-2) and the simian immunodeficiency viruses (SIV), and 4) the simian and human spumaviruses. Although SRV is in a separate genus from the primate lentiviruses (HIV and SIV) that cause acquired immunodeficiency in humans (AIDS) and simians (SAIDS), many aspects of the immunodeficiency and associated opportunistic infections are similar.

The Mason-Pfizer monkey virus (MPMV) was the original SRV to be isolated. SRV is currently subclassified into 5 subgroups based on serology (SRV 1–5). MPMV belongs to the SRV-3 subgroup.

Physical, Chemical, and Antigenic Properties

SRV is a Type D retrovirus. The Type D viruses are characterized by the formation of cytoplasmic Type A precursor core particles. Mature Type D viruses are pleomorphic in shape, spheroid, enveloped, and 80 nm to 100 nm in diameter. The nucleocapsid is isometric to spherical with an asymmetric, spherical nucleoid.

The RT of SRV has a preference for Mg^{2+} and uses $tRNA^{Lys}$ as a primer for negative-strand DNA reverse transcription.

SRV consists of at least five serotypes based on neutralization properties of the envelope.

Infectivity for Other Species and Culture Systems

SRV infects several species of monkeys. Serologic surveys have shown no conclusive evidence of SRV infection in animal handlers who work with monkeys.

SRV isolates replicate in both T and B lymphocytes and in macrophages. Various human and monkey cell lines of T and B cell, macrophage, and fibroblast origin support the growth of SRV. SRV induces syncytia in Raji cells, which can be used as a method to quantitate the virus.

A human counterpart of SRV — a human Type D retrovirus — has been reported. The distribution and clinical significance of this virus remains to be determined, as does its relationship to SRV.

HOST–VIRUS RELATIONSHIP

Distribution, Reservoir, and Transmission

SRV is indigenous and widespread in Asian macaques but does not naturally infect African monkey species. In one study, about 25% of captive macaques in U.S. primate centers were seropositive; however, the prevalence varies widely based on the location and the species studied.

SRV is transmitted primarily in the saliva by biting. Mortality has been estimated to be 30% to 50%, and often occurs at an early age. Inapparent carriers that are viremic but antibody negative may be an important reservoir for SRV.

Pathogenesis and Pathology

SRV infects both T and B lymphocytes in vivo and causes a profound depletion of both of these kinds of lymphocytes leading to fatal immunosuppressive disease. The absolute lymphocyte count decreases but the CD4/CD8 (helper lymphocyte to suppressor lymphocyte) ratio remains relatively stable. In the lymph nodes there is a depletion of lymphocytes and an absence of plasma cells. SRV also infects macrophages, but not granulocytes.

Host Response to Infection

Some infected monkeys die acutely 7 to 20 weeks after experimental inoculation, whereas some remain persistently infected, and some develop neutralizing antibody and become nonviremic and remain healthy.

LABORATORY DIAGNOSIS

Serologic screening methods include ELISA and Western immunoblots. Because infected monkeys may be seronegative, however, it is necessary to include virus culture as part of the screening process. Techniques based on antigen capture and polymerase chain reaction (PCR) have also been developed.

TREATMENT AND CONTROL

It is important to establish and maintain specific retrovirus-free breeding colonies, both for animal health as well as improving the quality of nonhuman primates used in biomedical research and, in the future, transplantation. A serial test and removal program can eliminate SRV infection in group-housed monkeys.

Vaccines against SRV have demonstrated effectiveness under experimental conditions.

AVIAN LEUKOSIS/SARCOMA COMPLEX

DISEASE

The avian leukosis/sarcoma complex of viruses (ALSV) induce a wide variety of diseases in chickens. These have been of great economic importance to the poultry industry, as well as being important research tools for the understanding of cancer. These diseases include lymphoid leukosis, erythroblastosis, myeloblastosis, myelocytomatoses, sarcomas, osteopetrosis, hemangiomas, and nephroblastoma. The signs of disease produced by the ALSVs are not specific, and differential diagnosis requires careful histopathologic examination and laboratory testing.

In lymphoid leukosis, the most common and economically important disease caused by ALSVs, the comb may be pale, shriveled, and occasionally cyanotic. Inappetence, emaciation, and weakness occur frequently. Enlargement of the liver, bursa of Fabricius, kidneys, and the nodular nature of the tumors can sometimes be detected on palpation.

ALSV also causes sporadic cases of nonlymphoid tumors, such as erythroblastosis, myeloblastosis, and myelocytomatoses. Clinical signs of these diseases include lethargy, general weakness, and slight paleness or cyanosis of the comb. In more advanced disease, weakness, emaciation, diarrhea, and occasionally profuse hemorrhage from feather follicles are observed.

Osteopetrosis, in which the long bones of the limbs are commonly affected, is also caused by ALSV. Thickening of the diaphyseal or metaphyseal region can be detected by inspection or palpation. Affected chickens are usually stunted, pale, and walk with a stilted gait or limp.

Reticuloendotheliosis virus (REV) is a retrovirus found in chickens and turkeys that is unrelated to the viruses of the leukosis/sarcoma group. REV is actually classified in the genus of mammalian Type C retroviruses based on nucleic acid homology and biochemical properties. REV causes neoplastic disease and nonneoplastic runting in several species of poultry.

ETIOLOGIC AGENT

Classification

ALSVs are classified into five subgroups, A to E, on the basis of differences in their viral envelope glycoprotein antigens that determine virus-serum neutralization properties and viral interference patterns with members of the same or different subgroups. Subgroup E viruses include ubiquitous endogenous leukemia viruses of low pathogenicity. Additional subgroups (F, G, H, I) comprise retroviruses from pheasants, quail, and partridges and have antigenic properties and host range distinct from that of the viruses in subgroups A to E.

It is important to note that many of the highly onco-genic avian type C retroviruses that are used in research studies are defective and require a helper virus to repli-cate. These viruses are packaged as pseudotypes using the envelope proteins of a helper virus. They therefore take on the interference and neutralization properties of their helper virus.

Physical, Chemical, and Antigenic Properties

In size, shape, and ultrastructural characteristics, viruses of the avian leukosis/sarcoma complex are Type C retro-viruses and are indistinguishable from one another. ALSVs within a subgroup cross-neutralize to varying extents. Viruses of different subgroups do not cross-neutralize except for partial cross-neutralization between subgroups B and D.

Resistance to Physical and Chemical Agents

The infectivity of ALSVs is abolished by treatment with lipid solvents such as ether or detergents such as sodium dodecyl sulfate. The thermal inactivation half-life of avian oncoviruses at 37°C ranges from 100 to 540 minutes. These viruses are rapidly inactivated at higher temperatures; the half-life for Rous sarcoma virus (RSV) at 50°C is 8.5 minutes, and at 60°C is 0.7 minutes. Viruses of this group can be preserved for long periods at tem-peratures below −60°C. The stability of viruses of this group changes little between pH 5 and pH 9. Outside this range, however, inactivation rates are markedly increased.

Infectivity for Other Species and Culture Systems

ALSVs occur in chickens and have also been isolated from pheasants, quail, and partridges. More distantly related retroviruses occur in turkeys. Experimentally, some of the ALSVs have a wide host range, especially RSV. Some strains of RSV induce tumors in other species of birds and even mammals, including monkeys. In general, very young or immunologically tolerant animals are required.

The avian oncoviruses, like many retroviruses, are not cytocidal for the cells in which they replicate. In chicken embryo fibroblast cell culture, RSV and other highly oncogenic members of the ALSV group induce rapid transformation of cells characterized by alterations in cell growth properties and cell morphology. These cells pro-liferate to produce discrete colonies or foci of transformed cells within a few days. The number of transformed foci is inversely proportional to the viral dilution and can be used as a gauge of viral concentration. Various strains of sarcoma virus can induce transformation in mouse, rat, and hamster embryo fibroblasts, as well as in chickens.

Although members of the weakly oncogenic ALSV group induce neoplastic disease, they produce no obvious cytopathic effects or detectable levels of transformation in chicken fibroblast culture. Their presence is assessed by an immunofluorescence focus assay with type-specific chicken antisera or by their ability to induce resistance to

transformation by RSV. This resistance occurs when the glycoproteins (attachment sites) of an identical or related virus block the cell receptors for the superinfecting virus. Stocks of leukosis virus originally detected by interference with RSV are referred to as *resistance-inducing factor* (*RIF*) strains.

HOST–VIRUS RELATIONSHIP

Distribution, Reservoir, and Transmission

ALSVs occur naturally in chickens and most flocks of chickens worldwide harbor various strains of avian leuko-sis virus, except for those derived from specific pathogen-free (SPF) flocks. Even in infected flocks, the frequency of lymphoid tumors is typically low and mortality is usually 2% or less, although sometimes losses can be much higher. The reservoir host for ALSV is the infected chicken.

Transmission can be either vertical (from hen through egg) or horizontal. Vertically infected chicks are immu-nologically tolerant to the virus and fail to produce neutralizing antibodies, and remain viremic for life. Horizontal infection is through infected saliva and feces and is characterized by transitory viremia followed by the development of persistent antibodies. Tumors are more frequent in vertical than horizontal infections.

Endogenous leukosis viruses, such as those of sub-group E, are usually transmitted genetically in the germ cells in the form of a DNA provirus. Many of these endogenous ALSVs are defective, but some (RAV-O) are released in an infectious form and can be transmitted horizontally, although most chickens are genetically resistant to infection.

Pathogenesis and Pathology

ALSVs induce a wide variety of neoplasms. A critical issue in the understanding of the pathogenesis of the ALSVs is whether the particular ALSV in question carries an onco-gene or not. ALSVs containing a v-oncogene are highly oncogenic retroviruses, transform cells in culture, are usually defective, and are most often products of the research laboratory that only occur sporadically in nature, if at all. ALSV strains that contain a particular v-oncogene usually cause a rapid and relatively reproducible type of neoplastic disease in a high percentage of infected chickens.

In contrast, naturally occurring ALSVs are weakly oncogenic, cause disease by insertional oncogenesis, do not transform cells at detectable levels in culture, are usually not defective, and are naturally transmitted. The oncogenic spectrum of non-oncogene-containing strains of ALSVs tends to overlap, so that a given strain of ALSV can induce many kinds of tumors depending on other factors, such as the amount of virus, age and genotype of chicken, and route of infection. This is consistent with the concept of insertional oncogenesis for these viruses in which the ALSV infects and replicates in a variety of cell types but, in order to produce neoplastic transformation, must integrate near an appropriate cellular proto-oncogene.

Under natural conditions, the most common disease caused by ALSV is lymphoid leukosis. Transformation of lymphocytes occurs in the bursa of Fabricius, usually at a few months after infection. Because lymphomagenesis is a multistage process, some of these early tumors regress while others enlarge and initiate metastatic foci in other visceral organs. Grossly visible tumors, variable in size and organ distribution, almost always involve the liver (a synonym for lymphoid leukosis is big liver disease), spleen, and bursa of Fabricius. Tumors are soft, smooth, and glistening and are usually miliary or diffuse, but may be nodular, or a combination of these forms. These tumors are composed of large B lymphocytes with IgM on their surfaces. The cells have a poorly defined cytoplasmic membrane, basophilic cytoplasm, and vesicular nucleus with marginated and clumped chromatin. There are often no consistent or significant hematologic changes in circulating blood, and frank lymphoblastic leukemia is rare. Fully developed lymphoid leukosis occurs at about 4 months of age and older.

Erythroblastosis occurs sporadically in ALSV-infected chicken flocks. The liver and spleen are enlarged by a diffuse intravascular infiltration of proliferating erythroblasts. The bone marrow is full of proliferating erythroblasts. Chickens become anemic and thrombocytopenic. Blood smears show an erythroblastic leukemia. Induction of erythroblastosis by naturally occurring, slowly transforming ALSV involves activation of the cellular oncogene c-erbB by insertional oncogenesis. Highly oncogenic, laboratory strains of ALSV carry the v-form of this oncogene and are termed *avian erythroblastosis virus* (AEV). Some strains of AEV can kill chickens by erythroblastosis within a week after experimental infection.

Myeloblastosis is relatively uncommon under natural conditions and tends to occur in adult chickens. The target organ in this disease is bone marrow and the first neoplastic alteration is in the form of multiple foci of proliferating myeloblasts in extrasinusoidal areas. These grow rapidly and spill over into the sinusoids. This is followed by leukemia and invasion of other organs, especially liver, kidney, and spleen. Microscopic examination reveals massive intravascular and extravascular accumulations of myeloblasts with variable proportions of promyelocytes. The v-myb gene is carried by the highly oncogenic avian myeloblastosis virus (AMV) strains. These laboratory strains produce mortality a few weeks after experimental infection.

Myelocytomatosis is another form of leukosis that occurs sporadically in chickens. In this disease, tumors characteristically occur on the surface of bones in association with the periosteum and near cartilage, and at the costochondral junctions, posterior sternum, and cartilaginous bones of the mandible and nares. They consist of compact masses of uniform myelocytes. Earliest changes occur in bone marrow in which there is crowding of intersinuosidal spaces by myelocytes,

destruction of sinusoid walls, and eventual overgrowth of the bone marrow. Tumors may crowd through the bone and extend through the periosteum. The v-myc oncogene is carried by the highly oncogenic avian myelocytomatosis virus.

Various benign and malignant connective tissue tumors occur sporadically in chickens, and many are caused by ALSV. There are a number of laboratory strains of avian sarcoma virus (ASV), the most famous of which is Rous sarcoma virus (RSV). ASVs induce sarcomas (tumors of connective tissue), including fibrosarcoma and fibroma; myxosarcoma and myxoma; histiocyte sarcoma, osteoma, and osteogenic sarcoma; and chondrosarcoma. These highly oncogenic ASVs carry an oncogene such as src (in RSV), fps, ros, or yes.

It has recently been realized that infection with ALSV is important in its own right and is probably even more important economically than tumors. Compared with specific pathogen-free chickens, ALSV-infected chickens have poorer growth and egg production even in the absence of tumor formation. The pathologic mechanisms of the subclinical syndrome are still poorly understood.

Host Response to Infection

Chickens exposed to ALSV virus fall into four classes: 1) no viremia, no antibodies; 2) no viremia, antibody; 3) viremia, antibody; and 4) viremia, no antibody. Category 1 consists of chickens that are in specific pathogen-free flocks or are genetically resistant.

Most chickens are in category 2. Antibody persists throughout the life of the animal and is passed via the yolk to progeny chicks. In general, passive immunity provided by such antibodies lasts for 3 to 4 weeks in chicks. In addition to the neutralizing antibodies directed against the envelope proteins, antibodies are produced to the internal group-specific antigens (Gag proteins), which are nonneutralizing and nonprotective. Although virus-neutralizing antibodies restrict the amount of virus in the animal, they have little direct effect on tumor growth.

Few chickens occur in the third category, which may represent chickens that are in the process of clearing an acute infection with ALSV.

Most chickens in category 4 acquired the ALSV vertically when in the egg and are immunologically tolerant to the virus. Hens in category 4 transmit virus to a high proportion of their progeny through the egg.

Since there are multiple subgroups (A to D) that commonly occur in chicken flocks and are not cross-neutralized by antibody, the status of a chicken for one subgroup of ALSV is independent of other viral subgroups.

LABORATORY DIAGNOSIS

ALSV can usually be isolated from plasma, serum, tumor tissue, and albumin, or from the embryo of infected eggs.

Since ALSV is generally not cytopathogenic, complement fixation, fluorescent antibody, or radioimmunoassay (RIA) tests must be used to detect and identify the viruses in cell culture. An ELISA test is used for direct detection of egg albumen or vaginal swabs. These tests have been used directly on test material (egg albumin) or indirectly on the cell cultures used for viral isolation. All tests require a source of chicken embryos free from endogenous ALSV.

Another means of identifying virus is based on phenotypic mixing of viruses. Chicken fibroblast transformed with envelope-defective strains of RSV are nonproducers (NP) of infectious RSV. Superinfection of NP cultures by another ALSV acting as a helper virus results in production of infectious RSV, which produces transformed foci on susceptible chicken embryo fibroblast.

TREATMENT AND CONTROL

Attempts to produce vaccine and immunization have generally been unsuccessful. Moreover, congenitally infected chicks, which constitute the major source of virus and are most likely to develop neoplasms, are immunologically tolerant and cannot be immunized.

It is possible to eradicate ALSV from chickens by establishing breeder flocks that are free of exogenous ALSVs. Hens are selected that are negative for ALSV antigens in their eggs. The fertile eggs laid by the selected hens are hatched and the chicks reared in isolation in small groups. The birds without leukosis virus antigen or antibody are used as the breeders for a leukosis virus-free flock. The flock must then be maintained in isolation from untested chickens.

BOVINE LEUKEMIA VIRUS

DISEASE

Bovine leukemia virus (BLV) causes malignant neoplasia of the lymphoreticular system (enzootic bovine leukosis [EBL]). The tumor-bearing animals are usually older than 3 years with the peak of tumor incidence between 5 and 8 years. Affected cattle develop lymphosarcoma with enlarged and firm superficial lymph nodes. Subsequent progression is often rapid toward emaciation and death. Chronic bloating, lameness, and paralysis occur in some affected cattle because of pressures of tumor growth on esophagus and nerves, respectively.

Another manifestation of BLV infection is a persistent lymphocytosis and occurs in about 50% of BLV-infected animals after incubation periods of 3 months to several years.

In many animals there may be no clinical signs of disease, but a low-level persistent infection and immune response develops; these animals are referred to as *aleukemic.*

ETIOLOGIC AGENT

Classification

Because of its genome structure, nucleotide sequence, and size and amino acid sequence of the structural and nonstructural viral proteins, BLV has recently been grouped in a genus with the human T cell leukemia/lymphoma viruses (HTLV-I and HTLV-II), and the closely related simian T-lymphotropic viruses (STLV). These viruses can induce diseases with similar pathologies, characterized by low viremia, long latency period, and a lack of preferred proviral integration sites in the tumors (i.e., the provirus is not necessarily found near an oncogene).

Physical, Chemical, and Antigenic Properties

Morphologically, BLV resembles other Type C retroviruses. Antibody to gp51 is neutralizing.

Resistance to Physical and Chemical Agents

The infectivity of BLV is abolished by lipid solvents, periodate, phenol, trypsin, and formaldehyde. Infectivity is rapidly destroyed at 56°C but can be retained for prolonged periods at less than 50°C.

Infectivity for Other Species and Culture Systems

BLV has been shown to be infectious for several animal species other than cattle, including sheep, goats, and pigs. Under natural conditions, the oncogenic potential of BLV appears to be expressed only in cattle and sheep. Since there are no significant antigenic or genetic differences between bovine and ovine isolates, the agent designated *ovine leukemia virus* is regarded as a bovine leukemia infecting a heterologous host. BLV-induced lymphosarcoma of sheep does occur, but persistent lymphocytosis is not seen as it is in cattle.

BLV replicates in cell culture from a wide variety of species, including bovine, human, simian, canine, caprine, and equine cells. Although BLV replicates in human cells, humans are not known to be infected. Seroepidemic studies among high-risk humans (veterinarians, farmers, animal keepers, and slaughterhouse personnel) revealed no infections. BLV has not been associated with human neoplastic disease.

HOST–VIRUS RELATIONSHIP

Distribution, Reservoir, and Transmission

The geographic distribution of BLV is worldwide. The reservoir is infected cattle. Disease is directly related to BLV prevalence, which can vary widely. Approximately 25% of the dairy cattle in the United States are infected with BLV, leading to large economic losses due to death of cattle, condemnation at slaughter, and veterinary expenses. There are additional monetary losses due to increased exportation restrictions by foreign countries that halt export of BLV-positive cattle or semen from infected bulls.

BLV is transmitted horizontally under conditions of close contact. The virus is highly cell-associated, and transmission is by blood or tissue containing lymphocytes between animals, usually trauma, or by contaminated veterinary equipment. Bovine leukemia virus is easily transmitted into susceptible calves or sheep by as few as 2500 lymphocytes from infected animals. Experimental transmission has also been accomplished with milk and colostrum, both of which contain lymphoid cells. In utero transmission of BLV has been documented, but occurs with estimates of frequency ranging from 3% to 20%. The transmission of BLV by hematophagous flies and ticks has been demonstrated experimentally; however, field observations do not support a major role for such vectors.

Pathogenesis and Pathology

Most BLV infections are asymptomatic. Some cattle develop only a transient viremia without seroconversion, and after 3 to 4 months virus can no longer be isolated. About one-third of infected cattle may develop persistent lymphocytosis within 3 months to several years after infection. The development of leukosis is a rare manifestation of BLV infection (rate less than 1%) and generally takes many years to become evident. Distribution of the tumor is unpredictable, but blood is often not involved.

Both T-lymphocytes and B-lymphocytes can be infected with BLV. The tumors are composed of B-lymphocytes.

Host Response to Infection

Most BLV-infected cattle develop antibodies to BLV structural proteins. A greater response is usually detected to the glycosylated proteins gp51 and gp30 than to the internal proteins p24, p15, p12, and p10 and to the reverse transcriptase.

Antibodies to BLV are also detected in the milk and colostrum and are partially protective against infection of calves. Antibodies do not provide protection against tumor development in infected animals, however, and do not prevent the spread of infectious BLV by carriers.

LABORATORY DIAGNOSIS

A variety of serologic tests (agar gel immunodiffusion [AGID], immunofluorescence, and ELISA) that detect BLV-specific antibody can be used. AGID is the official test used by the U.S. Department of Agriculture (USDA) to test animals for export. The animal usually becomes seropositive 4 to 12 weeks after viral exposure. A seronegative test is useful to rule out BLV as the cause of a case of leukosis.

Infected lymphoid cells and free BLV induce syncytia in target cells. This property has been used as a method for quantitation of BLV and identification of BLV-infected animals.

TREATMENT AND CONTROL

Infection, once established, appears to be lifelong. There is no treatment for leukosis or BLV infection in individual animals. BLV can be eliminated from a herd by repeated serologic testing and removal of positive animals immediately.

Subunit vaccines based on recombinant DNA technology appear to be promising.

VISNA/MAEDI/PPV VIRUS AND CAPRINE ARTHRITIS–ENCEPHALITIS VIRUS

DISEASE

These viruses produce chronic progressive disease of sheep and goats. In sheep, the virus mainly affects lungs and udder (maedi and progressive pneumonia) and/or the central nervous system (visna). In goats, the disease occurs mainly as a subacute paralysis starting early in life.

Initial signs of visna consist of a slight aberration of gait, especially of the hindquarters, trembling of the lips, unnatural tilting of the head, and in rare instances, blindness. The symptoms progress to paresis or even total paralysis. Fever is absent. Unattended animals die of inanition, hence the name *visna*, which means "wasting" in Icelandic. Most animals survive 1 to 2 years, but some die within a few weeks. In experimentally infected sheep, the incubation period ranges from 2 months to over 10 years.

Early manifestations of maedi include progressive loss of condition accompanied by dyspnea. Eventually, breathing requires the use of accessory muscles and is accompanied by rhythmic jerks of the head. There is sometimes a dry cough, but no nasal discharge. The clinical phase is variable from a few months to several years. Animals with maedi often die from secondary acute bacterial pneumonia.

Caprine arthritis–encephalitis virus (CAEV) induces a complex disease syndrome in domestic goats characterized by progressive arthritis, leukoencephalomyelitis, and occasionally interstitial pneumonia.

ETIOLOGIC AGENT

Classification

The agent of visna/maedi/progressive pneumonia and the closely related organism of CAEV are lentiviruses. The name designations are largely historical and refer to the site of virus isolation or the predominant pathology in an individual animal.

Physical, Chemical, and Antigenic Properties

The virion is composed of four structural proteins designated gp135, p30, p16, and p14. Neutralization tests have shown that variations in virus strains occur during infection in individual animals. If an animal is inoculated with plaque-purified virus, many months later a virus can be isolated that cannot be neutralized by antiserum that neutralizes the inoculum strain. Both the inoculum strain and the variant strains can be isolated simultaneously, indicating that new strains do not replace parental virus. With time, neutralizing antibodies are produced to the new strains.

The RT of these viruses has a preference for Mg^{2+} and uses $tRNA^{Lys}$ as a primer for negative-strand DNA reverse transcription.

Visna/maedi/progressive pneumonia virus and CAEV show extensive cross-reaction by immunodiffusion assays involving the major structural protein.

Resistance to Physical and Chemical Agents

Lentiviruses are relatively resistant to ultraviolet irradiation. Infectivity is abolished by lipid solvents, periodate, phenol, trypsin, ribonuclease, formaldehyde, and low pH (less than 4.2). Infectivity is relatively stable at 0°C to 4°C in the presence of serum and can be preserved for months at −50°C. Infectivity is rapidly destroyed at 56°C. At 37°C, one-half of the infectivity is lost in 6 to 8 hours.

Infectivity for Other Species and Culture Systems

Visna and maedi have been described only in sheep and goats. Experimental transmission to other species has failed. Some breeds of sheep appear to be more susceptible, especially Icelandic sheep, which are highly inbred.

The visna virus infects cells derived from many vertebrate species but replicates efficiently only in sheep cells. Primary isolates replicate best in macrophage cultures.

HOST–VIRUS RELATIONSHIP

Distribution, Reservoir, and Transmission

These viruses cause disease in sheep and goats throughout the world. The frequency of infection varies widely based on control programs, but can range to greater than 75% in some flocks in the United States. Infected sheep serve as the reservoir.

Transmission is via respiratory exudates and aerosol. Virus is excreted in the milk, and lambs raised on infected ewes develop disease at a young age. Infection rates are increased by practices that pool milk. Intrauterine transmission is infrequent.

Pathogenesis and Pathology

Visna and maedi infect cells of the monocyte-macrophage system. In visna, characteristic pathology is the destruction of tissue in inflammatory foci found principally in the neuroparenchyma bordering the ventricles, in the choroid plexus, and in the meninges. The choroid plexus is constantly and most intensely involved.

In maedi, an interstitial pneumonia, the most remarkable change is a twofold to threefold increase in the weight of the lung. The histopathologic lesion consists of thickening of the interalveolar septa as a result of infiltration of lymphocytes, monocytes, and macrophages. The thickening may be so pronounced as to obliterate the alveoli. Lymphoid accumulations with the formation of follicles and germinal centers are scattered throughout the lung parenchyma.

Host Response to Infection

Most infections are subclinical. In disease, severe, chronic, ongoing inflammation is the hallmark of lesions in affected tissues. Lesions may result in part from the cellular immune response of the host and not directly from viral damage.

In experimental infections, complement-fixing antibodies appear a few weeks after inoculation, rise to a maximum within 2 months, and remain constant throughout the course of disease. Neutralizing antibodies appear later, reach a maximum at about 1 year, and then remain constant. However, the virus persists despite a vigorous humoral immune response, possibly because most infected cells are not producing viral antigens and are therefore undetectable by the immune surveillance mechanisms.

LABORATORY DIAGNOSIS

In its early stages, visna can be confused with other central nervous system (CNS) diseases such as abscesses, trauma, or parasitic diseases. Later, the progressive protracted course, the absence of fever, and the pleocytosis in the cerebrospinal fluid (CSF) are indicative of visna. Tremor of the head, grinding of teeth, and itching are characteristic of scrapie (caused by a prion) but not visna.

Virus can be isolated from CNS, lung, spleen, peripheral blood leukocytes, and CSF, but because of the limited viral replication that occurs in vivo, tissue explanation and blind passage are often required. Since complement-fixing antibody appears early and is maintained throughout the disease, complement fixation is favored over serum neutralization for serologic diagnosis. Neutralization tests are of less value in diagnosis because they become positive much later in disease and are strain-specific. In addition, a variety of other serologic tests can be used to identify infected sheep and goats.

TREATMENT AND CONTROL

No effective vaccine currently exists and no useful therapeutic agents are available. Control of these viruses and their diseases is by serologic testing and the elimination of infected animals. Visna and maedi were eradicated in

Iceland as the result of a slaughter policy. Every animal in a flock where maedi or visna as recognized was killed. Restocking was from animals from a part of the island where the disease never had appeared. Between 1944 and 1965, it is estimated that 100,000 sheep died of visna or maedi and 650,000 sheep were killed in the eradication program.

Equine Infectious Anemia Virus

Disease

Equine infectious anemia virus (EIAV) causes a severe anemia in horses. The clinical presentation of EIA is highly variable. In the acute form, symptoms develop suddenly 7 to 21 days postinfection. Symptoms include fever, anorexia, thrombocytopenia, and severe anemia. There may also be profuse sweating and a serous discharge from the nose. Such attacks often last for 3 to 5 days, after which the animal appears to recover. Horses in the acute stage of the disease are still seronegative for EIA.

Subacute disease often follows the acute infection after a convalescence of 2 to 4 weeks. Acute symptoms are repeated along with weakness, edema, petechiae, lethargy, CNS depression, anemia, and ataxia. The animal again appears to recover and the cycle may then recur.

Chronic EIA is the classical presentation of "swamp fever." It is much the same as the subacute form but is milder and seldom leads to the death of the animal. The cycle of fever, weight loss, anorexia, and symptoms can recur six or more times. Each episode usually lasts 3 to 5 days, and the interval between cycles is irregular (weeks to months). The frequency and severity usually decrease after 6 to 8 episodes, usually within the first year. Most horses are then without symptoms but carry the virus for the remainder of their lives. EIA can be induced by stress or immunosuppressive drugs.

Foals exposed to EIAV have a high fatality rate, but generally the disease is not fatal. EIAV infection in most horses is either inapparent or a mild febrile episode. These horses remain asymptomatic but have antibody to the virus and are lifelong carriers of the virus. Asymptomatic but chronically viremic animals have been observed for periods in excess of 18 years.

Etiologic Agent

Classification

EIAV is a lentivirus, and was the first animal disease to be identified as caused by a filterable virus (1904).

Physical, Chemical, and Antigenic Properties

EIAV is composed of two envelope-encoded glycoproteins (gp 90 = SU and gp 45 = TM) and four major nonglyco-sylated proteins (p26 = CA, p15 = MA, p11 = NC, and p9). The p26 is the major core protein and demonstrates group specificity, while the envelope-associated glyco-proteins demonstrate hemagglutination activity and are type specific.

The EIAV genome is highly mutable. When the virus is placed under selective pressure by the host immune system, genomic point mutations produce novel new antigenic variants of the gp 45 and gp 90 envelope proteins. These antigenic variants cause EIA's characteristic episodic recurrence. In cell culture (where there is no immune selection), antigenic types remain stable and neutralizable by serum antibodies from the horse from which the virus was isolated. When introduced into a new horse, these same strains produce new antigenic viral variants that can no longer be neutralized by the original antibodies.

Resistance to Physical and Chemical Agents

EIAV is readily inactivated by common disinfectants that contain detergents. The virus is also inactivated by sodium hydroxide, sodium hypochlorite, most organic solvents, and chlorhexidine. EIAV heated in horse serum at 58°C for 30 minutes shows no infectivity for horses. However, at 25°C, EIAV remains infectious on hypodermic needles for 96 hours.

Infectivity for Other Species and Culture Systems

Horses, ponies, donkeys, and mules are susceptible to infection by EIAV. There is only one report of human infection, and no cases of EIA-like disease have been identified. Attempts to propagate the virus in lambs, mice, hamsters, guinea pigs, and rabbits have failed.

Primary isolates of EIAV can be propagated only in equine leukocyte cultures, where it grows in cells of the monocyte/macrophage lineage. Laboratory strains of EIAV can be propagated in a variety of cell lines from several species, including human fetal lung fibroblasts.

Host–Virus Relationship

Distribution, Reservoir, and Transmission

The distribution of EIAV is worldwide but is most prevalent in warm climates. In the United States, EIAV is most prevalent in the Southeast. Infection rates vary widely, but are probably on the order of 1% to 5% in the United States. Infection rates in some countries may be much higher.

Horses, donkeys, and mules are the only known reservoirs and natural hosts of the virus.

Mechanical inoculation of blood is considered the major mode of EIAV transmission. EIAV is naturally transmitted by hematophagous insects, especially deer and stable flies. EIAV does not replicate in the insect cells, but since 1 μL of blood can contain more than 10^3 horse infectious doses, individual flies can transmit the virus by simple mechanical transfer of infected blood. The transmission of EIAV via blood can also be through contaminated needles; thus it is important not to share needles or use unsterilized needles in veterinary procedures. Viral transmission to the nursing foal from a carrier mare is well documented. EIAV can also be transmitted in utero but this is probably rare.

Pathogenesis and Pathology

Acute EIA is related to massive viral replication. The primary cause of anemia is the reduced life span of red blood cells (RBCs) resulting from hemolysis and erythrophagocytosis by activated macrophages. A decrease in complement levels and the presence of complement-coated erythrocytes have been observed in EIAV-infected horses. Decreased erythropoiesis levels and defects in iron metabolism also contribute to anemia.

Microscopic lesions of EIA include degenerative changes in various organs, widespread hemorrhage, degeneration, and necrosis of lymphatic tissues, anemia, edema, and emaciation. Microscopic lesions include activation of the reticuloendothelial system in all lymphoid tissues, activation of Kupffer cells, and hemosiderin deposition in many organs. Immune complex-mediated glomerulonephritis and hepatic central necrosis are common. Granulomatous ependymitis, meningitis, choroiditis, subependymal encephalitis, and hydrocephalus are associated with ataxia.

Host Response to Infection

Horses infected with EIAV develop antibody titers within 45 days and antibody persists in the animals. Most animals become ELISA-positive within 12 days and AGID-positive within 24 days of infection.

LABORATORY DIAGNOSIS

Laboratory diagnosis depends on the detection of specific antibody using an agar gel immunodiffusion test (the Coggins test). A more sensitive ELISA test is also now available.

TREATMENT AND CONTROL

No specific treatments are available. Supportive therapy is the most important factor in recovery. Isoprinosine and ribovirine have been suggested as therapy, but no clinical data are available.

Affected animals should be either euthanized because the virus is contagious or physically isolated. Spread of EIAV can be reduced by control of stable flies and mosquitoes. Multiple use of hypodermic needles and transfusions from untested donors must be avoided.

Infected stallions should not be bred to seronegative mares, although the reverse need not be true. Uninfected foals can usually be obtained from positive mares and positive stallions if they are isolated from the infected mare and her milk.

A vaccine against EIAV is used in some countries (Cuba, China) but probably does not provide broad protection with variants of EIAV.

BOVINE IMMUNODEFICIENCY VIRUS

DISEASE

Infection with bovine immunodeficiency virus (BIV) is associated with immune dysregulation and chronic inflammation in cattle. Multiple organs can be affected after a prolonged period of clinical latency (months to years). Signs of the disease can include lethargy, mastitis, pneumonia, lymphadenopathy, and chronic dermatitis. When the brain is affected, disease is often accompanied by a substantial neuropathology.

ETIOLOGIC AGENT

Classification

BIV is a lentivirus that is not closely related to any other known lentivirus.

Physical, Chemical, and Antigenic Properties

The morphology and physical properties of BIV closely resemble those of other lentiviruses. BIV has an SU glycoprotein of 100 kd and a TM glycoprotein of 45 kd, and Gag proteins, MA, CA, and NC, of 16, 26, and 7 kd, respectively. BIV also produces several nonstructural proteins. The RT of BIV has a preference for Mg^{2+}.

Infectivity for Other Species and Culture Systems

Experimental infection of rabbits and sheep with BIV is possible, but these animals do not develop disease.

BIV can be cultured in cells from a variety of species, including bovine, rabbit, and canine, but not primates or human.

HOST–VIRUS RELATIONSHIP

Distribution, Reservoir, and Transmission

The distribution of BIV is probably worldwide. In the United States, the estimated prevalence of infected cattle is about 1% to 4%, although in some herds it might be higher than 50%. BIV infection is more common in the South. Herds infected with BIV are often also infected with BLV.

Pathogenesis and Pathology

The predominant cell type that is infected in vivo is cells of the monocyte/macrophage lineage.

Host Response to Infection

BIV infection in cattle results in a strong host antibody response. However, like most other lentiviruses, BIV induces a chronic lifelong infection. Most infections are probably subclinical.

LABORATORY DIAGNOSIS

Infected cattle can be detected by serologic tests for antibodies to BIV. BIV isolation from blood can also be used to detect infected animals.

TREATMENT AND CONTROL

There is no vaccine or treatment for BIV infection. The importance of BIV infection to the health of cattle has not been firmly established, but most infections appear to be without overt signs of disease.

FELINE IMMUNODEFICIENCY VIRUS

DISEASE

Feline immunodeficiency virus (FIV) infection of cats produces an acute fever and lymphadenopathy, followed by an asymptomatic carrier phase. In some cats, FIV disease progresses to a persistent generalized lymphadenopathy, secondary chronic infections of increasing severity, and ultimately profound immunodeficiency. Late stage signs of disease include weight loss, hematologic abnormalities, fever, chronic oral infections, persistent respiratory problems, and neurologic disorders.

Infection with FIV in cats has many characteristics in common with AIDS in humans, and FIV in cats is an important animal model for AIDS research.

ETIOLOGIC AGENT

Classification

FIV is a lentivirus that is not closely related to any other known lentivirus.

Physical, Chemical, and Antigenic Properties

The morphology and physical properties of FIV closely resemble those of other lentiviruses. FIV has an SU glycoprotein of 95 kd and a TM glycoprotein of 41 kd, and

Gag proteins, MA, CA, and NC, of 16, 27, and 10 kd, respectively. FIV also codes for several nonstructural proteins. The RT of FIV has a preference for Mg^{2+}.

Resistance to Physical and Chemical Agents

FIV is inactivated by appropriate concentrations of disinfectants such as chlorine, quaternary ammonium compounds, phenolic compounds, and alcohol. It survives at 60°C for only a few minutes.

Infectivity for Other Species and Culture Systems

FIV is a virus of cats. There is serologic evidence that FIV-like viruses infect wild *Felidae* in Africa (lions, cheetahs) and the Americas (puma, bobcats, jaguars).

FIV isolates replicate in primary cultures of feline mononuclear cultures stimulated to divide with mitogen and supplemented with IL-2 (T cell growth factor). Some isolates of FIV are also able to replicate in established feline cell lines. FIV does not replicate in nonfeline cell lines. There is no evidence of a link between FIV and any human disease, including AIDS.

HOST–VIRUS RELATIONSHIP

Distribution, Reservoir, and Transmission

FIV is endemic in cats throughout the world, with estimates of 0% to 12% of healthy cats and up to 44% of sick cats being seropositive to FIV.

FIV is shed in saliva and the most important route of transmission is probably through bites. Free-roaming male cats, which are most likely to fight, are most frequently infected with FIV. Casual, nonaggressive contact among cats does not appear to be an efficient route of spreading FIV. Sexual contact probably is not a primary means of spreading FIV. Transmission from an infected queen to her kittens can occur.

Cats remain infected with FIV for life, although the majority of cats probably have minimal disease problems.

Dual infection of FIV and FeLV is not uncommon. Cats infected with both FIV and FeLV appear to have a more severe disease course.

Pathogenesis and Pathology

There are no definitive gross or histologic changes in the tissues of FIV-infected cats, even in more advanced stages of disease. Following initial infection, the virus replicates in regional lymph nodes, then spreads to lymph nodes throughout the body, resulting in a generalized lymphadenopathy that eventually subsides. In most infected cats, the disease never progresses during the natural life of the animal. In some cats, however, there is lymphoid depletion and suppression of the immune system. In profoundly immunosuppressed cats, the pathology can vary greatly depending on the presence of secondary opportunistic infections.

FIV appears to infect both CD4+ lymphocytes and CD8+ lymphocytes, as well as macrophages in vivo. Many cats manifest an absolute decrease in the number of CD4+ lymphocytes with an inversion of the CD4/CD8 ratio.

Host Response to Infection

Infected cats respond with generally vigorous antibody responses and cell-mediated immune responses. These responses appear to be sufficient to limit the initial acute phase of infection in the cats. Like most lentiviruses, however, FIV is never eliminated. It probably produces various degrees of subclinical immune dysfunction in the majority of infected cats and clinically significant immunodeficiency and associated secondary infections in a minority of infected cats.

LABORATORY DIAGNOSIS

FIV infection is most easily diagnosed by detecting antibodies in the blood. Antibody to FIV can be detected using ELISA tests, Western immunoblots, and indirect fluorescent antibody (IFA). ELISA is often used as a first screening test, followed by Western blot as a confirmatory test.

FIV infection can also be diagnosed by virus isolation and PCR to detect FIV nucleic acid.

Young kittens may be antibody positive (and thus have a positive test result) without actually being infected with FIV due to passive transfer of FIV antibodies from a queen to her kittens.

TREATMENT AND CONTROL

Treatment of FIV-associated disease is largely supportive. Secondary and opportunistic infections are treated with appropriate antimicrobial therapy.

Control of FIV infection is by avoiding contact with stray cats and avoiding cat fights. Experimental vaccines appear promising.

SIMIAN IMMUNODEFICIENCY VIRUS

DISEASE

The simian immunodeficiency virus (SIV) comprises a number of lentiviruses indigenous in many simian species living in the wild in Africa. In their natural African simian hosts, these viruses apparently cause little or no disease. In contrast, the Asian macaques, which are not infected with SIV in the wild, are susceptible to a fatal immunosuppressive syndrome called *simian AIDS* (*SAIDS*) when infected by some strains of SIV.

SIV-infected macaques often develop a transient skin rash soon after infection. Lymph nodes and spleen may be initially enlarged. The architecture of lymph nodes becomes disrupted and eventually atrophies. The main clinical features of SAIDS in macaques are wasting and persistent diarrhea. Opportunistic infections occur and often persist in the immunocompromised monkey. Virtually all macaques infected with pathogenic SIV strains develop fatal SAIDS within 2 months to 3 years.

The fatal immunodeficiency disease caused by SIV in macaques is the major animal model for AIDS in humans. Further, an awareness of the biology of SIV is important for the occupational health of animal caretakers, technicians, and veterinarians who handle monkeys, as well as use of primates in biomedical research and medicine.

ETIOLOGIC AGENT

Classification

The primate lentiviruses exist as a broad continuum. For example, the prototype SIV isolate from macaques (designated SIVmac) is only about 50% related to HIV-1, but is 75% related to HIV-2 based on nucleic acid sequence. Other SIV isolates from chimpanzees (SIVcpz) are much more closely related to HIV-1 than to HIV-2. Further, some SIV isolates from other African primate species are even closer to HIV-2 than is SIVmac. Many isolates of SIV and HIV have been made and their nucleic acids sequenced and classified in phylogenetic trees of sequence relatedness in an effort to understand the origin of AIDS and the diversity and epidemiologic potentials of the primate lentiviruses.

Physical, Chemical, and Antigenic Properties

The morphology and physical properties of SIV closely resemble those of other lentiviruses. SIV has an SU glycoprotein of 120 kd and a TM glycoprotein of 32 kd, and Gag proteins, MA, CA, and NC, of 16, 28, and 8 kd, respectively. SIV also codes for several nonstructural proteins that function in regulation of viral expression and accessory functions.

The RT of SIV has a preference for Mg^{2+} and uses $tRNA^{Lys}$ as a primer for negative-strand DNA reverse transcription.

On the basis of seroepidemiologic data, as many as 30 distinct SIV strains may be harbored in their African monkey hosts. The prototype SIVmac strain is antigenically more closely related to HIV-2 than to HIV-1, in agreement with the sequence homology overall. SIV isolated from chimpanzees, SIVcpz, however, is more closely related to HIV-1 than to other SIV types.

Infectivity for Other Species and Culture Systems

SIV isolates replicate in primate (including human) lymphocyte cultures in stimulated cells that have a CD4 receptor. SIV isolates do not replicate in nonprimate cells.

Cross-species transmission of SIV to humans is possible and SIV has infected humans in laboratory accidents. HIV is able to infect chimpanzees, although it is not highly pathogenic.

HOST–VIRUS RELATIONSHIP

Distribution, Reservoir, and Transmission

SIV is carried as an apparently harmless infection in its natural hosts, species of African nonhuman primates (*Cercopithecus*, including African green monkeys, and *Cercocebus*, including sooty mangabeys). The prevalence of infection in both zoos and in the wild is variable, but can be over 50%. In macaques, in which the SIV is not found in nature, SIV produces a fatal immunodeficiency disease that has many features in common with AIDS.

Transmission of SIV is by biting and also by poor veterinary practices or intentionally by experimental protocol. Mother-to-infant and sexual transmission is thought to occur rather inefficiently in nature.

Pathogenesis and Pathology

Macaques in the initial stages of illness tend to have hyperplastic lymphoid tissues, whereas lymphoid depletion is frequent later in the disease. The types of lesions vary greatly depending on the presence of secondary infections and the stage of disease.

SIV persists in both macaques and its natural hosts despite a strong humoral and cellular immune response; however, fatal immunosuppression only ensues in macaques. Neutralization escape mutants arise and become the dominant phenotype. The kinetics of viral infection and alteration of CD4+ lymphocytes parallel those observed in human HIV-1 infection and provide reliable markers for disease progression.

Host Response to Infection

Infected monkeys generally respond with vigorous antibody responses and cell-mediated immune responses. These responses appear to be sufficient to limit the initial acute phase of SIV infection. Like most lentiviruses, however, SIV is never eliminated in either its natural hosts or in macaques. The reasons for the difference in pathogenesis between the natural African primates and the Asian macaques is not understood, but is the object of intense research.

LABORATORY DIAGNOSIS

SIV infection is most easily diagnosed by detecting antibodies in the blood. Antibody to SIV can be detected using indirect fluorescent antibody, Western blots, and ELISA tests. SIV infection can also be diagnosed by virus isolation, detection of viral antigen, and PCR to detect SIV nucleic acid.

TREATMENT AND CONTROL

Experimental vaccines and therapies are being evaluated as part of massive efforts in AIDS research and development.

SELECTED REFERENCES

Blacklaws BA, Bird P, Allen D, et al. Initial lentivirus-host interactions within lymph nodes: a study of maedi-visna virus infection in sheep. J Virol 1995;69:1400.

Clements JE, Zink MC. Molecular biology and pathogenesis of animal lentivirus infections. Clin Microbiol Rev 1996;9:100.

Coffin JM. Structure and classification of retroviruses. In: Levy JA, ed. The Retroviridae. New York: Plenum, 1992:19–49.

Darcel C. Lymphoid leukosis viruses, their recognition as "persistent" viruses and comparisons with certain other retroviruses of veterinary importance. Vet Res Commun 1996;20:83.

Gardner MB, Endres M, Barry P. The simian retroviruses SIV and SRV. In: Levy JA, ed. The Retroviridae. New York: Plenum, 1994:133–276.

Gonda MA. The lentiviruses of cattle. In: Levy JA, ed. The Retroviridae. New York: Plenum, 1994:83–109.

Hanson J, Hydbring E, Olsson K. A long term study of goats naturally infected with caprine arthritis–encephalitis virus. Acta Vet Scand 1996;37:31.

Hardy WD. Feline oncoretroviruses. In: Levy JA, ed. The Retroviridae. New York: Plenum, 1993:109–180.

Hofmann-Lehmann R, Holznagel E, Aubert A, et al. Recombinant FeLV vaccine: long-term protection and effect on course and outcome of FIV infection. Vet Immunol Immunopathol 1995;46:127.

Kettmann R, Burny A, Callebaut I, et al. Bovine leukemia virus. In: Levy JA, ed. The Retroviridae. New York: Plenum, 1994:39–81.

Lackner AA. Pathology of simian immunodeficiency virus induced disease. Curr Top Microbiol Immunol 1994;188:35.

Lerche NW, Yee JL, Jennings MB. Establishing specific retrovirus-free breeding colonies of macaques: an approach to primary screening and surveillance. Lab Anim Sci 1994;44:217.

Lichtenstein DL, Issel CJ, Montelaro RC. Genomic quasispecies associated with the initiation of infection and disease in ponies experimentally infected with equine infectious anemia virus. J Virol 1996;70:3346.

Montelaro RC, Ball JM, Rushlow KE. Equine retroviruses. In: Levy JA, ed. The Retroviridae. New York: Plenum, 1993:257–360.

Narayan O, Zink MC, Gorrell M, et al. The lentiviruses of sheep and goats. In: Levy JA, ed. The Retroviridae. New York: Plenum, 1993:229–255.

Payne LN. Biology of avian retroviruses. In: Levy JA, ed. The Retroviridae. New York: Plenum, 1992:299–404.

Pedersen NC. The feline immunodeficiency virus. In: Levy JA, ed. The Retroviridae. New York: Plenum, 1993:181–228.

Rasheed S. Retroviruses and oncogenes. In: Levy JA, ed. The Retroviridae. New York: Plenum, 1995:293–408.

Schwartz I, Levy D. Pathobiology of bovine leukemia virus. Vet Res 1994;25:521.

Snider T Jr, Luther DG, Jenny BF, et al. Encephalitis, lymphoid tissue depletion and secondary diseases associated with bovine immunodeficiency virus in a dairy herd. Comp Immunol Microbiol Infect Dis 1996;19:117.

75 Transmissible Spongiform Encephalopathies

Yuan Chung Zee

The transmissible spongiform encephalopathies (TSEs) are natural degenerative diseases of the central nervous system (CNS) that include Creutzfeldt–Jakob disease (CJD) and Gerstmann–Straussler syndrome (GSS) of humans, scrapie of sheep and goats, bovine spongiform encephalopathies of cattle, transmissible mink encephalopathy of mink, and chronic wasting disease of mule deer, elk, and antelope. The disease has also been reported in captive species of antelope in zoos and in domestic cats. Transmissible spongiform encephalopathies are progressive and invariably fatal diseases. The lesions are confined to the (CNS) and are characterized by neuronal vacuolation, reactive gliosis, and variable extracellular amyloid deposits. The causative agent for TSEs is yet to be definitively identified but most recent evidence indicates that prions play a major role in the disease (see Chapter 57).

SCRAPIE

DISEASE

Scrapie is an infectious neurologic disease of sheep and goats characterized by 1) a very long incubation period of 24 to 60 months, 2) a progressive and invariably fatal clinical course, 3) distinctive pathologic changes in the CNS, and 4) unique biochemical and biophysical properties of the infectious agent (prions). Clinical symptoms of scrapie are confined to the CNS; they include incoordination, pruritis, and paralysis.

ETIOLOGIC AGENT

The precise biophysical and biochemical nature of the scrapie agent is still uncertain. Available evidence indicates that the infectivity is associated with a sialoglycoprotein.

The scrapie agent is unusually resistant to heat, ultraviolet, and ionizing radiation as well as to disinfectants (e.g., formaldehyde, beta-propiolactone) and procedures that destroy nucleic acids. It is inactivated by most membrane-disrupting agents (e.g., phenol, Clorox, chloroform, urea).

In addition to sheep and goats, scrapie can be experimentally transmitted to hamsters, mice, ferrets, mink, and monkeys. It is not feasible at present to cultivate the scrapie agent in tissue culture.

HOST–VIRUS RELATIONSHIP

Scrapie is found throughout the world, with a few exceptions (e.g., Australia, New Zealand). The disease incidence is low in countries where the infection is known to exist. Adult sheep and goats are the natural reservoirs of the disease. The mode of transmission among animals is not known. Healthy sheep can develop scrapie when they are left on pastures that had been used by scrapie sheep but that were vacant for several years. The scrapie agent can be transmitted to laboratory animals by a number of routes of inoculation (e.g., intracerebral, intraperitoneal, intramuscular).

Pathologic lesions of scrapie are confined to the CNS. The most frequent feature of scrapie is the presence of neuronal vacuolation in the corpus striatum, cerebellar cortex, and brain stem. Amyloid plaques stained with Congo red dye are also a common occurrence in the brain of animals infected with the scrapie agent.

There is a lack of immunologic response throughout the course of scrapie disease. Antibodies to the scrapie protein have been produced by immunizing rabbits, but they do not neutralize the infectivity of the scrapie agent.

LABORATORY DIAGNOSIS

The diagnosis of scrapie is based on the histologic evidence of neuronal degeneration in the CNS. No laboratory test for scrapie is available at present.

TREATMENT AND CONTROL

There is no treatment or vaccine available for scrapie. Eradication of scrapie is by slaughtering all affected animals and by preventing contact between animals from different regions. Scrapie transmission in sheep may be prevented using embryo transfer, as experimental studies have shown that scrapie was not transmitted to the off-spring in the embryo or the uterus.

BOVINE SPONGIFORM ENCEPHALOPATHY

Bovine spongiform encephalopathy (BSE) or "mad cow disease" was first reported in Great Britain in 1986. Since then, a major epidemic of BSE affecting more than 160,000 cattle occurred in Great Britain and the disease has been reported in Northern Ireland and several European countries. The disease has a long incubation period and is presumably caused by a prion-like agent because of its unique characteristics. The infectious agent is extremely resistant to inactivation and may contain no nucleic acid. Some of the disease cases may be genetic in origin, but they are also transmissible.

Epidemiologic evidence indicates that BSE resulted from feed made of meat and bone meal prepared from rendered sheep and cattle offal. The onset of BSE in Great Britain appeared to coincide with the diminished use of hydrocarbon solvent in the rendering process of sheep offal allowing scrapie prions to pass into the meat and bone meal. The practice of feeding meat and bone meal from sheep and cattle offal has been banned in Great Britain since 1989 and in 1990 specified bovine offal was banned in pig and poultry feed. Now meat and bone meal is banned from all animal feed in Great Britain. This ban was prompted by the recent link between BSE and ten cases of a new form of Creutzfeldt–Jakob disease in young humans. Other European countries have banned the exportation of British beef and in Great Britain a ban on the consumption of British cattle more than 30 months of age has been imposed. Large scale culling of cattle in Great Britain has led to political and economic problems.

BSE has declined in cattle born subsequently, but more slowly than expected. Whether BSE will disappear with the ban on feeding animals rendered meat and bone meal remains to be seen.

Brain extracts from BSE cattle have produced disease in cattle, sheep, pigs, and mice after intracerebral inoculation. No laboratory diagnosis for BSE is available at the present time until the disease develops. Currently, BSE has not been detected in U.S. cattle. The U.S. Food and Drug Administration issued new rules on June 5, 1997, prohibiting the feeding of cattle and sheep offal to other cattle and sheep. However, the agency does allow pig, chicken, and horse remains to be used in animal feed. In addition, the agency does not prohibit the use of animals known to have TSEs such as sheep with scrapie for feeding to pigs or chickens. It would be a more appropriate practice for the U.S. government to institute a broad ban on the use of animal offal in animal feed.

SELECTED REFERENCES

Cohen FE, Pan KM, Huang Z, et al. Structural clues to prion replication. Science 1994;264:530.

Dealler SF, Lacey RW. Transmissible spongiform encephalopathies: the threat of BSE to man. Food Microbiol 1990;7: 253.

Hope J. The biology and molecular biology of scrapie-like diseases. Arch Virol 1993;7:201.

Parry HB. Scrapie disease in sheep. In: Oppenheimer DR, ed. Scrapie disease in sheep: historical, clinical, epidemiological, pathological and practical aspects of the natural disease. New York: Academic, 1983.

Prusiner SB. Molecular biology of prion diseases. Science 1991;252:1515.

Prusiner SB. The prion diseases. Sci Am 1995;272:48.

Wilesmith JW. An epidemiologist's view of bovine spongiform encephalopathy. Phil Trans R Soc Lond B 1994;343:357.

Index

Page numbers followed by f refer to figures; those followed by t refer to tables.

A

AAL-toxins, 276
Abortion
  in *Actinomyces* infection, 251
  in aflatoxin exposure, 275
  in *Arcanobacterium pyogenes* infection, 128
  in arteritis virus infection, equine, 428
  in *Aspergillus* infection, 266, 267
  in *Bacillus cereus* infection, 249
  in *Brucella* infection, 197, 198, 199, 200
  in *Campylobacter* infection, 193, 195
  in *Candida albicans* infection, 110
  in *Chlamydia* infection, 174, 175, 176
  in *Coxiella burnetii* infection, 292
  in *Ehrlichia* infection, 295
  in *Erysipelothrix* infection, 230
  in flavivirus infection and Japanese encephalitis, 388
  in *Flexispira rappini* infection, 97
  in herpes virus infection
    in cattle, 354
    in dogs, 358
    in horses, 351–352
    in pigs, 357, 358
  in *Leptospira* infection, 185, 187, 188
  in *Listeria* infection, 226, 227
  in *Mycobacterium* infection, 161
  in *Mycoplasma* infection of cattle, 168
  in orbivirus infection, 433
  in reproductive and respiratory syndrome virus infection of pigs, 429
  in *Salmonella* infection, 76
  virus isolation and identification in, 19t–20t
Abscess
  in anaerobic infection, 83–85
  in *Arcanobacterium pyogenes* infection, 128
  in *Corynebacterium pseudotuberculosis* infection, 130, 132
  in *Mycoplasma* infection, 166
  in *Staphylococcus* infection, 117, 118, 119
  in *Streptococcus* infection, 123, 124

Absidia, 268
Acholeplasma, 165, 166, 170, 171
Acne in *Corynebacterium pseudotuberculosis* infection, 130
Actidione in *Brucella* infection, 200
Actinobacillus, 141–143
  capsulatus, 141
  equuli, 141, 142
  lignieresii, 141, 142
  pleuropneumoniae, 141, 142, 143
  salpingitidis, 141
  seminis, 141, 142
  suis, 141, 142
Actinomyces, 250–253
  bovis, 250, 251
  characteristics of, 250, 251t
  hordeovulneris, 251
  israelii, 250, 251
  morphology and staining of, 250, 251f
  naeslundii, 251
  pyogenes, 127–129, 128f
  sulfur granules of, 251, 252, 252f
  viscosus, 250, 251
Actinomycetes, 250–255
  Actinomyces, 250–253
  Nocardia, 250, 253–255
Adenosine diphosphate-ribosylation, 5
Adenoviridae, 346–349
Adenovirus, 346–349
  diseases caused by, 346, 347t
  structure of, 346, 347f
    cubic symmetry in, 313, 314, 314f
Adherence
  of bacteria, 61
  of neutrophils, 8, 9f
Adhesin, bacterial, 4, 7, 64, 65
  of *Bordetella*, 148
  and colonization resistance, 4, 7
  of *Escherichia coli*, 4, 64, 65, 69, 70, 71
  and fibronectin receptors, 49
  mannose-resistant, 65, 70
  of *Pasteurella*, 135
  of *Salmonella*, 75, 76
  virulence-associated, 61, 65
Adsorption, selective, 61
Aegyptianella, 304, 305

pullorum, 305
Aerobic bacteria, 16
Aflatoxin, 274–275, 279
African heartwater disease, 296
African horsesickness virus, 433, 435–436
African swine fever virus, 340–342, 341f
Agar gel immunodiffusion test
  in *Mycobacterium paratuberculosis* infection, 107
  in viral infections, 26
    in avian species, 21t
    in mammalian species, 19t, 20t
Agglutination reaction, 61–63
AIDS
  feline, 448
  simian, 449, 459
Airborne infection, 4
Aleutian disease in mink, 337–338
Alimentary tract
  anaerobes in, 61–64, 62t–63t
  Aspergillus in, 267
  bovine, normal flora of, 62t
  Campylobacter in, 89–91, 192
  Candida albicans in, 109, 110, 111
  chicken, normal flora of, 62t
  Chlamydia in, 174, 175
  Clostridium perfringens in, 234, 235
  colonization resistance in, 4, 7, 49, 64
  coronavirus in
    bovine, 421, 422
    canine, 422–423
    equine, 427
    feline, 424–425
    in pigs, transmissible gastroenteritis in, 418–420
    in turkeys, enteritis in, 426–427
  direct smear of, 47
  dog, normal flora of, 63t
  enterococcus in, 61–64
  enterovirus in, in pigs, 374, 375
  Escherichia coli in, 69–74
  Helicobacter in, 93–98
  horse, normal flora of, 62t
  Listeria in, 226
  microbial flora of, 61–64
    regulation of population size, 63, 64

Alimentary tract (*continued*)
  Mycobacterium paratuberculosis in, 104, 105, 105f
  non-spore-forming obligate anaerobes in, 83–85
  normal flora of, 61–64
  orthoreovirus in, mammalian, 430, 431
  parvovirus in, in dogs, 334, 335–336
  pestivirus in, bovine diarrhea in, 390f, 390–392
  pig, normal flora of, 63t
  rinderpest virus in, 407
  rotavirus in, 436, 437
  Salmonella in, 75–79
  Shigella in, 80–82
  Streptococcus in, 123
  virus isolation and identification in, 18t–19t, 21t
  yeast in, 61–64
  Yersinia pseudotuberculosis in, 283
Allantoic fluid factors in *Brucella* infection, 198
Alpha toxin
  of *Clostridium perfringens*, 234, 234t
  of *Staphylococcus*, 115
Alphavirus, 385–387
Alternaria, toxins of, 276
Aminoglycosides, 36–37
  adverse effects of, 37
Amoxicillin in *Helicobacter* infection, 98
Amphotericin B, 43
Anaerobic bacteria, 16–17, 47
  in alimentary canal, 62t, 63, 63t
    antimicrobials affecting, 64
    non-spore-forming obligate, 83–85
  culture of, 16–17
Anaeroplasma, 165
Anaplasma, 304
  caudatum, 304
  centrale, 304
  marginale, 304–305, 305f
Anemia
  equine infectious, 456–457
  feline infectious, 305–306
  hemolytic, in *Leptospira* infection, 187
Anthrax, 246–248
Antibiotics, 28–43, 46–49, 321
  in *Actinobacillus* infection, 141, 143
  in *Actinomyces* infection, 252, 253
  in anaerobic infection, 85
  in *Arcanobacterium pyogenes* infection, 127, 129
  in *Arcobacter* infection, 91
  in *Bartonella* infection, 301
  in *Bordetella* infection, 148, 150
  in *Brucella* infection, 202
  in *Burkholderia* infection, 156, 157
  in *Campylobacter* infection, 91, 194, 195
  in *Chlamydia* infection, 175, 176
  and colonization resistance, 49, 64
  combinations of, 40
  in *Corynebacterium pseudotuberculosis* infection, 130, 132
  in *Dichelobacter nodosus* infection, 207, 208

discovery of, 28, 30
dosage of, 38, 39
duration of treatment with, 40
in *Erysipelothrix* infection, 229, 231
in *Escherichia coli* infection, 74
in *Haemophilus* infection, 147
in *Helicobacter* infection, 98
historical development of, 28, 29f, 30
indications for, 46–47, 47t
in *Leptospira* infection, 188
mechanisms of action, 28–38, 30f
minimum inhibitory concentration of, 38, 38t, 39
in *Mycobacterium* infection, 159, 163–164
  paratuberculosis, 107
  of skin, 209–210
in *Nocardia* infection, 255
in obligate anaerobic bacterial infections, non-spore-forming, 85
in *Pasteurella* infection, 136, 139
and postantibiotic effect, 39
in *Pseudomonas aeruginosa* infection, 101
ramifications of misuse, 47–49
rational use of, 46–47, 47t
resistance to, 38, 40–43, 48–49
in *Rhodococcus equi* infection, 132, 134
routes of administration, 39
in *Salmonella* infection, 78
selection of, 47
selective toxicity of, 28
in *Serpulina* infection, 87
in *Shigella* infection, 82
spectrum of action, 28
in *Staphylococcus* infection, 116, 119
in *Streptococcus* infection, 123, 125
susceptibility of pathogens to, 38
in *Taylorella equigenitalis* infection of horses, 204, 205
in urinary tract infection of dogs, 181, 181t
in *Yersinia enterocolitica* infection, 103
Antibodies, 11–13, 51
  cell mediated cytotoxicity dependent on, 12, 13
    in African swine fever, 342
  and virus interactions, 12–13, 329
  measurement of, 25
Antifungal drugs, 43
  in dermatophyte infections, 217–218
  systemic, 43
  topical, 43
Antigens, 11
  antibody response to, 11, 12f
Antimicrobial drugs, 28–44
  antibiotic, 28–43. *See also* Antibiotics
  antifungal, 43, 217–218
  antiviral, 43–44, 44t, 321
  resistance to. *See* Resistance to antimicrobials
Antitoxin, 56
  tetanus, 244
Antiviral drugs, 43–44, 44t, 321
  systemic, 44, 44t

topical, 44, 44t
Aphthovirus, 371–373, 372t
Aquabirnavirus, 439
Aquareovirus, 430, 431t, 437–438
Arachidonic acid, 5
Arcanobacterium pyogenes, 127–129, 128f
Arcobacter, 89–91, 192–195
  in alimentary tract, 89–91
  butzleri, 89, 90, 192
  cryaerophilus, 89, 192, 193
  in genital tract, 192–195
  nitrofigilis, 192
  skirrowii, 89, 192
Arteritis virus, equine, 428–429
Arterivirus, 418, 427–429
Arthritis
  in *Actinobacillus* infection, 141, 142
  in *Brucella* infection, 199
  in *Chlamydia* infection, 174, 175, 176
  in *Erysipelothrix* infection, 229, 230, 231
  in lentivirus infection of goats, 454, 455
  in *Mycoplasma* infection, 168, 169
  in orthoreovirus infection, avian, 432
Ascites, viral, 440
Aspergillus, 265–268
  clavatus, 266f
  deflectus, 267, 268
  flavus, 274
  fumigatus, 265, 266, 268
  parasiticus, 274
  terreus, 267, 268
  toxins of, 265, 274, 276, 278, 279
Asteroplasma, 165
Atrophic rhinitis, in pigs, 136t, 137–138, 149, 150
Attachment
  in bacterial infections, 4, 7
  in viral infections, 321
Attenuated vaccines, 53t, 53–54, 56
Aujesky's disease in herpes virus infection, 357–358
Avian conditions. *See* Birds
Avibirnavirus, 439
Avipoxvirus, 366t, 368

B
B cells, 11, 52
Bacillary angiomatosis, 299, 300, 301
Bacille Calmette-Guérin vaccine, 159, 162
Bacillus, 246–249
  anthracis, 246–248, 247f, 247t
  cereus, 246, 247t, 249
  piliformis, 239–240
Bacitracin
  in *Brucella* infection, 200
  in *Streptococcus* infection, 125
Bacteria
  aerobic, 16
  anaerobic. *See* Anaerobic bacteria
  and antibiotic drugs, 28–43, 46–49. *See also* Antibiotics
  antibody response to, 12
  attachment to host surfaces, 4, 7

cell wall synthesis in, antibiotics inhibiting, 28–32
endotoxins of, 5, 56, 65, 69
exotoxins of, 4–5, 56. *See also* Exotoxins
in genital tract, 190
Group EF-4, 139
host defenses against, 4
laboratory diagnosis of infection, 15–17
    and indications for antimicrobial drugs, 46–47
in normal flora, 7, 48–49
    of alimentary tract, 61–64
    antimicrobials affecting, 49
    of genital tract, 190
    of respiratory tract, 113–114
    of skin, 206
    of urinary tract, 178–179
phagocytosis of, 8, 10
resistance to antimicrobial drugs, 38, 40–43, 48–49
on skin, 206
susceptibility to antimicrobials, 38
in urinary tract, 178–183
vaccines against, 55–56
Bactericidal drugs, 28, 38
    in combination with bacteriostatic drugs, 40
Bacterin, 51, 56
Bacteriocins, 63
Bacteriostatic drugs, 28
    in combination with bactericidal drugs, 40
Bacteriuria in dogs, 180, 181
Bacteroides
    fragilis, 83, 84, 85
    nodosus, 207–208
Bartonella, 299–302
    bacilliformis, 299, 300
    clarridgeiae, 299, 300, 301
    doshiae, 299, 300
    elizabethae, 299
    grahamii, 299, 300
    henselae, 299, 300, 301, 302
    peromysci, 299, 300
    quintana, 299, 300, 301
    talpae, 299, 300
    taylorii, 299, 300
    vinsonii, 299, 300, 301
Basidiobolus, 270
BCG vaccine, 159, 162
Beach's form of Newcastle disease, 408
Beaudette's form of Newcastle disease, 408
Beta-lactam antibiotics, 28, 29, 30, 32
Beta-lactamase enzymes, 30, 31
Beta toxin
    of *Clostridium perfringens*, 234, 234t
    of *Staphylococcus*, 115
Bighead of sheep in *Clostridium novyi* infection, 236
Birds
    Actinobacillus in, 141
    adenovirus in, 349
    Aegyptianella in, 305
    aflatoxin sensitivity of, 275

alimentary canal microbial flora of, 62t
alphavirus in, 385, 386, 387
Aspergillus in, 266, 267, 267f, 268
avipoxvirus in, 368
Bordetella in, 148, 149, 150
Borrelia in, 287–289
bronchitis virus in, infectious, 425–426
bursal disease virus in, 439–440
Campylobacter in, 90
Candida albicans in, 109, 110, 111
Chlamydia in, 175, 176
Clostridium in
    botulinum, 242
    colinum, 240
    perfringens, 234
colibacillosis in, 72
coronavirus in
    and bronchitis, 425–426
    and enteritis of turkeys, 426–427
Cryptococcus neoformans in, 264, 265
enterovirus in, 375–377
    and encephalomyelitis, 376–377
    and hepatitis of ducks, 375–376
Erysipelothrix in, 229, 230, 231
erythroblastosis virus in, 452
flavivirus in, 388, 389
    and meningoencephalitis in turkeys, 387, 389
Haemophilus in, 144, 145, 146, 146t, 147
Helicobacter in, 93, 94t, 97
hepatitis in
    in adenovirus infection, 349
    in enterovirus infection of ducks, 375–376
    vibrionic, 97
herpes virus in, 361–363
    and laryngotracheitis, 362–363
    and Marek's disease, 361–362
Histoplasma capsulatum in, 260
influenza virus in, 400–401, 402
Microsporum in, 215t, 216t
Mycobacterium in, 158, 159, 162, 163, 164
Mycoplasma in, 166, 167t, 167–168, 170
    detection of, 171, 172
    treatment and control of, 172
myeloblastosis virus in, 452
myelocytomatosis virus in, 452
orthoreovirus in, 431f, 432–433
paramyxovirus and Newcastle disease in, 407–409
Pasteurella in, 135, 136, 136t, 137, 138, 139
Riemerella anatipestifer in, 153
Salmonella in, 77, 78–79
sarcoma virus in, 446, 452
    and leukosis complex, 450–453
Serpulina in, 86, 87
Staphylococcus in, 117, 119
Trichophyton in, 215t, 216t
virus isolation and identification in, 21t
    in embryonating chicken eggs, 22–23, 23f

Birnaviridae, 439–440
Bismuth subsalicylate in *Helicobacter* infection, 98
Black disease in *Clostridium novyi* infection, 236
Blackleg in *Clostridium chauvoei* infection, 238
Blastomyces, 256
    dermatitidis, 261–263, 262f
Bluetongue virus, 433–435
Border disease virus, 392–393
Bordetella, 148–150
    avium, 148, 149, 150
    bronchiseptica, 137, 139, 148, 149
    parapertussis, 148
    pertussis, 148
Borrelia, 287–289
    afzelii, 288
    anserina, 287–288
    burgdorferi, 287, 288–289
    coriaceae, 287
    garinii, 288
    theileri, 287, 288
Botryomycosis, 118
Botulism, 240–242
Bovine conditions. *See* Cattle
Bradsot disease in *Clostridium septicum* infection, 237
Braxy disease in *Clostridium septicum* infection, 237
Bronchitis virus, avian infectious, 425–426
Brucella, 196–202
    abortus, 196, 197, 198, 199
        immunologic aspects of, 200
        laboratory diagnosis of, 201
    canis, 196, 197, 198, 199
        immunologic aspects of, 200
        treatment and control of, 202
    melitensis, 196, 197, 198, 199
        immunologic aspects of, 200
        laboratory diagnosis of, 201
        treatment and control of, 202
    in milk, 201, 201f
    neotomae, 196, 197, 199
    ovis, 196, 197, 198f, 199
        immunologic aspects of, 200
        laboratory diagnosis of, 201
        treatment and control of, 202
    suis, 196, 197, 198, 199
        immunologic aspects of, 200
Bubonic plague, 282
Budding process in virus replication, 323f, 323–324, 413f
Buffalopox, 365, 366
Bumblefoot, 117
Burkholderia, 155–157
    mallei, 155–156
    pseudomallei, 155, 156–157
Bursal disease, infectious, 439–440, 440f

C
C-reactive protein, 8
Caliciviridae, 379–383
Calicivirus, 379–383
    structure of, 379, 380f

Camelpox, 365, 366
CAMP reaction
    in *Listeria* infection, 227, 227f
    in *Streptococcus* infection, 120, 122f,
        125
Campylobacter, 89–91, 192–195
    in alimentary tract, 89–91, 192
    coli, 89, 91
    concisus, 89
    descriptive features of, 89–90, 192
    ecology of, 90–91, 192–193
    fetus, 192, 194
        fetus, 192, 193, 194f
        venerealis, 192
    in genital tract, 192–195
    helveticus, 89, 90
    hyointestinalis, 89
    immunologic aspects of, 91, 193
    jejuni, 89, 90, 91, 192, 193
    laboratory diagnosis of, 91, 193–194
    lari, 89, 90
    mucosalis, 89
    sputorum, 192
    treatment of, 91, 194–195
    upsaliensis, 89, 90
Candida, 109–111
    albicans, 109–111
    chlamydospore of, 109, 110f, 111
    germ tube formation, 109, 110f
    laboratory diagnosis of, 111, 111f
Canine conditions. *See* Dogs
Capping in *Mycoplasma* infection, 170
Capripoxvirus, 366t, 368–369
Capsid, 311
Capsomeres, 311
Carbohydrates, viral, 317
Cardiovirus, 372t, 377
Cat scratch disease, 299, 300, 301
Catarrhal fever, malignant, in herpes
        virus infections, 356
Cats
    anemia in, infectious, 305–306
    Bartonella in, 300–301, 302
    Bordetella in, 149
    calicivirus in, 382–383
    Campylobacter in, 89, 90
    Candida albicans in, 111
    Chlamydia in, 175, 176, 176f
    Clostridium in
        difficile, 239
        perfringens, 234, 235
    coronavirus in, enteric, 424–425
    Cryptococcus neoformans in, 263, 264,
        265
    Haemobartonella felis in, 305–306,
        306f
    Helicobacter in, 93, 94t, 95, 96, 97, 98
    herpes virus in, 359–360
    Histoplasma capsulatum in, 259, 260
    immunodeficiency virus in, 458–459
    leukemia virus in, 447–449
    Microsporum in, 215, 215t, 216t, 217f,
        219
    Mycobacterium in, 161, 164, 209–210
        leprae, 209
    Mycobacterium lepraemurium in, 209
    Mycoplasma in, 167t, 169

Nocardia in, 253, 254
orthoreovirus in, 430
parvovirus and panleukopenia in,
        333–334
Pasteurella in, 136t, 138
peritonitis in, infectious, 423–424
Prototheca in, 270
rabies virus in, 412, 413, 414
    diagnosis of, 415
    treatment and control of, 415
respiratory syncytial virus in, 411
Salmonella in, 77
sarcoma virus in, 447–449
Sporothrix schenckii in, 220, 221f
Streptococcus in, 121t, 123
Trichophyton in, 215, 215t, 216t
urinary tract infections in, bacterial,
        182
Yersinia in
    pestis, 282, 283
    pseudotuberculosis, 283
Cattle
    Actinobacillus in, 142
    Actinomyces in, 251, 252
    adenovirus in, 348
    aflatoxin sensitivity of, 275
    alimentary canal microbial flora in,
        62t
    Anaplasma in, 304, 305
    aphthovirus and foot-and-mouth
        disease in, 371, 373
    Arcanobacterium pyogenes in, 128
    Arcobacter in, 89
    Aspergillus in, 266, 267, 268
    Bacillus in
        anthracis, 247, 248
        cereus, 249
    Borrelia in, 287, 288
    Brucella in, 197, 198, 199, 200
        diagnosis of, 200, 201
        treatment and control of, 202
    Campylobacter in, 91, 192–193,
        194–195
    Candida albicans in, 109, 110, 111
    Chlamydia in, 173, 175
    Clostridium in
        botulinum, 242
        chauvoei, 238–239
        haemolyticum, 236
        novyi, 236
        perfringens, 234
        septicum, 238
    Coccidioides immitis in, 256, 258
    coronavirus in, 419f, 421–422
    Corynebacterium in
        pseudotuberculosis, 129f, 130, 131
        renale, 182f, 182–183
    Cowdria ruminantium in, 296
    Cryptococcus neoformans in, 264
    Dermatophilus congolensis in, 211
    dicumarol exposure of, 278
    Ehrlichia in, 295, 296
    encephalopathy in, spongiform, 312,
        461, 462
    enterovirus in, 375
    ephemeral fever virus in, 417
    Escherichia coli in, 70

fescue toxicosis in, 277
footrot in, 208
Haemophilus in, 144, 145, 146, 146t
herpes virus in, 353–356
    herpesvirus-1, 354–355
    herpesvirus-2, 355–356
    herpesvirus-4, 356
    herpesvirus-5, 356
immunodeficiency virus in, 457–458
Leptospira in, 185, 186, 187
    diagnosis of, 188
    vaccination against, 188
leukemia virus in, 453–454
Listeria in, 226, 227
Moraxella in, 151, 152, 152f
Mycobacterium in, 159, 161, 162, 164
    paratuberculosis, 104, 105, 105f, 106
    and ulcerative lymphangitis, 210
Mycoplasma in, 166, 167, 167t, 168
    detection of, 171
    immune response to, 170
    mastitis from, 166, 168, 168f
    treatment and control of, 172
Nocardia in, 253, 254, 255
ochratoxin exposure of, 278
orbivirus in, 434, 435
    and bluetongue disease, 433, 434,
        435
papillomavirus in, 343–344
parainfluenza virus in, 409, 410–411
Pasteurella in, 136, 136t, 137, 137t,
        139
pestivirus in
    and border disease, 392, 393
    and diarrhea-mucosal disease, 390f,
        390–392
poxvirus in, 366–368, 369
Prototheca in, 270, 270f
pseudocowpox in, 367–368
Pseudomonas aeruginosa in, 100
rabies virus in, 412, 414
respiratory syncytial virus in, 411
rhinovirus in, 378
rinderpest virus in, 406, 407
rotavirus in, 431f, 436, 437
Salmonella in, 76, 77
shipping fever in, 137, 137t, 409,
        410–411
slaframine exposure of, 277
sporidesmin exposure of, 279
Staphylococcus in, 115, 117, 118, 119
Streptococcus in, 120, 121t, 123–124
Trichophyton in, 215, 215t, 216t
trichothecene mycotoxin exposure of,
        275
Ureaplasma in, 165
vesicular stomatitis virus in, 416–417
Yersinia pseudotuberculosis in, 283
zearalenone exposure of, 277
CD4 cells, 51, 52
    functions of, 13t
CD8 cells, 51, 52
    functions of, 13t
Cell membrane function, antibiotics
        affecting, 32–33
Cell wall synthesis, antibiotics affecting,
        28–32

Centrifugation techniques in viral purification, 319–320
Cephalosporins, 32
    adverse effects of, 32
    mechanism of action, 28, 29, 30, 32
Chemiluminescence, 8
Chemotaxis of neutrophils, 8, 10
Chickens
    alimentary canal microbial flora of, 62t
    bronchitis virus in, 425–426
    bursal disease virus in, 439–440
    and embryonated chicken eggs. *See* Embryonated chicken eggs
    enterovirus and encephalomyelitis in, 376–377
    herpes virus in, 361–363
        and laryngotracheitis, 362–363
        and Marek's disease, 361–362
    Microsporum in, 216t
    Mycobacterium in, 159
    Mycoplasma in, 167t, 167–168
    orthoreovirus in, 432–433
    paramyxovirus and Newcastle disease in, 407–409
    poxvirus in, 368
    Salmonella in, 78
    sarcoma virus in, 446
        and leukosis complex, 450–453
    Trichophyton in, 216t
Chlamydia, 173–176
    elementary bodies of, 173, 174, 174f
    pecorum, 173, 175
    pneumoniae, 173
    psittaci, 173, 174f, 175, 176
    staining of, 175, 176f
    structure and composition of, 173, 174f
    trachomatis, 173
Chlamydoconidium of *Candida albicans*, 109, 110f
Chlamydospore of *Candida albicans*, 109, 110f, 111
Chloramphenicol, 35–36
    adverse effects of, 36
Chloriridovirus, 340
Cholera
    hog virus, 393–395
    in *Pasteurella* infection of fowl, 138, 139
Chorodopoxviridae, 365–370
    genera of, 366t
Chromoblastomycosis, 222–223, 223f
Chromosomal mutations, antibiotic resistance in, 41, 48
Circulation, 13f, 13–14
    of lymphocytes, 13f, 13–14
Citrinin, 279
Claviceps
    paspali, 276
    purpurea, 277
Clindamycin, 37–38
Clostridium, 233–244
    botulinum, 233, 240–242
        types of, 241, 241t, 242
    chauvoei, 238–239
    colinum, 240

difficile, 239
haemolyticum, 236–237
novyi, 235–236
perfringens, 233–235
    types of, 234, 234t
piliforme, 239–240
septicum, 237–238
sordellii, 240
spiroforme, 240
tetani, 233, 242–244, 243f
Coagulase in *Staphylococcus* infections, 115, 117, 119
Coccidioides, 256
    immitis, 3, 256–259, 257f, 258f
Coccidioidomycosis, 256
Cold exposure, virus reactions to, 320
Colibacillosis of fowl, 72
Colonization, 7
    resistance to, 4, 7, 48–49, 61, 64
        antimicrobials affecting, 49, 64
        in respiratory tract, 113
        in *Salmonella* infection, 76, 77
        in *Shigella* infection, 80
Colostrum, 64, 72
Commensal, 3
Competitive exclusion of *Salmonella*, 77
Complement system, 7–8
    activation of, 5, 7–8, 12
    alternate pathway in, 8
    classical pathway in, 12
    fixation test in viral infections, 26
        in avian species, 21t
        in mammalian species, 18t, 19t, 20t
    in inflammatory response, 10
Conidiobolus, 270
Conjugation, antibiotic resistance in, 41, 48
Conjunctivitis
    in *Chlamydia* infection, 175
    in herpes virus infection
        in cats, 359, 360
        in cattle, 354, 355
Contagious ecthyma (sheep), 367
Coronaviridae, 418–429
    arterivirus, 418, 427–429
    coronavirus, 418–427
    torovirus, 418
Coronavirus, 418–427
    in birds, 425–427
    bovine, 419f, 421–422
    canine, 422–423
    diseases caused by, 418, 419t
    equine, 427
    feline, 423–425
    morphology of, 418, 419f
    in pigs, 418–421, 423
Corynebacterium
    cystidis, 183
    diphtheriae, 127
    pilosum, 183
    pseudotuberculosis, 127, 129–132
        inhibition of staphylococcal beta toxin, 129f, 131
        synergy with *Rhodococcus equi*, 130f, 131, 132
    renale, 127, 182f, 182–183

Coryza
    in *Bordetella* infection of turkeys, 149, 150
    in *Haemophilus* infection of fowl, 144, 145, 146, 147
Counterimmunoelectrophoresis in Aleutian disease of mink, 338
Cowdria ruminantium, 294, 296
Cowpox, 365, 366, 366f
Coxiella, 291–293, 292t
    burnetii, 291, 292, 292t, 293
Creutzfeldt-Jakob disease, 461, 462
Cryptococcus neoformans, 263f, 263–265
    var. *gattii*, 264
    var. *neoformans*, 264
Cultures
    of bacteria and fungi, 15–17
        Enterobacteriaceae, 67–68
        sample collection and transport for, 15
        technique in, 16
        of urinary tract, 180–181
    of viruses, 20–22, 318
        cytopathic effect in, 22, 22f, 318
Cystitis
    in cattle, 183
    in dogs, 181
Cytokines, 10, 11
Cytopathic effect, viral, 22, 22f, 318, 325
    in serum neutralization test, 25
Cytotoxic necrotizing factors of *Escherichia coli*, 69, 70
Cytotoxicity, antibody dependent cell mediated, 12, 13
    in African swine fever, 342

D
Deer, orbivirus in, 433, 434, 435
Defense mechanisms of host, 4, 7, 48–49, 63, 64
    in alimentary tract, 61, 63, 64
    antimicrobials affecting, 49, 64
    colonization resistance in. *See* Colonization, resistance to
    in genital tract, 190
    immune response in, 7–14
    in respiratory tract, 113–114
    in skin, 206
    in urinary tract, 178
Delta toxin of *Staphylococcus*, 115
Dengue fever, 387, 388
Deoxynivalenol (DON), 274, 275–276, 279
Dermatitis, in *Mycobacterium* infection of cats, 209
Dermatophilus congolensis, 211–212, 212f
Dermatophytes, 214–219
    descriptive features of, 214, 215t
    ecology of, 214–215, 215t
Detergents, virus reactions to, 320
Diacetoxyscirpenol (DAS), 275
Diagnostic procedures, 15–27
Diarrhea
    in *Campylobacter* infection, 89, 90, 91
    in *Clostridium* infection
        difficile, 239

Diarrhea (*continued*)
  perfringens, 234, 235
  piliforme, 239
  in coronavirus infection
    bovine, 421, 422
    canine, 422, 423
    feline, 424–425
  in *Escherichia coli* infection
    enterohemorrhagic, 72
    enterotoxigenic, 70–71, 73
    nonenterotoxigenic, 71–72
  in orthoreovirus infection,
      mammalian, 430, 431
  in parvovirus infection of dogs, 334,
      335
  in pestivirus infection, bovine, 390f,
      390–392
  in rinderpest virus infection, 407
  in rotavirus infection, 436, 437
  in *Salmonella* infection, 76, 77
  in *Serpulina* infection, 87
  in *Shigella* infection, 81
  in *Yersinia enterocolitica* infection, 103
Dichelobacter nodosus, 207f, 207–208
Dicumarol toxicosis, 278
Diffusion antimicrobial tests, 38
Dilution antimicrobial tests, 38
Dissemination of infection, 4
  viral, 328–329, 329f
Distemper
  canine, 328, 330f, 403–406
  phocine, 406
DNA
  in antibiotic resistance, 41, 48
  drugs inhibiting function of, 33–35
  probe techniques, 17, 24–25
    in *Mycobacterium paratuberculosis*
        infection, 107
  in vaccines, 52, 55
  in viruses, 311, 313t, 315, 316, 317
    and oncogenesis, 447
    in replication cycle, 321, 322
    restriction endonuclease cleavage
        site analysis of, 326, 326f
    retroviral, 443, 444f, 445–446
Dogs
  Actinomyces in, 251, 252
  adenovirus in, 346–348
    and hepatitis, 346–348
    type 1, 346–348
    type 2, 346, 348
  alimentary canal microbial flora of,
      63t
  Aspergillus in, 267, 268
  Bartonella in, 300, 301
  Blastomyces dermatitidis in, 261, 262,
      262f
  Bordetella in, 149, 150
  Borrelia in, 288
  Brucella in, 197, 198, 199, 200
    diagnosis of, 200, 201
    treatment and control of, 202
  Burkholderia in, 155, 156
  Campylobacter in, 89, 90
  Candida albicans in, 111
  Clostridium in
    difficile, 239

  perfringens, 234, 235
  Coccidioides immitis in, 256, 257f, 258
  coronavirus in, 422–423
  Cryptococcus neoformans in, 264, 265
  distemper virus in, 328, 330f, 403–406
  Ehrlichia in, 294–295, 296
  Erysipelothrix in, 230
  Haemophilus in, 146, 146t
  Helicobacter in, 95, 96, 97, 98
  herpes virus in, 358–359
  Histoplasma capsulatum in, 259, 260
  Leptospira in, 185, 186–187
  Microsporum in, 214, 215, 215t, 216t
  Mycobacterium in, 161, 162
  Mycoplasma in, 167t, 168–169
  Neorickettsia helminthoeca in, 297, 297f
  Nocardia in, 253, 253f, 254, 255
  orthoreovirus in, 430
  otitis externa in, 210f, 210–211
    in *Pseudomonas aeruginosa* infection,
        100, 210
    in *Staphylococcus* infection, 115,
        117, 118, 210
  papillomavirus in, 343, 345
  parainfluenza virus in, 409–410
  parvovirus in, 334–336, 335f
  Pasteurella in, 136t, 138
  Prototheca in, 270
  Pseudomonas in, 100, 182t
    aeruginosa, and otitis externa, 100,
        210
    in urinary tract, 179t, 182t
  rabies virus in, 412, 413, 414
    diagnosis of, 415
    treatment and control of, 415–416
  Rickettsia in, 292, 292t, 293
  Salmonella in, 77
  Serpulina in, 86, 87
  Staphylococcus in, 115, 117
    and otitis externa, 115, 117, 118,
        210
    in urinary tract, 179t, 181t
  Streptococcus in, 121t, 123, 124
  Trichophyton in, 215, 215t, 216t, 217f
  urinary tract in, 178–179
    bacterial infections of, 179t,
        179–181, 181t, 182t
Dosage of antimicrobials, 38, 39
Doxycycline in *Bartonella* infection, 301
Doyle's form of Newcastle disease, 408
Drugs
  antibiotic. *See* Antibiotics
  antifungal, 43, 217–218
  antiviral, 43–44, 44t, 321
  interactions between, 40
  resistance to, 38, 40–43. *See also*
      Resistance to antimicrobials
Ducks
  enterovirus hepatitis in, 375–376
  Riemerella anatipestifer in, 153
Dysentery
  in *Serpulina* infection, 86, 87
  in *Shigella* infection, 80, 81

E
Eastern equine encephalitis, 385–387

Eclipse period in virus replication, 321
Ecthyma, contagious, 367, 367f
Ectothrix, 215
Eczema, facial, in sporidesmin exposure,
      279
Edema
  in *Clostridium septicum* infection, 237
  in *Escherichia coli* infection of pigs, 72,
      73
Eggs, embryonated chicken. *See*
      Embryonated chicken eggs
Ehrlichia, 294–296
  bovis, 294, 296
  canis, 294–295
  chaffeensis, 294
  equi, 294, 295, 295f, 296
  ewingii, 294
  human granulocytic ehrlichiosis
      (HGE) agent, 294
  muris, 294
  ondiri, 294, 296
  ovina, 294, 296
  phagocytophila, 294, 295–296
  platys, 294, 295
  risticii, 294, 296
  sennetsu, 294, 296
Ehrlichieae, 294–297
Electron microscopy
  immune technique, 23–24
  virus identification in, 23–24, 318
    in mammalian species, 18t, 19t, 20t
Elementary bodies
  of *Chlamydia*, 173, 174, 174f
  of ehrlichiae, 294
Embryonated chicken eggs
  cultivation of viruses in, 318
  isolation of viruses in, 22–23, 23f
    in avian species, 21t
    in mammalian species, 18t, 19t, 20t
    in serum neutralization test, 25
Encephalitis
  in alphavirus infection, 385–387
  equine, 385–387
  in flavivirus infection, 387, 388–389
  Japanese, 387, 388–389
  in lentivirus infection of goats, 454,
      455
  in *Listeria* infection, 226, 227
Encephalomyelitis
  in *Chlamydia* infection of cattle, 175
  in coronavirus infection of pigs,
      420–421
  in distemper virus infection, canine,
      405
  in enterovirus infection of birds,
      376–377
Encephalomyocarditis virus, 377
Encephalopathy
  in mink, 312, 461
  spongiform, 461–462
    bovine, 312, 461, 462
Encephalosis virus, equine, 433, 436
Endocarditis
  in *Bartonella* infection, 299, 300, 301
  in *Erysipelothrix* infection, 229, 230
Endometritis in *Campylobacter* infection,
      193

Endomycotoxins, 274
Endonucleases, restriction, in analysis of viral DNA, 326, 326f
Endothrix, 215
Endotoxins, 5, 56, 65
    compared to exotoxins, 4, 5t
    of *Escherichia coli*, 69
    of fungus, 274
    of *Salmonella*, 76
Enteric tract. *See* Alimentary tract
Enteritis
    in *Campylobacter* infection, 89, 90, 91
    in *Clostridium* infection
        perfringens, 234, 235
        spiroforme, 240
    in coronavirus infection
        equine, 427
        of turkeys, 426–427
Enterobacteriaceae, 62t, 63t, 65–68
    cellular anatomy and composition of, 65, 66f
    cellular products of, 65, 66
    Escherichia coli, 69–74. *See also* *Escherichia coli*
    genera in, 65, 66t
    growth characteristics of, 66
    laboratory diagnosis of, 67–68
    overgrowth of, 64
    regulation of population size, 63
    resistance to antimicrobials, 66
        of *Escherichia coli*, 41–42, 74
    Salmonella, 75–79. *See also* *Salmonella*
    Shigella, 80–82. *See also* *Shigella*
    variability of, 66–67
    Yersinia, 102–103, 281–283. *See also* *Yersinia*
Enterococcus
    in alimentary canal, 62t, 63t
    faecalis, 124
    in urinary tract of dogs, 179t, 181t
Enterotoxins
    of *Clostridium perfringens*, 234, 235
    of *Escherichia coli*, 69–70, 73
    of *Salmonella*, 75
    of *Shigella*, 80, 81
    of *Staphylococcus*, 115
    of *Yersinia enterocolitica*, 102, 103
Enterovirus, 372t, 373–377
Entomobirnavirus, 439
Entomopoxviridae, 365
Enzyme-linked immunosorbent assay. *See* Immunosorbent assay, enzyme-linked
Enzymes, retroviral, 443–444
Eperythrozoon, 304, 305
    suis, 305
Ephemeral fever virus, bovine, 417
Epidermophyton, 214
    features of, 215t
    floccosum, 214
Epididymis, *Brucella* infection of, 198, 198f, 199
Equine conditions. *See* Horses
Ergot, 277–278
Erysipelas, 229–231
Erysipelothrix, 229–231
    rhusiopathiae, 229, 230, 231

tonsillarum, 229, 230, 231
Erythroblastosis, in avian leukosis/sarcoma complex of viruses infection, 450, 452
Erythromycin, 37
Escherichia coli, 3, 69–74
    adhesin of, 4, 64, 65, 69, 70, 71
    antimicrobial resistance of, 41–42, 74
    attaching and effacing strains, 71–72, 73
    cellular anatomy and composition of, 65, 66f, 69
    cellular products of, 69–70
    colibacillosis of fowl from, 72
    edema disease from, 72, 73
    enterohemorrhagic, 72
    enteropathogenic, 71–72, 73
    enterotoxigenic, 70–71, 73
    growth characteristics of, 66
    immunologic aspects of, 72
    invasive, 71, 71f, 73, 74
    laboratory diagnosis of, 67, 73
    nonenterotoxigenic, 71–72
    reservoir and transmission of, 70
    treatment and prevention of, 73–74
    in urinary tract infection of dogs, 179, 179t, 180, 181t
Ether susceptibility of viruses, 320
Eubacterium suis, 183
Exanthema
    equine coital, 353
    of swine, vesicular, in calicivirus infection, 379–380, 380f, 381f
Exfoliative toxins of *Staphylococcus*, 115, 117
Exochelins of *Mycobacterium paratuberculosis*, 104
Exomycotoxins, 274
Exotoxins, 4–5, 56, 65
    compared to endotoxins, 4, 5t
    of *Corynebacterium pseudotuberculosis*, 129, 130
    of fungus, 274
    of *Pseudomonas aeruginosa*, 100, 101
    of *Salmonella*, 75
    of *Streptococcus*, 120
Extravasation of neutrophils, 8

F
Farcy
    in *Burkholderia* infection, 155
    in *Nocardia* infection, 254
Fatty acid excretion by anaerobic bacteria, 64
Fc receptors, 8, 12
Feed, mycotoxins in, 274–279
Feline conditions. *See* Cats
Ferrets, *Helicobacter* infection in, 93, 94t, 95, 97, 98
Fescue foot, 277
Fibronectin, 4, 49, 64
Fibrosarcoma, in feline sarcoma virus infection, 447
Fimbriae, 61–63, 64, 65
    type 1, 63, 65
    virulence-associated, 65

Fish
    aflatoxin sensitivity of, 275
    aquareovirus in, 438
    lymphocystis disease virus in, 340
    pancreatic necrosis in, infectious, 439, 440
    Streptococcus in, 124
    Yersinia ruckeri in, 283
Flaviviridae, 387–395
    flavivirus, 387–389
    pestivirus, 390–395
Flavivirus, 387–389
Flexispira rappini, 94t, 97
Flora, microbial
    of alimentary tract, 61–64
    antimicrobials affecting, 49
    of genital tract, 190
    of respiratory tract, 113–114
    of skin, 206
    of urinary tract, 178–179
Florida horse leeches, 223
Fluconazole, 43
Flucytosine, 43
Fluoroquinolones, 33–34
Folliculitis in *Corynebacterium pseudotuberculosis* infection, 130
Foot-and-mouth disease in aphthovirus infection, 371–373
Footrot, 207–208, 211
Forages, mycotoxins in, 276–278
Formaldehyde, virus reactions to, 321
Fouls, and footrot of cattle, 208
Fowl. *See* Birds
Fowlpox, 368
Francisella tularensis, 285–286
Fumonisin, 276, 279
Fungi
    and antifungal drugs, 43, 217–218
    laboratory diagnosis of infection, 15–17
    mycotoxins of, 274–279
    in normal flora, 7
    in subcutaneous mycoses, 220–223
    in systemic or deep mycoses, 256–270
Fusarium
    moniliforme, 276
    proliferatum, 276
    roseum, 277
    semitectum, 278
    solani, 278
    toxins of, 274, 275, 276, 277, 278, 279
Fusobacterium necrophorum, 83, 207, 208

G
Gamma toxin of *Staphylococcus*, 115
Gastroenteritis in coronavirus infection
    in dogs, 422, 423
    in pigs, 418–420
Gastrointestinal tract. *See* Alimentary tract
Genetics
    in antibiotic resistance, 41, 48, 49
        to multiple drugs, 41, 48
    of *Escherichia coli*, 70, 71, 72, 73
    of *Salmonella*, 75, 76
    of *Serpulina*, 86

Genetics (*continued*)
  of *Shigella*, 80
  of viruses, 315–317, 325–326
    influenza, 396, 398
    and mapping of genomes, 324–325
    oncogenetic, 446–447
    in replication cycle, 321–324, 322t
    restriction endonuclease cleavage
      site analysis of, 326, 326f
    retroviral, 443, 446–447
    and vaccines, 53–54, 55
  of *Yersinia*, 281–282
Genital tract
  Actinobacillus in, 141, 142
  Arcobacter in, 192–195
  Brucella in, 197, 198, 199
  Campylobacter in, 192–195
  Candida albicans in, 109, 110, 111
  Chlamydia in, 173, 174
  Haemophilus in, 144, 146
  herpes virus in
    in cattle, 354, 356
    in dogs, 358, 359
    in horses, 353
  microbial flora in, 190
  Mycoplasma in, 168, 169
  reproductive and respiratory syndrome
    virus in, in pigs, 429
  Taylorella equigenitalis in, 204–205
  virus isolation and identification in,
    19t–20t
Gentamicin in *Chlamydia* infection,
    175
Getah virus, 385, 386, 387
Ghon complex in *Mycobacterium*
    infection, 161
Glanders, 155–156
Glässer's disease, 144, 145, 146
Glycoproteins, viral, 317
  of retroviruses, 443, 446
Goatpox, 368–369
Goats
  arthritis-encephalitis virus in, 454,
    455
  Brucella in, 197, 198–199
    diagnosis of, 201
    treatment and control of, 202
  Burkholderia in, 155, 156
  Campylobacter in, 192, 193, 194, 195
  Chlamydia in, 175
  Clostridium perfringens in, 234, 235
  Corynebacterium pseudotuberculosis in,
    130, 131, 132
  Dermatophilus congolensis in, 211
  ecthyma in, contagious, 367
  footrot in, 207–208
  herpes virus in, 357
  leukemia virus in, 453
  maedi virus in, 454–456
  Mycobacterium in, 161
    paratuberculosis, 105, 106f, 107
  Mycoplasma in, 166, 167, 167t, 169
    treatment and control of, 172
  Pasteurella in, 137
  pestivirus in, 391
    and border disease, 392
  poxvirus in, 368–369

  and ecthyma, contagious, 367
  scrapie in, 461–462
  visna virus in, 454–456
Gram stain, 16
Granuloma formation, 13
  in *Actinobacillus* infection, 142
  in *Mycobacterium* infection, 158, 159
    paratuberculosis, 104, 105
  in *Rhodococcus equi* infection, 132
Grasses, mycotoxins in, 276–278
Grease heel of horses, 211
Green beans, moldy, 278
Griseofulvin, 43
Group EF-4 bacteria, 139
Guinea pigs, *Burkholderia* in, 156

H
H-antigens
  of *Salmonella*, 75
  of *Yersinia enterocolitica*, 102
Haemobartonella, 304, 305–306
  felis, 305–306, 306f
Haemophilus, 144–147
  agni, 144, 146, 146t
  haemoglobinophilus, 145, 146, 146t
  influenzae, 144, 146t
  paragallinarum, 144, 145, 146, 146t
  parasuis, 144, 145–146, 146t, 400
  satellitism of, 144, 145f
  somnus, 144, 145, 146, 146t, 147
Hairy shakers, in pestivirus infection of
    sheep, 392
Hamsters
  Burkholderia in, 156
  Helicobacter in, 94t, 97, 98
Haverhill fever in *Streptobacillus
    moniliformis* infection, 290
Heat stability of viruses, 320
Hektoen enteric agar, 67
Helicobacter, 93–98
  bilis, 94t, 96, 97
  bizzozeronii, 93, 94t, 95, 96, 97
  canis, 94t, 96, 97, 98
  cholecystus, 94t, 97
  cinaedi, 94t, 97, 98
  diagnosis of, 93, 95, 95f
  felis, 93, 94t, 95, 96, 97
  fennelliae, 94t, 97
  heilmannii, 93, 94t, 95, 96, 97
  hepaticus, 94t, 96, 97, 98
  host sites of, 94t
  muridarum, 94t, 97
  mustelae, 93, 94t, 96, 97
  pametensis, 94t, 97
  pullorum, 93, 94t, 97, 98
  pylori, 93, 94t, 95, 96, 97, 98
  rodentium, 93, 94t, 97
  species of, 93, 94t
  suis, 94t, 97
  trogontum, 94t, 97
Hemadsorption in virus infections, 318
  assay of, 26
  in avian species, 21t
  in mammalian species, 19t, 20t
Hemagglutinating encephalomyelitis
    virus, 420–421

Hemagglutinins of viruses, 318
  influenza, 396
  inhibition test of, 25
    in avian species, 21t
    in mammalian species, 18t, 19t, 20t
Hemoglobinuria in *Clostridium
    haemolyticum* infection, 236,
    237
Hemolysins
  of *Escherichia coli*, 69, 70, 71
  of *Shigella*, 81
Hemolysis
  in *Streptococcus* infection, 120, 125
  synergistic, by *Corynebacterium
    pseudotuberculosis* and
    Rhodococcus equi, 130f, 131
Hemolytic anemia in *Leptospira*
    infection, 187
Hemolytic uremic syndrome, 72
Hemorrhage in *Leptospira* infection, 187
Hemorrhagic disease
  in calicivirus infection of rabbits, 383
  in orbivirus infection, 433–435
  virus isolation and identification in,
    20t, 21t
Hepatitis
  in adenovirus infection
    of birds, 349
    of dogs, 346–348
  in birds
    in adenovirus infection, 349
    in enterovirus infection of ducks,
      375–376
    vibrionic, 97
Herpesviridae, 350–363
Herpes virus, 350–363
  in birds, 361–363
  in cats, 359–360
  in cattle, 353–356
  in dogs, 358–359
  in goats, 357
  in horses, 350–353
  in monkeys, 360–361
  in pigs, 357–358
  in sheep, 356–357
  structure of, 350, 351f
Herpesvirus-1
  alcephaline, 356
  bovine, 354–355
  caprine, 357
  cercopithecine, 360–361
  equine, 351–352
  feline, 359–360
  gallid, 362–363
  ovine, 356
Herpesvirus-2
  alcephaline, 356
  bovine, 355–356
  equine, 352–353
  gallid, 361
  ovine, 356–357
Herpesvirus-3
  equine, 353
  gallid, 361
Herpesvirus-4
  bovine, 356
  equine, 353

Herpesvirus-5
  bovine, 356
  equine, 353
Herpesvirus B, simian, 360–361
Histocompatibility complex, major, 11
  class I, 11, 13, 51, 52
  class II, 11, 51–52
  restriction process, 11
Histophilus ovis, 144, 145, 146, 146t
Histoplasma, 256
  capsulatum, 259f, 259–261, 261f
    var. *capsulatum*, 222, 259–261
    var. *farciminosum*, 221–222
Hitchner's form of Newcastle disease,
    408
Horsepox, 130, 365, 366
Horses
  Actinobacillus in, 141, 142, 143
  Actinomyces in, 251
  adenovirus in, 348–349
  alimentary canal microbial flora of, 62t
  alphavirus and encephalitis in,
      385–387
  anemia in, infectious, 456–457
  arteritis virus in, 428–429
  Aspergillus in, 267, 268
  Bacillus anthracis in, 247, 248
  Borrelia in, 287, 288
  Brucella in, 197, 199
  Burkholderia in, 155, 156
  Candida albicans in, 110
  Clostridium in
    botulinum, 240, 242
    difficile, 239
    sordellii, 240
    tetani, 242, 243, 244
  coronavirus in, 427
  Corynebacterium pseudotuberculosis in,
      129f, 130, 131, 132
  Dermatophilus congolensis in, 211, 212f
  Ehrlichia in, 295, 295f, 296
  exanthema in, coital, 353
  fescue toxicosis in, 277
  flavivirus and Japanese encephalitis in,
      388
  fumonisin toxicosis in, 276
  herpes virus in, 350–353
    herpesvirus-1, 351–352
    herpesvirus-2, 352–353
    herpesvirus-3, 353
    herpesvirus-4, 353
    herpesvirus-5, 353
  Histoplasma capsulatum in, 221–222
  influenza virus in, 398–399
  Leptospira in, 185, 186, 187
  Listeria in, 225, 226
  Microsporum in, 215, 215t, 216t
  Mycobacterium in, 161
  Mycoplasma in, 167t, 169
  Nocardia in, 253, 254
  orbivirus in
    and African horsesickness, 433,
        435–436
    and encephalosis, 436
  papillomavirus in, 343, 344f, 344–345
  Pasteurella in, 136t, 138
  Potomac fever in, 296

Pseudomonas aeruginosa in, 100
Pythium insidiosum in, 223
rhinovirus in, 378
Rhodococcus equi in, 132–134, 133f
Salmonella in, 77
slaframine exposure of, 277
Staphylococcus in, 118
Streptococcus in, 121t, 123
Taylorella equigenitalis in, 204–205
Trichophyton in, 215t, 216t
vesicular stomatitis virus in, 416
Horsesickness fever, 435
Hospital-acquired infections,
        antimicrobial resistance in, 42
Host
  and bacteria interactions, 61–64
  defense mechanisms of. *See* Defense
      mechanisms of host
  and parasite interactions, 3
  and virus interactions, 328–332
    consequences of, 328, 328t
Humans
  Actinomyces in, 252
  alphavirus in, 387
  Arcanobacterium pyogenes in, 128
  Aspergillus in, 265
  Bacillus in
    anthracis, 246–247, 248
    cereus, 249
  Bartonella in, 299, 300, 301
  Bordetella in, 148, 149
  Borrelia in, 287, 288
  Brucella in, 199
  Burkholderia in, 155, 156
  Campylobacter in, 89, 90, 193
  Candida albicans in, 109
  Chlamydia in, 173
  Clostridium in
    botulinum, 241, 242
    difficile, 239
    novyi, 236
    perfringens, 234
    piliforme, 239
    septicum, 237
    tetani, 243
  Coxiella burnetii in, 292, 292t
  Cryptococcus neoformans in, 264
  Ehrlichia in, 294
  Erysipelothrix in, 229, 230
  Francisella tularensis in, 285
  Helicobacter in, 93, 94t, 95, 97–98
  Histoplasma capsulatum in, 259, 260
  immunodeficiency virus in, 459, 460
  influenza virus in, 399, 401–402
  Leptospira in, 187, 188
  Listeria in, 225, 226
  Mycobacterium in, 159, 160, 161–162
  paramyxovirus and Newcastle disease
      in, 408
  parapoxvirus in, 367
  Pasteurella in, 136t, 138
  poxvirus in, 365, 366
  rabies virus in, 412, 413, 414
    diagnosis of, 415
  Rhodococcus equi in, 132, 133
  Salmonella in, 77
  Serpulina in, 86, 87

Shigella in, 80, 81
Sporothrix schenckii in, 220, 221
Staphylococcus in, 115, 118
Streptobacillus moniliformis in, 290
Streptococcus in, 120, 121t, 124
vesicular stomatitis virus in, 416
Yersinia in
  enterocolitica, 103
  pestis, 282
Hydrogen peroxide, 8
Hypergammaglobulinemia in Aleutian
    disease of mink, 338
Hypersensitivity reactions, 12, 13
  cell-mediated, 5, 51
  to cephalosporins, 32
  to *Coccidioides immitis*, 258
  to *Mycobacterium*, 158, 162, 163
    paratuberculosis, 104, 107
  to penicillins, 32
  to sulfonamides, 34

I
Ibaraki virus, 433, 434
Icterus in *Leptospira* infection, 187
Imidazoles, 43
  mechanism of action, 33
Immune electron microscopy, virus
    identification in, 23–24
Immune response, 5, 7–14
  antibodies in, 11–13
    in virus infections, 329
  in *Campylobacter* infection, 193
  cell-mediated, 11, 13, 51
    in virus infections, 329–330
  in *Coccidioides immitis* infection,
      257–258
  in *Escherichia coli* infection, 72
  generation of, 11
  in genital tract infection, 190
  in *Helicobacter* infection, 98
  in *Mycobacterium* infection, 158, 159,
      161, 162
    paratuberculosis, 105, 106
  in *Mycoplasma* infection, 170
  in *Salmonella* infection, 77
  in *Shigella* infection, 81
  of skin, 206
  in urinary tract infection, 178
  to vaccines, 51–52
    bacterial, 56
    viral, 55
  in virus infections, 329–330
    suppression of, 331–332
Immunity, 7–14, 51
  acquired, 7, 11–13
  innate, 7–11
Immunodeficiency disorders in viral
    infections, 331–332
  bovine, 457–458
  feline, 448, 458–459
  lentivirus, 447
  simian, 449, 450, 459–460
Immunodeficiency virus, 457–460
  bovine, 457–458
  feline, 458–459
  simian, 449, 459–460

Immunodiffusion test in viral infections, 26
  in avian species, 21t
  in mammalian species, 19t, 20t
Immunofluorescence techniques, virus detection and identification in, 24, 24f
  in avian species, 21t
  in mammalian species, 18t, 19t, 20t
Immunoglobulins
  hypergammaglobulinemia in Aleutian disease of mink, 338
  IgA, 56
    functions of, 11t, 12–13
    secretory, 12, 13
  IgE, functions of, 11t, 12
  IgG, 11, 12f
    functions of, 11t, 12
  IgM, 11, 12f, 56
    functions of, 11t, 12
Immunologic diagnostic techniques in bacterial and fungal infections, 17
Immunosorbent assay, enzyme-linked
  in *Mycobacterium paratuberculosis* infection, 107
  in viral infections, 25, 26–27
    in mammalian species, 18t, 19t, 20t
    parvovirus, 336, 337
Immunosuppression in viral infections, 331–332
Inclusion bodies, 325
Induction period in feline leukemia virus infection, 448
Inflammation, 5, 10–11
Influenza virus, 396–402
  avian, 400–401
  equine, 398–399
  in humans, 399, 401–402
  morphology of, 396, 397f
  swine, 399–400
Inoculation of animals, for study of viruses, 23, 318
Integration complex in retroviruses, 445
Integrins, 14
Interference mechanisms in virus infections, 324–325
Interferons
  alpha, 330, 331t
  beta, 330, 331t
  gamma, 12, 13, 51, 330, 331t
  in innate immunity, 8
  in virus infections, 330, 331f, 331t
Interleukins, 11
  IL-1, 11, 51
  IL-2, 11, 51
  IL-4, 11, 51
  IL-12, 13
Iridoviridae, 340–342
Iridovirus, 340
Iron
  bacteria requirements for, 65
  as limiting factor in virulence, 4, 8
Iron-binding proteins, 4
Israel turkey meningoencephalitis, 389
Itraconazole, 43

J
Johne's disease, 104, 105f, 106f, 158
Johnin of *Mycobacterium paratuberculosis*, 104, 107

K
K-antigens, 65
  of *Escherichia coli*, 69
Kauffman-White classification of *Salmonella*, 75
Kennel cough of dogs
  in adenovirus infection, 348
  in *Bordetella* infection, 149
  in herpes virus infection, 358
  in parainfluenza virus infection, 409–410
Keratitis, in herpes virus infection of cats, 359, 360
Keratoconjunctivitis
  in *Moraxella* infection of cattle, 151, 152
  in *Mycoplasma* infection, 169
Keratomycosis in *Aspergillus* infection, 267, 268
Ketoconazole, 43
Klebsiella, in urinary tract infection of dogs, 179t, 182t
Koch criteria on pathogenicity, 3–4
Koch phenomenon in *Mycobacterium* infection, 162

L
Laboratory diagnosis, 15–27
  of bacterial and fungal infections, 15–17
    of urinary tract, 180–181
  and indications for drug therapy, 46–47
  of viral infections, 17–27
β-Lactam antibiotics, 28, 29, 30, 32
β-Lactamase enzymes, 30, 31
Lactobacillus in alimentary canal, 62t
Lactoferrin, as limiting factor in virulence, 4, 8, 65
Lame disease in *Clostridium botulinum* infection, 242
Lancefield groups of streptococci, 120, 121t, 125
Langhans giant cell in *Mycobacterium* infection, 159, 160f
Laryngotracheitis, in herpes virus infection of chickens, 362–363
Larynx, defense mechanisms of, 113
Lawsonia, 89–91
  intracellularis, 89, 90
Lelystad virus, 429
Lentiviruses, 442, 443t, 454–460
  immunodeficiency from, 447, 449, 457–460
Leprosy in cats, 209
Leptospira, 185–188
  bratislava, 185, 186, 187, 188
  canicola, 185, 186, 187, 188
  dinger zone of, 185

  grippotyphosa, 185, 186, 187
  hardjo, 185, 186, 187, 188
  icterohaemorrhagiae, 185, 186, 187, 188
  interrogans, 185, 186
  pomona, 185, 186, 186f, 187
  staining of, 185, 186f
Leukemia virus
  bovine, 447, 453–454
  feline, 447–449
  ovine, 453
Leukocytes, 8
Leukoencephalomalacia in horses, 276
Leukopenia in parvovirus infection of cats, 333–334
Leukosis/sarcoma complex of viruses, avian, 450–453
Leukotoxin of *Pasteurella*, 135
Limberneck disease in *Clostridium botulinum* infection, 242
Lincomycin, 37–38
  in *Bartonella* infection, 301
Lincosamides, 37–38
Lipids
  of endotoxins, 65
  of viruses, 317
    retroviral, 443
Lipopolysaccharide, 5, 56, 65
  of *Actinobacillus*, 141, 142
  of *Escherichia coli*, 69, 71f
  of *Pasteurella*, 135
Listeria, 225–227
  grayi, 225
  innocua, 225
  ivanovii, 225, 227
  monocytogenes, 225, 226, 227, 227f
  seeligeri, 225
  welshimeri, 225
Lockjaw in *Clostridium tetani* infection, 244
Louping-ill virus, 387, 389
Lumpy jaw in *Actinomyces* infection of cattle, 251, 252
Lumpy skin disease in poxvirus infection, 369
Lumpy wool of sheep, 211
Lungs, defense mechanisms of, 113–114
Lyme disease, 287, 288–289
Lymphadenitis
  in *Corynebacterium pseudotuberculosis* infection, 130, 131, 131f
  in *Streptococcus* infection, 123, 124, 125
Lymphangitis
  in *Histoplasma capsulatum* infection, 221, 222
  ulcerative
    in *Corynebacterium pseudotuberculosis* infection, 130, 131
    in *Mycobacterium* infection of cattle, 210
Lymphocystis disease virus, 340
Lymphocytes
  B cells, 11, 52
  circulation of, 13f, 13–14
  T cells. See T cells
Lymphoid tissue, mucosa-associated, 113

Lymphosarcoma in leukemia virus
  infection
    bovine, 453
    feline, 447, 448, 449
Lysozyme, 8

M
MacConkey agar, 16, 67, 73
Macroconidia, 214, 215t
Macrolide antibiotics, 37
  adverse effects of, 37
Macrophage activating factor, 12
Macrophages, 10
  activation of, 12, 13, 51
    in virus infections, 330
  in inflammatory response, 10, 11
  pulmonary alveolar, 113, 114
Mad cow disease, 462
Maedi virus, 454–456
Malassezia pachydermatis, 210f, 210–211
Mammillitis in herpes virus infection of
  cattle, 355–356
Mannose-resistant adhesin, 65, 70
Marek's disease, 350, 361–362
Margination process, 8, 9f
Mason-Pfizer monkey virus, 449
Mastitis
  in Actinomyces infection, 251
  in Arcanobacterium pyogenes infection,
    128
  in Aspergillus infection, 267
  in Bacillus cereus infection, 249
  in Brucella infection, 198–199
  in Candida infection, 110
  in Cryptococcus neoformans infection,
    264
  in Mycoplasma infection, 166, 168,
    168f, 169
  in Nocardia infection, 253, 254
  in Pasteurella infection, 137
  in Prototheca infection, 270, 270f
  in Staphylococcus infection, 115, 117,
    118, 119
  in Streptococcus infection, 123–124, 125
Melioidosis, 156
Membrane attack complex, 8, 12
Meningitis in Streptococcus infection,
  123
Meningoencephalitis
  in flavivirus infection of turkeys, 387,
    389
  in Haemophilus infection, 146
  in herpes virus infection
    in cattle, 354, 355, 356
    in pigs, 358
  in Listeria infection, 226, 227
Meningoencephalomyelitis in canine
  distemper virus infection, 405
Metabolism of antimicrobials, 39
  of aminoglycosides, 36–37
  of cephalosporins, 32
  of chloramphenicol, 36
  of macrolide antibiotics, 37
  of penicillins, 31
  of sulfonamides, 34

and trimethoprim, 35
Metritis in Taylorella equigenitalis
  infection of horses, 204–205
Metronidazole in Helicobacter infection,
  98
Mice. See Rodents
Miconazole, 43
Microcins, 63
Microconidia, 214, 215t
Microscopy
  electron. See Electron microscopy
  in urine examination, 180
Microsporum, 214–219
  audouinii, 214, 216
  canis, 214, 215, 215t, 216, 216t
    laboratory diagnosis of, 217f
  distortum, 214
  equinum, 216t
  features of, 215t
  gallinae, 215t, 216t
  gypseum, 215, 215t, 216t, 218f
  nanum, 215, 215t
Milk
  Brucella in, 201, 201f
  Mycobacterium in, 161–162
Milk drop syndrome in Leptospira
  infection, 187
Milker's nodules, 368
Mink
  Aleutian disease in, 337–338
  Clostridium botulinum in, 240, 242
  encephalopathy in, 312, 461
  Staphylococcus in, 117
Molecular diagnostic techniques, 17
  in Mycobacterium paratuberculosis
    infection, 107
  in viral infections, 24–25
Mollicutes, 165–172
Monkeys
  Helicobacter in, 94t, 97
  herpes virus in, 360–361
  immunodeficiency virus in, 459–460
  retrovirus type D in, 449–450
  Streptococcus in, 123
Monoclonal antibodies in viral
  diagnosis, 27
Monocytes, 10
Moraxella, 151–152
  bovis, 151, 152f
Morbillivirus, 403–407, 404t
Mortierella, 268
  wolfii, 269
Mouth
  microbial flora of, 61, 63
    antimicrobials affecting, 64
  papillomavirus infection of, in dogs,
    345
Mucociliary apparatus, 114
Mucor, 268
  toxins of, 274
Mucous membrane infections, viral, 19t,
  21t
Mutations
  antibiotic resistance in, 41, 48
  viral vaccines from, 53
Mutualism, 3

Mycelium, 214
Mycetomas, 223, 268
  in Nocardia infection, 254
Mycobacterium, 158–164
  avium, 158, 159, 161, 162
    paratuberculosis, 104–108, 158
  avium-intracellulare complex, 162
  bovis, 158, 159, 161, 162
  in cats, 161, 164, 209–210
  fortuitum, 209
  genavense, 162
  haemophilum, 162
  leprae, 158
  lepraemurium, in cats, 209
  marinum, 162
  microti, 158, 162
  phlei, 209
  simiae, 162
  in skin infections, 164, 209–210
  smegmatis, 209
  thermoresistible, 209
  tuberculosis, 158–164
  ulcerans, 209
  xenopi, 209
Mycobactin, 158
  of Mycobacterium paratuberculosis, 104,
    105, 107
Mycolic acids of Mycobacterium, 158
Mycoplasma, 165–172
  agalactiae, 167t, 169, 170
  alkalescens, 167t, 168
  arthritidis, 167t, 169, 170
  bovigenitalium, 167t, 168
  bovis, 167t, 168, 170, 171
  californicum, 167t, 168
  canadense, 167t, 168
  canis, 167t, 169
  capricolum, 167t, 169, 170
  conjunctivae, 167t, 169
  cynos, 167t, 169
  diseases associated with, 167t
  dispar, 167t, 168, 170
  felis, 167t, 169
  gallisepticum, 167, 167t, 170, 172
  gatae, 167t, 169
  hyopneumoniae, 167t, 169, 170, 171
  hyorhinis, 167t, 169, 170
  hyosynoviae, 167t, 169
  iowae, 167t, 168
  laboratory diagnosis of, 170–172, 180
  meleagridis, 167t, 168, 172
  mycoides, 166, 167, 167t, 168, 169,
    170
  neurolyticum, 165, 167t, 169
  ovipneumoniae, 167t, 169
  pulmonis, 167t, 169
  putrefaciens, 167t, 169
  spumans, 167t, 169
  staining of, 171, 171f
  synoviae, 167t, 168, 170, 172
Mycoses, 274
  subcutaneous, 220–223
  systemic or deep, 256–270
Mycothecium, toxins of, 275
Mycotoxicosis, 274
Mycotoxins, 274–279

Myeloblastosis, in avian leukosis/
    sarcoma complex of viruses
    infection, 450, 452
Myelocytomatosis, in avian
    leukosis/sarcoma complex of
    viruses infection, 450, 452
Myeloencephalitis in herpes virus
    infection of horses, 351, 352
Myeloperoxidase, 8

N
Nanophyetus salmincola, 296, 297
Nasopharynx
    defense mechanisms of, 113
    microbial flora of, 113
Natural kills cells, 10, 11
Navel ill in *Actinobacillus* infection, 142
Necrosis of pancreas, infectious, 439,
    440
Negri bodies in rabies virus infection,
    414, 415
Neomycin, 36, 37
Neophytodium, 276, 277
    coenophialum, 277
    lolia, 276, 277
Neoplasia
    oncogenesis in. *See* Oncogenesis
    virus isolation and identification in,
    20t, 21t
Neorickettsia helminthoeca, 294, 296–297,
    297f
Nephritis in *Leptospira* infection, 187
Neuraminidase of influenza virus, 396
Neutralization test, serum virus, 25
Neutrophils, 8
    compared to macrophages, 10
    in inflammatory response, 10
    in phagocytosis, 8, 9f
Newborn
    Actinobacillus in, 141, 142
    Clostridium perfringens in, 234, 235
    Escherichia coli in, 70, 72
    microbial flora in, 61, 64
    rotavirus in, 436
    Salmonella in, 77
    Streptococcus in, 123, 124
    susceptibility to enteric disease, 64
Newcastle disease, 407–409
Nitric oxide, 10
Nitrofurans, 33
Nitroimidazoles, 33
Nocardia, 250, 253–255
    asteroides, 253, 253f, 254, 255
    brasiliensis, 253, 254
    characteristics of, 251t
    nova, 253, 255
    otitidiscaviarum, 253, 254
Nose
    defense mechanisms of, 113
    microbial flora of, 113
Nucleic acid
    drugs inhibiting function of, 33–35
    hybridization techniques for virus
        identification, 24–25
    of retroviruses, 443, 444f
Nucleocapsid, 311

Nucleoprotein of influenza virus, 396
Nystatin in *Chlamydia* infection, 175

O
O-antigens
    of *Enterobacteriaceae*, 65, 66f
    of *Salmonella*, 75, 76t
    of *Yersinia enterocolitica*, 102
Ochratoxin, 278
Oncogenes, 446–447
Oncogenesis, 442, 446–447
    avian leukosis/sarcoma complex of
        viruses in, 450–453
    bovine leukemia virus in, 453–454
    DNA viruses in, 447
    feline leukemia and sarcoma viruses
        in, 447–449
    insertional, 447, 451
    transactivation mechanism in, 447
Oncoviruses, 442
Ondiri disease, 296
Opsonins, 8, 12
Optochin sensitivity of *Streptococcus*, 125
Orbivirus, 430, 431t, 433–436
Orchitis in *Brucella* infection, 198, 199,
    200
Orientia, 291
    tsutsugamushi, 292t
Ornithosis in *Chlamydia* infection of
    birds, 175
Oroya fever, 299
Orthomyxoviridae, 396–402
Orthomyxovirus, 316
    helical symmetry of, 313
Orthopoxvirus, 365–366
Orthoreovirus, 430–433, 431t
    avian, 431f, 432–433
    mammalian, 430–432
Osteoarthropathy, hypertrophic
    pulmonary, 161
Otitis externa, 210f, 210–211
    in *Pseudomonas aeruginosa* infection,
        100, 210
    in *Staphylococcus* infection, 115, 117,
        118, 210
Overeating, *Clostridium perfringens*
    infection in, 234, 235
Oxidation reduction potential, 4

P
Paecilomyces, 268
Pancreatic necrosis, infectious, 439, 440
Panleukopenia virus in cats, 333–334
Papillomavirus, 343–345, 344f
Papovaviridae, 343–345
Paracoccidioides, 256
Parainfluenza virus, 409–411
    type 2, 409–410
    type 3, 404f, 409, 410–411
Paralysis in enterovirus infection of pigs,
    374
Paramyxoviridae, 403–411
    morbillivirus, 403–407, 404t
    paramyxovirus, 404t, 407–411
    pneumovirus, 404t, 411

    structure of, 403, 404f
    subgroups of, 404t
Paramyxovirus, 404t, 407–411
Parapoxvirus, 366t, 366–368
Parasites, 3
    relationship with host, 3
Paratyphoid, 78
Parinaud's oculoglandular syndrome in
    Bartonella infection, 300
Parvoviridae, 333–338
Parvovirus, 333–338
    diseases caused by, 333, 334t
Pasteurella, 135–139
    caballi, 136t, 138
    canis, 136t, 138
    dagmatis, 136t, 138
    epidemiology of, 138, 138t
    gallinarum, 136t, 138
    haemolytica, 135, 136, 136t, 137, 139
    multocida, 135, 136, 136t, 137, 138,
        139
    pneumotropica, 136t, 138
    species of, 135, 136, 136t
    trehalosi, 136, 136t, 137
Pathogenesis
    criteria in, 3–4
    direct damage in, 4–5
    immune-mediated damage in, 5
    of viral diseases, 328–332
Peliosis hepatis, bacillary, 300
Penicillin-binding proteins, 29, 30
Penicillin G, 30, 31
Penicillins, 30–32
    absorption, distribution, and excretion
        of, 31
    adverse effects of, 32
    antimicrobial activity of, 31
    in *Brucella* infection, 201
    discovery of, 30
    mechanism of action, 28, 29, 30–32
    resistance to, 31, 40, 41
Penicillium, 268, 268f
    toxins of, 274, 278, 279
Peptidoglycan of *Mycobacterium*, 158
Peristalsis in host defense of alimentary
    canal, 64
Peritonitis, feline infectious, 423–424
Pestivirus, 390–395
Petechial fever in *Ehrlichia* infection, 296
pH
    in host defenses, 4, 7
    of skin, 206
    of urinary tract, 178
    virus reactions to, 320
Phaeohyphomycosis, 222–223
Phagocytosis, 5, 8
    macrophages in, 10, 51
    neutrophils in, 8
    process in, 8, 9f
Phagolysosome, 8
Pharynx
    defense mechanisms of, 113
    microbial flora of, 113
Phocine distemper virus, 406
Photodynamic inactivation of viruses,
    320
Picornaviridae, 371–378

Picornavirus, 316, 371–378
  genera of, 371, 372t
Pigs
  Actinobacillus in, 141, 142, 143
  Actinomyces in, 251
  aflatoxin sensitivity of, 275
  African fever virus in, 340–342
  alimentary canal microbial flora in,
      63t
  aphthovirus and foot-and-mouth
      disease in, 371, 372, 373
  Arcobacter in, 89, 193, 194, 195
  Bacillus anthracis in, 247
  Bordetella in, 149, 150
  Brucella in, 197, 198, 199
    diagnosis of, 201
  calicivirus and vesicular exanthema in,
      379–382, 380f, 381f
  Campylobacter in, 89, 90, 193, 194
  cardiovirus in, 377
  Chlamydia in, 173
  Clostridium in
    perfringens, 234
    tetani, 242, 244
  Coccidioides immitis in, 256, 258
  coronavirus in, 423
    and hemagglutinating
        encephalomyelitis, 420–421
    and transmissible gastroenteritis,
        418–420
  enterovirus in, 374–375
    and vesicular disease, 374, 375
  Erysipelothrix in, 229, 230, 231
  Escherichia coli in, 70
    and edema disease, 72
  flavivirus and Japanese encephalitis in,
      388, 389
  fumonisin toxicosis in, 276
  Haemophilus in, 144, 145–146, 146t,
      400
  Helicobacter in, 94t, 97
  herpesvirus and pseudorabies in,
      357–358
  influenza virus in, 399–400, 401, 402
  Leptospira in, 185, 186, 186f, 187
    vaccination against, 188
  Microsporum in, 215, 215t
  Mycobacterium in, 161, 163
  Mycoplasma in, 167t, 169, 170
    detection of, 171
  ochratoxin exposure of, 278
  parvovirus in, 336–337
  Pasteurella in, 136t, 137–138
  pestivirus in, 391
    and cholera, 393–395
  polioencephalomyelitis in, 374–375
  poxvirus in, 369–370
  reproductive and respiratory syndrome
      virus in, 429
  Rhodococcus equi in, 132, 133
  Salmonella in, 76–77
  Serpulina in, 86, 87
  Staphylococcus in, 115, 117, 118, 118t
  Streptococcus in, 121t, 123, 124
  Teschen disease in, 374–375
  trichothecene mycotoxin exposure of,
      275

  urinary tract infections of, 183
  vesicular stomatitis virus in, 416
  zearalenone exposure of, 277
Pink eye in equine arteritis virus
    infection, 428
Pithomyces chartarum, 278
Pizzle rot in *Corynebacterium* infection of
    sheep, 183
Plague
  in influenza virus infection of birds,
      400
  in *Yersinia pestis* infection, 282–283
Plaque in virus infections, 319, 319f,
      320
Plasmids
  in antibiotic resistance, 41, 42, 48
  of *Salmonella*, 75
  of *Shigella*, 80
  of *Yersinia*, 281
    enterocolitica, 102
Pleuropneumonia in *Mycoplasma*
    infection, 168, 169
Pneumocystis carinii, 270
Pneumonia
  in *Actinobacillus* infection, 142
  in *Chlamydia* infection, 175
  enzootic, 169
  in *Mycobacterium* infection, 161
  in *Mycoplasma* infection, 168, 169
  in *Pasteurella* infection, 137–138, 139
  in *Pneumocystis carinii* infection, 270
  in respiratory syncytial virus infection,
      411
  in *Rhodococcus equi* infection, 132–133
  in *Streptococcus* infection, 123, 124
  in visna/maedi/progressive virus
      infection, 454, 455
  in *Yersinia pestis* infection, 282
Pneumovirus, 404t, 411
Pododermatitis in cattle, 208
Polioencephalomyelitis
  in enterovirus infection of pigs,
      374–375
  in rabies virus infection, 414
Polyenes, mechanism of action, 33
Polymerase chain reaction techniques,
      17, 25, 47
  in *Bartonella* infection, 299, 301
  in *Mycobacterium paratuberculosis*
      infection, 107
Polymyxins
  in *Brucella* infection, 200
  mechanism of action, 33
Polyomavirus, 343
Polyserositis in *Riemerella anatipestifer*
    infection, 153
Postantibiotic effect, 39
Posthitis in *Corynebacterium* infection of
    sheep, 183
Potomac horse fever, 296
Poultry. See Birds
Poxviridae, 365–370
Poxvirus, 365–370
  complex structure of, 313, 314
Prions, 312–313
Proteins
  acute phase, 8

  antibiotics inhibiting synthesis of,
      35–38
  viral, 315
    of influenza virus, 396–398
    interferon affecting, 330, 331f
    of retrovirus, 443–445, 445f, 446
    synthesis of, 323, 323t
Proteus
  laboratory diagnosis of, 67
  mirabilis, in urinary tract infection of
      dogs, 179t, 180, 182t
Prototheca, 270, 270f
  wickerhamii, 270
  zopfii, 270
Providencia, laboratory diagnosis of, 67
Pseudallescheria boydii, 223, 268
Pseudocowpox, 367–368
Pseudolumpy skin disease in herpes
    virus infection of cattle,
      355–356
Pseudomonas
  aeruginosa, 100–101, 182t
    in otitis externa, 100, 210
  laboratory diagnosis of, 67, 68
  in urinary tract infection of dogs,
      179t, 182t
Pseudorabies
  in herpes virus infection, 357–358
  vaccine, 53–54
Pseudotuberculosis, 283
Psittacosis in *Chlamydia* infection of
    birds, 175, 176
Public health issues, in antimicrobial
    resistance of animal pathogens,
      42–43
Pullorum disease, 78
Purification of viral particles, 319–320
Pus formation, 10
Pyelonephritis
  in cattle, 182, 182f, 183
  in dogs, 180, 181
Pyocyanin of *Pseudomonas aeruginosa*,
      100, 101
Pyoderma in *Staphylococcus* infection,
      117, 118, 119
Pyolysin of *Arcanobacterium pyogenes*,
      127, 128
Pythium, 269
  insidiosum, 223

Q
Q fever, 292, 292t, 293

R
R plasmids (factors) in antibiotic
    resistance, 41, 42, 43, 48
Rabbits
  Actinobacillus in, 141
  calicivirus and hemorrhagic disease in,
      383
  Clostridium spiroforme in, 240
  Pasteurella in, 138
  Staphylococcus in, 118
Rabies, 412–416
Radiation, virus reactions to, 320

Radioimmunoassay, virus detection and
identification in, 26
in avian species, 21t
in mammalian species, 20t
Rain scald or rot of horses, 211, 212f
Ranavirus, 340
Rat bite fever, 290
Redmouth in *Yersinia ruckeri* infection,
283
Redwater disease in *Clostridium
haemolyticum* infection, 236,
237
Reoviridae, 430–438
aquareovirus, 430, 431t, 437–438
genera of, 430, 431t
orbivirus, 430, 431t, 433–436
orthoreovirus, 430–433, 431t
rotavirus, 430, 431t, 436–437
Replication of viruses, 321–324
in different families, 322t
and dissemination, 328
effects on cells, 325, 325t
events in, 324, 324t
interference with, 324–325
interferon affecting, 330, 331f
retroviral, 445f, 445–446
Resistance to antimicrobials, 38, 40–43,
48–49
acquired, 40–41
to aminoglycosides, 36
to antifungal agents, 43
to cephalosporins, 32
to chloramphenicol, 36
clinical importance of, 41–42
constitutive, 40
control of, 42–43
of Enterobacteriaceae, 66
Escherichia coli, 41–42, 74
genetic factors in, 41, 48, 49
in hospital-acquired infections, 42
to macrolide antibiotics, 37
to multiple drugs, 41, 48
to penicillins, 31, 40, 41
public health issues in, 42–43
of *Salmonella typhimurium*, 42
of *Staphylococcus*, 116
to sulfonamides, 34
and trimethoprim, 35
to tetracyclines, 35
Respiratory burst, 8
in *Mycoplasma* infection, 170
Respiratory syncytial virus
bovine, 411
feline, 411
Respiratory tract
Actinobacillus in, 141, 142, 143
adenovirus in, 348, 349
aphthovirus in, 371, 373
arteritis virus in, equine, 428
Aspergillus in, 266, 267
Blastomyces dermatitidis in, 262
Bordetella in, 148, 149
bronchitis virus in, avian, 425–426
Burkholderia in, 155
calicivirus in, in cats, 382–383
Chlamydia in, 173, 174, 175
Coccidioides immitis in, 256–259

Cryptococcus neoformans in, 264
Haemophilus in, 144–145, 146
herpes virus in
in cats, 359–360
in cattle, 354
in chickens, 362–363
in dogs, 358, 359
in horses, 350, 352, 353
in sheep, 356
Histoplasma capsulatum in, 260
influenza virus in
avian, 400–401
equine, 398–399
swine, 399–400
microbial flora in, 113–114
Mycobacterium in, 159, 161
Mycoplasma in, 166–167, 168, 169
orbivirus in, African horsesickness in,
435, 436
orthoreovirus in, mammalian, 430, 431
parainfluenza virus in, 409–411
paramyxovirus in, Newcastle disease
in, 408
Pasteurella in, 137t, 137–138
Pneumocystis carinii in, 270
pneumovirus in, 411
reproductive and respiratory syndrome
virus in, in pigs, 429
rhinovirus in, 378
Rhodococcus equi in, 132–134, 133f
rinderpest virus in, 407
Streptobacillus moniliformis in, 290
Streptococcus in, 123, 124
virus isolation and identification in,
18t, 21t
visna/maedi/progressive pneumonia
virus in, 454, 455
Restriction endonuclease cleavage site
analysis of viral DNA, 326,
326f
Reticuloendotheliosis virus, 450
Retroviridae, 442–460
genera of, 442, 443t
lentivirus, 442, 443t, 447, 454–460
Retrovirus, 442–454
avian, 450–453
bovine, 453–454
classification of, 442
feline, 447–449
general features of, 442–445
immunologic characteristics of, 446
morphology of, 442, 444f, 445f
oncogenesis by, 442, 446–447
replication of, 445f, 445–446
simian type D, 449–450
Rhabdoviridae, 412–417
morphology of, 412, 413f
subgroups of, 414t
Rhabdovirus, 316
Rhinitis
in *Bordetella* infection, 149, 150
in *Pasteurella* infection, 137–138, 139
Rhinopneumonitis in herpesvirus-4
infection of horses, 353
Rhinosporidium seeberi, 269, 269f
Rhinotracheitis in herpes virus infection
of cats, 359–360

Rhinovirus, 372t, 377–378
Rhizopus, 268, 269f
toxins of, 274
Rhodococcus equi, 127, 132–134
synergy with *Corynebacterium
pseudotuberculosis*, 130f, 131,
132
Rickettsia, 291–293, 292t
felis, 292t
prowazekii, 292t
rickettsii, 292, 292t, 293
typhi, 292t
Riemerella anatipestifer, 153
Rifampin, 34
in *Brucella* infection, 201
Rinderpest virus, 406–407
Ringworm, 215, 216, 218
RNA in viruses, 311, 313t, 315, 316–317
influenza, 396, 398
negative-strand, 321
positive-strand, 321
in replication cycle, 321–324, 322t
retroviral, 443, 444f, 445–446
Rocky Mountain spotted fever, 292,
292t, 293
Rodents
Brucella in, 197
Helicobacter in, 94t, 96, 97, 98
Mycoplasma in, 167t, 169
Pasteurella in, 138
Streptobacillus moniliformis in, 290
Yersinia in
pestis, 282
pseudotuberculosis, 283
Rolling disease in *Mycoplasma* infection,
169
Romanowsky-type stain, 16
Rotavirus, 430, 431t, 436–437
bovine, 431f, 436, 437
Rous sarcoma virus, 446, 451, 452
Rubivirus, 385

S
Salmon disease, 296–297
Salmonella, 75–79
anatum, 77
arizonae, 78–79
cellular anatomy and composition of,
65, 75
cellular products of, 75
cholerae-suis, 77
dublin, 76, 77
ecology of, 75–77
enteriditis, 77
gallinarum, 78
growth characteristics of, 66
host specificity of, 3
immunologic aspects of, 77
invasive, 76
laboratory diagnosis of, 67, 68, 77–78
newport, 76, 77
in poultry, 78–79
pullorum, 77, 78
treatment and prevention of, 78
typhimurium, 76, 77
antimicrobial resistance of, 42

typhisuis, 77
Salt stabilization of viruses, 320
Samples in laboratory diagnosis. *See*
        Specimens, clinical
San Miguel sea lion virus, 380
Saprophytes, 3
Sarcoma virus
    avian, 446, 452
        and leukosis complex, 450–453
    feline, 447–449
Satellitism of *Haemophilus*, 144, 145f
Scalded skin syndrome, staphylococcal,
        115
Scedosporium apiospermum, 223, 268
Scrapie, 312–313, 461–462
Sea lions
    calicivirus in, 380
    Leptospira in, 185, 186, 187
Seals, distemper virus in, 406
Septicemia
    in *Actinobacillus* infection, 142, 143
    in *Haemophilus* infection, 144
    in *Leptospira* infection, 187
    in *Listeria* infection, 226, 227
    in *Pasteurella* infection, 137, 139
    in *Riemerella anatipestifer* infection,
        153
    in *Salmonella* infection, 76, 77
    in *Streptococcus* infection, 123
Serologic tests
    in *Mycobacterium paratuberculosis*
        infection, 107
    virus detection in, 25–27
Serpulina, 86–87
    hyodysenteriae, 86, 87
    innocens, 86, 87
    intermedius, 86
    murdochii, 86
    pilosicoli, 86, 87
Shaker foal syndrome in *Clostridium
        botulinum* infection, 242
Sheep
    Actinobacillus in, 141, 142
    adenovirus in, 349
    aflatoxin sensitivity of, 275
    Bacillus anthracis in, 247, 248
    Borrelia in, 288
    Brucella in, 197, 198, 198f, 199
        diagnosis of, 201
        treatment and control of, 202
    Burkholderia in, 155, 156
    Campylobacter in, 192, 193, 194, 194f,
        195
    catarrhal fever associated with,
        malignant, 356
    Chlamydia in, 173, 175, 176
    Clostridium in
        chauvoei, 238, 239
        hemolyticum, 236
        novyi, 236
        perfringens, 234, 235
        septicum, 237
    Coccidioides immitis in, 256, 258
    Corynebacterium pseudotuberculosis in,
        130, 131, 131f, 132
    Cowdria ruminantium in, 296
    Dermatophilus congolensis in, 211

    ecthyma in, contagious, 367
    Ehrlichia in, 295, 296
    Erysipelothrix in, 229, 230
    Escherichia coli in, 70
    Flexispira in, 97
    footrot in, 207–208, 211
    herpes virus in, 356–357
    leukemia virus in, 453, 454
    Listeria in, 226, 227
    louping-ill virus in, 389
    maedi virus in, 454–456
    Mycobacterium in, 161
        paratuberculosis, 105, 107
    Mycoplasma in, 167t, 169
    orbivirus in, 434
        and bluetongue disease, 433, 434,
            435
    orthoreovirus in, 430
    Pasteurella in, 137
    pestivirus in, 391
        and border disease, 392–393
    poxvirus in, 368–369
        and contagious ecthyma, 367
    Salmonella in, 76
    scrapie in, 461–462
    sporidesmin exposure of, 279
    Staphylococcus in, 117–118
    Streptococcus in, 120, 121t
    urinary tract infections in, bacterial,
        182, 183
    visna virus in, 454–456
    Wesselsbron virus in, 389
Sheeppox, 368–369
Shiga-like toxins
    in *Campylobacter jejuni* infection, 89
    in *Escherichia coli* infection, 69, 70, 72
Shiga toxin, 70, 80, 81
Shigella, 80–82
    boydii, 80, 81
    dysenteriae, 80, 81
    flexneri, 80, 81
    laboratory diagnosis of, 67, 68, 81
    serotypes of, 80, 81t
    sonnei, 80, 81
Shipping fever, 137, 137t, 139, 409
    in parainfluenza virus infection of
        cattle, 409, 410–411
Siderophores, 65
    of *Bordetella*, 148
    of *Escherichia coli*, 69, 70, 71
    of *Pasteurella*, 135
    of *Pseudomonas aeruginosa*, 100
    of *Salmonella*, 75, 76
    of *Staphylococcus*, 115
    of *Yersinia*, 281
        enterocolitica, 102, 103
Sindbis virus, 317, 317f
Skin, 206–212
    antifungal agents for, 43
    antimicrobial properties of, 206
    aphthovirus infection and foot-and-
        mouth disease of, 371–373
    calicivirus infection and vesicular
        exanthema of, 379–382, 380f,
        381f
    Corynebacterium pseudotuberculosis
        infection of, 130, 131

    Erysipelothrix infection of, 229, 230
    herpes virus infection of, in cattle,
        355–356
    Histoplasma capsulatum infection of,
        221–222, 260
    microbial flora of, 206
    Microsporum infection of, 214–219
    Mycobacterium infection of, 164,
        209–210
    papillomavirus infection and warts of,
        343–345
    poxvirus infection of, 365–370
    Staphylococcus infection of, 115, 117,
        118, 118f
    sterilization of, 206–207
    and subcutaneous mycoses, 220–223
    Trichophyton infection of, 214–219
    virus isolation and identification in,
        19t, 21t
Slaframine, 277
Sleepy foal disease in *Actinobacillus*
        infection, 142
Smears, in diagnosis of bacterial
        infections, 15–16, 46, 47
    of alimentary tract, 47
    of urinary tract, 180
SMEDI enterovirus, 374
Snuffles, 138
Specimens, clinical
    in bacterial and fungal infections, 15
        collection of, 15
        transport of, 15
        of urinary tract, 180
    in viral infections, 17, 20–25
        in avian species, 21t
        collection of, 22
        in mammalian species, 18t–20t
Spectinomycin, 37
Spiroplasma, 165
Spleen, 14
Splicing in virus replication, 322
Spongiform encephalopathy, 312,
        461–462
Sporidesmin, 278–279
Sporothrix schenckii, 220–221, 221f
Spumavirus, 442, 443t, 449
Stachybotryotoxin, 275
Stachybotrys atra, toxins of, 275
Staggers in mycotoxin exposure,
        276–277
Staining methods in bacterial infections,
        16
Staphylococcus, 115–119
    aureus, 115, 116, 116f, 117, 118, 119
    epidermidis, 115, 117
    hyicus, 115, 117, 118, 119
    intermedius, 115, 117, 119
    morphology and staining of, 115, 116f
    in otitis externa, 115, 117, 118, 210
    schleiferi, 115, 117, 119
    sciuri, 117
    toxins of, 115, 116f
        inhibition by *Corynebacterium
            pseudotuberculosis*, 129f, 131
    in urinary tract infection of dogs,
        179t, 181t
    xylosus, 117

Sterilization of skin, 206–207
Stiff lamb disease in *Chlamydia* infection, 175
Stomatitis
    in herpes virus infection of cattle, 355
    in parapoxvirus infection of cattle, 367
    vesicular virus, 314, 315f, 319f, 416–417
        budding of, 323f, 413f
Strangles, 123, 124, 125
Strawberry footrot, 211
Streptobacillus moniliformis, 290
Streptococcus, 3, 120–125
    agalactiae, 120, 121t, 122, 123, 124, 125
    in alimentary canal, 62t, 63t
    alpha-hemolytic, 120, 125
    beta-hemolytic, 120, 125
    CAMP phenomenon from, 120, 122f, 125
    canis, 121t, 123, 124
    dysgalactiae, 121t, 123, 124
    equi, 120, 121t, 122, 123, 124
        host specificity of, 3
    equisimilis, 121t, 123
    gamma nonhemolytic, 120
    Lancefield groups of, 120, 121t, 125
    pneumoniae, 120, 121t, 123, 124, 125
    pyogenes, 120, 121t, 123, 124, 125
    suis, 121t, 123, 124
    uberis, 121t, 123, 124
    viridans group, 120, 123
    zooepidemicus, 121t, 122f, 123, 124
Streptomyces, toxins of, 274
Streptomycin, 36, 37
    resistance to, 41
Streptothricosis, 211
Stress, susceptibility to disease in, 64
Struck in *Clostridium perfringens* infection of sheep, 234
Suipoxvirus, 366t, 369–370
Sulfonamides, 34
    adverse effects of, 34, 35
    and trimethoprim, 34–35
Summer syndrome in fescue toxicosis, 277
Susceptibility
    to antibiotics, 38
    to antifungal drugs, 43
Swamp cancer in *Pythium insidiosum* infection, 223
Swamp fever in lentivirus infection of horses, 456
Sweet potatoes, moldy, 278
Swine. *See* Pigs
Swine fever, 393–395
Swinepox, 369–370
Symbiosis, 3
Syncytia formation in virus infections, 325

T

T cells, 11
    cytotoxic, 13, 13t, 51, 52
    gamma-delta, 10
    helper, 11, 51
T-lymphotropic virus

human, 449
simian, 449
Talfan disease in enterovirus infection of pigs, 374–375
Target cells, 61
    of *Salmonella*, 75, 76, 77
    of *Shigella*, 80
Taylorella equigenitalis, 204–205
Temperature of body, in host defenses, 4
Teschen disease in enterovirus infection of pigs, 374–375
Tetanus, 242–244
Tetracycline, 35
    adverse effects of, 35
    in *Chlamydia* infection, 176
    minimum inhibitory concentration of, 38t
Tick-borne fever, 295
Tiger heart, in aphthovirus infection and foot-and-mouth disease, 373
Tissue culture of viruses, 20–22, 318
Togaviridae, 385–387
    alphavirus, 385–387
    rubivirus, 385
Togavirus, 316
Tongue, wooden, in *Actinobacillus* infection, 142, 143
Torovirus, 418
Toxic shock syndrome, 115
Toxins, 51, 56
    of *Actinobacillus*, 141, 142
    of *Aspergillus*, 265, 274
    of *Bacillus*
        anthracis, 246, 247
        cereus, 249
    of *Clostridium*
        botulinum, 240, 241, 241t, 242
        chauvoei, 238
        difficile, 239
        novyi, 236
        perfringens, 234, 234t, 235
        tetani, 243, 244
    endotoxins. *See* Endotoxins
    exotoxins. *See* Exotoxins
    mycotoxins, 274–279
    of *Pasteurella*, 135–136
    shiga, 70, 80, 81
    shiga-like
        of *Campylobacter jejuni*, 89
        of *Escherichia coli*, 69, 70, 72
    of *Staphylococcus*, 115, 116f
Toxoids, 51, 55, 56
Trachea, defense mechanisms of, 113
Tracheobronchitis of dogs
    in adenovirus infection, 348
    in *Bordetella* infection, 149, 150
    in parainfluenza virus infection, 409–410
Transduction, antibiotic resistance in, 41, 48
Transferrin, as limiting factor in virulence, 4, 8, 65
Transformation, antibiotic resistance in, 41, 48
Transmission of infectious agents, 4
Transposons in antimicrobial resistance, 41, 48

Trench fever, 299, 300
Trichophyton, 214–219
    equinum, 215t, 216t
    features of, 215t
    mentagrophytes, 215, 215t, 216t, 217f, 219f
    rubrum, 214, 215
    simii, 215t, 216t
    tonsurans, 214
    verrucosum, 215, 215t, 216, 216t, 219
Trichothecene mycotoxins, 275–276
Trichothecium roseum, toxins of, 275
Trimethoprim, 34
    and sulfonamide, 34–35
Tubercle formation in *Mycobacterium* infection, 159–160, 160f, 161
Tuberculin, 158
    in immunodiagnosis of *Mycobacterium* infection, 163, 163f
Tuberculosis, 158–164
    miliary, 161
    pneumonia in, 161
    reinfection, 161
Tularemia, 285–286
Tumors
    oncogenesis in. *See* Oncogenesis
    virus isolation and identification in, 20t, 21t
Turkeys
    Bordetella in, 149, 150
    Chlamydia in, 175, 176
    coronavirus and enteritis in, 426–427
    Erysipelothrix in, 230, 231
    flavivirus and meningoencephalitis in, 387, 389
    influenza virus in, 400, 401
    Mycoplasma in, 167t, 167–168
    paramyxovirus and Newcastle disease in, 408
    Salmonella in, 78, 79
    Staphylococcus in, 117, 119
Typhoid in fowl, 78
Tyzzer's disease in *Clostridium piliforme* infection, 239

U

Ulcers, gastric and duodenal, in *Helicobacter* infection, 96, 97, 98
Ureaplasma, 165, 166
    diversum, 168
    laboratory diagnosis of, 171, 181
Urinary tract, 178–184
    antimicrobial defenses of, 178
    Candida albicans in, 111
    in cats, bacterial infection of, 182
    in cattle, bacterial infection of, 182f, 182–183
    in dogs, 178–179
        bacterial infection of, 179t, 179–181, 181t, 182t
    laboratory diagnosis of infections, 180–181
    Leptospira in, 186, 186f, 187
    microbial flora in, 178–179
    in pigs, bacterial infection of, 183
    Streptococcus in, 124

Urine
  antimicrobial properties of, 178
  collection of sample, 180
  cultures of, 180–181
  microscopic examination of, 180
Urolithiasis
  in dogs, 180
  in *Staphylococcus* infection, 117
Urological syndrome of cats, 182
Uterus, microbial flora of, 190

V
Vaccines, 51–56
  adenovirus, 348
  adjuvants to, 52
  African horsesickness virus, 436
  alphavirus, 387
  anemia virus, equine, 457
  Bacillus anthracis, 248
  bluetongue virus, 435
  Bordetella, 149, 150
  Borrelia, 288–289
  bronchitis virus, avian, 426
  Brucella, 200, 202
  bursal disease virus, 440
  Campylobacter, 193, 195
  Chlamydia, 175, 176
  comparison of, 54t
  coronavirus
    bovine, 422
    canine, 423
    in transmissible gastroenteritis of
      pigs, 420
  Corynebacterium pseudotuberculosis, 131
  distemper virus, canine, 405–406
  DNA, 52, 55
  Erysipelothrix, 231
  herpes virus, 358
    bovine, 355
    equine, 352
    feline, 360
    gallid, 362, 363
  immunodeficiency virus, 458, 459, 460
  inactivated viral, 53t, 54t, 54–55
  influenza virus
    avian, 401
    equine, 399
    swine, 400
  Leptospira, 188
  leukemia virus, feline, 449
  Listeria, 226, 227
  live attenuated viral, 53t, 53–54, 54t
  Mycobacterium, 159, 162
  Mycoplasma, 170
  Newcastle disease virus, 409
  orthoreovirus, avian, 433
  papillomavirus, 344
  parainfluenza virus, 410–411
  parvovirus, 336, 337
  Pasteurella, 139
  pestivirus, 392, 395
  rabies virus, 414, 415–416
  respiratory syncytial virus, 411
  rinderpest virus, 407

  rotavirus, bovine, 437
  Salmonella, 77, 78
  Staphylococcus, 118
  Streptococcus, 124, 125
  synthetic peptide, 55
  Trichophyton, 216, 219
  types of, 53t
  vesicular stomatitis virus, 417
  virulence of, 53, 54
Vaccinia virus, 365, 366
Vacuoles, phagocytic, 8
Vagina, microbial flora of, 190
Vancomycin in *Chlamydia* infection, 175
Venezuelan equine encephalitis, 385–387
Vesicular disease
  in enterovirus infection of pigs, 374,
    375
  susceptibility to, 381, 382t
Vesicular exanthema of swine in
    calicivirus infection, 379–380,
    380f, 381f
Vesicular stomatitis virus, 314, 315f,
    319f, 416–417
  budding of, 323f, 413f
Virion, 311
Viroids, 312
Viropexis, 321
Virulence, 3
  of viral vaccine, 53, 54
Viruses
  antibody response to, 12–13, 329
    measurement of, 25
  and antiviral drugs, 43–44, 44t, 321
  chemical composition of, 315–317
  classification of, 311–313, 313t
  culture of, 20–22, 318
  cytopathic effect of, 22, 22f, 318, 319,
    325
    in serum neutralization test, 25
  defective, 311
  direct damage from, 5
  dissemination of, 328–329, 329f
  electron microscopy of, 23–24, 318
  in embryonated chicken eggs
    cultivation of, 318
    isolation and identification of,
      22–23, 23f
  families of, 312, 313t
  general properties of, 311–326
  genetics of. *See* Genetics, of viruses
  and host interactions, 328–332
    consequences of, 328, 328t
    immune response to, 329–330
      suppression of, 331–332
  immunofluorescence of, 24, 24f
    in avian species, 21t
    in mammalian species, 18t, 19t, 20t
  immunosorbent assay of, enzyme-
    linked, 25, 26–27
    in mammalian species, 18t, 19t, 20t
    of parvovirus, 336, 337
  inoculation procedure for study of, 23,
    318
  isolation and identification of, 17–27,
    318–320

  in avian species, 21t, 22–23, 23f
  in mammalian species, 18t–20t
  monoclonal antibodies in, 27
  nucleic acid hybridization in, 24–25
  polymerase chain reaction in, 25
  purification in, 319–320
  pathogenesis of diseases from, 328–
    332
  in persistent or latent infections, 332
  physical conditions and chemical
    agents affecting, 320–321
  replication of. *See* Replication of viruses
  serologic assays of, 25–27
  structure of, 311, 312f, 313–314, 316f
    complex, 314
    symmetry in, 313–314, 314f
  vaccines against, 52–55
Visna virus, 454–456
Vomiting and wasting disease in
    coronavirus infection of pigs,
    420, 421
Vomitoxin (deoxynivalenol), 274,
    275–276

W
Warts in papillomavirus infection,
    343–345
Weak calf syndrome in *Leptospira*
    infection, 187
Weil-Felix reaction, 291, 293
Wesselsbron virus, 387, 388, 389
Western equine encephalitis, 385–387
Western immuno-blot assay, 26f, 27
Wildebeests, malignant catarrhal fever
    associated with, 356
Wooden tongue, in *Actinobacillus*
    infection, 142, 143
Wounds, *Clostridium* infection of
  botulinum, 241, 242
  chauvoei, 238
  perfringens, 234
  septicum, 237
  tetani, 243, 244

X
Xylose lysine deoxycholate agar, 67

Y
Yeasts
  in alimentary canal, 62t, 63t
  Candida, 109–111
Yellow fever, 387–388
Yersinia, 281–283
  enterocolitica, 102–103, 281
  pestis, 3, 281, 282–283
  pseudotuberculosis, 281, 283
  ruckeri, 281, 283

Z
Zearalenone, 277
Zygomycetes, 268